Gastrointestinal symptoms in advanced cancer patients

Gastrointestinal symptoms in advanced cancer patients

Edited by

Carla Ripamonti
Rehabilitation and Palliative Care Division, National Cancer Institute, Milan, Italy

and

Eduardo Bruera
Department of Palliative Care and Rehabilitation, The University of Texas, M.D. Anderson Cancer Center, Texas, USA

OXFORD
UNIVERSITY PRESS

OXFORD
UNIVERSITY PRESS

Great Clarendon Street, Oxford OX2 6DP

Oxford University Press is a department of the University of Oxford. It furthers the University's objective of excellence in research, scholarship, and education by publishing worldwide in

Oxford New York

Auckland Bangkok Buenos Aires Cape Town Chennai Dar es Salaam Delhi Hong Kong Istanbul Karachi Kolkata Kuala Lumpur Madrid Melbourne Mexico City Mumbai Nairobi São Paulo Shanghai Taipei Tokyo Toronto

and an associated company in Berlin

Oxford is a registered trade mark of Oxford University Press in the UK and in certain other countries

Published in the United States
by Oxford University Press Inc., New York

First published 2002

British Library Cataloging in Publication Data

Data available

Library of Congress Cataloging in Publication Data

ISBN 0 19 263284 1
10 9 8 7 6 5 4 3 2 1

Typeset by Cepha Imaging Pvt Ltd, India
Printed in Great Britain
on acid-free paper by TJ International, Padstow, Cornwall

For Maria, Felice, Dario, Fausto, Maddalena, and Francesco Ripamonti

and

Maria, Ed, Sofia, and Sebastian Bruera

Preface

Gastrointestinal symptoms are among the most frequent and devastating in patients with advanced cancer. Approximately one in three adults will be diagnosed with cancer during their lives and approximately 50% of them will die because of malignancy. More than 80% of patients who die of cancer will present severe gastrointestinal symptoms before death. Until now there has been no specific book addressing the multiple and complex gastrointestinal symptoms brought about by malignancy.

This book provides a comprehensive scholarly review of the epidemiology, assessment, diagnosis, and treatment of gastrointestinal symptoms in advanced cancer patients. It has been written from a clinical perspective but with an effort to provide scholarly and evidence-based information that will serve not only clinicians, but also researchers in this field.

The appropriate assessment and management of gastrointestinal symptoms in patients with advanced cancer requires the participation of professionals from multiple disciplines. Our book reflects this complexity—contributors are from medical and non-medical disciplines and come from many countries around the world.

Gastrointestinal symptoms in advanced cancer patients is intended primarily for physicians and nurses with a primary interest in oncology and palliative care. Specifically, hospice and palliative care specialists, medical, radiation, and surgical oncologists, and selected family physicians and internists with an interest in the care of advanced cancer patients will benefit from its contents. Oncology and academic nurses, nutritionists, clinical psychologists, and other health care professionals regularly involved in oncology and/or palliative care will also find this book useful.

Various chapters address such diverse areas as epidemiological findings, physical and psychosocial assessment and support, sophisticated techniques (eg endoscopic management or radiation therapy), and pharmacological, nutritional, and ethical considerations. Because of the great diversity of the body of knowledge for each of these areas, we have chosen to allow our different contributors flexibility to address each of these issues in the most effective way possible. We believe that this will help readers better apppreciate the diversity of issues involved in the management of gastrointestinal symptoms in advanced cancer.

We are grateful to the many contributors for their excellent work and timeliness. We also thank Oxford University Press for expressing great faith in this project and providing support during the publication process. It is our hope that this book will contribute in improving the care of our advanced cancer patients and their families.

Milan, Italy — C. R.
Houston, Texas USA — E. B.
March 2002

Contents

List of Contributors

Dr Matthew Ballo
Department of Radiation Oncology
University of Texas, M.D. Anderson
Cancer Center
Houston, Texas
USA

Dr Jean-Jacques Body
Institut Jules Bordet
Brussels, Belgium

Dr C. Borreani
Psychology Unit
National Cancer Institute
Milan, Italy

Dr Frederico Bozzetti
National Cancer Institute
Milan, Italy

Dr Eduardo Bruera
Professor of Medicine
Department of Symptom Control and
Palliative Care
University of Texas, M.D. Anderson
Cancer Center
Houston, Texas
USA

Dr Nathan I. Cherny
Director of Cancer Pain and
Palliative Care Service
Department of Medical Oncology
Shaare Zedek Medical Center
Jerusalem, Israel

Dr Christopher Crane
Department of Radiation Oncology
University of Texas, M.D. Anderson Cancer Center
Houston, Texas
USA

Dr Mellar P. Davis
Medical Director
The Harry Horvitz Center for
Palliative Medicine
The Cleveland Clinic Foundation
Cleveland, Ohio
USA

Dr Marc Delclos
Department of Radiation Oncology
University of Texas, M.D. Anderson
Cancer Center
Houston, Texas
USA

Dr Robin L. Fainsinger
Director of Palliative Care Program
Royal Alexandra Hospital,
Edmonton, Alberta
Canada

Dr Marie T. Fallon
Senior Lecturer and Honorary Consultant
Department of Palliative Medicine
University of Edinburgh
Western General Hospital
Edinburgh, UK

Dr Cecilia Gavazzi
Nutrition Unit
National Cancer Institute
Milan, Italy

Dr Brett T. Gemlo
Clinical Assistant Professor of Surgery
Division of Colon and Rectal Surgery
University of Minnesota
St Paul, Minnesota,
USA

Dr Alain Hendlisz
Institut Jules Bordet
Brussels, Belgium

Professor Irene Higginson
Department of Palliative Care and Policy
GKT School of Medicine
King's College London
Weston Education Centre
London, UK

Dr Nora Janjan
Department of Radiation Oncology
University of Texas, M.D. Anderson Cancer Center
Houston, Texas
USA

Dr Aminah Jatoi
Assistant Professor
Division of Medical Oncology
Mayo Clinic
Rochester, Minnesota
USA

Dr J. C. Keen
Consultamt in Palliative Medicine
St Columba's Hospice
Edinburgh, UK

Dr Charles Loprinzi
Division of Medical Oncology
Mayo Clinic
Rochester, Minnesota
USA

Professor Neil MacDonald
Director, Cancer Ethics Program
Center for Bioethics
Clinical Research Institute of Montreal
Montreal, Quebec
Canada

Dr Isabelle Mancini
Institut Jules Bordet
Brussels, Belgium

Dr Mary-Ellen Mazuryk
Department of Medicine
Tom Baker Cancer Center
Calgary, Alberta
Canada

Dr Sebastiano Mercadente
Clinica La Maddelena
Palermo, Italy

Dr G Miccinesi
Epidemiology Unit
Center for Study and Prevention of Cancer
Florence, Italy

Dr Jean Potter
Department of Palliative Care and Policy
GKT School of Medicine
King's College London
Weston Education Centre
London, UK

Dr Carla Ripamonti
Rehabilitation and Palliative Care Division
National Cancer Institute
Milan, Italy

Dr Alberto Sbanatto
Medical Oncology Division
European Institute of Oncolgy
Milan, Italy

Dr Pasquale Spinelli
Division of Endoscopy
National Cancer Institute
Milan, Italy

Dr Florian Strasser
Department of Symptom Control and Palliative Care
University of Texas, M.D. Anderson Cancer Center
Houston, Texas
USA

Dr M. Tamburini
Psychology Unit
National Cancer Institute
Milan, Italy

Dr Paul Walker
Assisant Professor
Division of Anesthesiology
Department of Symptom Control and Palliative Care
University of Texas, M.D. Anderson Cancer Center
Houston, Texas
USA

Dr Declan Walsh
Professor and Director
The Harry Horvitz Center for Palliative Medicine
The Cleveland Clinic Foundation
Cleveland, Ohio
USA

Chapter 1

Frequency and severity of gastrointestinal symptoms in advanced cancer

Jean Potter and Irene Higginson

Introduction

Knowledge of the prevalence of symptoms is important for the care of patients. Symptoms are prerequisite to making diagnoses, and the identification of symptoms is an essential part of medical and nursing training. The prevalence of symptoms contributes to the identification of patients' needs in terms of symptom control, and therefore provision of services. Furthermore, such information can direct research, audit, and care planning, especially since the development of new symptoms can herald disease progression, which in turn may be a prognostic indicator for determining survival.

Prevalence is a measure of frequency. Perhaps the simplest definition of prevalence is the number of people at risk of a disease or symptoms divided by the number of people that actually have the disease or symptoms.

Prevalence, or *point prevalence*, is determined at a single point in time. *Period prevalence* is based on the percentage of people with the disease or symptoms during a defined period of time. This therefore includes new and existing cases that occur within the defined time period. *Period prevalence* values are usually greater than those calculated for *point prevalence.* Studies usually measure one and sometimes both of these types of prevalence.

Studies measure the prevalence of various symptoms in a particular population; for example, all cancer patients referred for terminal care to a hospice in-patient unit or all patients with pancreatic cancer. Others calculate *point* or *period prevalence* for a specific symptom; for example, nausea and vomiting in patients receiving chemotherapy. In studies measuring *period prevalence*, the designated time period varies: it may be as short as the last three days or much longer, up to the last year of life.

Prevalence of gastrointestinal symptoms

Gastrointestinal symptoms are common in advanced cancer patients. 'Gastrointestinal symptoms' in the fullest sense can encompass a wide range of symptoms from xerostomia to haemorrhoids. Certainly, this term includes the problems of anorexia, nausea and vomiting, weight loss, and constipation, all of which are a major source of physical and emotional morbidity to patients and their families. Several symptoms may occur in the same patient simultaneously. This may be either because they are interrelated; for example, nausea and anorexia, or because they have arisen independently of each other. In addition, different symptoms may develop over time. The majority of patients suffer from multiple symptoms.

The results of studies assessing the prevalence of a range of symptoms in cancer patients in various settings give highly variable results. Table 1.1 shows the range and median values found for gastrointestinal symptom prevalence in cancer patients in 27 studies. Studies were identified from a Medline search (MeSH) (1966–2000) and hand-searching relevant journals. The MeSH yielded few studies, largely because the word 'symptom' is not a MeSH heading. Hand-searching all issues of the journals, *Palliative Medicine, Journal of Pain and*

Table 1.1 Prevalence of symptoms

Symptom	Prevalence range (%)	Median (%)	Number of studies that assess symptom
Dry mouth[a]	40–81	59	9
Anorexia[b]	30–92	57	22
Weight loss[c]	33–93	51	8
Early Satiety[d]	33–62	43	6
Nausea	11–54	25	24
Vomiting	10–32	21	16
Dysphagia	3–46	23	14
Constipation[e]	5–64	40	21
Diarrhoea	3–25	8	9
Hiccups	3–15	12	3
Dyspepsia	2–17	10	6
Taste change	2–36	26	5
Bloating	6–11	11	5
Belching	5–7	5	5

[a] Despite the high prevalence of dry mouth found in studies of groups of symptoms, there are few studies that have addressed dry mouth in particular. Oral candidal infections may be asymptomatic, but more often cause problems with taste change, dry and sore mouth, and dysphagia. Forbes found symptomatic oral candidal infections in 18/38 (47%) patients suffering from head and neck cancer (4), whilst Redding found the prevalence of candidal infections to be 27% in 30 head and neck cancer patients undergoing radiotherapy (50).

[b] The term 'cancer–cachexia syndrome' encompasses many symptoms including anorexia, early satiety, loss of body protein and fat, anaemia and marked asthenia (51). This has also become known as the 'cancer anorexia–cachexia syndrome'. It has been cited as one of the most common causes of death among cancer patients, and is present in 80% at death (18).

[c] Despite high prevalence, no specific studies found on this subject.

[d] Despite high prevalence, few studies of this symptom have been carried out. It appears that this symptom is related to another relatively poorly studied symptom: taste change. Neilson *et al.* (52) found that 80% of patients with taste aversions experience early satiety compared with 49% without early satiety.

[e] Definitions of constipation vary. Prevalence is likely to be an underestimate as some patients will be successfully treated with laxatives (53). Constipation is more common in patients who are terminally ill with cancer than those dying from other causes (54).

Symptom Management, and the *Journal of Palliative Care* for relevant articles, reviewing the relevant chapters in *The Oxford Textbook of Palliative Medicine* (1), *The Oxford Textbook of Oncology* (2), and *Gastrointestinal Disease* (3) and then reviewing the reference lists from both these sources proved more fruitful. Three studies of patients with particular cancers (4–6) were excluded from Table 1.1. Further details of these 30 studies appear in Table 1.2, and are discussed in more detail in the following sections.

Factors affecting the prevalence of specific gastrointestinal symptoms

The data from prevalence studies will be considered in terms of tumour type, tumour stage, age and gender of patient, and symptoms caused by treatment rather than by disease.

Tumour type

On occasion, a particular symptom may be the presenting complaint of a malignancy, and may be due to the physical mass of the primary lesion. Despite optimal treatment, it may not be treated successfully. Dysphagia, for example, is a common presenting complaint in patients diagnosed to have oropharyngeal or oesophageal malignancies. It has also been found to be more common in patients suffering from advanced head and neck and oesophageal malignancies than any other cancer type (7,8). In a study of 38 patients suffering from head and neck malignancies and referred to a palliative care team, Forbes found that 74% of these patients had dysphagia (4).

Many studies indicate a relationship between primary site and symptom prevalence, and this cannot be explained fully by anatomical factors alone. Grond found that 'the primary cancer site had major influence on symptom prevalence… only frequency of insomnia, dyspepsia, pruritus and dermatological symptoms showed no significant differences between the subgroups' (9). Vainio found that only constipation, weakness, and insomnia did not show a predilection for a particular primary site (10).

The exact relationship varies between studies, but various patterns emerge. Most notably, nausea and/or vomiting have been shown to be more common in gynaecological malignancies than other cancers (10–13). Furthermore, anorexia (13), dry mouth (13), dyspepsia (7,13), and early satiety (13) also have been shown to be more common in this group of diseases.

Other studies, however, have found that nausea and/or vomiting predominate in gastrointestinal malignancies (10,13–15), along with constipation (13) and anorexia (13,14).

Tumour stage

Most studies of symptom prevalence took their sample of patients from hospice or palliative care teams, and it may be supposed that these patients on the whole have further advanced disease. Schuitt, however, found in a study of all cancer patients attending an oncology out-patient department (including, therefore, patients under routine follow up) that 30%–40% of all patients reported constipation, nausea and/or anorexia, which is broadly comparable with other studies summarized in Table 1.1(16). These values in Schuitt's study fell to around 50% of the original value of each symptom prevalence when only symptoms graded three or more on the Symptom Distress Scale were considered.

Table 1.2 Prevalence of symptom studies

Author	Sample size	Study details	Outcome measures	Notes
Twycross (37)	6677	Cancer patients referred to PCT	Data collected from medical notes 1975–1984	Six symptoms recorded Data quoted in text, not published in journal
Wachtel (14)	1119	Terminally ill cancer patients receiving hospice care	Two-weekly questionnaire Spitzer QOL	Eight symptoms recorded Patient or proxy Period prevalence: 2 weeks
Reuben (25)	1592	Terminally ill cancer patients expected prognosis less than six months	Two-weekly questionnaire KPS scale	Fourteen symptoms recorded Patient or proxy Period prevalence: 2 weeks
Hockley (36)	26 15 cancer	Hospital patients with expected prognosis less than three months	Questionnaire including mood	Sixteen symptoms recorded Patient or proxy
Dunlop (26)	50	Cancer patient referred to hospital PCT or in-patient hospice	'Symptom cards' severity scale	Twenty-seven symptoms recorded Period prevalence: 3 days No proxy
McIllmurray (30)	256	Cancer patients admitted for terminal care to a hospice	Questionnaire on admission then weekly until death or discharge	Three symptoms recorded Patient or proxy
Lichter (27)	200	All patients in hospice Last 48 hours of life	Questionnaire	Thirteen symptoms recorded Patient or proxy
Ventafridda 1990 (61)	120	Cancer patients referred to hospice home care team. Assessment of symptoms requiring sedation	Review of medical notes	Four symptoms that needed sedation
Coyle (20)	90	Cancer referred to SCP	Review of medical notes at 4,3,2,1 weeks prior to death	Twenty-three symptoms recorded (only those actively volunteered by patient)

Brescia (12)	1103	Cancer patients admitted to oncology hospital and dying within six months of admission	Review of medical records	Six symptoms recorded
Dunphy (55)	547	Cancer patients referred to PCT	Review of medical records	Seven symptoms recorded Patient or proxy
Addington-Hall (23)	80	Carers of cancer patients who died between 1987 and 1989	Questionnaire	Fifteen symptoms recorded Only proxy
Seale (56)	800 216 cancer	Carers of patients who died in 1987	Questionnaire	Twenty-three symptoms recorded Only proxy
Krech (5)	39	Pancreatic cancer patients referred to PCT	Questionnaire Severity scale	Twenty-five symptoms recorded Patient only?
Fainsinger (11)	100	Cancer patients in last week of life in hospice	Multiple VASs	Eight symptoms recorded Patient or proxy
Curtis (24)	100	Cancer patients referred to hospital PCT	Questionnaire Severity scale	Thirty symptoms recorded Patient only?
Krech (6)	100	Lung cancer patients referred to PCT	Questionnaire Severity scale	Thirty symptoms recorded Patient only?
Sebastian (62)	312	All cancer patients attending oncology OPD	Questionnaire	Nine symptoms recorded Patient only
Grond (9)	1635	Cancer patients referred to pain clinic	Questionnaire Activity on VRS	Fifteen symptoms recorded Patient or proxy
Addington-Hall (22)	2074	Carers of cancer patients who died in UK in 1990	Questionnaire Severity score	Sixteen symptoms recorded Period prevalence: last year and last week of life Only proxy
Donnelly (13)	1000	Cancer patients referred to PCT. Last week of life?	Questionnaire Severity scale	Twenty symptoms recorded Period prevalence: one week Patient or proxy

Table 1.2 (Continued) Prevalence of symptom studies

Author	Sample size	Study details	Outcome measures	Notes
Ellershaw (42)	125	Cancer patients referred to hospital PCT	PACA McCorkle symptom distress scale	Eight symptoms recorded Patient only
Vainio (10)	1640	Cancer patients referred to PCT	Questionnaire Severity scale	Nine symptoms recorded Patient only
Conill (57)	176	Cancer patients referred to PCT in last week of life	Questionnaire	Eighteen symptoms recorded Period prevalence: one week Patient only?
Forbes (4)	38	Head and neck cancer patients referred to PCT	Review of medical notes	Twelve symptoms recorded Patient or proxy
Jenkins (58)	96	Cancer patients admitted to palliative care unit	ESAS Multiple VASs	Nine symptoms recorded Patient or proxy
Ng 1998 (59)	100 59 cancer	Cancer and non-cancer admissions to hospital Palliative Care Unit	Questionnaire	Sixteen symptoms recorded Patient or proxy
Schuitt (16)	151	All patients attending oncology OPD	Questionnaire Symptom distress scale	Nine symptoms recorded Patient only Data collected on general population
Edmonds (60)	352 324 cancer	All patients referred to hospital PCT	Modified STAS Repeated measure every 2 weeks until death	Eleven symptoms reported Period prevalence: 2 weeks Patient only
Desbiens (41)	1582 452 cancer	'Seriously ill' (with definition) patients admitted to hospital	Questionnaire Duke activity status index Severity score	Nine symptoms recorded Patient or proxy

Notes: QoL: Quality of Life; KPS: Karnofsky Performance Status; PCT: Palliative Care Team; VAS: Visual Analogue Scale; OPD: Out-patients Department; VRS: Verbal Rating Scale; PACA: Palliative Care Assessment; ESAS: Edmonton Symptom Assessment Scale; STAS: Support Team Assessment Schedule; SPC: Supportive Care Programme.

The National Hospice Survey in 1988 suggested a 'Terminal Common Pathway' based on their study of 1119 patients that found that the prevalence of symptoms in the last four to six weeks of life remained essentially the same towards death. Fever, dyspnoea, anorexia, and weight loss increased by 12%–15% during the last six weeks of life, but pain, nausea and/or vomiting, constipation, and diarrhoea changed very little (14).

Grond *et al.* also found little evidence that stage impacts on symptoms: they found that only the prevalence of dyspnoea increased in advancing disease, and that some symptoms; for example, dysphagia and dyspepsia, decreased with worsening condition (9). Others have found that the prevalence of anorexia changed as the disease progressed: from 40% at diagnosis, to 70% in advanced disease (7,17). The 'cancer anorexia—cachexia syndrome' has been found to be present in 80% of patients at death (18).

Conversely, others have found that dyspnoea, problems eating, dry mouth, difficulty swallowing, and weight loss independently predict poor prognosis (15,19). Reuben also found that pain, nausea and vomiting, constipation, diarrhoea, fever, dizziness, and haemorrhage did not have any impact on survival.

In general, studies that find no change in the prevalence of symptoms suffered by patients as their diseases progress do not assess the severity of symptoms. It may be that those who do suffer from a particular symptom find this more troublesome as their disease progresses. Certainly, the National Hospice Study showed that function and quality of life decrease towards the end of life. Krech found that in patients with pancreatic cancer, those with the fewest symptoms lived the longest (5).

The fact that certain symptoms appear to be more common in particular types of malignancy suggests that any 'common pathway' does not occur in the earlier stages of disease. In terms of prognosis, Vigano's systematic review of predictors of survival in terminal cancer patients found that performance status was the most important indicator of survival, better than any particular symptom. However, the strength of association between performance status and survival appears to be time dependent, being more evident in the short–medium term (3–12 weeks) rather than in the long term (3–6 months) (19).

Studies have been carried out to assess the period prevalence of patients' symptoms in different stages of disease as evidenced by their time to death; for example, the last 6 months (12), last month (20), last week (11), or last 48 hours of life (21). However, these studies are difficult to compare. Some studies used responses from proxies (usually nursing staff or nearest relative involved in care) when patients became too ill to answer for themselves, whereas other studies did not compile data on patients that were too ill to perform this task. Other studies interviewed carers about prevalence of symptoms after the patient's death (22,23).

Coyle interviewed patients at four, three, two, and one week before death, and found no difference in the prevalence of anorexia, nausea, constipation, or dysphagia over this period of time (20). This study, however, only noted symptoms about which patients actively volunteered information, and did not use a proxy when a patient was too ill to respond to questioning. Furthermore, severity was not studied in this group.

Age and gender of patients

There is no clear relationship between symptom prevalence and age. The National Hospice Study found little evidence of any relationship between age and most symptoms. It does, however, describe a curvilinear relationship between the prevalence of nausea and/or vomiting symptoms and age, lower in the 65–74-year-old age group (14). Grond found an increase in the prevalence of dysphagia in those under the age of 58 years, with an increase in constipation, nausea and vomiting in older patients (9).

It would appear that there is a clearer relationship between certain symptoms and gender. Several studies have shown that nausea and/or vomiting is more common in women (6,9,13,14,24,25) and there is evidence to suggest that women find nausea more distressing than men (26). Where severity has been assessed, more women than men have been found to suffer 'severely' (13). This may in part at least be explained by the prevalence of these symptoms in gynaecological malignancies. Other studies have found constipation (9), anorexia (24), early satiety (7,13), and taste change (24) more common in women.

Men, conversely, have been shown to suffer more often with dysphagia (7,13,26) (which may be explained in part by the male predominance in head and neck and oesophageal malignancies), xerostomia (24), and hiccup (7).

Symptoms caused by treatment rather than by disease

All therapeutic interventions have side-effects, and it may well be that some 'symptoms' are actually the side effects of treatments given with the aim of cure, prolongation of life, or relief of other symptoms. Most studies have calculated the prevalence of symptoms without attempting to ascertain the underlying cause. Of those that have looked at possible iatrogenic causes for symptoms, opioids, chemotherapy, and radiotherapy are most commonly under scrutiny.

Opioids

Lichter ascertained that in their group of 100 hospice in-patients in the last 48 hours of life, 13% had nausea and/or vomiting due to drugs (27). It has been estimated that about 30% of patients starting morphine feel nauseated during the first week of treatment (28). Studying specifically the use of strong opioids, Grond found that the administration of opioids in cancer patients referred to a pain clinic was associated with an increase in anorexia, constipation, nausea and vomiting (9). Campora found a similar trend in 260 cancer patients referred to a pain clinic, and also noted a sex distribution: men had more nausea and/or vomiting with buprenorphine, morphine, codeine, and oxycodone (29).

In general, it may be that these side effects are short-lived if medications are prescribed with the appropriate skills and knowledge. McIllmurray found that of the 30% of patients experiencing nausea and/or vomiting on admission to a hospice, the majority were taking opioids (30). However, despite an increase in the use of opioids during a hospice stay, there was a marked reduction in nausea or vomiting to only 9% of patients by the time of discharge or death. This may be attributable to the use of antiemetic drugs, and the development of tolerance to this particular side-effect over time.

Chemotherapy

Chemotherapy can produce side-effects or symptoms in a range of severity. The most common gastrointestinal symptoms are nausea and vomiting, stomatitis, and diarrhoea. Husain followed 624 patients with gynaecological malignancies receiving placitaxel chemotherapy, and found that 24% were hospitalized for gastrointestinal toxicity (31).

Nausea and vomiting associated with chemotherapy has been extensively studied, and has been shown to be of major significance. Four studies carried out in the same centre with similar study design between 1978 and 1990 have shown the prevalence of post-chemotherapy nausea and vomiting despite antiemetics to be 62%–72% (32). The prevalence did not decrease with time or the introduction of more effective antiemetic agents. It is postulated that more recent chemotherapy regimens involve higher doses of more severely emetogenic drugs, which contribute to this continued high prevalence. Pre-chemotherapy or anticipatory nausea and vomiting has a prevalence of approximately 23% (33).

Radiotherapy

Radiotherapy can cause side-effects that produce symptoms for the treated patients in the acute and late phase after treatment. Late side effects are more likely to be permanent. Increasing the total dose given, the dose per fraction, and/or the total volume treated, will increase the chance of side-effects.

Side-effects are more likely after radical radiotherapy. This is illustrated by several studies. Wang studied 220 patients who received radical radiotherapy for cervical carcinoma. Of these patients, 65% experienced moderate or severe diarrhoea, and 47% suffered from radiation proctitis from one to four years later (34). Benk studied the prevalence of late rectal bleeding after radiotherapy for prostate carcinoma by following patients for a median of 3.7 years. Rectal bleeding occurred in 16%–34% of patients depending on the type of treatment: those who received a higher total dose were more likely to suffer side effects. None required hospitalization, however (35).

Methodological considerations

Sample size and setting

The sample size varied between studies, from 26 (36) to 6677 (37). The samples studied represent diverse populations of patients, as evidenced by the broad range of inclusion criteria. For example, whilst most studied patients with cancer in general, some studied all patients referred to a hospital palliative care team with cancer and non-cancer diagnoses, or patients with a severe illness, or those with a particular cancer diagnosis (see Table 1.2).

Moreover, patients are studied in many different settings; for example, in in-patients units in hospital or in hospice, or in oncology out-patients or pain clinics (see Table 1.3). The setting may have an impact on prevalence of symptoms. First, it is possible that in-patients are in general more unwell than out-patients, although many patients will end their lives at home. Certainly, in a study of patients attending an oncology out-patients service, 15% of patients had no symptoms at all (16).

It may also be possible that the symptom mix, severity, or associated distress are affected by the study setting. For example, patients discharged home and trying to 'return to normal', may find anorexia more distressing and therefore report it more often.

Symptom measurement

Symptoms are inherently subjective, therefore patient self-report must be a primary source of information. Thus the subjective nature of symptoms has other important implications. There is often a wide overlap between patients in terms of understanding what is meant: heartburn in one patient may be abdominal pain in another. Studies of the epidemiology of symptoms are further complicated by the use of different symptom

Table 1.3 Site of patients at time of study

Sample setting	Number of studies
Hospital	11
Hospice/palliative care unit	9
Oncology out-patient clinic	2
Pain out-patient clinic	1
Home	4
Carers interviewed after patient's death	3

definitions by health care professionals. For example, over 20 definitions of dyspepsia have been identified (38).

It is also important to note that symptoms are not specific to cancer, nor indeed necessarily to an identifiable pathological condition. Dyspepsia accounts for 3%–4% of all general practice consultations (38). The 6-month prevalence of dyspepsia in a community study has been found to be 38% (39), but no organic lesion has been found in 34% of published cases (40).

The source of the information varies greatly: some studies used ready-made tools, e.g. the Edmonton Symptom Assessment Scale (ESAS), others formulated their own questionnaires or symptom checklists, others still drew information from the medical notes. Information that is included or excluded in questionnaires and notes will have a significant effect on the ultimate value of prevalence.

Some studies questioned only the patient about symptoms experienced. Some only recorded information actively volunteered by the patient (20). Others included information given by a surrogate (usually a relative or nurse directly involved in the patient's care). It may be that surrogates give less accurate information, but this approach facilitates the study of patients too unwell to answer questions.

Some studies quote point prevalence, others period prevalence of a symptom over a variable length of time; for example, the last year to the last 48 hours of life, making the prevalence values difficult to compare.

The reporting of a symptom does not in itself imply burden, nor the degree of any burden. Some studies have measured severity of symptoms. The prevalence of symptoms suffered 'severely' is less than overall prevalence (24,41,42).

Measurement tools

To understand a patient's experience more fully, it is necessary to measure symptom severity, or symptom impact in terms of function or quality of life. The use of global constructs may be useful in this respect. Global symptom distress may be an indicator of overall symptom burden in a population. The following tools have been used for symptom assessment in advanced cancer.

Symptom Distress Scale (43)

This scale was developed for patients with either cancer or heart disease. Eleven symptoms are measured using a five-point Likert scale in relation to quality of life.

Rotterdam Symptom Checklist (RSCL) (44)

This tool includes 30 physical and psychological symptoms measured on a four-point Likert scale and, in addition, eight items specifically attempt to define the impact of symptoms on physical activity and function.

Edmonton Symptom Assessment Scale (ESAS) (45)

The ESAS was developed for quick assessment of outcomes of routine clinical practice. It consists of visual analogue scales related to eight symptoms.

The Support Team Assessment Schedule (STAS) (46)

STAS is a validated measure of the effectiveness of palliative care. The effect of the items on the daily life of the patient over the last week is scored on a five-point Likert scale. Extended or adapted versions assess individual symptoms that can include nausea, vomiting, constipation, diarrhoea, dysphagia, anorexia, and oral discomfort.

European Organization for Research and Treatment of Cancer (EORTC QLQ C30) (47)

This is a 30-item questionnaire composed of multi-item and single items that reflect the multidimensionality of the quality of life construct. It includes seven items on specific symptoms.

Memorial Symptom Assessment Scale (48)

This instrument characterizes 32 physical and psychological symptoms in terms of intensity, frequency, and distress. It also includes a Global Distress Index.

Palliative Care Assessment (PACA) (42)

This measure was developed to assess the outcome of interventions made by a hospital palliative care team. Eight symptoms are scored on a four-point scale assessing severity.

Palliative Care Outcome Scale (POS) (49)

This is an 11-item scale designed to cover more than either physical symptoms or quality of life. Extended versions now include a core of symptoms with the same rating scales as for STAS symptoms.

Future research questions

Systematic symptom assessment is a cornerstone of clinical practice and research. The measurement of symptom prevalence is a prerequisite. The severity and impact of symptoms need to be more fully studied. The relationships between symptoms and tumour types have been investigated. The identification of any relationship between individual symptom types would also be useful. Any such relationships may give an indication of pathophysiological mechanisms, and thus contribute to improved symptom control. Further statistical evaluation of data would prove useful; for example, multivariate analysis would determine whether gender or cancer type is the predominant cause of increased nausea and/or vomiting in women. The majority of studies have assessed populations in in-patient units. It may be that the experience of cancer patients is different when they are at home, especially in terms of symptom burden, and this needs to be formally assessed.

Conclusions

The results of studies assessing the prevalence of a range of symptoms (6–23 symptoms, see Table 1.2) in cancer patients in various settings give highly variable results. The wide range of prevalence reflects differences in definition, survey methods, and sample population. It is also the result of differing time periods over which prevalence was measured.

Nevertheless, several studies show certain trends. Gender affects the type of symptoms experienced. Most notably, nausea and vomiting appear to be more common in women. The primary site of a cancer has a major influence on symptom prevalence. This suggests that any 'terminal common pathway' does not occur in the earlier stages of disease, although some symptoms do have prognostic value in more advanced disease. Performance status and quality of life are the most important prognostic indicators.

Information on symptom prevalence is most useful when it is coupled with data on symptom severity and measures of quality of life of function. This gives a clearer picture of patients experience of advancing malignant disease.

References

1. **Doyle D; Hanks GWC; Macdonald N.** *Oxford Textbook of Palliative Medicine.* 2nd edn. Oxford: Oxford University Press, 1998.
2. **Peckham M; Pinedo HM; Veronesi U.** *The Oxford Textbook Of Oncology.* Oxford: Oxford University Press, 1995.
3. **Sleisinger MH; Fordham JS.** *Gastrointestinal Disease.* Philadelphia: Saunders, 1993.
4. **Forbes K.** Palliative care in patients with cancer of the head and neck. *Clinical Otolaryngology* 1997;22:117–22.
5. **Krech R; Walsh D.** Symptoms of pancreatic cancer. *Journal of Pain and Symptom Management* 1991;6:360–7.
6. **Krech R; Davis J; Walsh D; Curtis EB.** Symptoms of lung cancer. *Palliative Medicine* 1992;6:309–15.
7. **Donnelly S; Walsh D.** The symptoms of advanced cancer. *Seminars in Oncology* 1995;22(2 Suppl.3):67–72.
8. **Sykes N; Baines M.** Clinical and pathological study of dysphagia conservatively managed in patients with advanced malignant disease. *The Lancet* 1988; 28(613):726–8.
9. **Grond S; Zech D; Diefenbach C; Bischoff A.** Prevalence and pattern of symptoms in patients with cancer pain: a prospective evaluation of 1635 cancer patients referred to a pain clinic. *Journal of Pain and Symptom Management* 1994;9:372–82.
10. **Vainio A; Auvinen A.** With members of the symptom prevalence group. Prevalence of symptoms among patients with advanced cancer. *Journal of Pain and Symptom Management* 1996;12:3–10.
11. **Fainsinger R; Miller MJ; Bruera E; Hanson J; Macheachern T.** Symptom control during the lastweek of life on a palliative care unit. *Journal of Palliative Care* 1991;7(1):5–11.
12. **Brescia FJ; Adler D; Gray G; Ryan MA; Cimino J; Mamtani R.** Hospitalised advanced cancer patients: a profile. *Journal of Pain and Symptom Management* 1990;5:221–7.
13. **Donnelly S; Walsh D.** The symptoms of advanced cancer: identification of clinical research priorities by assessment of prevalence and severity. *Journal of Palliative Care* 1995;11(1):27–32.
14. **Wachtel T; Allen-Masterston A; Reuben D; Goldberg R; Mor V.** The end stage cancer patient: terminal common pathway. *The Hospice Journal* 1998;4(4):43–81.
15. **Reuben DB; Mor V; Hiris J.** Clinical symptoms and length of survival in patients with terminal cancer. *Archives of Internal Medicine* 1988;148:1586–91.

16. **Schuit KW; Sleijfer DT; Meijler WJ; Otter R; Schakenraad J; van de Bergh FCM; Meyboon-de Jong B.** Symptoms and functional status of patients with disseminated cancer visiting outpatients departments. *Journal of Pain and Symptom Management* 1998;16:290–7.
17. **Lelli G; Angelelli B; Giambiasi ME.** The anabolic effect of high dose medroxyprogesterone acetate in oncology. *Pharmacological Research Communications* 1983;15:561–8.
18. **Nelson KA.** The cancer anorexia–canchexia syndrome. *Seminars in Oncology* 2000;27(1):64–8.
19. **Vigano A; Dorgan M; Buckingham J; Bruera E; Suarez-Almazar ME.** Survival prediction in terminal cancer patients: a systematic review of the literature. *Palliative Medicine* 2000;14:363–74.
20. **Coyle N; Adelhardt J; Foley KM, Portenoy RK.** Character of terminal illness in the advanced cancer patient: pain and other symptoms during the last four weeks of life. *Journal of Pain and Symptom Management* 1990;5:83–93.
21. **Lichter I; Hunt E.** The last 48 hours of life. *Journal of Palliative Care* 1990;6:7–15.
22. **Addington-Hall J; McCarthy M.** Dying from cancer: results of a national population-based investigation. *Palliative Medicine* 1995;9:295–305.
23. **Addington-Hall J; Macdonald LD; Anderson HR; Freeling P.** Dying from cancer: the views of bereaved family and friends about the experiences of terminally ill patients. *Palliative Medicine* 1991;5:207–14.
24. **Curtis EB; Krech R; Walsh D.** Common symptoms in patients with advanced cancer. *Journal of Palliative Care* 1991;7(2):25–9.
25. **Reuben D; Mor V.** Nausea and vomiting in terminal cancer patients. *Archives of Internal Medicine* 1986;146:2021–3.
26. **Dunlop GM.** A study of the relative frequency and importance of gastrointestinal symptoms and weakness in patients with far advanced cancer. *Palliative Medicine* 1989;4:37–43.
27. **Lichter I.** Results of antiemetic management in terminal illness. *Journal of Palliative Care* 1993;9(2):19–21.
28. **Baines M.** Nausea and vomiting in the patient with advanced cancer. *Journal of Pain and Symptom Management* 2000;3(2):81–5.
29. **Campora E; Merlini L; Pace M; Bruzzone M; Luzzani M; Gottlieb A; Rosso R.** The incidence of narcotic induced emesis. *Journal of Pain and Symptom Management* 1991;6:428–30.
30. **McIllmurray MB; Warren MR.** Evaluation of a new hospice: the relief of symptoms in cancer patients in the first year. *Palliative Medicine* 1989;3:135–40.
31. **Husain A; Aptaker L; Spriggs DR; Barakat RR.** Gastrointestinal toxicity and clostridium difficile diarrhea in patients treated with placitaxel-containing chemotherapy. *Gynaecologic Oncology* 1998;71(1);104–7.
32. **Morrow GR.** Behavioural factors influencing the development and expression of chemotherapy induced side effects. *British Journal of Cancer* 1992;66(Suppl. XIX):S54–S61.
33. **Watson M; McCarron J; Law M.** Anticipatory nausea and emesis, and psychological morbidity: assessment of prevalence among outpatients on mild to moderate chemotherapy regimens. *British Journal of Cancer* 1992;66:862–6.
34. **Wang CJ; Leung SW; Chen HC; Sun LM; Fang FM; Huang EY; Hsiung CY; Changchien CC.** The correlation of acute toxicity and late rectal injury in radiotherapy for cervical carcinoma: evidence suggestive of consequential late effect (CQLE). *International Journal of Radiation Oncology* 1998;40(1):85–91.
35. **Benk VA; Adams JA; Shipley WU; Urie MM.** Late rectal bleeding following combined X ray and proton high dose irradiation for patients with stage T3-T$ prostate carcinoma. *International Journal of Radiation Oncology, Biology, Physics* 1993;26(3):551–7.

36. **Hockley JM; Dunlop R; Davies RJ**. Survey of distressing symptoms in dying patients and their families in hospital and the response of the symptom control team. *British Medical Journal* 1988;296:1715–7.

37. **Twycross RG; Lack SA. Diarrhoea**. In: Control of Alimentary Symptoms in Far Advanced Cancer. London: Churchill Livingstone, 1986: pp. 208–29.

38. **Grainger SL; Klass HJ; Rake MO; Williams JG**. Prevalence of dyspepsia: the epidemiology of overlapping symptoms. *Postgraduate Medical Journal* 1994;70:154–61.

39. **Jones R; Lydeard S**. Prevalence of symptoms of dyspepsia in the community. *British Medical Journal* 1989;298:30–2.

40. **Grant Thompson W**. Non-ulcer-dyspepsia. *Canadian Medical Association Journal* 1984;130:565–9.

41. **Desbiens NA; Mueller Ritzner N; Connors AF; Neil S; Wenger MD; Lynn J**. The symptom burden of seriously ill hospitalised patients. *Journal of Pain and Symptom Management* 1999;17:248–55.

42. **Ellershaw J; Peat SJ; Boys LC**. Assessing the effectiveness of a hospital palliative care team. *Palliative Medicine* 1995;9:145–52.

43. **McCorkle R; Young K**. Development of a symptom distress scale. *Cancer Nursing* 1978;101:373–8.

44. **de Haes JCJM; van Knippenberg FCE; Neijt JP**. Measuring psychological and physical distress in cancer patients: structure and application of the Rotterdam Symptom Checklist. *British Journal of Cancer* 1990;62:1034–8.

45. **Bruera E; Kuehn N; Miller MJ; Selmer P; Macmillan K**. The Edmonton Symptom Assessment System (ESAS): a simple method for the assessment of palliative care patients. *Journal of Palliative Care* 1991;7(2):6–9.

46. **Higginson I; Higginson IJ**, editors. *Clinical Audit in Palliative Care. A community schedule.* Oxford: Radcliffe Medical Press, 1993: pp. 34–7.

47. **Aaronson NK; Ahmedzai S; Bergman B; Bullinger M; Cull A; Duez N; Filiberti A**. The European Organization for Research and Treatment of Cancer QLQ-C30: A quality of life instrument for use in international clinical trials in cancer. *Journal of the National Cancer Institute* 1993;85(5):365–76.

48. **Portenoy RK; Thaler HT; Kornblith AB; Lepore JM; Friedlander KH; Kiyasu E**. The memorial symptom assessment scale: an instrument for the evaluation of symptom prevalence, characteristics and distress. *European Journal of Cancer* 1994;30A:1326–36.

49. **Hearn J; Higginson IJ**. Development and validation of a core outcome measure for palliative care: the palliative care outcome scale. *Quality in Health Care* 1999;8:219–27.

50. **Redding SW; Zellars RC; Kirkpatrick WR; McAtee RK; Caceres MA; Fothergill AW; Lopez-Ribot JL; Bailey CW; Rinaldi MG; Patterson TF**. Epidemiology of oropharyngeal Candida clonization and infection in patients receiving radiation for head and neck cancer. *Journal of Clinical Microbiology* 1999;37(12):3896–900.

51. **Armes PJ; Plant HJ; Allbright A; Silverstone T; Slevin ML**. A study to investigate the incidence of early satiety in patients with advanced cancer. *British Journal of Cancer* 1992;65:481–4.

52. **Neilson SS; Theologides A; Vickers ZM**. Influence of food odours on food aversions and preferences in patients with cancer. *American Journal of Clinical Nutrition* 1980;33:2253–61.

53. **Cartwright A; Hockley JM; Anderson JL**. *Life before Death.* London: Routledge & Kegan Paul, 1973:23p.

54. **Sykes NP; Doyle D; Hanks GWC; Macdonald N**, editors. Constipation and diarrhoea. In: *Oxford Textbook of Palliative Medicine.* 2nd edn. Oxford: Oxford University Press, 1998; 9.3.3: pp. 513–25.

55. **Dunphy KP.** A comparison of hospice and homecare patients: patterns of referral, patient characteristics and predictors of death. *Palliative Medicine* 1990;4:105–111.
56. **Seale C.** Death from cancer and death from other causes: the relevance of the hospice approach. *Palliative Medicine* 1991;**5**:12–19.
57. **Conill C; Verger E; Henriquez I.** Symptom prevalence in the last week of life. *Journal of Pain and Symptom Management* 1997;14(6):328–31.
58. **Jenkins CA; Taube AW; Turner K; Hanson J.** Initial demographic, symptom and medication profiles in patients in continuing palliative care units. *Journal of Pain and Symptom Management* 1998;16(3):163–70.
59. **Ng K; von Gunten CF.** Symptoms and attitudes of 100 consecutive patients admitted to an acute hospice/palliative care unit. *Journal of Pain and Symptom Management* 1998;16(5):307–16.
60. **Edmonds PM; Stuttaford JM; Penny J; Lynch A.** Do hospital palliative care teams improve symptom control? Use of a modified STAS as an evaluation tool. *Palliative Medicine* 1998;12:345–51.
61. **Ventafridda V; Ripamonti C; de Conno F; Tamburini M.** Symptom prevalence and control during cancer patients' last days of life. *Journal of Palliative Care* 1990;6(3):7–11.
62. **Sebastian P; Varghese C; Sankaranarayanan R; Zaina CP.** Evaluation of symptomatology in planning palliative care. *Palliative Medicine* 1993;7:27–43.

Chapter 2

The clinical assessment of the patient with gastrointestinal symptoms

Mary-Ellen Mazuryk

Introduction

Gastrointestinal symptoms are a common source of distress in advanced cancer patients. A survey of 1000 palliative care patients has revealed that four of the 10 most frequently observed symptoms were gastrointestinal in nature. These included anorexia, weight loss, constipation, and early satiety (1). Other common gastrointestinal symptoms included in the 21 overall most common symptoms were nausea, vomiting, taste change, and dysphagia. Furthermore, these symptoms were rated as clinically significant in 60%–80% of cases. Symptom severity tended to vary according to tumour type for some symptoms. For example, dysphagia was most prevalent in patients with oesophageal or head and neck tumours and nausea and vomiting was most prevalent in patients with gynaecological malignancies. The median number of symptoms experienced at a given time was 10–12, implying that the majority of patients will be suffering with several different gastrointestinal symptoms.

It is essential that gastrointestinal symptoms be recognized and properly assessed in order to provide patients with interventions to relieve symptoms and improve quality of life. Many gastrointestinal symptoms are related. In other words, improvement in one symptom may have positive effects on another. An example of this would be successful management of constipation that could also improve symptoms of nausea, vomiting, and anorexia as well as non-gastrointestinal symptoms of confusion or psychological distress/anxiety.

This chapter focuses on common gastrointestinal symptoms and problems, which develop in advanced cancer patients. A clinically based approach to assessment of these problems will be presented.

Assessment of symptoms

Health care professionals are constantly assessing and evaluating patients, sometimes even unconsciously. It is important to bring mindfulness and discipline to this process so that the patient's needs can be met most effectively. A comprehensive assessment should incorporate an awareness of the multidimensional nature of symptoms. It is helpful to consider each symptom separately, but then to relate it to other symptoms and to other aspects of the patient's life (spiritual, psychological, social, etc.).

Assessment begins with communication. Symptoms are purely subjective and therefore the patient is the best person to describe them (2–4). The patient should be made aware that open communication about symptoms is encouraged and that relief of symptoms is a major endpoint goal. A detailed history should be obtained regarding every symptom and the symptoms should be reassessed at each patient visit.

In addition to questioning the patient about symptoms, there is value in administering measurement or assessment tools that can help to quantify patient perceptions about symptoms in a reliable way. These tools can be used to document the intensity of a symptom over time, allowing the health care professional and the patient to gauge the therapeutic effect of interventions and make ongoing clinical decisions. Tools also allow for ongoing evaluation of practice for quality assurance and/or research.

The visual analog scale (VAS) has been validated as a tool to assess a variety of physical and psychological symptoms (5). It is simple and quick to administer, and provides a numerical score for a given symptom that can be followed over time. To provide a more multidimensional view of a given symptom, the VAS has been expanded into a broader system, the Edmonton Symptom Assessment System or ESAS (3,6). The ESAS consists of nine VASs, 0–100 mm, for pain, activity, nausea, depression, anxiety, drowsiness, appetite, shortness of breath, and sensation of well-being. In addition, an extra VAS is reserved for the assessment of a less frequent symptom that might be particularly important to a given patient and is not otherwise specified (3). For practical purposes, the ESAS may be favoured over other more complex assessment tools because of its ease of administration, a factor that is particularly important in the advanced cancer population, where there is a high prevalence of fatigue, distress, and cognitive impairment (2).

Other potential symptom assessment tools include standardized toxicity scales such as those recommended by the World Health Organization or National Cancer Institute (7,8). While these tools may be useful in the context of research studies, they provide very limited practical information to clinicians. Assessment of global quality of life may also be performed to supplement specific symptom assessment, but, up to now, the use of these tools has not been incorporated into routine patient care (2). There are no other validated tools for the assessment of specific gastrointestinal symptoms in advanced cancer patients. This is an important area, which could be developed through research.

Clinically, symptom assessment consists of obtaining a detailed history, targeted physical examination, ancillary investigations where appropriate, and administration of validated measurement tools. In the absence of a gold standard tool for the assessment of gastrointestinal symptoms, the VAS or ESAS may be the most useful tool to administer. Once symptoms are identified and assessed, the information obtained should be shared with the patient and prioritized according to their overall impact on the patient's situation. A management plan can then be developed that is appropriate to the patient's needs.

Assessment of specific gastrointestinal symptoms/problems

Abdominal pain

Epidemiology

Pain of any type is present in 30%–60% of cancer patients during active treatment, and in greater than 65% of those with advanced disease (9). The differential diagnosis of abdominal pain in advanced cancer patients is extensive (10). Generally, it can be broken down into tumour-related causes and benign non-tumour-related causes. Common potential causes are covered elsewhere in this textbook. Although tumour-related causes tend to be emphasized, it is important to consider non-cancer causes of pain as well. Advanced cancer patients are not immune to developing serious non-cancer-related abdominal pain emergencies and, in fact, the symptoms of an acute abdomen may be blunted or masked in these patients (11).

History

It is important to ask about the character of the pain. What words would the patient use to describe it? Its distribution, intensity, and temporal course can provide valuable clues as to the classification and aetiology of the pain. Somatic pain tends to be well localized and described as sharp, aching, or throbbing. Visceral pain is usually diffuse and described as gnawing or cramping if due to obstruction of a hollow viscus and aching or sharp if due to involvement of mesentery or organ capsule. Neuropathic pain may be described as burning, tingling, stabbing or lancinating (9). Exacerbating and alleviating factors should be elicited, as well as response of the pain to any interventions (pharmacological and non-pharmacological) that the patient has tried. The effect of the pain on physical, psychological, and social function should be queried. The pain should also be assessed in the context of other existing symptoms. Pain may affect the patient's perception or ability to describe other symptoms or vice versa (12). ESAS may be particularly useful in this regard by allowing the simultaneous study of other symptoms.

There are other specific multidimensional tools for pain assessment including the McGill Pain Questionnaire (13), the Memorial Pain Assessment Card (14) and the Brief Pain Inventory (15). This may be helpful in selected clinical situations.

Physical examination

Abdominal examination is required. Inspection of the abdomen should be carried out for any obvious masses that may be indicative of tumour, organomegaly, or faeces. Scars indicative of previous surgeries may be helpful. Auscultation of the abdomen for bowel sounds should be performed. These may be absent in the setting of ileus or peritonitis. High-pitched, tinkling bowel sounds may be present with bowel obstruction. Palpation of the abdomen for tender areas and associated masses or organomegaly is useful. The typical signs associated with peritonitis, e.g. from a perforated viscus, may be masked in the advanced cancer patient. A high index of suspicion is required (16).

Ancillary tests

Occasionally, additional investigations may be helpful. A plain abdominal radiograph can document severe constipation or ileus. A recumbent and upright abdominal radiograph will show partial or complete bowel obstruction or perforation. Ultrasound or abdominal computerized tomography (CT) scan may be appropriate in some cases to document extent/location of tumour or acute problems such as haemorrhage. A complete blood count can identify associated or contributing features such as leukocytosis, anaemia, or thrombocytopenia. Extensive investigations are not always appropriate in advanced cancer patients. Before ordering any tests, the health care professional should consider whether or not the result of the test will benefit the patient in terms of symptom relief or opening up useful treatment options. Whenever possible, the patient and/or family should also be part of this decision.

Constipation

Epidemiology

Constipation has been defined in various ways including passage of small, hard stool infrequently and with difficulty, passing stool less than three times per week, straining at stool during more than 25% of bowel movements, or bowel movements lasting greater than 10 minutes (17). There can be major interindividual differences in what constitutes abnormality in a given patient. Constipation is present in more than 50% of patients on a palliative care unit or hospice (17,18). This may actually underestimate the problem as many of these patients will already be on an effective laxative regimen. Opioids are the major cause of constipation in advanced cancer patients with constipation occurring in 90% of patients on opioids (19).

History

It is helpful to use the patient's prior stool pattern as a basis for comparisons. Useful questions include:

1 When was the last bowel movement?
2 What were the characteristics of the bowel movement? Was straining necessary? Was there pain on defaecation?
3 Does the patient feel an urge to move bowels but is unable to? This may suggest rectal obstruction or the presence of hard stool.
4 Has the patient lost urge to move bowels? This may suggest the presence of a spinal cord problem.
5 Does the patient have easy access to the toilet or commode? Impaired mobility or reliance on care-givers to assist in toileting may predispose to the development of constipation (20).
6 Are there other associated symptoms? These may include flatulence, abdominal pain, nausea and/or vomiting, bloating, or anorexia (17). The presence of additional symptoms may also suggest possible causes for constipation. For example, constipation in the context of abdominal pain and vomiting may suggest the presence of partial or complete bowel obstruction.
7 Is the patient taking any medications, that could predispose to constipation? These include opioids, anticholinergics, many antidepressants, chemotherapy (particularly the vinca alkaloids), 5HT3 antagonist antiemetics, iron preparations, and others.
8 Is the patient using laxatives? What is the particular laxative regimen?

Physical examination

Palpation of the abdomen may reveal faecal masses, particularly in the region of the descending colon. Several features help to distinguish a faecal mass from tumour. Faeces will usually indent with deep palpation. The mass may have a crepitus-like feel due to entrapped gas. Over time, a faecal mass will move (17). Rectal examination is essential in the assessment of constipation. It may reveal impacted, hard stool that should then be removed to facilitate bowel movement. Other rectal pathology such as tumour, rectocele, or ulceration may also be palpable. Anal sphincter tone and sacral nerve root sensation should be assessed to rule out a spinal cord lesion. The actual stool can be examined. Small, hard pellets suggest slowed colonic transit, commonly present in advanced cancer patients.

Ribbon-like stool suggests bowel stenosis or haemorrhoids. The presence of blood or mucus is suggestive of haemorrhoids, tumour, or inflammation.

Ancillary tests

A plain abdominal radiograph can be extremely useful in the assessment of constipation. Diagnosis of constipation by history and physical examination alone has been shown to be inaccurate, unreliable, and often omitted by health care professionals (21). An abdominal radiograph can provide an objective assessment of faecal load. A constipation scoring system has been proposed based on the amount of stool visible in each quadrant (ascending colon, transverse colon, descending colon, and rectum). Each quadrant is assigned a score from 0 to 3 where 0 = no stool, 1 = stool < 50%, 2 = stool > 50% but < 100%, and 3 = stool occupies 100% of lumen. A score of greater or equal to 7/12 is considered to reflect severe constipation (21,22). The abdominal radiograph is a non-invasive and relatively inexpensive test. It allows an accurate and rapid diagnosis of constipation, leading to timely treatment. Other more sophisticated tests including radio opaque marker studies of colonic transit time, defaecography, and anal sphincter electromyogram are arduous and generally inappropriate for use in the advanced cancer population.

An important laboratory test to obtain in any patient with constipation is a serum calcium, since malignant hypercalcaemia is an easily reversible cause of constipation and other gastrointestinal complaints. Thyroid hormone studies to rule out hypothyroidism may also be helpful in selected patients.

The specific causes and management of constipation are addressed in Chapter 9.

Nausea and vomiting

Epidemiology

Nausea and/or vomiting affects 50%–60% of advanced cancer patients (23) and up to 70%–80% of patients receiving chemotherapy (24). A basic understanding of the emetic pathway and the primary neurotransmitters involved is essential for accurate assessment and management of nausea. Antiemetic drugs are effective at different neurotransmitter receptor sites and therefore are more or less effective, depending on the cause of the nausea (25,26). This pathophysiology is covered elsewhere in this textbook (Chapter 8).

History

It is important to ascertain the onset and duration of nausea symptoms, the intensity (using a VAS or related scale), the frequency, and any exacerbating or relieving factors. The quantity of emesis is useful. Large volumes of emesis may suggest the presence of gastric outlet or proximal small bowel obstruction. Small volumes suggest gastroparesis (25). The character of the emesis including the presence of blood or undigested food is helpful. Undigested food suggests gastroparesis or proximal gastrointestinal obstruction. Other features that suggest the presence of gastroparesis or autonomic aetiology of nausea include syncopal symptoms, anorexia, and early satiety (25,27). Anorexia, asthenia, and weight loss, along with chronic nausea, suggest the cancer anorexia–cachexia syndrome (25,28). The specific cancer diagnosis may provide clues as to the aetiology of nausea. For example, a diagnosis of a cancer that frequently metastasises to the brain, such as small cell lung cancer, may lead one to consider the possibility of brain metastasis and increased intracranial pressure as a possible aetiology. The presence of an intra-abdominal cancer may suggest obstruction as a factor. A review of medication may identify a contributing factor. Knowledge of other co-morbidities such as peptic ulcer disease or diabetic gastroparesis may identify other causes for nausea.

Physical examination

An abdominal examination is essential to rule out causes such as bowel obstruction, ileus, constipation, or 'squashed stomach' due to compression by tumour or hepatomegaly. A succussion splash indicative of a large, fluid-filled stomach may be present with gastric outlet obstruction (29). Rectal examination as part of the routine screen for constipation is helpful. Postural hypotension, a fixed heart rate, and tachycardia may be indicative of autonomic neuropathy. These features can be quantified more precisely using standardized tests for diabetic autonomic neuropathy including postural blood pressure measurement (positive test is failure to increase systolic blood pressure when standing from a supine position), measurement of diastolic blood pressure during hand grip manoeuvre (positive test is pressure increase of less than 5 mm Hg), and heart rate change during deep breathing in supine position (rate variation of less than 10 beats per minute is abnormal) (30).

Ancillary tests

A plain abdominal radiograph is helpful, particularly if constipation is suspected. In addition, an upright abdominal radiograph may show bowel obstruction or ileus. There are several ways to assess gastric emptying if autonomic neuropathy is suspected. These include the saline load test (which requires placement of a nasogastric tube), radiographic barium studies, ultrasound (useful to assess gastric emptying of liquids only), and radionuclide studies (27). Cardiac features of autonomic neuropathy can be identified using electrocardiogram recordings to measure best-to-beat heart rate variation with Valsalva manoeuvre and postural changes (30). Many of these tests are invasive and arduous and are generally inappropriate in the majority of advanced cancer patients except in the setting of research studies. Laboratory tests to rule out metabolic causes for nausea include assessment of serum electrolytes, creatinine, blood urea nitrogen, calcium, albumin, and liver enzymes. A CT scan of the brain is useful if increased intracranial pressure is suspected. In resistant cases, upper gastrointestinal endoscopy or barium studies may be useful to document the presence of peptic ulcer disease or esophagitis as a cause for nausea. The causes and management of chronic nausea are discussed in Chapter 8.

Malignant bowel obstruction

Epidemiology

Malignant bowel obstruction is a diagnosis rather than a symptom, but deserves separate comment. It is most commonly associated with ovarian or gastrointestinal cancer. It can develop anytime in the illness trajectory but is more common in the advanced stages. It can occur in up to 45% of advanced-stage ovarian cancer patients (31,32) and 10%–30% of advanced-stage gastrointestinal cancer patients (32,33). However, any cancer that spreads into the abdomen can cause obstruction. The site of obstruction varies with the tumour type. Obstruction due to pancreas cancer tends to localize to duodenum or stomach; colon cancer tends to block jejunum and ileum; prostate or bladder cancer may contribute to more distal blockages. Ovarian cancer causes small bowel obstruction more commonly than large bowel (32). There may be multiple sites of obstruction in a single patient. The cause of bowel obstruction in advanced cancer patients is usually tumour related, either via extrinsic compression or intrinsic or intramural occlusion. Paraneoplastic autonomic neuropathy or severe constipation may cause a 'pseudo-obstruction'. Occasionally, non-cancer-related causes are found such as adhesions.

History

Bowel obstruction is less likely to be an acute presentation in advanced cancer patients compared with non-cancer patients. Usually, blockage is slowly progressive and passes through a partial obstruction phase. It is important to ask about associated symptoms of nausea and vomiting, abdominal pain, constipation, or diarrhoea. Large volume emesis, often biliary in nature, develops early in the course of gastric outlet or proximal small bowel obstruction. Late onset emesis, sometimes of faecaloid material, is more characteristic of large bowel obstruction. The presence and character of abdominal pain is important information. Pain may be particularly colicky and intense in the setting of proximal bowel obstruction. Large bowel obstruction tends to produce pain that is deeper, less intense, and more constant. An acute onset of pain is suspicious for perforation or strangulation (32,33). The presence of medications such as corticosteroids can mask symptoms and contribute to increased risk of perforation (34).

Physical examination

Abdominal examination is essential. This includes inspection for abdominal distension and visible loops of bowel or peristalsis. Auscultation of bowel sounds is helpful. High pitched, tinkling bowel sounds are characteristic of obstruction. Absence of bowel sounds suggests ileus or peritonitis. Percussion of the abdomen may demonstrate hypertympany. Palpation may reveal tumour masses contributing to obstruction. A rectal examination is important to rule out faecal impaction. There may be hyperdynamic instability due to dehydration, electrolyte imbalance, or sepsis.

Ancillary tests

Radiographically, multiple views of the abdomen can be helpful. These radiographs can differentiate between bowel obstruction and severe constipation. In patients with clinical evidence of bowel obstruction and who would be candidates for surgery, radiographs can confirm the presence of obstruction and determine its site (35). In patients who are not surgical candidates, radiographs may still be of use to confirm the diagnosis in difficult cases. This allows for the application of medical management for bowel obstruction. Contrast studies may be considered in selected cases, particularly those with non-diagnostic plain radiographs, atypical clinical presentation, or protracted courses of obstructive symptoms. A contrast enema can confirm the presence of large bowel obstruction. If a partial obstruction is suspected clinically, water soluble contrast such as gastrografin should be used rather than barium since the water content of the barium can be absorbed by the colon and the barium can become inspissated above the partially obstructing lesion, sometimes worsening the obstruction (36). The causes and management of bowel obstruction are discussed in Chapter 12.

Diarrhoea

Epidemiology

Diarrhoea is difficult to define in an individual patient, since normal bowel function can vary significantly. However, it is generally accepted that diarrhoea is present if there is an increase in one or more of daily stool weight, water content, or frequency (37). Diarrhoea is present in approximately 5% of advanced cancer patients and in up to 10% of hospice patients (37). The most common cause of diarrhoea in palliative medicine is imbalance of laxatives. This generally settles within a day or two if the laxatives are stopped and subsequently restarted at a lower dose (38). Diarrhoea can be further classified into either osmotic or secretory forms. Osmotic diarrhoea is caused by the addition of an unabsorbed solute into the gastrointestinal tract. Examples include diarrhoea secondary to excessive lactulose use, or carbohydrate malabsorption (17). Secretory diarrhoea is caused by the active secretion of fluid and electrolytes by the bowel that is greater than normal absorptive capacity. Examples include diarrhoea secondary to endocrine tumours such as gastrinoma, VIPoma, and carcinoid (39).

History

It is helpful to use the patient's prior stool pattern as a basis for comparison. The onset, duration, frequency, and nature of stools should be assessed. Pale, fatty, greasy stools suggest malabsorption. Sudden onset of diarrhoea following a period of constipation suggests 'overflow' diarrhoea, related to leakage of fluid material around impacted hard stool (17). Relation of diarrhoea to eating and the presence or absence of nocturnal diarrhoea are important distinctions as osmotic diarrhoea typically stops with fasting whereas secretory diarrhoea does not (39). History of recent antineoplastic therapy including chemotherapy, radiation, or surgery is important since these may be contributing factors. Use of medications, particularly laxatives, antibiotics, and antacids may suggest a cause. Excessive intake of a stimulating laxative such as senna may cause colicky pain and faecal urgency. Excessive intake of a softening laxative such as docusate may cause watery stools and faecal oozing (17). Other associated symptoms may suggest diagnostic entities. These include the presence of hypotension, diaphoresis, flushing, palpitations, and wheezing in carcinoid syndrome and post-prandial nausea, abdominal distension, diaphoresis, and tachycardia in gastric 'dumping syndrome' (37).

Physical examination

Complete abdominal examination and rectal examination is indicated. It is important to exclude a hard faecal mass on rectal examination which may be contributing to overflow diarrhoea.

Ancillary tests

Stool samples can be sent for a variety of tests including occult blood, culture and sensitivity (particularly for clostridium difficile), stool electrolytes and stool osmolality. Stool anion gap is defined as stool osmolality −2 (stool potassium + stool sodium). Values of greater than 50 mmol per litre are consistent with osmotic diarrhoea and values of less than 50 mmol per litre are consistent with secretory diarrhoea (17). In extreme or resistant cases, colonoscopy may be indicated to assess for the presence of colitis, graft versus host disease in selected patients, or other etiologies. The causes and management of diarrhoea are discussed in Chapter 10.

Dysphagia

Epidemiology

Dysphagia is defined as difficulty in transferring solids or liquids from the mouth to the stomach (40). It can be associated with odynophagia (painful swallowing), vomiting, and aspiration. Dysphagia is particularly prevalent in patients with oesophageal or head and neck cancers. Patients with head and neck cancers have an incidence of 40% on presentation and up to 80% in advanced diseases (41). Dysphagia is present in up to 90% of new oesophageal cancer patients, with odynophagia coexisting in 50% of these patients (42). Overall, dysphagia is present in 12%–23% of hospice patients (43).

History

The patient's description of where food or liquid seems to 'stick' is very important since patient localization corresponds to the anatomical site of the problem in the vast majority of cases (40). Onset of dysphagia, progression of symptoms over time, and problems with solids, liquids, or both helps to clarify possible etiologies. Obstructing lesions often produce difficulty with solids initially, then liquids as the degree of obstruction increases. Neuromuscular disorders usually produce difficulty with solids and liquids simultaneously. Dysphagia symptoms that progress over weeks to months are suggestive of cancer, while transient acute dysphagia and/or odynophagia is suggestive of inflammatory causes (40,44). It is important to ask about associated symptoms. Weight loss is generally due to decreased oral intake or, in some cases, anorexia/cachexia from advanced malignancy. Hoarseness may develop in advanced oesophageal cancer as the recurrent laryngeal nerve becomes involved. In that case, hoarseness usually follows the onset of dysphagia (44). Nasal regurgitation suggests the presence of a tracheoesophageal fistula or oropharyngeal weakness. Unilateral wheezing can develop from an associated mediastinal mass. Hiccoughs may be indicative of a lesion in the distal oesophagus contributing to dysphagia.

Physical examination

Physical examination may clarify possible causes of dysphagia. In patients without a prior diagnosis of malignancy, examination should focus on looking for signs of malignancy, including head and neck lesions, peripheral adenopathy, presence of cachexia and wasting, etc. Examination of the cranial nerves may reveal weakness or sensory changes that could be contributing to dysphagia. Examination of the lungs to rule out coexisting aspiration pneumonia is also helpful.

Ancillary tests

Specific diagnostic tests may be useful in the setting of dysphagia in order to determine the underlying cause and to make subsequent recommendations for treatment or rehabilitation options. The appropriateness of testing a given patient must first be assessed on the basis of the overall condition of the patient and the expected benefit that might be derived from the test. Involvement of a speech and language pathologist to perform a simple bedside swallowing evaluation may be helpful, particularly in cases where the dysphagia is mainly related to oral or pharyngeal problems. A modified barium swallow allows for a more extensive evaluation of dysphagia and assesses all four phases of swallowing. It can aid in identifying all potential causes of dysphagia, including obstruction from tumour. More sophisticated studies have been developed, including a videofluroscopic swallowing study and flexible endoscopic evaluation of swallow, but these are less widely used in advanced cancer patients (45). Upper endoscopy can be useful to diagnose the cause of dysphagia, particularly malignancy or esophagitis. If necessary, biopsies can be performed. Endoscopy may also help to guide the choice of therapy such as stents or laser therapy (42,46).

The assessment of dysphagia is further discussed in Chapter 7; endoscopic management of dysphagia is discussed in Chapter 17.

Ascites

Epidemiology

Ascites is a clinical sign rather than a symptom, but deserves separate mention as it is often associated with distressing symptoms of abdominal distension, bloating, abdominal discomfort, nausea and vomiting, anorexia, acid reflux, and dyspnea. There are many potential causes of ascites but this section will focus on malignant ascites. Ascites is defined as a collection of intraperitoneal fluid. Malignant ascites is most commonly associated with either gynaecologic or gastrointestinal malignancies. Of women who present with malignant ascites, 75% of these will be related to a gynaecologic malignancy (ovarian, uterus, or cervix). In men, more than 50% of cases are related to a gastrointestinal malignancy (colorectal, gastric, or pancreatic) (47).

History

The onset of symptoms related to ascites is generally insidious. It is important to ask specifically about associated symptoms of abdominal bloating, pain or discomfort, nausea, anorexia, weight gain, increased abdominal girth, and gastrointestinal reflux. Dyspnea and orthopnea can develop in advanced cases due to elevation of the diaphragm and/or leakage of ascitic fluid into the pleural space (47,48). Questions about the recent development of ankle edema, weight gain, and increased abdominal girth may be particularly helpful in diagnosing ascites (49).

As with any symptom in advanced cancer patients, it is important to assess the severity of the symptom in the context of overall function, distress, and quality of life.

Physical examination

Abdominal findings associated with ascites include flank dullness, bulging flanks, shifting dullness, fluid wave, and puddle sign. None of these tests have been found to be both highly specific and sensitive for the presence of ascites except in advanced cases that are readily apparent clinically even without these tests. In addition, these tests are dependent on the free flow of ascitic fluid, which can be limited in situations where loculation has occurred (50). Extra abdominal findings associated with ascites include pleural effusions in approximately 5% of cases, and ankle oedema are felt to be related to hypoalbuminaemia and/or lymphatic obstruction (48).

Ancillary tests

Ultrasound is considered the gold standard for diagnosing the presence of ascites. It can detect as little as 100 ml of ascitic fluid (50). Once a patient is known to have malignant ascites, there is little need to perform repeated ultrasound examinations. A plain abdominal radiograph may be suggestive of ascites with a generalized 'ground glass' appearance, dimming of the psoas shadow, and the presence of air-filled small bowel loops in a central distribution. However, a radiograph alone is not generally recommended for diagnosis of ascites (47). Abdominal paracentesis can be performed for both diagnostic and therapeutic purposes. Fluid can be sent for a variety of studies including complete cell count and differential, chemistry (including protein and LDH levels), microbiology, tumour markers (including CEA or CA-125), and cytology. These studies are most important if the diagnosis has not yet been made. Features suggestive of malignant ascites include >10 000 erythrocytes per microlitre, >1000 leukocytes per microlitre, increased ascitic/serum ratios of protein (>0.4), increased ascitic/serum ratios of LDH (>1.0), positive cytology, and positive tumour markers (47). If paracentesis is being performed purely for therapeutic reasons, then special testing of the fluid is not routinely necessary. The causes and management of ascites are discussed in depth in Chapter 15.

Conclusion

Gastrointestinal symptoms and syndromes are commonly encountered in advanced cancer patients. A comprehensive approach to assessment is essential if a patient's symptoms are to be categorised and relieved. An appropriate blend of subjective and objective information must be obtained around each symptom. Whenever possible, a multidimensional assessment focusing on each symptom in the context of other physical, emotional, social, and spiritual concerns should be performed. There is a need for ongoing research in order to develop more effective and reliable ways of assessing gastrointestinal symptoms.

References

1. **Donnelly S; Walsh TD.** The symptoms of advanced cancer. *Seminars in Oncology* 1995; 22(Suppl. 3):67–72.
2. **Ingham J; Portenoy RK.** The measurement of pain and other symptoms. In: Doyle D; Hanks GWC; MacDonald N., editors. *The Oxford Textbook of Palliative Medicine.* 2nd edn. Oxford: Oxford University Press, 1998: pp. 203–19.
3. **Bruera E; Kuehn N; Miller MJ., *et al.*** The Edmonton symptom assessment system (ESAS): a simple method for the assessment of palliative care patients. *Journal of Palliative Care* 1991;7:6–9.
4. **Nekolaichuk CL; Bruera E; Spachynski K., *et al.*** A comparison of patient and proxy symptom assessments in advanced cancer patients. *Palliative Medicine* 1999;13:311–23.
5. **Price DD; McGrath P; Rasffi A., *et al.*** The validation of a visual analog scale or ratio scale for pain. *Pain* 1983;17:45–6.
6. **Chang VT; Hwang SS; Feuerman M.** Validation of the Edmonton symptom assessment scale. *Cancer* 2000;88:2164–71.
7. **Miller AB; Hoogstraten B; Staquet M., *et al.*** Reporting results of cancer treatment. *Cancer* 1981;47:207–14.
8. US Department of Health and Human Services, National Institutes of Health, National Cancer Institute. *Investigator's Handbook: A Manual for Participants in Clinical Trials of Investigational Agents Sponsored by DCTD, NCI.* Bethesda, MD: National Cancer Institute, 1998.
9. **Chemiy NI.** Cancer pain: principles of assessment and syndromes. In: Berger AM; Portenoy RK; Weissman DE., editors. *Principles and Practice of Supportive Oncology.* Philadelphia: Lippincott-Raven, 1998: pp.3–42.
10. **Schwartzentuber DJ.** Abdominal pain. In: DeVita VT; Hellman S; Rosenberg SA., editors. *Cancer: Principles and Practice of Oncology.* 5th edn. Philadelphia: Lippincott-Raven, 1997: pp. 2500–1.
11. **Amigo P; Mazuryk M; Watanabe S; Bruera E.** Recent onset of abdominal pain in a patient with advanced breast cancer. *Journal of Pain and Symptom Management* 2000;20:77–80.
12. **Bruera E; Watanabe S.** New development in the assessment of pain in cancer patients. *Supportive Care in Cancer* 1994;2:312–18.

13. **Melzack R**. The McGill pain questionnaire: major properties and scoring methods. *Pain* 1975;1:277–99.
14. **Fishman B; Pasternak S; Wallenstein SL., *et al.*** The memorial pain assessment card: a valid instrument for the evaluation of cancer pain. *Cancer* 1987;60:1151–8.
15. **Daut RL; Cleeland CS; Flanery RC**. Development of the Wisconsin brief pain questionnaire to assess pain in cancer and other diseases. *Pain* 1983;17:197–210.
16. **Turnbull ADM**. *Surgical Emergencies in the Cancer Patient.* Chicago: Yearbook Medical Publishers, 1987: pp. 47–52.
17. **Sykes NP**. Constipation and diarrhea. In: Doyle D; Hanks GWC; MacDonald N., editors. *The Oxford Textbook of Palliative Medicine.* 2nd edn. Oxford: Oxford University Press, 1998: pp. 513–26.
18. **Curtis EB; Krech R; Walsh TD**. Common symptoms in patients with advanced cancer. *Journal of Palliative Care* 1991;7:25–9.
19. **Mancini I; Bruera E**. Constipation in advanced cancer patients. *Supportive Care in Cancer* 1998;6:356–64.
20. **Fallon M; O'Neill B**. ABC of palliative care: constipation and diarrhoea. *BMJ* 1997;315:1293–6.
21. **Bruera E; Suarez-Almazor M; Velasco A., *et al.*** The assessment of constipation in terminal cancer patients admitted to a palliative care unit: a retrospective review. *Journal of Pain and Symptom Management* 1994;9:515–19.
22. **Starreveld JS; Pols MA; Van Wijk HJ., *et al.*** The plain abdominal radiograph in the assessment of constipation. *Gastroenterology* 1990;28:335–8.
23. **Baines MJ**. ABC of palliative care: nausea, vomiting and intestinal obstruction. *BMJ* 1997;315:1148–50.
24. **Berger A; Clark-Snow RA**. Nausea and vomiting. In: DeVita VT; Hellman S; Rosenberg SA., editors. *Cancer: Principles and Practice of Oncology.* 5th edn. Philadelphia: Lippincott-Raven, 1997: pp. 2705–12.
25. **Pereira J; Bruera E**. Chronic nausea. In: Bruera E; Higginson I., editors. *Cachexia–Anoxrexia in Cancer Patients.* Oxford: Oxford University Press, 1996: pp. 23–37.
26. **Lichter I**. Which antiemetic? *Journal of Palliative Care* 1993;9:42–50.
27. **Nelson KA; Walsh TD; Sheehan FG., *et al.*** Assessment of upper gastrointestinal motility in the cancer-associated dyspepsia syndrome. *Journal of Palliative Care* 1993;9:27–31.
28. **Watanabe S; Bruera E**. Anorexia and cachexia, asthenia, and lethargy. *Hematology/Oncology Clinics of North America* 1996;10:189–205.
29. **Fallon BG**. Nausea and vomiting unrelated to cancer therapy. In: Berger AM; Portenoy RK; Weissman DE., editors. *Principles and Practice of Supportive Oncology.* Philadelphia: Lippincott-Raven, 1998: pp. 179–90.
30. **Bruera E; Catz Z; Hooper R., *et al.*** Chronic nausea and anorexia in advanced cancer patients: a possible role for autonomic dysfunction. *Journal of Pain and Symptom Management* 1987;2:19–21.
31. **Beattie GJ; Leonard R; Smyth JF**. Bowel obstruction in ovarian carcinoma: a retrospective study and review of the literature. *Palliative Medicine* 1989;3:275–80.
32. **Ripamonti C**. Bowel obstruction. In: Berger AM; Portenoy RK; Weissman DE., editors. *Principles and Practice of Supportive Oncology.* Philadelphia: Lippincott-Raven, 1998: pp. 207–16.
33. **Feuer DJ; Broadley KE; Shepherd JH., *et al.*** Systematic review of surgery in malignant bowel obstruction in advanced gynaecological and gastrointestinal cancer. *Gynecologic Oncology* 1999;75:313–22.
34. **ReMine SG; Mcllrath DC**. Bowel perforation in steroid-treated patients. *Annals of Surgery* 1980: 192:581–6.

35. **Baines MJ**. The Pathophysiology and management of malignant intestinal obstruction. In: Doyle D; Hanks GWC; MacDonald N., editors. *The Oxford Textbook of Palliative Medicine*. 2nd edn. Oxford: Oxford University Press, 1998: pp. 526-34.
36. **Schwartzentruber DJ**. Surgical emergencies. In: DeVita VT; Hellman S; Rosenberg SA., editors. *Cancer: Principles and Practices of Oncology*. 5th edition. Philadelphia: Lippincott-Raven, 1997: pp. 2500–11.
37. **Mercadente S.** Diarrhoea in terminally ill patients: pathophysiology and treatment. *Journal of Pain and Symptom Management* 1995;10:298–309.
38. **Twycross RG; Lack SA.** Diarrhea. In: *Control of Alimentary Symptoms in Far Advanced Cancer*. London: Churchill Livingstone, 1986: pp. 208–29.
39. **Mercadente S.** Diarrhea, malabsorption, and constipation. In: Berger AM; Portenoy RK; Weissman DE., editors. *Principles and Practice of Supportive Oncology*. Philadelphia: Lippincott-Raven, 1998: pp. 191–205.
40. **Twycross R; Regnard C.** Dysphagia, dyspepsia, and hiccup. In: Doyle D; Hanks GWC; MacDonald N., editors. *The Oxford Textbook of Palliative Medicine*, 2nd edn. Oxford: Oxford University Press, 1988: pp. 499–512.
41. **Aird DW; Bihari J; Smith C.** Clinical problems in the continuing care of head and neck cancer patients. *Ear Nose and Throat Journal* 1983;62:10–30.
42. **Roth JA; Putnam JB; Rick Ta., *et al.*** Cancer of the esophagus. In: DeVita VT; Hellman S; Rosenberg SA., editors. *Cancer: Principles and Practice of Oncology*. 5th edn. Philadelphia: Lippincott-Raven, 1997: pp. 980–1020.
43. **Sykes NP; Baines M; Carter RL.** Clinical and pathological study of dyspahgia conservatively managed in patients with advanced malignant disease. *The Lancet* 1988;2:726–8.
44. **Goyal RK.** Dysphagia. In: Isselbacher KJ; Braunwald E; Wilson JD., *et al.*, editors. *Harrison's Principles of internal Medicine*. 13th edn. New York: McGraw-Hill, 1996: pp. 206–8.
45. **Leder SB.** Dysphagia. In: Berger AM; Portenoy RK; Weissman DE., editors. *Principles and Practice of Supportive Oncology*. Philadelphia: Lippincott-Raven, 1998: pp. 153–64.
46. **Lewis-Jones CM; Sturgess R; Ellershaw JE.** Laser therapy in the palliation of dysphagia in esophageal malignancy. *Palliative Medicine* 1995;9:327–30.
47. **Marincola FM; Schwartzentruber DJ.** Malignant ascites. In: DeVita VT: Hellman S; Roseberg SA., editors. *Cancer: Principles and Practice of Oncology*. 5th edn. Philadelphia: Lippincott-Raven, 1997: pp. 2598–606.
48. **Bain VG.** Jaundice, ascites, and hepatic encephalopathy. In: Doyle D; Hanks GWC; MacDonald N., editors. *The Oxford Textbook of Palliative Medicine*. 2nd edn. Oxford: Oxford University Press, 1998: pp. 557–72.
49. **Williams JW; Simel DL.** Does this patient have ascites? How to divine fluid in the abdomen. *The Journal of the American Medical Association* 1992;267:2645–68.
50. **Cattau EL; Benjamin SB: Knuff TE., *et al.*** The accuracy of the physical examination in the diagnosis of suspected ascites. *The Journal of the American Medical Association* 1982;247:1164–6.

Chapter 3

Assessment and psychosocial support of patients with advanced GI malignancies

C. Borreani, G. Miccinesi, and M. Tamburini

Quality of life assessment

In the advanced stages of oncological diseases a quality of life (QoL) assessment becomes necessary for the monitoring of the quality of assistance or the evaluation of the efficacy of a specific treatment, and it is useful in facilitating communication between patient and caring staff regarding specific problems and symptoms.

Thanks to the 1980s, which marked an important period for the definition of QoL theories in cancer patients and the development of instruments for QoL assessment, the use of self-rated, cancer-specific, and concise questionnaires is now recommended. The questionnaires set out to prove psychometric properties and assess the functional, physical, psychological, and social conditions of the patient as well as his/her global health.

More recently, it has been found that it is necessary to consider (in the case of longitudinal results) the psychological action of coping mechanisms (response shift), which can radically mature the interpretation of QoL measurements (1). Also important is the indication that distinguishes the questionnaire items into 'causal variables', i.e. symptoms and similar items assessed in QoL scales that probably could cause a change in QoL, and 'indicator variables', which reflect the latent variable to be measured (QoL) while being a manifestation of that variable, without causing change in it. This affects both the instrument development and the analysis and interpretation of QoL scores. It is clear from the above that the QoL assessment is structured to measure both overall QoL and its components—so as to monitor assistance quality and find more effective treatments for the patient's QoL—also to make the clinician aware of symptom and side-effect problems. Indicator variables are not enough to improve the management of patients: clinicians on the whole try to relieve symptoms despite their patients coping well with them and claiming to have a good QoL (2).

The histology and the initial location of the tumour do not seem to have any predictive value in terms of survival in terminally ill patients, and often have no relevance to the treatment of symptoms (3).

On the other hand, regarding gastrointestinal advanced cancers, the suggestion to have standardized measures was proposed for specific symptoms such as disphagya in patients with cancer of the oesophagus (4).

Recently, many instruments for the evaluation of QoL have been developed for advanced cancer patients. Table 3.1 shows the principal questionnaires concerning QoL specifically for gastrointestinal cancers and/or for advanced cancer patients. Some of these also show gastrointestinal symptoms as well; others do not. For example, the Support Team Assessment Schedule (STAS) only refers to problems met when 'other symptoms' are treated, i.e. any symptom other than pain, while the Edmonton Symptom Assessment System (ESAS) dedicates two out of nine items to this symptom area: nausea and lack of appetite (5,6). The Therapy Impact Questionnaire (TIQ), composed of a good 36 items, includes 10 that refer to this area: loss of appetite, dry mouth, difficulty swallowing, nausea, vomiting, stomach ache, indigestion, diarrhoea, constipation and hiccups (7).

In a multicentric assessment study that analysed 601 patients under palliative care, it was shown that an average gastrointestinal symptom score indicated a sense of good control by these patients during the whole period of care; also in the final stages of life (8).

In addition, a debate has just been opened on 'neoplastic' patients in the advanced stages of the disease and on the utility of the QoL results not gleaned directly from patients (9).

The agreement between 'by proxy' and self-related questionnaires was found to be generally better for physical symptoms and functional capacities than for psychological states. In the case of TIQ the agreement for the 10 gastrointestinal symptoms gives a result of between 53% and 94% with a higher tendency to underestimation than overestimation regarding the symptom by proxy (10). It has recently been proposed to consider (by, for example, utilizing concise and easy-to-use instruments like ESAS) the utility of an integrated QoL assessment by the carer and—where possible—by the patient (11).

Psychiatric assessment: controversial issues

Depression constitutes a specific problem for patients with cancer of the pancreas, and there are many unanswered questions regarding its role in all advanced-stage tumours and the problems of differential diagnosis.

An association between diseases of the pancreas and depression has been suspected since medieval times. An association between depression and cancer of the pancreas in the initial phases of disease has been confirmed. In a prospective study on suspected intra-abdominal neoplasia patients, a good 76% of those who were shown to be affected by cancer of the pancreas (but only 20% of the others, who had other types of intra-abdominal neoplasia) showed a heightening of the level of depression at the Minnesota Multiphasic Personality Inventory, and half of the former were shown already to have had psychiatric symptoms for an average of six months. Also, the association between advanced cancer of the pancreas and depression has been confirmed. The hypothesized aetiology was based on neuroendocrine, immunologic or metabolic mechanisms. The concurrence of pain with variable clinical gravity and intensity (present in most of the patients with cancer of the pancreas) is difficult to evaluate in the pathogenesis of the depression (4,12).

The problem of differential diagnosis of depression in patients with advanced cancer is two-fold. On the one hand, if there is a definite relationship between a symptom and the physical condition present, then that symptom should not be used in the diagnosis of depression. A high portion of the criteria for major depression in DSM IV are made up of somatic items. To screen patients who risk depression, self-rated questionnaires such as the Hospital Anxiety and Depression Scale (based on the anhedonic nucleus of depressive symptoms) are recommended (13,14).

Table 3.1 Assessment tools used for gastrointestinal advanced cancer patients and in palliative care

Instrument	Author	Description
M. D. Anderson Symptom Assessment System (ASAS)	Eduardo Bruera (5)	Derived from the Edmonton Symptom Assessment System (ESAS) the tool consists of 10 numerical scales numbered from 0 to 10 used to rate the patient's perception of pain, fatigue, nausea, depression, anxiety, drowsiness, shortness of breath, appetite, sleep and feeling of well-being. The scale is a series of horizontal lines each 100 mm in length and numbered from 0 for the least to 10 for the worst perception of each of the sysmptoms. The scores for each symptom can easily be marked on a graph that is updated daily to follow the patient's progress. More information (Assessment Tool section): www.mdanderson.org/departments/palliative/
EORTC Quality of Life Questionnaire Core 30 Items (QLQ-C30)+modules	EORTC Study Group on Quality of Life (25)	The EORTC Quality of Life Questionnaire (QLQ-C30) is an integrated system for assessing the quality of life of cancer patients participating in clinical trials. The QLQ-C30 is designed for use with a wide range of cancer patient populations, and is intended to be supplemented by cancer-specific questionnaire modules. At present, the validated modules are Lung (LC13), Breast (BR23) and Head & Neck (H&N35). Phase III modules that are available include the Bladder, Brain, Colorectal, Gastric, Multiple myeloma, Ophthalmic, Pancreatic, Prostate and Satisfaction with Care modules. The modules that are (presently being field tested are the) Oesophageal and Ovarian. More information: www.eortc.be/home/qol/
Functional Assessment of Chronic Illness Therapy (FACIT) Measurement System	David F. Cella (26)	The FACIT has multiple disease-, treatment-, and condition-specific subscales to complement the FACT-G: a Generic core set of questions for cancer patients, which can be used with patients of any tumour type, and which constitutes the core of the specific scales. The FACT-G is comprised of 27 items. Some FACIT specific scales are: FACT-C (Colorectal), FACT-E (Oesophageal), FACT-Pa (Pancreatic), FACT-Pal (Palliative). More information: www.facit.org
Hospice Quality of Life Index (HQLI)	Susan C.McMillan (28)	The Hospice Quality of Life Index (HQLI) is designed to measure overall quality of life for persons receiving palliative care. It has 28 items measured on 11 point (0–10) numeric rating scales. Total scores may range from 0 (worst possible quality of life) to 280 (best possible quality of life). The HQLI includes three subscales: Psychophysiological Well-being, Functional Well-being, and Social/Spiritual Well-being. More information: www.QLMed.org/HQLI/

(Continued)

Table 3.1 (Continued) Assessment tools used for gastrointestinal advanced cancer patients and in palliative care

Instrument	Author	Description
Palliative Outcome Scale (POS)	Irene Higginson (6)	The POS measure has taken components that have appeared to work well in earlier measures and includes aspects concerned with pain and symptom control, patient and family psychosocial needs and communication and information. The POS. has been piloted now in over 400 patients over six months. Early testing suggests that it appears to be valid, can be used by patients and if patients become too unwell to complete the form, by trained staff. It is responsive to change, can detect service failings and successes, and is reliable in a small group of patients whose condition remains stable.
Support Team Assessment Schedule (STAS)	Irene Higginson (27)	The STAS is a standardized evaluation instrument for clinical auditing designed for use in palliative care. It is a multidimensional tool, to be compiled by the team, and is designed to evaluate the quality of care, the quality of the patient's life, the effectiveness of organizational aspects. More information: www.QLMed.org/STAS/
Therapy Impact Questionnaire (TIQ)	Marcello Tamburini (7)	The Therapy Impact Questionnaire (TIQ) is especially designed for palliative care settings. If the patient was unable to fill in by him/herself or to dictate the questionnaire (self-compiled questionnaire), the nurse—or the doctor—was asked to compile it immediately after the home visit and to register the reason (proxy-complied questionnaire). The TIQ is a questionnaire on four major components of quality of life of oncological patients: physical symptoms resulting from disease or therapies (24 items), functional conditions (capacity to work, to enjoy one's free time, to look after oneself; three items), concomitant psychological conditions (emotional and cognitive; six items), family and social relationships (two items) and one item for the patient's global judgement of 'not feeling well'. Answers are classified as 'not at all', 'slight', 'severe', 'very severe'. More information: www.QLMed.org/Tiq/

Willing to die is another difficult diagnostic issue. In various countries, thanks to the availability of a Cancer Registry, suicide rates in populations afflicted with cancer have been studied and have been found higher than in the general population. The act of contemplating suicide in itself does not justify a depression diagnosis, but is one of the criteria for major depression analysed in DSM IV. To set up studies concerning the relationship between suicide and depression, a set of criteria would be needed for depression that excludes suicidal ideation. This issue remains at present still open to debate and study (15).

Specific psychological issues: indications for psychological support

Patients with gastrointestinal cancer present a series of problems with a specific psychological relapse concerning, on the one hand, psychological significance connected to the loss of corporal integrity (mutilations) and, on the other hand, the relational and emotive significance of alimentation.

The psychological effects of stoma surgery have been described in terms of 'significant loss' (16,17) in as much as it is necessary for the patient to undertake a real process of separation from the perception of integrity of his/her own image and his/her own functions to obtain some form of adaptation to his/her new condition.

This process could take place during a crisis in self-esteem and thus become complicated by the necessity of dealing with those problems of a physical character connected to stoma (change of bag, washing, odours).

These aspects intervene above all in the interpersonal sphere shown among those patients who have compromised the most (18).

It is the psychological characteristics (and personalities) of each single patient, the quality and type of support he/she has received during the disease, as well as the evolution the disease will follow, which determines the quality of adaptation to the stoma. Even the adaptation times are variable: terminal-stage patients may have reached a good psycho-physical adaptation to stoma, but they could also still not have managed to overcome the first phase of refusal and negation of the change.

It is always important to evaluate the patient's adaptation to stoma also in relation to the quality of internal (psychological and emotive) and external (family members, social relations) resources.

With regard to the relational and emotive significance of alimentation, the term anorexia in the case of oncological patients should be utilized with caution. This term usually denotes a disturbance: anorexia nervosa, characterized by a refusal of the required food and a strong emotive confliction that is more or less unconscious. If such a psychological unease (often emphasized) is present in these patients, then the prevalence of physical and metabolic disturbances connected to the tumour and its treatment will render any specific psychological approach difficult to undertake.

It is important to note the symbolic value that food takes on for patients and (especially) their families. Feeding is a vital function, it represents 'life'; stopping eating is considered a 'bad sign', a point of no return. The continuous encouragement of patients to eat becomes a way of avoiding death. Food becomes a therapy administered to patients by their families or doctors, an act that allows the carrying out of an extreme form of control on the disease (19).

Also, nausea and vomiting and constipation are symptoms that can be characterized by the presence of a psychological component connected above all to feelings of anxiety or fear (20). Even though there exists a wide range of literature on the psychological and psychotherapeutic aspects of some of these symptoms, considered as side-effects of oncological therapies (21), it is not possible to apply such psychological literature to terminal diseases without considering the globality of the patient's experience.

Cachexia in the terminal oncological patient is, in fact, considered to be the paradigm of a syndrome with determinant bio-psychosocial characteristics. It represents one of the most distressing symptoms and can be seen as a metaphor for the advancement of the disease that arrives to seriously threaten survival (22). From this viewpoint, the symptoms that characterize it could be interpreted also as emotional replies to the perception of this threat.

When patients reach the terminal stage of their disease, they experience mainly a condition of tiredness; a psychological tiredness rather than a physical one.

This symptom represents the results of life's journey, disease, therapies, side effects, delusions, struggles, hopes, defeats, good and bad relationships, all of which strongly contribute to determining and characterizing the psychological conditions of the last stage.

The existence of a psychological adaptation process to disease (23), which presupposes a constant and, at times, unconscious re-adaptation of one's own existential parameters (response shift) (1) mitigates the perception of changes linked to the advancement of the disease and allows the individual to slowly mobilize his/her own resources. The fragmentation of care in therapeutic objectives of symptom control, re-evaluated day by day, is functional for this adaptation process.

Awareness of clinical, therapeutic, and existential methods and of how patients adapt themselves in time can be useful in providing the instruments for understanding and treating the symptoms more adequately. It is important to listen to the patient, to get to know his/her 'story' with the objective of adapting the right therapeutic proposal to his/her constructed 'plot' (24). It is important to try to comprehend the 'story' in which the patient is living—whether it is a story of struggle, of resignation, or of hope—to try to see which spaces and possibilities are available so as to build together with the patient the last page of his/her story.

References

1. **Wilson IB**. Clinical understanding and clinical implications of response shift. *Social Science and Medicine* 1999;48:1577–88.
2. **Fayers P; Machin D**. *QoL Assessment, Analysis and Interpretation.* John Wiley & Sons, Chichester, 2000.
3. **Toscani F**. Classification and staging of terminal cancer patients: rationale and objectives of a multicentre cohort prospective study and methods used. The Italian Co-operative Research Group on Palliative Medicine. *Supportive Care in Cancer* 1996;4:56–60.
4. **Hurny BJ**. Gastrointestinal cancer. In: Holland J., editor. *Psycho-oncology.* New York: Oxford University Press, 1998: pp.324–39.
5. **Bruera E; Kuehn N; Miller MJ; Selmser P; Macmillan K**. The Edmonton Symptom Assessment System (ESAS): a simple method for the assessment of palliative care patients. *Journal of Palliative Care* 1991;7:6–9.
6. **Hearn J; Higginson IJ**. Development and validation of a core outcome measure for palliative care: the palliative care outcome scale. Palliative Care Core Audit Project Advisory Group. *Quality Health Care* 1999;8:219–27.
7. **Tamburini M; Rosso S; Gamba A., *et al.*** A therapy impact questionnaire for quality of life assessment in advanced cancer research. *Annals of Oncology* 1992;3:565–70.

8. **Paci E; Miccinesi G; Toscani F; Tamburini M; Brunelli C; Costantini M; Peruselli C; DiGiulio P; Gallucci M; Addington-Hall J; Higginson IJ.** Quality of life assessment and outcome of palliative care. *Journal of Pain and Symptom Management* 2001;21:179–88.
9. **Sprangers MA; Sneeuw KC.** Are healthcare providers adequate raters of patients' quality of life—perhaps more than we think? *Acta Oncologica* 2000;39:5–8.
10. **Brunelli C; Costantini M; Di Giulio P; Gallucci M; Fusco F; Miccinesi G; Paci E; Peruselli C; Morino P; Piazza M; Tamburini M; Toscani F.** Quality-of-life evaluation: when do terminal cancer patients and health-care providers agree? *Journal of Pain and Symptom Management* 1998;15:151–8.
11. **Nekolaichuk CL; Maguire TO; Suarez-Almazor M; Rogers WT; Bruera E.** Assessing the reliability of patient, nurse, and family caregiver symptom ratings in hospitalized advanced cancer patients. *Journal of Clinical Oncology* 1999;17:3621–30.
12. **Passik SD; Breitbart WS.** Depression in patients with pancreatic carcinoma. Diagnostic and treatment isues. Review. *Cancer* 1996;78 (Suppl. 3):615–26.
13. **Kathol RG; Mutgi A; Williams J; Clamon G; Noyes R Jr.** Diagnosis of major depression in cancer patients according to four sets of criteria. *American Journal of Psychiatry* 1990;147(8):1021–4.
14. **Hopwood P; Howell A; Maguire P.** Psychiatric morbidity in patients with advanced cancer of the breast: prevalence measured by two self-rating questionnaires. *British Journal of Cancer* 1991;64:349–52.
15. **Brown JH; Henteleff P; Barakat S; Rowe CJ.** Is it normal for terminally ill patients to desire death? *American Journal of Psychiatry* 1986;43:208–11.
16. **Model G.** A new image to accept: psychological aspects of stoma care. *Professional Nurse* 1990;5:310–16.
17. **Kelly MP; Henry P.** Open discussion can lead to acceptance. The psychosocial effects of stoma surgery. *Professional Nurse* 1993;9:101–6.
18. **Thomas C; Madden F; Jehu D.** Psychological effects of stomas. Factors influencing outcome. *Journal of Psychosomatic Research* 1987;31:317–23.
19. **Fleishman SB.** Cancer cachexia. In: Holland J., editor. *Psycho-oncology*. New York: Oxford University Press, 1998: pp.468–75.
20. **Komurcu S; Nelson KA; Walsh D.** The gastrointestinal symptoms of advanced cancer. *Supportive Care in Cancer* 2001;9:32–9.
21. **Morrow GR; Roscoe JA; Hickok JT.** Nausea and vomiting. In: Holland J., editor. *Psycho-oncology*. New York: Oxford University Press, 1998: pp. 476–84.
22. **Glauss A.** Fatigue and cachessia in cancer patients. *Supportive Care in Cancer* 1998;6:77–78.
23. **McCaul KD; Sandgren AK; King B., *et al.*** Coping and adjustment to breast cancer. *Psycho-oncology* 1999;8:230–36.
24. **Mattingly C.** The concept of therapeutic 'emplotment'. *Social Science and Medicine* 1994;38:811–22.
25. **Aaronson NK; Ahmezai S; Bergman B., *et al.*** The European Organization for Research and Treatment of Cancer QLQ-C30: a quality-of-life instrument for use in international clinical trials in oncology. *Journal of the National Cancer Institute* 1993;85:365–76.
26. **Cella DF; Tulsky DS; Gray G., *et al.*** The Functional Assessment of Cancer Therapy Scale: development and validation of the general measure. *Journal of Clinical Oncology* 1993;11(3):570–9.
27. **Higginson IJ; McCarthy M.** Validity of the Support Team Assessment Schedule: do staff's ratings reflect those made by the patient or their families? *Palliative Medicine* 1993;7:219–28.
28. **McMillan SC; Weitzner M.** Quality of life in cancer patients: use of a revised hospice index. *Cancer Practice* 1998;6:282–8.

Chapter 4

Cancer anorexia/cachexia syndrome: epidemiology, pathogenesis, and assessment

Florian Strasser and Eduardo Bruera

Introduction

Anorexia/cachexia is a frequent problem in patients with advanced cancer, and is distressing for both patients and families (1). However, since many cachexia-associated symptoms, such as anorexia and asthenia, are 'silent' symptoms, as compared with pain or shortness of breath, its importance is often underestimated and therefore underdiagnosed (2). Cachexia can be separated into primary (metabolic) and secondary (starvation) cachexia, which occur often together, and are often confused with each other (Table 4.1). Since treatments for them are frequently different, the paraneoplastic, metabolic cancer cachexia syndrome (the 'primary cachexia') needs to be distinguished from impaired nutritional intake secondary to obstacles in the gastrointestinal (GI) tract, and other causes for 'secondary cachexia' (Table 4.2). Anorexia is, besides weight loss, a leading symptom of the paraneoplastic, metabolic cachexia syndrome, therefore we use the term cancer anorexia/cachexia syndrome (ACS). ACS is one of the most important causes for the symptom complex of asthenia, weakness, and fatigue, which, beside pain, is the most common symptom in patients with advanced cancer (3). This chapter focuses on the three areas of epidemiology, pathogenesis, and assessment of ACS, providing a basis for understand actual and future treatments.

The epidemiology of ACS will be described under the premiss that several different definitions of ACS have been used and starvation/secondary cachexia and ACS have been mixed.

In the section on pathogenesis the complex interactions between the tumor and the host on several levels will be highlighted, supporting a new view of the paraneoplastic metabolic alterations associated with anorexia/cachexia, and other symptoms.

The diagnosis of ACS is based on the simple assessment of weight loss and anorexia, but there are no established tools to distinguish starvation/secondary cachexia from ACS. The multidimensional assessment of both primary and secondary cachexia includes measurement of the impact of cachexia on the symptom profile, quality-of-life (QoL) and function, nutritional status, and body composition, among others.

Table 4.1 Metabolic alterations in primary and secondary cachexia

	Primary cachexia (metabolic)	**Secondary cachexia (starvation)**
Protein synthesis	⇑	⇓
◆ muscle proteins	⇓	⇓
◆ acute phase proteins	⇑	⇔
Lipogenesis	⇓	⇓
Proteolysis	⇑⇑	⇔
Lipolysis	⇑	⇑⇑
Glucose turnover	⇑	⇓

Note: Clinically both forms of cachexia are identical.

Table 4.2 Mechanisms of secondary cachexia

Impaired oral intake
◆ Stomatitis, taste alterations
◆ Dry mouth (xerostomia)
◆ Dysphagia, odynophagia
◆ Bowel obstruction
◆ Vomiting
◆ Severe constipation
◆ Severe pain, dyspnea, depression
◆ Cognitive impairment/delirium
◆ Social and financial obstacles
Impaired GI absorption
◆ Malabsorption
◆ Exocrine pancreatic insufficiency
◆ Chronic severe diarrhea
Catabolic states
◆ Hyperthyroidism
◆ Chronic and acute infections
Significant loss of proteins
◆ Frequent drainage of ascites or pleural fluid punctions
◆ Nephrotic syndrome

Definition of cachexia

Usually cachexia is primarily defined (Table 4.3) by the presence of involuntary weight loss (4). However, different definitions for weight loss have been used in several clinical trials. Common definitions are a weight loss of >5% compared with stable preillness weight (5,6)

Table 4.3 Definitions of anorexia/cachexia

Weight loss (4)	>5% compared with stable pre-illness weight (5,6)
	>5% during the previous 6 months (7)
	>2% within a one-month period (8)
	>2–3 kg during the last two months (9,10)
	<20 cal kg^{-1} day^{-1} oral intake and a weight loss problem (9,10)
	decrease of 11 kg in the previous 2 months (11)
Anorexia	visual analog scale >3/10 (288)
Reduced caloric intake	
Asthenia	
Chronic nausea	
Loss of muscle and fat tissue	
Changes in body image	
Low serum albumin	
Peripheral edema	
Anemia	

or during the previous 6 months (7). Other actual clinical trials use a definition of 'weight loss >2% within a one month period' (8), 'loss of 2.3 kg during the last two months OR less than 20 calories per kg per day oral intake and a weight loss problem' (9,10), or 'nonvolitional weight loss between 6%–9% of usual body weight over past 6 months OR decrease of 5 pounds in the past 2 months or less' (11). These definitions describe different patient populations. Some of them lost weight many months ago, perhaps even after surgery, rather than from an active cancer. Others have a very recent weight loss, but to a very low degree. The concept of ongoing, significant weight loss, reflecting an active wasting process, is therefore difficult to catch in clinical reality (12). Therefore, since there is still a clinical instrument missing to separate primary and secondary cachexia, the reported frequency of weight loss often includes both forms.

The second most important element in defining cancer cachexia is anorexia. The frequency of anorexia is lower than that of weight loss due to several reasons. Patients losing weight due to secondary cachexia often present without concurrent anorexia (13,14). Patients suffering from primary metabolic cachexia will probably experience different manifestations with more pronounced muscle weakness, anorexia, or constitutional symptoms, respectively. Research is ongoing to define these potential subtypes and their underlying pathogenesis. The assessment of anorexia is a less common practice than the assessment of weight loss, and the diagnostic criteria are not standardized. In some studies anorexia is part of the inclusion criteria (5,6), i.e. at visual analog scale for loss of appetite >3/10.

Other parameters, such as hypoalbuminemia (13), the presence of asthenia (15–17), chronic nausea (18,19), changes in body image (20), reduced caloric intake (21), or clinical judgment of reduced muscle and fat mass (22) can serve as additional criteria, i.e. 'minor criteria', for the presence of cachexia (3) (Table 4.3). These additional criteria can be helpful in patients with relevant fluid retention (pleural effusion, ascites, edema), where the extent of weight loss due to cachexia is masked by the accumulation of fluids (23). At the present time there is no gold standard for the diagnosis of cachexia.

Epidemiology of cachexia

Weight loss affects the vast majority of patients with neoplastic disease reaching >80% in the terminal stage (24,25). The classic study by DeWys *et al.* (16) showed that 54% of 3074 patients with a variety of different tumors recruited by the Eastern Cooperative Oncology Group (ECOG) for chemotherapy trials had weight loss (46% of patients 0% weight loss, 22% 0%–5%, 17% 5%–10%, 15% >10%), which was assessed for the six months before study entry by patient interviews and expressed as a percent weight loss compared with the patient's weight before illness (except for pancreatic cancer, where weight loss referred to the previous two months) (26). Numerous other studies document a high frequency of weight loss, ranging from 24% to 83%, at diagnosis of a cancer, i.e. prior to chemotherapy or surgery (27–30), and with increasing frequency at more advanced disease (31–36). However, the reported frequencies vary widely, even for an individual primary tumor (13).

Since it is not possible to discuss all primary tumors, the example of pancreatic cancer can highlight both the frequency of weight loss as well as the problems of the new outcome measurement 'clinical benefit'. The reported frequencies of weight loss from patients with advanced pancreatic cancer enrolled recently in Phase II and Phase III studies (the number of patients at baseline is in parentheses) have a wide range, from 36% (n=25) (37), 47% (n=90) (38), 58% (n=43) (39), 87% (n=27) (40) to 93% (n=42) (41). One reason is the inclusion criteria, since data from prospective Phase II and III studies may include patients less likely to be cachectic (a classic oncological design to assess tumor response rates and survival) or need to be symptomatic and therefore likely to be cachectic (a modern design to assess symptomatic outcomes) the true frequency of weight loss. Another reason is a 'publication bias', since from several Phase II and Phase III studies the extent of weight loss or symptoms in the patient characteristics (42–45) has not been communicated. This is somewhat surprising, since the concept of 'clinical benefit' to measure the efficacy of an antineoplastic treatment by symptomatic benefit (improvement in weight loss, pain, analgesics use, anorexia, and QoL, among others) rather than by classic response criteria based on tumor measurements, has been developed in patients with pancreatic cancer, among others (20,22,46). However, the initial Phase III study, pioneering the concept of 'clinical benefit', which compared gemcitabine and 5-FU for patients with advanced pancreatic cancer, had as 'symptomatic' inclusion criteria the presence of at least one or more of the following conditions: a baseline karnofsky performance status of less than 80, a baseline analgesic consumption of $\geq 10\,\mathrm{mg\,d^{-1}}$ morphine equivalent daily dose (MEDD), and a baseline pain intensity score of ≥ 20 mm per 100 mm (47). Therefore instead of weight loss at baseline, numbers of patients with progressive disease two months before study entry (48), and performance status are reported, assuming a reliable correlation with weight loss.

The study by DeWys *et al.*(16) compared *different primary tumors* and found a higher frequency of weight loss for patients with solid tumors (pancreas 83%, gastric 83%–87%, colon 54%, non-small-cell lung cancer 61%, small-cell lung cancer 57%, prostate 56%) compared with hematological malignancies (non-Hodgkin lymphoma 36%), except for breast cancer (36%) (10). Newer studies comparing, in a large number of patients, the frequency of weight loss among different primaries are scarce, and the available data from single cancer studies are variable, as shown above for pancreatic cancer (49) (Table 4.4).

Table 4.4 Frequency of cachexia/weight loss and anorexia in different tumor types

Reference	**DeWys (21)**	**SCH (42)**	**SPG (23)**		**Various (ref. no)**
patients	**3074**	**608**	**1640**		
	Weight loss	**Cachexia**	**Weight loss**	**Anorexia**	**Malnutrition**
Lung NSCLC	61%	89%	49%	35%	50%–66% (289,290)
Lung SCLC	57%	89%	49%	35%	50% (291)
Breast	36%	53%	22%	26%	9% (292)
Colorectal	54%	75%	53%	43%	40*–60%
Pancreas	83%	82%	N/A	N/A	—
Prostate	56%	89%	26%	33%	—
Gastric	85%	87%	45%	42%	—
Lymphoma	36%	86%	33%	28%	55% (293)
Ovarian	N/A	95%	22% (Gyn)	25% (Gyn)	—
H&N	N/A	N/A	33%	20%	72% (294)
Esophageal	N/A	96%	62%	32%	79% (292)

The available data describing the association of the frequency of weight loss with the *disease stage* are conflicting, probably since the populations are not well described, and primary and secondary causes have been mixed. Overall, there is limited evidence of an association between weight loss and the extent of the cancer, which is surprising (50). The study from DeWys *et al.* (16) showed that patients with breast cancer had more weight loss when more than one organ (bone, liver or lungs) was involved, probably reflecting the changed biology of visceral metastatic breast cancer compared with bone metastasis. Similarly, in patients with sarcoma, when more than one organ was involved, weight loss was more prominent. No association was seen for prostate, lung, pancreas or gastric cancer.

These observations reflect that in early oncology studies the TNM staging systems were less elaborate. Since then the association between stage with prognosis as well as of weight loss with prognosis (18) has been established for numerous tumor types.

However, the metabolic effects of a certain individual tumor can only incompletely be detected by traditional staging systems. Many patients teach us that the biology of an individual tumor (growth dynamics, differentiation, metastatic behavior, genetics) is more important than the crude tumor mass or number and sites of metastases. The independent prognostic value of the simple clinical estimation of performance status in many tumor types highlights also that the complexity of the neoplastic disease is incomplete by describing the tumor mass and spreading pattern.

Besides the metabolic (primary) effects of a tumor the local effects vary widely within the same stage, when additional causes of (secondary) cachexia develop.

Weight loss is a well-known adverse event of many *antineoplastic treatments*, i.e. high-dose chemotherapy, bone marrow transplantation, immunotherapy, i.e. interleukin-2, and radiotherapy, among others (51). Many surgical procedures lead transiently to weight loss or, as a long-term adverse event, to persistent secondary cachexia.

The *epidemiology* of *symptoms*, rather than weight loss, associated with cachexia is more complex, since their measurement is subjective and more prone to influencing factors, i.e. mostly multifactorial (30,52). The description of the frequency of symptoms, which can be a cause of secondary cachexia, such as depression, but can also be part of the symptomatic manifestations of primary cachexia (21), is more complicated. Careful assessment specifically to clarify individual symptom interactions (53), is therefore necessary, although the quality of the assessment is mainly dependent on the skills of the investigator.

Among the *symptoms* leading to a *new cancer diagnosis* the most common are pain, cough, jaundice, etc. reflecting more visible events. However, if symptoms are assessed systematically patients presenting with a new cancer diagnosis develop a number of common symptoms such as weakness, fatigue, weight loss, and anorexia, among others (54). There are tumor- and site-specific symptoms, such as jaundice for tumors of the head or pancreas, or dysphagia for esophageal tumors, but the more the tumor is biologically active, as reflected by growth dynamics, differentiation, and tumor mass, respectively, the more it manifests with the common general symptoms leading to cachexia.

In patients with *advanced cancer* the number of symptoms increases with the disease progression, whereas the frequency of symptoms shows a wide variation in several studies: pain is present in >50% (55–58), anorexia varies from 6%–74%, fatigue 13%–91%, nausea and vomiting 4%–44%, insomnia 7%–28%, delirium 4%–85%; weight loss is reported to be present in >50% (58%–77%) (27–33,49).

In a prospective, systemic analysis of the prevalence and severity of 37 symptoms, 1000 patients, seen on consecutive consultations by a single palliative care hospital service, were assessed by ranking the 37 symptoms. The three symptoms—anorexia, pain, and easy fatigue—were associated with cancer at all sites, and were also among the 10 most prevalent symptoms, ranging from 50% to 85%. The other seven most frequent or most severe symptoms were weakness, lack of energy, dry mouth, constipation, early satiety, dyspnea, and greater than 10% weight loss (59,60).

The prospective study by Portenoy *et al.* to develop the Memorial Symptom Assessment Scale evaluated 33 symptoms for prevalence, characteristics, and distress in 218 cancer patients (61). Anorexia (lack of appetite) was present in 45% of patients, with 83% moderate to severe intensity, 55% frequent to constant frequency, and 30% moderate to severe distress. Numbers for lack of energy were 73%, 77%, 55%, and 33%, respectively.

Another study assessed the symptom patterns of patients with 'terminal phase of the disease' suffering from different tumors, measured by the ESAS and the EORTC-QLQ-c30 (62). At the time of assessment patients experienced an average of six symptoms. Fatigue, anorexia, poor feeling of well-being as well as impaired cognitive function showed the worst scores.

The Symptom Prevalence Group, consisting of seven palliative care centers in different countries, collected in the early 1990s prospective data about symptom occurrence from 1640 patients with advanced or terminal cancer, no longer receiving any specific cytoreductive cancer treatment, referred to a palliative care service (49). Pain was the leading symptom, present in 57% of all patients at the time of admission, followed by weakness (51%), anorexia (30%), constipation (23%), and nausea (21%); weight loss was present in 39% of patients.

A majority of the most frequent and most distressing symptoms are related to the GI tract (63), even for many patients with other than GI solid tumors, with the exception of breast cancer (31).

These data underline that many symptoms associated with ACS occur together, but that anorexia is less frequent than weight loss and weakness/fatigue. However, the methodology often does not apply common criteria towards a definition of the threshold for a 'positive' symptom, nor does it allow good insight into the symptom interactions in an individual patient on a longitudinal basis. For example, it is not well known when and in what patients anorexia occurs, and which patients with weight loss experience anorexia.

The frequency of anorexia varies also between different tumor types (Table 4.4). Data from several Phase III trials in individual tumors, such as colorectal (64) or non-small-cell lung cancer (65), often report changes in anorexia scores in association with antineoplastic treatment, among other QoL measurements, but report neither the baseline values for anorexia nor the relation between anorexia and weight loss, respectively.

Weight loss is a well recognized *prognostic factor* (12,31), but anorexia and asthenia are predictive of limited survival, too (66). In 1115 patients with advanced colorectal or lung cancer, anorexia, assessed by patient questionnaire, predicted limited survival, even after multivariate analysis, including performance status and psychological parameters, respectively (67). In 1753 patients involved in the National Hospice Study, shortness of breath, problems eating or anorexia, trouble swallowing, dry mouth, and weight loss had independent predictive value besides performance status, independent of patient age, sex, primary tumor type, or site (68). In a recent study from Spain of 200 patients with advanced cancer, defined as 'no further antineoplastic treatment, as per consistent judgement of the physician and the oncological nurse', asthenia was found to be an independent prognostic factor (69) in patients with different tumor types. The frequency of similar symptoms among patients with cancer of various primary and metastatic sites highlights the concept of a common pathogenetic mechanism in patients with advanced malignant neoplasms leading to malnutrition/cachexia and associated symptoms.

The measurements of the *impact of cachexia on QoL* is challenging and probably requires specific assessment instruments. As an example, a recent study of 48 patients with head and neck cancer examined cross-selectional QoL by the EORTC-QLQ-c30 questionnaire, nutritional status, energy intake, severity of disease, and two-year-survival (70). The study found better QoL in two-year survivors, but was unable to detect a correlation of QoL with the severity of the disease as well as with malnutrition. This reflects that 'comprehensive' QoL assessments can be insensitive in detecting the relative contribution of specific symptoms, such as anorexia, to global QoL, both due to interfering factors and a heterogeneous patient population. Another study examined the association between weight loss, anorexia, QoL, skinfold anthropometry, C-reactive protein, and albumin in 119 patients with advanced GI cancer, 97 of them experiencing weight loss >5% compared with preillness weight (13). Appetite scores and EORTC-QLQ-c30 scores were lower in the weight loss group.

In order to provide optimal care for patients with advanced cancer, and their families, it is paramount to acknowledge the *emotional impact* of anorexia/loss of appetite, weight loss, and declining function (71). Although anorexia probably is pathophysiologically an epiphenomenon, rather than a primary mechanism leading to malnutrition/cachexia, its presence affects QoL to a major extent (72), both in combination with weight loss, as well as an independent distressing symptom (73). Anorexia is often perceived as a barometer of overall condition and finally, i.e. when clinical signs of cachexia are apparent, as a sign of impending death, by both the patient and family. Anorexia also represents a source of conflict between the patient and the family, when a patient becomes unwilling to eat (74).

Anorexia/cachexia leads to asthenia, with aspects of fatigue, weakness, and poor physical functioning, which often represents a leading distressing symptom complex (75,76). An important element can be the change in body image, which is a recognizable and distressing sign of serious illness, but also contributes to self-confidence, a sense of body integrity, and attractiveness (20). An important contributor to emotional distress of the patient with progressive cachexia, and the family, can be the misunderstanding of the avoidance of nutritional support, which has profound philosophical and sometimes religious connotations. It is important to provide adequate counselling of patients and families by addressing the anxiety of family members that a relative is 'starving to death'. Reframing families' understanding of cachexia from 'starving to death' towards an understanding of metabolic abnormalities of the cancer is a useful strategy. It is helpful that the family understands that the administration of more food to patients with metabolic cachexia will not result in additional fat or muscle synthesis because of the generally irreversible underlying abnormalities. This reframing can decrease the emotional distress in both patients and families and can maintain the social benefits of meal times. When progressive disease occurs and oral intake is likely to decrease to almost nothing, adequate mouth care and small amounts of ice chips or sips of cold beverages may be adequate for some patients. In other patients with symptoms related to dehydration, the use of hypodermoclysis can be very useful in maintaining adequate hydration at home at little costs and with minimal invasiveness (77).

We can summarize this section with the following points:

- Weight loss is frequent in cancer patients and is of poor prognostic significance.
- Weight loss is more frequent in solid than hematologic neoplasia, except breast cancer.
- Weight loss correlates with the tumor stage, tumor biology, and tumor location.
- Anorexia and asthenia are frequent in cancer patients, can occur independently of weight loss, and are of poor prognostic value.
- Declining function as a consequence of malnutrition/cachexia is a major, contributor to discomfort for patients and their families and impairs the patient's ability to express her optimal physical and psychosocial potential as long as possible. It no longer has to be accepted as an indispensable part of advanced cancer, as pain had been rejected to be unavoidable (78).

Mechanism of cachexia

Primary versus secondary cachexia

The impairment of nutritional intake (by obstacles or damage to any segment of the GI tract) or loss of nutritients (malabsorption, fluids, catabolism) results in malnutrition/cachexia, or secondary cachexia, which can be treated successfully by returning the lost nutritients. In contrast, patients with advanced cancer often suffer from cachexia despite intact GI tract, 'sufficient' nutritional intake and the lack of nutrient losses, i.e. in the context of the metabolic, paraneoplastic anorexia/cachexia syndrome, or primary cachexia (Table 4.1, Table 4.2, Figure 4.1).

The controversial data about nutritional support in weight-losing cancer patients underline the importance of a better understanding of the metabolic, paraneoplastic mechanism

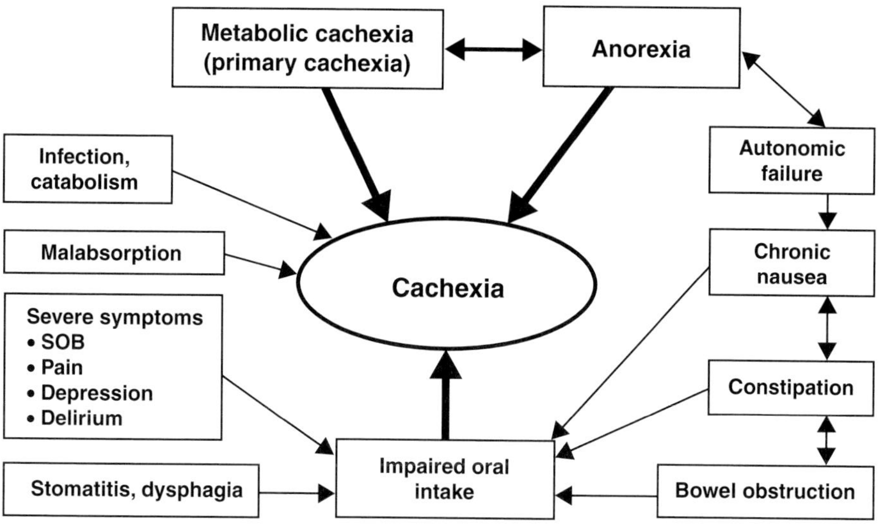

Figure 4.1 Causes of cachexia in cancer.

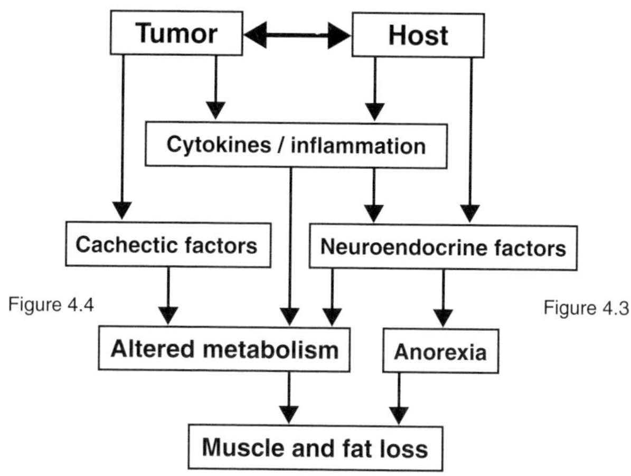

Figure 4.2 Main elements of the pathogenesis of metabolic/primary cachexia in cancer.

leading to primary cachexia, as well as the identification of patients with 'true' secondary cachexia who potentially would profit from nutritional support.

Primary cachexia

Anorexia/cachexia syndrome (ACS) is a paraneoplastic syndrome in which complex metabolic alterations occur, mediated partly by tumor-produced cachectic factors, in the context of a chronic inflammatory state as well as of central and GI-mediated anorexia, resulting in loss of skeletal muscle and fat, leading to many symptoms and impaired QoL (Figure 4.2).

Until recently, cachexia in the context of cancer was believed to be the result of a nutrition as deficit caused by the combination of increased energy consumption by the tumor and decreased energy intake due to tumor-related factors which acted at the satiety center in the central nervous system (the traditional model of cachexia). However, until the early 1990s attempts were made to increase nutrition intake including aggressive nutritional therapies which failed to reverse ACS, without significant improvements in most clinical outcomes (79–81). Data derived from more than 70 prospective randomized controlled trials reveal that in fact a heterogenic patient population has been studied, including patients with both primary or secondary cachexia, as well as different types and stages of antineoplastic treatments. In addition, there are various outcome measurements reported, such as body composition, including weight, assessment of metabolism (protein metabolism, other nutritients), survival, response rate to antineoplastic treatment, tolerance to these nutritional treatment, as well as QoL (82–84).

Aggressive nutritional therapy neither significantly influences the outcome (improvement of survival, tumor response, chemotherapy-toxicity) of patients with advanced cancer nor has been shown to improve symptom control and performance status, i.e. QoL (83,85,86).

In patients with primary cachexia due to progressive cancer, invasive artificial nutrition is usually not beneficial (87) or have a negative impact on QoL (88,89). The European Association for Palliative Care published guidelines on artificial nutrition versus hydration in terminal cancer patients (90). The guidelines concluded that part of the controversy related both to the definition of terminal cancer patients as a group with different needs, expectations, and potential for medical intervention, as well as to the prediction of life expectancy and the patient's likely response to nutritional support.

An interesting comparison from non-cancer cachexia is shown by patients with chronic obstructive pulmonary disease, where a high caloric oral nutritional therapy over eight weeks was unsuccessful in patients with elevated systemic inflammatory response and relative anorexia (91). The concept of providing parenteral or enteral nutrition was based on the observation that weight-losing cancer patients really have a decreased caloric intake (92), and on the observation that patients lose fat tissue. However, in contrast to simple starvation, where more than 75% of weight loss is from body fat, in cancer weight loss is due to approximately equal losses of fat and body-cell mass, particularly skeletal muscle (93–95).

Therefore, a new view of cancer cachexia emerged where in contrast to starvation, where the patient undergoes adaption to reduce energy expenditure, conserve protein and utilize fatty acids and ketone bodies from fat as an energy source, in cancer cachexia there is an accelerated catabolism, despite declining food and energy intake with normal or increased resting energy expenditure, mobilization of peripheral proteins and lipid stores, and augmented liver gluconeogenesis (96–98).

Metabolism

Increased metabolism is probably an important feature of the paraneoplastic primary cachexia in the contrast to secondary cachexia (99,100). The already published studies of resting energy expenditure did not divide patients into these two forms of cachexia and also did not define the patients at advanced disease or terminal disease. The latter point proved important since studies in a cachetic rat model suggested that animals or preterminal hypometabollic in contrast to initially hypermetabolic (101). In addition, resting energy expenditure has to be described in relation to the actual weight or, better, through the lean body mass rather than through the ideal body weight, which is sometimes described (102).

In correlation to the accelerated catabolism there is a change in carbohydrate metabolism (103) in that patients have relative glucose intolerance and insulin resistance with increased rates of glucose production and recycling via lactate, there is an association of these changes with progressive cachexia (104,105).

Lipid metabolism also is altered with reduced lipogenesis, but with inconsistent reports about lipolysis rates, lipoprotein lipase is probably working at reduced levels (106).

Probably the most important metabolic change is in increased whole body protein turnover. Several data compare these rates with non-weight-losing cancer patients and weight-losing non-cancer patients. As with the carbohydrate changes, there is an association with progressive disease too (107,108). Protein synthesis shifts from normal muscle protein and other tissue protein synthesis to increased liver protein synthesis; this reprioritization has often been seen in other inflammatory states such as trauma, inflammation, and infection (109). On the other hand, muscle breakdown is increased, as shown by the activated ubiquitine–proteasome pathway (110,111). The muscle fibrillar synthesis is shown to be reduced at the mRNA level [NF-κB induced loss of the MyoD messenger (112–114).] Feeding without modification of the complex metabolic alterations can increase muscle protein synthesis (115) but does not influence its breakdown. The acute phase protein synthesis has shown to be accelerated by feeding, compared with healthy controls, while not influencing albumin synthesis rate (116).

Cytokines

Since the above-mentioned changes are seen to a certain extent in other inflammatory states, assessment of the impact of pro-inflammatory cytokines in the pathogenisis of primary cachexia is suggested. Tumor necrosis factor (TNFα) administration can promote weight loss, anorexia, acute phase protein response, protein and fat breakdown, increasing levels of cortisone and glucagon, and insulin resistance, but it also reduced insulin levels, fever, and elevation of energy expenditure in animals and humans. Since TNFα is a short-lived molecule in the blood, its detection has been hampered for technical reasons, but a new assessment of the TNFα receptors (sTNF-R55&75) has improved our understanding of this cytokine. There is a positive correlation between resting energy expenditure and sTNF-55, as shown in patients with non-small-cell lung cancer (117). In tumor-bearing mice, a soluble pegylated 55-kDA TNFα receptor construct improved food intake and led to weight gain compared with a vehicle treated group (118). In contrast, in rats bearing the Yoshida AH-130 acites hepatoma treatment with goat anti-mTNFα lgG did not effect weight loss but decreased protein degradation rates in heart, liver, and gastrognemius muscle (119). TNFα concentrations in the serum of cancer cachexia patients are not elevated in some studies (120–122), which cannot be explained by methodological issues since increased concentrations were detected in cachetic patients with parasitic infections (123).

Recently it has been shown that TNF, which activates NF-κB, prevented immature myoblasts from differentiating into major myotubes capable of synthesizing myosin, suppressed myosin synthesis by differentiated myotubes, and showed suppression of the mRNA encoding myogenenic transcription factor, myo-D, in muscle (112). The effects of NF-κB in regulating muscle loss and gain are complicated; for example, insuline-like growth factor, which probably promotes the accrual of muscle protein, also activates NF-κB which then increases nitric oxide production with stimulation of the transformation of myoblasts to myotubes, which were also capable of synthesizing myosin (124).

These data suggest that TNFα is an epiphenomenon of the inflammatory state rather than a directly causal factor. *In vivo* data from gene knockout mice showed that weight loss from implanted experimental tumors was not improved by knocking out the host cytokines TNFα, Interleukin-12 (IL-12), or interferon-γ, but that the host cytokine IL-6 could play a role. Therefore host cytokines are less important than tumor-derived factors in explaining cachexia and, probably, anorexia (125).

IL-6 is probably an epiphenomenon of the host cytokine cascade mediating increased acute phase protein production rather than being the key element of mediating muscle wasting and cachexia: In mice bearing the colon-26 adenocarcinoma, it was shown that increased serum IL-6 was associated with the progression of cachexia and that administration of anti-IL-6 immunogloblin reduced the loss of GI muscle, but had in one trial suppressed the progression of the cachexia and in another did not affect overall loss of body weight or adipose tissue (126,127). IL-6 did not cause weight loss in normal mice, but is associated with an increased acute phase protein production (128,129). Several studies with patients suffering from different cancers had shown that increases in serum IL-6 correlate with weight loss (130), but nevertheless IL-6 is probably a manifestation of the metabolic disturbances with increased inflammatory mediators rather than a direct cause of weight loss, and specifically muscle catabolism. Moreover, TNFα and IL-6 studies examining IL-1 and Interferon-γ both failed to find a significant role for these two cytokines in protein catabolism and weight loss in cancer cachexia (131,132).

PIF/LMF

Recently, two tumor-derived catabolic factors, the lipid-mobilizing factor (LMF) (133) and the proteolysis-inducing factor (PIF) (134) were detected, which directly mobilize fatty acids and amino acids from adipose tissue and skeletal muscle, respectively (135,136). However, since loss of skeletal muscle and its sequale, namely fatigue and asthenia, are more predominant in morbidity, rather than loss of fat tissue, interest has focused more on monitoring PIF.

PIF is a sulfated glycoprotein of 24 kDA, which is chemically and immunologically identical both from the human and viewing forms (137–140). PIF initiates muscle protein degradation directly, causing rapid weight loss associated with a significant decrease in the weight of the spleen and soleus and gastrognemic muscle, but with no effect on the weight of the heart or kidney, finally resulting in a decrease in lean body mass which was accounted for by an increase (50%) in protein degradation and a decrease (by 50%) in protein synthesis. These effects are reversible by antibody treatment against PIF (141–144). The direct effect of PIF in inducing protein catabolism *in vitro* as well as muscle catabolism *in vitro* (rat model of cachexia) follows a bell-shaped dose–response curve with a decrease in the effect at higher doses of PIF and tumor burden, respectively (145,146). Recently a study showed that PIF was associate with an accelerated rate of weight loss in patients with tumors of the pancreatic head, in comparison with patients where PIF was not detectable in urine, which had less weight loss. The PIF expression and the association with weight loss was found to be independent of the acute phase response (147).

The exact site of PIF-induced protein degradation is controversial. PIF induces an accumulation of ubiquitine protein conjugates in weight-losing mice (143) but also (*in vitro* data from C_2C_{12} myoblasts) an increased release of arachnidoic acid with a dose–response curve parallel to that of protein degradation (145). This direct idonic acid was shown to be rapidly metabolized to the prostaglandins E_2, $F_2\alpha$ and hydroxyeicosatetraaenoic acid (HETES). The role of prostaglandin E_2 is controversial, showing increased protein degradation of extremity muscles (148) as well as no change in the proteolytic rate due to inhibition of PG_2 in septic rats (145,149,150). Since 15-HETE produced *in vitro* a significant increase in protein degradation with the same bell-shaped dose curve as that produced by PIF, it is hypothesized that the effect of PIF could be mediated by an increased synthesis of 15-HETE (114). The ubiquitine–proteasome pathway is the major pathway for the breakdown of intracellular protein and skeletal muscle. Among them, the ATP–ubiquitine-dependent proteolytic pathway is probably responsible for the accelerated protolysis seen in a variety of wasting conditions including cancer cachexia, sepsis, as well as fasting (151). Data from experimental cachexia models show an increase in the amount of ubiquitine protein E_2, as well as proteasome subunits (143,152,153); this process is independent of the amount of protein consumed.

Beside the PIF, LMF has been demonstrated in the serum and urine of cachetic cancer patients which caused the immediate release of glycerol when intubated with epididymal adipodicytes (154–156), which correlated with the extent of weight loss (157) as well with the response to chemotherapy (158). LMF is believed to counteract the two major mechanisms proposed to account for the decrease in body lipids in cancer cachexia, mainly the inhibition of the clearing enzyme lipoprotein lipase, which prevents adipocytes from extracting fatty acids from plasma lipoproteins for storage as well as the direct stimulation of triglyceride hydrolysis in adipocytes by activation of triglyceride lipase.

The role of *cortisol* in the propagation of malnutrition/cachexia is not well established. An infusion of cortisol can cause protein loss, acute phase protein response, increased energy expenditure, and glucose intolerance (159,160); elevated levels of cortisone and glucagone have been shown in patients with cancer (161–165). *In vivo* data from a mice model failed to show an improvement in weight loss with treatment of mifepristone\RU486, an anticortisol medication (166).

Mechanism of anorexia

The pathogenesis of anorexia, or reduction in appetite, as well as its relation to weight loss is matter or further investigation. Anorexia can occur without weight loss, but with clinical features of malnutrition/cachexia as well (32). Whether anorexia and weight loss are two different presentations of the same syndrome or whether they present two different pathogenetical mechanisms needs to be revealed. As discussed above, proinflammatory cytokines can have anorexic effects (295) (hormones in the hypothalamus could contribute to anorexia, since serotonergic activity in the hypothalamus can be anorectic). Free tryptophan, the precursor of serotonin, has been found to be increased in cancer patients and correlated with reduced food intake (167). Neuropeptid-Y is probably low in anorectic cancer patients compared with healthy controls. Experimental data from tumor-bearing rats (296) failed to show that Neuropeptid-Y injected into the hypothalamic region could simulate feeding (168). The significance of leptine, a hormone that suppresses appetite and increases energy expenditure to maintain weight stability, which is produced by fat tissue, is unclear. Leptin is the primary signal through which the hypothalamus senses

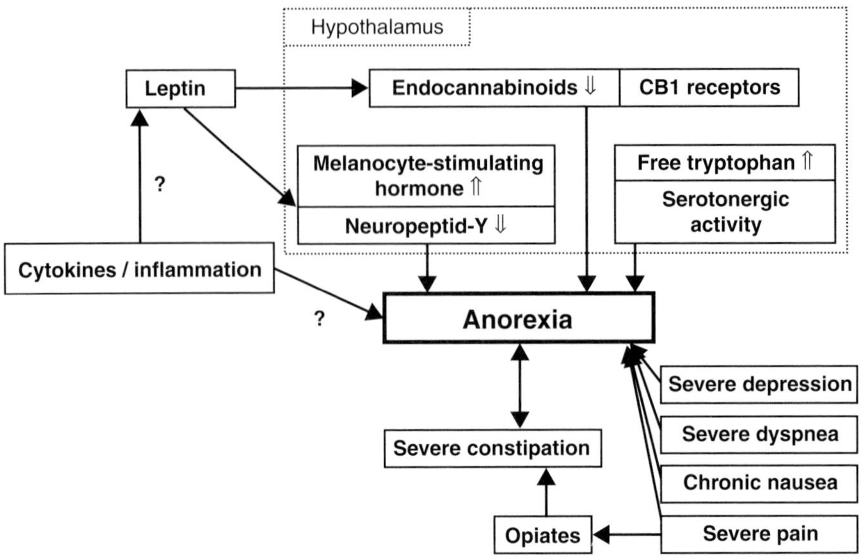

Figure 4.3 Potential mechanisms (the role of leptin and other hypothalamic factors has not been demonstrated for cancer-related cachexia).

nutritional state and modulates food intake and energy balance. Leptin reduces food intake by downregulating appetite-stimulating factors, primarily neuropeptide Y4, and by upregulating appetite-reducing neuropeptides, such as melanocyte-stimulating hormones. Leptin levels are increased in some models of inflammation (169,170). However, initial data in patients with cancer and weight loss found low levels of leptin (171).

Recently it was shown that cannabinoid CB1 receptor knockout mice eat less than their wild-type littermates, and the CB1 antagonist SR141716A reduces food intake in wild-type but not knockout mice. Since it is known that defective leptin signalling is associated with elevated hypothalamic, but not cerebellar, levels of endocannabinoids (in obese db/db and ob/ob mice and Zucker rats) and that acute leptin treatment of normal rats and ob/ob mice reduces anandamide and 2 arachidonoyl glycerol in the hypothalamus, these findings indicate that endocannabinoids in the hypothalamus may tonically activate CB1 receptors to maintain food intake and form part of the neural circuitry regulated by leptin (172). These findings strengthen the potential role of endocannabinoids in the pathogenesis of anorexia. See Figures 4.3, and 4.4.

Chronic nausea/autonomic failure

Chronic nausea, early satiety, and anorexia can be manifestations of autonomic failure, which can occur as a consequence of malnutrition/cachexia, but probably represent also a distinct paraneoplastic syndrome [autonomic neuropathy (173)] in patients with advanced cancer, and finally can occur as an adverse effect of neurotoxic treatments or neuropathic conditions (diabetes mellitus, spinal cord compression, etc.). Whether the GI [chronic nausea, early satiety, anorexia, pseudo-bowel obstruction (174)], cardiovascular [postural hypotension

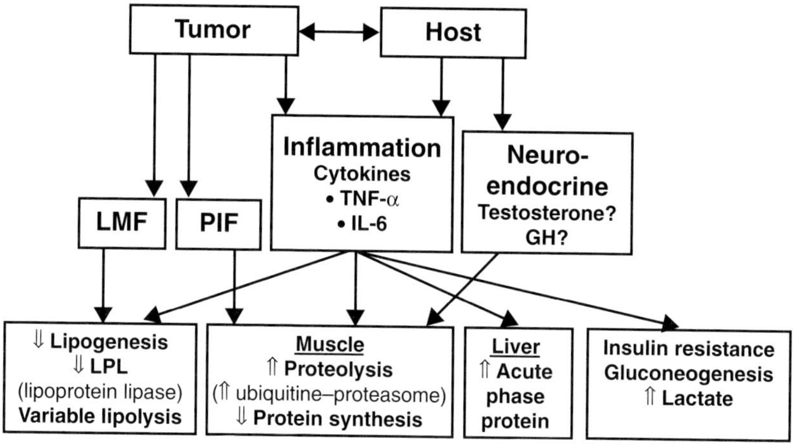

Figure 4.4 Metabolic abnormalities in primary cachexia.

(175), fixed heart rate (176)] and constitutional [asthenia, chronic fatigue (177)] symptoms of autonomic insufficiency represent the same underlying mechanism remains unknown.

Mechanism of asthenia/fatigue

Asthenia (178), easy fatigue (62), weakness (49,59,60), loss of energy (59,60), lack of energy (30), or tierdness all describe one of the most frequent symptoms in advanced and terminal cancer. The distinction between fatigue as a beneficial physiological phenomenon protective against over exertion and fatigue as a pathological finding causing distress is important and needs to be educated to our patients. At the present time there is a growing awareness of the frequency and importance of fatigue in the trajectory of the cancer illness (179). Fatigue is described as a multidimensional phenomenon, that develops over time, diminishing energy, mental capacity, and the psychologic condition (180). Cancer-related fatigue is often seen in the context of fatigue as a common side-effect of cancer treatment, even in cancer survivors without evidence of disease (181). This understanding of fatigue contrasts with fatigue in the context of advanced and progressive cancer, where probably considerably different major causes apply, i.e. primary cachexia. Fatigue may represent a final common pathway to which many predisposing or etiologic factors contribute, whose importance changes during the course of the illness.

Asthenia means absence or loss of strength (from the Greek *Asthenos*) and can be characterized as profound tiredness occurring after usual or minimal effort activities accompanied by a sensation of generalized weakness (182). Asthenia can be seen as having three components (183).

1 Fatigue or lassitude, defined as easy tiring and a decreased capacity to maintain performance;

2 Generalized weakness, defined as anticipatory sensation or difficulty in initiating a certain activity;

3 Mental fatigue(184), defined as the presence of impaired mental concentration with or without loss of memory or emotional lability.

However, in patients with advanced cancer the clinical distinction in the different characteristics of asthenia/fatigue remains to be established.

Usually, multiple causes coexist in patients with advanced cancer suffering from asthenia/fatigue. It may result from one clearly dominant abnormality or from a combination of other lesser abnormalities.

Given the high frequency of cancer anorexia/cachexia syndrome (ACS) and asthenia/fatigue in the same patients it is likely that the latter can be an epiphenomenon of ACS, which pathogenesis is discussed in detail above. As shown above, cytokines play an important role in ACS. TNF-α, IL-1, IL-6, and interferon-α have been shown to cause profound asthenia in animal models and humans (185,186), even in the absence of cancer. To what extent the recently identified tumor byproducts LIF and PIF are associated with asthenia/fatigue remains to be established. In contrast to these arguments there are clinical situations where the relationship between ACS and asthenia/fatigue is not as close as has been assumed. For example, asthenia/fatigue is frequent and severe in patients with advanced breast cancer (178) or lymphomas (187), who have a low frequency of ACS. In patients with non-malignant conditions, such as the chronic fatigue syndrome (188) or psychologic depression (189), fatigue can be very important in the absence of cachexia. In contrast, severe cachexia can be observed in patients with anorexia nervosa without the important presence of fatigu (190,191). The fatigue observed in chronic infections, such as tuberculosis, leprosy, or AIDS, could reflect a common pathway of inflammatory mediated asthenia/fatigue, which is present in patients with ACS too. Data from patients enrolled in the development of the Brief Fatigue Inventory (BFI) support the probably high contribution of anorexia/cachexia as a cause of asthenia/fatigue in patients with advanced cancer. Both in the hematologic group ($n = 253$) including 53% lymphoma, 42% leukemia, and 5% multiple myeloma, and the solid tumor group ($n = 107$), including 60% GI cancer, 27% breast cancer, 6% gynecologic and genitourinary cancers, 4% with sarcoma, and 3% with other cancers, fatigue severity was significantly correlated with appetite, sleep disturbances, albumine level ($r = -0.40$ for solid tumors, $r = -0.49$ for the hematologic group) and hemoglobin (192).

Autonomic failure, as discussed above , is a paraneoplastic syndrome, which is probably involved as a cofactor in fatigue/asthenia, but its importance remains to be established.

Besides the common paraneoplastic anorexia/cachexia syndrome, and autonomic failure, several rare paraneoplastic neurologic and neuromuscular syndromes are associated with asthenia/fatigue. They occur most commonly in patients with lung cancer: dermatomyositis, polymyositis, Eaton–Lambert syndrome, myasthenia gravis, ascending acute polyneuropathy (Guilain–Barre), paraneoplastic encephalomyelitis, and progressive multifocal leucencephalopathy, among others (193). Patients with lymphoma can also present with some of these syndromes, but most often asthenia/fatigue is caused by constitutional symptoms, fever, sweating, weight loss, reflecting immune activation (194).

Psychological distress is considered to be the final cause of asthenia/fatigue in patients without cancer in almost 75%, including depression, anxiety, and other psychologic disorders (195). In patients with cancer the presence of major psychiatric disorders has been reported to be low (196,197). However, in patients with advanced cancer, mild to severe, fluctuating and often transient mood alterations are common, but their relative contribution to the cause of fatigue/asthenia in advanced cancer patients remains to be established. Since fatigue/asthenia is common in patients with advanced cancer, it has been replaced as a criterion for major depression by other criteria, such as loss of joy and pleasure (198).

In patients with cancer a positive correlation between the level of hemoglobin/anemia (180,199) and fatigue, energy level, ability to do daily activities, and QoL scores has been well documented through data from clinical trials of epoetin alfa as supportive treatment during antineoplastic treatment (200–202). This was shown in an older placebo-controlled trial in cancer patients with and without cytotoxic chemotherapy (203). A recent randomized (2 : 1), double-blind, placebo-controlled multicenter trial of epoetin alfa three times per week enrolled 375 patients with solid or non-myeloid hematologic malignancies undergoing non-platinum chemotherapy and with hemoglobin levels $\leq 10.5\,\mathrm{g\,dl^{-1}}$ or $\leq 12.0\,\mathrm{g\,dl^{-1}}$ after a decrease of $\geq 1.5\,\mathrm{g\,dl^{-1}}$ per cycle since starting chemotherapy. Baseline hemoglobin was $9.9\,\mathrm{g\,dl^{-1}}$ and $9.7\,\mathrm{g\,dl^{-1}}$, respectively; there are no baseline values for symptoms reported, nor the performance status. Patients were assessable for efficacy after completion of 28 study days; study duration was a maximum of 28 weeks. The patients were mostly in 'late-stage disease', i.e. for the three most common cancer types, stage III or IV was 59% for breast cancer, 76% for non-Hodgkin's lymphoma, and 65% for myeloma, but many patients with these disease stages can be treated with curative intent. A strong positive correlation was found between change in hemoglobin and linear–analogue scales (LASA) for energy level, ability to do daily activities, and overall QoL, as well as for the FACT-An (Functional Assessment of Cancer Therapies) fatigue subscale, the FACT-General, and finally both the physical and mental component summary of the SF-36 (Medical Outcomes Study Short Form-36) (204). Another recent prospective, community-based, multicenter, open-label, non-randomized study of once-weekly epoetin alfa enrolled 3012 patients with non-myeloid malignancies undergoing chemotherapy and with hemoglobin levels $< 11.0\,\mathrm{g\,dl^{-1}}$, mean hemoglobin at baseline was $(9.5 \pm 0.9)\,\mathrm{g\,dl^{-1}}$. 2869 patients were assessable (defined as having at least two hemoglobin measurements, which were done monthly), 58.8% completed the study after four months. Baseline symptom burden, assessed with LASA was 39.2/100 (± 21.2) for energy level, 40.5 ± 23.9 for ability to perform daily activities, and 46.6 ± 23.5 for overall QoL, the fatigue subscale of the FACT-An score was $24.9/52 \pm 11.6$, and the ECOG performance status was 1 (Median). Percentage changes from baseline were significant ($p < 0.001$ for all changes) with 30% for energy level, 26% for ability to perform daily activities, and 19% for overall QoL, respectively. The correlation between the increase in QoL and the increase in hemoglobin from baseline was positive and significant; the correlations with activity and energy level were not shown. Interestingly, patients with no increase in hemoglobin levels had no corresponding improvement of LASA scores (199). In patients with advanced, progressive as well as terminal cancer not undergoing chemotherapy, who suffer from loss of energy and fatigue, it remains to be established which contribution to the overall symptom burden is caused by anemia.

Fatigue/asthenia often occurs during infections, particularly when the course is protracted. Even chronic infections such as the Ebstein–Barr virus, which are often not apparent, can cause resistant fatigue/asthenia. In patients with advanced cancer intercurrent bacterial or fungal infections are more common and contribute to the severity of fatigue, even though systematic prospective research is missing to quantify the importance of that factor.

Electrolyte disorders, such as hypercalcemia, low sodium, low potassium, or low magnesium, can contribute to fatigue/asthenia and can be treated easily. Uncontrolled diabetes mellitus can contribute to the symptom burden too. Hypocortisolismus/Addison's syndrome also needs to be considered as an endocrine cause for fatigue/asthenia. Symptomatic hypothyroidism is rare in patients with advanced cancer; most common is probably the sick euthyreot syndrome, whose contribution to fatigue/asthenia remains to be investigated.

Dehydration is fairly common in patients with advanced cancer, i.e. out-patients with limited social and financial resources, and can contribute to asthenia/fatigue. Severe hypoxemia can be a contributory factor in fatigue/asthenia, and in addition can also cause over-exertion.

Over-exertion is probably the most common cause of fatigue in non-cancer patients. In contrast, patients suffering from cancer and its treatment frequently experience several anatomical and functional changes (anemia, reduction of vital capacity, impairment of left ventricular function, loss of muscle mass and of plasma volume, increased production of inflammation mediators), which may result in a severe loss of physical performance (205,206). The empirical advise to avoid physical effort and to reduce the level of physical activity then generates a more severe loss of muscle mass and a further impairment of cardiorespiratory function. Aerobic exercise programmes have been shown to improve the physical performance and QoL of patients undergoing surgery or antineoplastic treatment for hematological neoplastic diseases (207–209) and also to improve fatigue, psychologic status (210) and accelerate bone marrow regeneration of patients undergoing high-dose chemotherapy (207), probably in association with increased production of hematopoietic active cytokines (211). The importance of prolonged bedrest and deconditioning in patients with advanced, progressive cancer as a cause of asthenia/fatigue remains to be elaborated.

Antineoplastic treatments such as surgery, radiotherapy, chemotherapy, and biological response modifiers, i.e. interferon-α, are well-known causes of fatigue/asthenia (212). On the other hand, there is a growing body of literature documenting the symptomatic effect of antineoplastic treatments, in addition to the 'classical' oncological outcome measurements of response rate, survival, etc. as well as toxicity and adverse events (213,214). However, the indication and monitoring of antineoplastic treatments for alleviating symptoms and improvement of QoL is difficult. Even though a careful design was implemented in several of the Phase III studies assessing chemotherapy for patients with advanced cancer, several factors can contribute to a biased conclusion regarding symptomatic endpoints. For several reasons the control arms were never placebo-controlled, therefore the high symptomatic placebo effect of many interventions in patients with advanced cancer, reaching 30%–50% improvement of several symptoms, such as pain (215), anorexia (216), tiredness (as recently seen in a prospective placebo-controlled trial evaluating fish oil in cancer patients, data submitted), among others, could contribute to a biased interpretation of the symptomatic benefit. The quality of the accompanying symptom control interventions, often referred to as 'best supportive care', has not been controlled for in most trials, mostly due to a lack of prospective definitions and of trained palliative care teams, respectively. Nevertheless, a careful tailored and monitored antineoplastic treatment can be of important symptomatic benefit, and newer antineoplastic treatments aiming at stabilizing (217), rather than reducing the cancer, will strengthen this approach. Many new antineoplastic treatment modalities are under active development, such as angiogenesis inhibitors, molecular targeted agents (i.e. inhibition of EGFR, c-KIT, m-TOR), targeting ras/MAP kinases, single transduction inhibitors, cell-cycle-based strategies, or monoclonal antibodies, the symptomatic effects of which, besides their antineoplastic activity, remain to be shown.

Many of the medications administered to patients with advanced canced can aggreviate asthenia/fatigue. It is crucial in any patient with advanced cancer that we have a good understanding of the actual pharmacological treatment: justification of the actual indication, typical side-effects, metabolism including excretion, influence on liver metabolism and renal function, and pharmacological interactions. The most common drugs contributing to fatigue are psychoactive substances, including opioids, but also the long-term use of corticosteroids (218,219). On the other hand, preliminary data showed that patients with chronic fatigue syndrome could benefit from low-dose corticosteroid treatment (220,221).

Patients with advanced cancer often suffer from multiple symptoms (see above), which can contribute to asthenia/fatigue.

In addition to all these factors, any other chronic disease or organ failure can cause asthenia/fatigue, including chronic fatigue syndrome, chronic heart failure, chronic obstructive pulmonary disease, and renal and hepatic failure, among others.

Since prospective studies systematically evaluating the different causes of asthenia/fatigue in patients with advanced, progressive as well as terminal cancer are missing, and the present research on cancer-related fatigue often focuses on patients undergoing active antineoplastic treatment, judgment of the relative contribution of the above-mentioned possible causes of asthenia/fatigue relies on a careful and continuous clinical assessment.

Hypogonadotropic hypogonadism/growth hormone deficiency

Chronic (inflammatory) diseases can be associated with complex neuroendocrine alterations (222,223). Endogenous opioids play an important role in the regulation of gonadotropins (i.e. LH) as well as in neuromodulation of growth hormone(GH) and thyroid stimulating hormone (TSH) (224). In patients with non-malignant chronic pain (mainly failed back surgery) long-term intrathecal administration (27 ± 16 months) of opoids was related to the development of hypogonadotropic hypogonadism, as well as central hypocorticism and GH deficiency (225). Treatment with GH resulted in several non-cancer cachexia situations (cardiac cachexia (226,227), aging (228), chronic obstructive pulmonary disease (229), to an increase in lean body mass, and to an improvement of function in HIV wasting (230). Because of concerns about tumor growth stimulation there are no clinical trials with GH for cachexia treatment reported in cancer patients. Several studies with anabolic steroids showed an increase in fat-free mass in patients with HIV wasting (231), end-stage renal disease (232), and chronic obstructive pulmonary disease (233). Low testosteron levels were found in HIV patients, and replacement therapy was beneficial (234–236). In summary, these data from non-cancer wasting situations suggest a considerable role of hormonal abnormalities, which in cancer anorexia/cachexia syndrome are probably hidden behind the effects of predominant inflammatory alterations and tumor-related cachectic factors.

Taste alterations

Whether taste alterations are an independent symptom in the context of progressive cancer, or whether they are sequelae or paraneoplastic treatment of complications in the oral cavity, is controversial. There is a positive correlation between weight loss or the presence of the normal taste sensation(237). The role of zinc deficiency requires further research: Plasma zinc levels are reduced in patients with bronchial carcinoma as well as in leukemic cells compared with a healthy population and normal blood cells, respectively (238).

Mechanism/pathogenesis of starvation or secondary cachexia

Several conditions leading to impaired caloric intake or loss of nutrients occur in patients suffering from cancer and can be summarized in four groups (see Table 4.1).

1 Impaired oral intake: stomatitis, dysphagia, odynophagia, bowel obstruction, vomiting, severe constipation (239), intractable pain (240), severe dyspnea, severe depression, delirium and social obstacles, etc.

2 Impaired GI absorption: malabsorption, exocrine pancreatic insufficiency, chronic severe diarrhea, etc.

3 Catabolic states: hyperthyroidism, chronic and acute infections, chronic active inflammation, etc.

4 Significant loss of proteins: body fluids, i.e. frequent ascites or pleural fluid punctions, nephrotic syndrome, etc.

In patients with secondary cachexia and terminal diseases nutritional support needs to be considered when the estimated life expectancy from the underlying disease in longer than the average time to die from starvation. Healthy adults die from starvation after a nitrogen loss of 35% of the ideal weight, i.e. after 60–75 days, despite adequate adipose reserves, since the protein mass is the major determinant of starvation (241). In patients with advanced cancer there are no similar data available, since the population is very heterogeneous to study. An estimate for dying from starvation equals about 15–30 days for patients with progressive, terminal cancer. The average nitrogen loss per day of $3\,g\,day^{-1}$ for a healthy adult increases to $15–20\,g\,day^{-1}$ in the setting of systemic inflammatory response syndrome, as seen in sepsis or severe trauma, leading to a 30% reduction of muscular mass after 10–13 days, and of body cell mass after 20 days, respectively (242).

GI surgery leading to malnutrition/cachexia

Patients undergoing GI surgery (esophagectomy, gastrectomy, gastrointestinal bypass, pancreatoduodenectomy, colectomy, etc.) are at risk for developing secondary cachexia/starvation. After the post-operative phase, weight can usually be maintained using nutritional supplements, and enteral or even parenteral nutrition (see below). However, when progressive cancer is present causing ACS, or complications occur such as infections, spinal cord injury potentiating autonomic failure, symptomatic brain metastasis, hypercalcemia, among others, the impaired GI integrity aggravates the possibility of malnutrition/cachexia.

In summary the following issues are relevant in the pathogenesis of ACS:

- The difference between primary (metabolic) and secondary (starvation) malnutrition/cachexia
- Primary cachexia is a paraneoplastic metabolic syndrome with increased metabolism in the context of chronic inflammation
- Alterations in the cytokine milieu play a major role in the perpetuation of metabolic, neuroendocrine, and symptomatic manifestations of primary cachexia
- Primary cachexia increases muscle proteolysis but also acute phase protein synthesis. Nutritients can increase protein synthesis but do not reduce proteolysis

- Cachectic factors produced by the tumor, such as PIF and LMF, play an increasing role in mediating malnutrition/cachexia
- The symptoms of anorexia and asthenia/fatigue correlate incompletely with weight loss

Assessment of malnutrition/cachexia

Basics of malnutrition/cachexia assessment

In addition to all the sophisticated diagnostic tests, the most important tool is clinical suspicion. Since malnutrition/cachexia is a 'silent' syndrome it is paramount to assess actively ('look, listen, ask') for it.

The assessment of the nutritional status includes different domains, as mentioned below, and there is a wide variation in what is meant by nutritional status, ranging from pure anthropometrics to function to QoL. Nutritional assessment using laboratory and technical data alone has failed to consistently identify patients at risk for nutritionally mediated complications and symptomatic impact (243). Clinical judgment was equivalent to objective measurements in 59 patients admitted to a surgical ward (244), leading to the development of the Subjective Global Assessment (SGA) tool, which was predictive of nutrition-associated complications of patients undergoing GI surgery. This tool has been of value in different populations for predicting nutrition-related complications such as in geriatric patients (245), chronic renal failure (246), AIDS (247), as well as cancer (27). [A study of 87 patients with GI and urological tumors showed independent contributions to the overall classification by weight loss in the previous six months, level of food intake, problems with eating, physical activity, and muscle wastage. Survival was significantly higher in SGA A than in SGA B+C, $P<0.001$) but failed to be prognostic of survival in liver transplantation (248).]

Components of malnutrition/cachexia assessment

Different domains need to be differentiated for a comprehensive assessment of malnutrition/cachexia (Table 4.5).

Body composition/anthropometrics: static tests

The hallmark of body composition assessment is a thorough, careful history of *weight* and skillful weight measurement using scales that are standardized and avoidance of variability due to clothes. *Weight loss* should be quantified in percent during the previous two or six months as well as to pre-illness weight and assessment of unvoluntary weight loss should be done. The presence of fluid retention needs to be assessed as being clinically relevant or not. In very rapidly progressing tumors, sometimes the tumor mass can contribute to weight gain. The *body mass index* (BMI), even if independent of age, gender, and height, does not tell us about the body's energy storage compartments and therefore is not very useful as a reflection of the functional body composition.

Serum albumin reflects, to quite a good extent, the protein content: its half-life is 19 days and there are numerous studies showing the correlation of serum albumin with weight loss in cancer cachexia patients. Pre-albumin is often used by nutritionists. Its advantage is a shorter half-life of a few days which allows closer monitoring of nutritional interventions. However, it probably is not a good assessment tool for baseline rather than longitudinal monitoring.

Table 4.5 Assessment of cachexia

Clinical assessment
◆ Weight and weight loss (% during previous 2 and 6 months, comparison with pre-illness weight)
◆ Subjective global assessment
◆ Performance status
◆ Serum albumin
◆ Symptom assessment including anorexia, fatigue, nausea: ASAS, others
◆ Any cause for secondary cachexia
◆ Oncological situation, prognosis
Additional assessments
◆ Bioimpedance analysis (BIA)
◆ Midarm circumference, skinfold thickness
◆ Dual energy X-ray absorptiometry (DEXA)
◆ Dynamometer: grip strength, elbow flexor muscles, knee extensor muscles
◆ Edmonton Functional Assessment Tool (EFAT)
◆ Functional Assessment of Appetite Cachexia Therapy (FAACT)
◆ QoL tools (EORTC-QLC-c30)
◆ Estimation of caloric intake

The *skinfold thickness* is helpful in estimating body fat, usually measured by pinching a sample of skin and subcutaneous fat between a pair of calipers with standard area and pressure. The recommended sites for sampling are the triceps, biceps, subscapular, and suprailliacal. This method is prone to errors, second to observer variability, which goes up to 7%. Other interfering factors are edema and excessive water content of the examined tissues with an over-estimation of body fat. There are few prospective data from a cancer/cachexia population; the prediction equations have been developed in young and fit populations (249).

The *midarm circumference* correlates with the muscle mass, which can be calculated by a formula (250); however, the two methods of skinfold thickness and midarm circumference rely on the assumptions that there is a constant relationship between the subcutaneous fat mantel and total body fat. However, these measurements are easy to use and therefore useful for longitudinal follow-up of individual patients with advanced cancer.

Bioimpedance analysis (BIA) is based on the fact that different body tissues possess characteristic conductive and resistive properties. It is assumed that resistance is the pure opposition of a conductor to an alternating current and a reactant is the capacitive effect of cell membranes, tissue interfaces, and non-ionic tissues. The measurements are difficult to compare between individuals since the actual conductive path through the body is unknown and the small measured electrical resistance is primarily influenced by the limbs, therefore BIA may be relatively insensitive to differences in tissue composition of the trunk, which is an important body fat store. In addition, changes in the electrolyte millieu may affect conductivity through the body, changes in hydration status, and fluctuating body fluids in the context of fluid retention can alter the results. With fast-growing tumors there can also be a mismatch of left- and right-sided measurements, i.e. in the context of liver metastases (251). However, there are few prospective data evaluating the validity and reliability of BIA in cachexia monitoring (252,253).

Dual photon absorptiometry/dual energy X-ray absorptiometry (DEXA) is based on the fact that the ratio for the absorbance of two different energy level photons (applied by X-ray source) is linearly related to the percentage of fat and soft tissue of the body and therefore the body fat and fat-free mass can be predicted. Its value in cancer cachexia/malnutrition has not been fully established (254). DEXA is also prone to alterations and variations, but is less observer dependent and probably more comparable between individuals than BIA (255,256). Total body potassium, total body monitor, and *in vivo* neutron activation analysis can be used as additional research methods to assess further body cell mass and hydration status (257).

Functional assessments: dynamic

Grip strength (258) as a dynamometric assessment has been shown to be a prognostic tool in post-operative patients (259,260). In a recent study (261) dynamometric measurements were used as a primary assessment for the pharmacological treatment of primary cachexia. Treatment with ATP seemed to be associated with an improvement in weight loss and muscle strength (262). However, these tools are not standard practice and their value has not been demonstrated to be independent of a subjective assessment of function (see below).

In addition to dynamometrics the performance status can reflect the function and activity of daily living. These tools, such as ECOG, Karnofsky performance status and the Edmonton functional assessment tools (263), are common practice in oncology. Several QoL tools, such as the EORTC-QLC30 questionnaire, assess the subjective assessment of function by the patient. The data showing reliable estimation of symptoms by care-givers suggest that third-party assessment of function can be useful for monitoring patients too, as reflected by the good reliability of performance status as an independent prognostic marker.

Symptomatic impact/QoL

Part of a comprehensive cachexia assessment is measurement of the symptomatic impact of cachexia (Table 4.6). The assessment of the most common symptoms can be achieved by using a questionnaire such as the Edmonton Symptom Assessment Scale which measures the severity of nine symptoms (including anorexia, nausea, and fatigue) and overall well-being [ESAS (264)], or by using the memorial symptom assessment scale [MSAS(61)], which measures the perceived distress of an individual symptom. The application of instruments designed to measure different domains of QoL, such as the EORTC-QIQ-c30 questionnaire (265) or the FACT (266), also provide adequate symptom screening.

Which instrument is available to assess the different characteristics typical for anorexia/cachexia? There is only one published (Abstract) assessment tool designed for anorexia/cachexia, namely the Functional Assessment of Appetite Cachexia Therapy (FAACT) (267), which has not been evaluated in prospective trials. Some of the questions provide additional information, such as: 'The amount I eat is sufficient to meet my needs', 'I enjoy eating breakfast', 'My interest in food drops as soon as I try to eat', 'I have difficulty eating rich or heavy foods', 'My family or friends are pressuring me to eat', 'I am

Table 4.6 Assessment of cachexia: common concerns of patients

When I eat I seem to get full quickly
The amount I eat is not sufficient to meet my needs
My interest in food drops as soon as I try to eat
I have difficulty eating rich or heavy foods
My family or friends are pressuring me to eat
I don't enjoy the mealtime because of tension and stress to eat enough
I am concerned about how thin I look
I avoid social contacts because of my appearance
I am worried about the meaning of my weight loss (i.e. starving to death)
Because I don't eat enough, I am so tired and fatigued

concerned about how thin I look', 'I avoid social contacts because of my appearance'. An ad hoc-module-anorexia/cachexia-EORTC-QLC30 for is actually under evaluation in a prospective multicentric phase III study comparing placebo to 9-d-THC to a for 9-d-THC standardized cannabis extract reference (7).

In addition to the information about individual symptoms associated with anorexia/cachexia, i.e. fatigue, from the symptom-screening tools, additional specialized assessment tools are necessary. A number of instruments have been developed, such as the Pearson–Byars Fatigue Feeling Checklist (assessment of 13 energy level descriptors), the Brief Fatigue Inventory (187) (see below), the Fatigue-subscale of the FACT (Functional Assessment of Cancer Treatment) assessment system (268) (see below), or longer instruments assessing more than the dimension of fatigue [Piper Fatigue Self-Report Scale (269), Rhoten Fatigue Scale (270), Multidimensional Fatigue Inventory (271), Multidimensional Fatigue Symptom Inventory (272), Fatigue Assessment Instrument (273), Fatigue Symptom Inventory (274), Fatigue Symptom Checklist (275), and the Asthenia Questionnaire (276)]. However, it remains to be established which domains of fatigue are most prevalent in patients with advanced cancer (in contrast to chemotherapy-associated fatigue), i.e. fatigue or lassitude, generalized weakness, or mental fatigue.

The brief fatigue inventory [BFI (187)] was developed comparing 290 controls (healthy members of service groups) with 305 cancer patients, and was reported to be a reliable instrument for rapid fatigue assessment capable of identifying patients with severe fatigue. The BFI asks for rating of fatigue or weariness or tiredness now, both usual and worst level during the past 24 hours, and interference by fatigue in general activity, walking ability, normal work, mood, enjoyment of life, and relations with other people. It was tested against two validated measures of fatigue, the POMS—vigor and the POMS—fatigue (277), which measure subjective mood states (Profile Of Mood States), and the fatigue subscale and the anemia specific items of the FACT assessment system (268). Patients were not eligible 'if their clinical status was felt to be too poor', resulting in a sample of 55 patients fully active (ECOG performance status 0), 87 patients restricted, but ambulatory (ECOG 1), 128 patients ambulatory, capable of self-care (ECOG 2), two patients capable of only limited self-care (ECOG 3), no patients completely disabled (ECOG 4), and 33 patients' data missing for performance status. The BFI, like the two other instruments (POMS, FACT), showed discriminant validity both for hemoglobin levels and for ECOG performance status. Interestingly, a significant inverse correlation was found between the BFI and serum albumin, both in patients with hematological malignancies and solid tumors. The clinical utility of the BFI in patients with advanced cancer, i.e. ECOG performance status 3 and 4, remains to be established.

The FACT-F, the fatigue subscale of the FACT, was developed together with the FACT-An, the anemia-subscale of the FACT (268,278,279). These subscales are based on the 28-item FACT-G (general) questionnaire and add 13 fatigue items and 7 anemia-related, but non-fatigue, items. This subscales were constructed based on an item pool from 14 anemic oncology patients and five oncology experts. The validation sample consisted of 50 cancer patients, reflecting the most common tumors, with performance status 0, 36%, 1, 44%, and 2 and 3, 20%. As discussed for the BFI, the FACT-F should be evaluated more in patients with advanced cancer, i.e. poorer performance status. In addition, the FACT-F is based on both the FACT-G and the FACT-An and has not been evaluated separately.

Given the wide distribution in patients with advanced cancer and extensive experience with the FACT-G, the use of FACT-F for assessment of fatigue seems reliable in clinical practice.

In order to facilitate progress in the treatment of cancer-related fatigue a set of diagnostic criteria have been developed, leading to the proposal for ICD-10 criteria (280). The criteria consist of criterion A, which includes 11 common clinical manifestations reported by cancer patients who complain of fatigue, criterion B, which is a requirement that fatigue causes significant distress or disrupts the patients social or occupational role, criterion C, which ensures that fatigue is a consequence of cancer or cancer therapy, and finally criterion D, which excludes fatigue related to a larger psychiatric condition, such as major depression or delirium. To meet the diagnostic criteria, symptoms must be present nearly every day for a period of two weeks over a period of a month. Further development of the ICD-10 proposal for fatigue led to the adaption of the criterion A, which now requires 'main' criteria (significant fatigue, diminished energy, or increased need to rest, disproportionate to any recent change in activity level), and five (or more) additional criteria (complaints of generalized weakness or limb heaviness, diminished concentration or attention, decreased motivation or interest in engaging in usual activities, insomnia or hypersomnia, experience of sleep as unrefreshing or non-restorative, perceived need to struggle to overcome inactivity, marked emotional reactivity (e.g. sadness, frustration, or irritability) to feeling fatigued, difficulty completing daily tasks attributed to feeling fatigued, perceived problems with short-term memory, post-exertional malaise lasting several hours)(180). It remains to be demonstrated if this proposal for criteria for cancer-related fatigue is useful both in patients with early disease, undergoing or completed antineoplastic treatments, and also in patients with advanced, progressive or terminal disease.

In summary, it is more important in the clinical situation (outside clinical research questions) to perform a thorough symptoms screening and careful palliative assessment than use the right tool. As for pain, it seems likely that the assessment of anorexia or fatigue by a patient-based visual analog scale of fatigue severity can serve as a simple uniscale of high sensitivity. In patients with advanced cancer the assessment of symptom interference should include any of the, at a given time obvious, important individual symptoms.

Measurement of caloric intake and appetite

The measurement of appetite by a visual analog scale has been well established, and is part of many symptom assessment and QoL tools. The assessment of caloric intake can be made at the bedside by a nutritionist or trained nurse; other methods include dietary records, prospective records, as well as recalled records. The recalled records are of limited accuracy in patients with cognitive failure/delirium, depression, or asthenia (281). Prospective third-person assessment is a simple method of food intake measurement by the percentage calculation of food products consumed at each meal by the patient, that can be done by a nurse or volunteer by observation, and has been shown to correlate well with actual weighing of the food (282).

Secondary cachexia

It is crucial to assess patients for the presence of secondary cachexia, as mentioned above. There are several tests for assessing digestive function, for general assessment of malabsorption/maldigestion, pancreatic/small bowel function, bile salt loss or gastric emptying, as well as newer tests (PABAX tests of the digestive function), which are still research tools and should not be used to screen for inappercept digestive malfunction (283). In patients with suspected autonomic failure, presenting with orthostatic intolerance, early satiety, or secretomotor dysfunction, a fixed heart rate can be measured with a simple electrocardiogram (177). In addition, a new assessment questionnaire has recently been published for patients with neurological disorders (284).

Since the frequency or the role of secondary compared with primary cachexia in weight-losing cancer patients has not been assessed prospectively, it is not possible to give clear recommendations to what extent assessments are justified. Often there is a need for a thorough internal medical assessment of a patient and of a surgical assessment to weigh the probability of secondary cachexia causes.

Extent of primary cachexia

At the present time the diagnosis of primary cachexia is based on the exclusion of causes for secondary cachexia. In the future the assessment of the proteolysis inducing factor (90), measurable in the urine, will be part of routine practice, both for assessment at baseline and for monitoring. The value of other factors, as discussed in the pathogenesis section, such as the lipid-mobilizing factor, neuropeptid-Y, leptine, TNF-receptors (STNF-R55 or 75), among others, is not established. Several studies found an association of IL-6 with weight loss, which reflects unspecific inflammation, but does not allow a distinction of primary in contrast to secondary cachexia. However, in a cohort of well-defined patients in whom causes of secondary cachexia have been excluded, IL-6 could become a more important parameter. The measurement of other parameters of altered carbohydrate, fat or protein metabolisms such as triglycerides or the cortisol/insulin ratio, as well as measurement of resting energy expenditure, are not of proven clinical value.

Immunological tests

Anergy or cutaneous reactions as well as absolute lymphocyte counts, among other immunological tests, have been of some prognostic value for nutritional status in the non-cancer population (285). However, as discussed in the pathogenesis section, the value of these tests is probably difficult to interpret in the population with progressive weight loss in the context of cancer.

Oncological situation—prognosis

An estimation of the prognosis can guide further assessments as well as guide further decision-making. The estimation of survival in patients with advanced cancer is, even for experienced healthcare professionals, accurate only in 20%–70%, with an over-estimation from physicians by a factor of 2–5, and a reliable survival prediction is possible only in very ill patients (286,287). Some of the possible predictive factors of survival may be counteracted to some extent by appropriate nutritional support, i.e. causes of secondary cachexia such as dysphagia, complicating the clinical decision-making.

In summary, the above-mentioned seven different domains of malnutrition/cachexia assessment reflect available methods for further assessment (Table 4.5). In clinical practice the assessment of weight loss, function (by performance status and questionnaire), symptomatic impact assessed by an easy screening tool including appetite, albumin and, in future, PIF, as well as a thorough exclusion or documentation of causes of secondary cachexia, will reach a high level of quality. Most sophisticated tests need to be proven to add improvement of that quality.

References

1. **Hockley JM; Dunlop R; Davies RJ.** Survey of distressing symptoms in dying patients and their families in hospital and the response to a symptom control team. *British Medical Journal* (Clinical Research Edition) 1988;296(6638):1715–17.
2. **Velikova G; Wright P; Smith AB., *et al.*** Self-reported quality of life of individual cancer patients: concordance of results with disease course and medical records. *Journal of Clinical Oncology* 2001;19(7):2064–73.
3. **Costantini M; Mencaglia E; Giulio PD; Cortesi E; Roila F; Ballatori E; Tamburini M., *et al.*** Cancer patients as 'experts' in defining quality of life domains. A multicentre survey by the Italian Group for the Evaluation of Outcomes in Oncology (IGEO). *Quality of Life Research* 2000;9(2):151–9.
4. **Bruera E; Fainsinger R.** Clinical management of cachexia and anorexia In: Doyle D; Hanks GWC; MacDonald N., editors. *The Oxford Textbook of Palliative Medicine*, 2nd edn. Oxford: Oxford University Press, 1998: pp. 548–56.
5. **Scotia (Chairman, Fearon KCH).** A Double Blind, Placebo Controlled, Randomised, Parallel Group, Multicentre Phase II Dose Response Study of EPA 95% Diester Capsules in Patients with Cancer Cachexia. Stirling: Scotia.
6. **Bruera E; Neumann CM; Pituskin E; Calder K; Ball G; Hanson J.** Thalidomide in Patients with Cachexia due to Terminal Cancer: Preliminary report. *Annals of Oncology* 1999;10(7):857–9.
7. European Institute for Oncological and Immunological Research, Berlin, Germany (Chairmen, Schnelle M; Strasser F; Cerny T.). Double-blind, Placebo Controlled Parallel Study to Compare the Efficacy of a for THC Standardized Cannabis Sativa Extract and Delta-9-thc on Appetite and Weight in Cancer Patients. Berlin: European Institute for Oncological and Immunological Research.
8. CLB-9473, NCI-P97-0097 (Chairman, Burns P). Phase I/II Study of Omega-3 Fatty Acids in Advanced Cancer Patients with Cachexia.
9. NCCTG-959255, NCI-P96-0075 (Chairman, Loprinzi C.). Phase III Randomized, Double-Blind Study of Megestrol vs Dronabinol vs Both in Patients with Cancer-Related Anorexia and Cachexia.
10. **Loprinzi CL; Kugler JW; Sloan JA., *et al.*** Randomized comparison of megestrol acetate versus dexamethasone versus fluoxymesterone for the treatment of cancer anorexia/cachexia. *Journal of Clinical Oncology* 1999;17(10):3299–306.
11. NU-98CC6, NCI-G00-1705 (Chairman, Hayden Von Roenn J.). Phase II Study of Megestrol and Progressive Resistance Training in Patients with Cancer Related Weight Loss.
12. **Strasser F; Schnelle M; Kuechler T; Reif M; Cerny T.** How to Study Patients with Cancer Anorexia/cachexia Syndrome (CCS). 'Work in progress report' from a placebo-controlled phase

III trial with emphasis on the difficulties to define an adequate patient population and on the development of outcome measurement instruments. Berlin: 1st Congress of the Research Network of the Eurpoean Association for Palliative Care—EAPC Onlus, 7–9 December 2000. Abstract 145.

13. **O'Gorman P; Mcmillan DC; McArdle CS.** Longitudinal study of weight, appetite, performance status, and inflammation in advanced gastrointestinal cancer. *Nutrition and Cancer* 1999;35(2):127–9.
14. **Fordy C; Glover C; Henderson DC; Summerbell C; Wharton R; Allen-Mersh TG.** Contribution of diet, tumour volume and patient-related factors to weight loss in patients with colorectal liver metastases. *British Journal Surgery* 1999;86(5):639–44.
15. **MacDonald N; Alexander HR; Bruera E.** Cachexia–anorexia–asthenia. *Journal of Pain and Symptom Management* 1995;10(2):151–5.
16. **Bruera E; Beattie-Palmer L.** Pharmacologic management of nonpain symptoms in surgical patients. *Surgical Oncology Clinics of North America* 2001;10(1):89–107.
17. **Watanabe S; Bruera E.** Anorexia and cachexia, asthenia, and lethargy. *Hematology and Oncology Clinics of North America* 1996;10(1):189–206.
18. **Pereira J; Bruera E.** Chronic nausea. In: Bruera E; Higginson I. editors. *Cachexia–Anorexia in Cancer Patients.* Oxford: Oxford Medical Publications, Oxford University Press, 1996, pp. 23–37.
19. **Bruera E; Catz Z; Hooper R; Lentle B; MacDonald N.** Chronic nausea and anorexia in advanced cancer patients: a possible role for autonomic dysfunction. *Journal of Pain and Symptom Management* 1987;2(1):19–21.
20. **Hopwood P; Fletcher I; Lee A; Al Ghazal S.** A body image scale for use with cancer patients. *European Journal of Cancer* 2001;37(2):189–97.
21. **Bruera E; Carraro S; Roca E; Cedaro L; Chacon R.** Association between malnutrition and caloric intake, emesis, psychological depression, glucose taste, and tumor mass. *Cancer Treatment Reports* 1984;68(6):873–6.
22. **Persson C; Sjoden PO; Glimelius B.** The Swedish version of the patient-generated subjective global assessment of nutritional status: gastrointestinal vs urological cancers. *Clinical Nutrition* 1999;18(2):71–7.
23. **Strasser F.** Impact of fluid retention on evaluation of cancer cachexia (Abstract #33). *Supplement to Care in cancer* 2000;8(3):249.
24. **Bruera E; MacDonald RN.** Nutrition in cancer patients: an update and review of our experience. Issues in symptom control. Part 3. *Journal of Pain and Symptom Management* 1988;3(3):133–40.
25. **Tchekmedyian NS.** Costs and benefits of nutrition support in cancer. *Oncology* (Huntingt), 1995;9(Suppl. 11):79–84.
26. **Dewys WD; Begg C; Lavin PT., *et al.*** Prognostic effect of weight loss prior to chemotherapy in cancer patients. Eastern Cooperative Oncology Group. *American Journal of Medicine* 1980;69(4):491–7.
27. **Muller JM; Brenner U; Dienst C; Pichlmaier H.** Preoperative parenteral feeding in patients with gastrointestinal carcinoma. *The Lancet* 1982;1(8263):68–71.
28. **Andreyev HJ; Norman AR; Oates J; Cunningham D.** Why do patients with weight loss have a worse outcome when undergoing chemotherapy for gastrointestinal malignancies? *European Journal of Cancer* 1998;34(4):503–9.
29. **Terwee CB; Nieveen Van Dijkum EJ; Gouma DJ., *et al.*** Pooling of prognostic studies in cancer of the pancreatic head and periampullary region: the Triple-P study. Triple-P Study Group. *European Journal of Surgery* 2000;166(9):706–12.
30. **Portenoy RK; Thaler HT; Kornblith AB., *et al.*** Symptom prevalence, characteristics and distress in a cancer population. *Quality of Life Research* 1994;3(3):183–9.

31. **Reuben DB; Mor V; Hiris J.** Clinical symptoms and length of survival in patients with terminal cancer. *Archives of Internal Medicine* 1988;148(7):1586–91.
32. **Grosvenor M; Bulcavage L; Chlebowski RT.** Symptoms potentially influencing weight loss in a cancer population. Correlations with primary site, nutritional status, and chemotherapy administration. *Cancer* 1989;63(2):330–4.
33. **Brescia FJ; Adler D; Gray G; Ryan MA; Cimino J; Mamtani R.** Hospitalized advanced cancer patients: a profile. *Journal of Pain and Symptom Management* 1990;5(4):221–7.
34. **Ventafridda V; De Conno F; Ripamonti C; Gamba A; Tamburini M.** Quality-of-life assessment during a palliative care programme. *Annals of Oncology* 1990;1(6):415–20.
35. **Coyle N; Adelhardt J; Foley KM; Portenoy RK.** Character of terminal illness in the advanced cancer patient: pain and other symptoms during the last four weeks of life. *Journal of Pain and Symptom Management* 1990;5(2):83–93.
36. **Curtis EB; Krech R; Walsh TD.** Common symptoms in patients with advanced cancer. *Journal of Palliative Care* 1991;7(2):25–9.
37. **Rauch DP; Maurer CA; Aebi S., *et al.*** Activity of gemcitabine and continuous infusion fluorouracil in advanced pancreatic cancer. *Oncology* 2001;60(1):43–8.
38. **Hoffman K; Glimelius B.** Evaluation of clinical benefit of chemotherapy in patients with upper gastrointestinal cancer. *Acta Oncology* 1998;37(7–8):651–9.
39. **Ulrich-Pur H; Kornek GV; Raderer M., *et al.*** A phase II trial of biweekly high dose gemcitabine for patients with metastatic pancreatic adenocarcinoma. *Cancer* 2000;88(11):2505–11.
40. **Martin JL; Harvey HA; Lipton A; Martin R.** Combined chemoradiotherapy for unresectable pancreatic cancer. *American Journal of Clinical Oncology* 1999;22(3):309–14.
41. **Feliu J; Lopez Alvarez MP; Jaraiz MA., *et al.*** Phase II trial of gemcitabine and UFT modulated by leucovorin in patients with advanced pancreatic carcinoma. The ONCOPAZ Cooperative Group. *Cancer* 2000;89(8):1706–13.
42. **Burch PA; Block M; Schroeder G., *et al.*** Phase III evalution of octreotide versus chemotherapy with 5-fluorouracil or 5-fluorouracil plus leucovorin in advanced exocrine pancreatic cancer: a North Central Cancer Treatment Group study. *Clinical Cancer Research* 2000;6(9):3486–92.
43. **Cantore M; Pederzoli P; Cornalba G., *et al.*** Intra-arterial chemotherapy for unresectable pancreatic cancer. *Annals of Oncology* 2000;11(5):569–73.
44. **David AK; Vaughn DJ; Holroyde CP; Armstead B; Haller DG.** A phase II trial of 5-fluorouracil, leucovorin, and interferon alpha 2A (IFN-alpha 2a) in metastatic pancreatic carcinoma: a Penn Cancer Clinical Trials Group (PCCTG) trial. *American Journal of Clinical Oncology* 2000;23(1):37–9.
45. **Berlin JD; Adak S; Vaughn DJ., *et al.*** A phase II study of gemicitabine and 5-fluorouracil in metastatic pancreatic cancer: an Eastern Cooperative Oncology Group study (E3296). *Oncology* 2000;58(3):215–8.
46. **Burris H; Storniolo AM.** Assessing clinical benefit in the treatment of pancreas cancer: gemcitabine compared to 5-fluorouracil. *European Journal of Cancer* 1997;33(Suppl 1):S18–S22.
47. **Burris HA 3rd; Moore MJ; Andersen J., *et al.*** Improvements in survival and clinical benefit with gemcitabine as first-line therapy for patients with advanced pancreas cancer: a randomized trial. *Journal of Clinical Oncology* 1997;15(6):2403–13.
48. **Cascinu S; Silva RR; Barni S., *et al.*** A combination of gemcitabine and 5-fluorouracil in advanced pancreatic cancer, a report from the Italian Group for the Study of Digestive Tract Cancer (GISCAD). *British Journal of Cancer* 1999;80(10):1595–8.
49. **Vainio A; Auvinen A.** Prevalence of symptoms among patients with advanced cancer: an international collaborative study. Symptom Prevalence Group. *Journal of Pain and Symptom Management* 1996;12(1):3–10.

50. **Dunlop R.** Clinical epidemiology of cancer cachexia. In: Bruera E; Higginson I. editors. *Cachexia-anorexia in Cancer Patients.* Oxford: Oxford Medical Publications, Oxford University Press, 1996; pp. 76–82.
51. **Verweij J; Nooter K; Stoter G.** Principles of systemic therapy of cancer. In: Cavalli F; Hansen H; Kaye SB., editors. *Textbook of Medical Oncology.* 2nd edn. London: Martin Dunitz, 2000, pp. 67–98.
52. **Bruera E; Sweeney C.** Cachexia and asthenia in cancer patients. *The Lancet Oncology* 2000;1:138–147.
53. **Ingham J; Portenoy R.** Cachexia in context: the interactions among anorexia, pain and other symptoms. In: Bruera E; Higginson I. editors. *Cachexia–Anorexia in Cancer Patients.* Oxford: Oxford Medical Publications, Oxford University Press, 1996, pp.158–71.
54. **Gullo L; Migliori PT; Casadei R; Marrano D.** Do early symptoms of pancreatic cancer exist that can allow an earlier diagnosis? *Pancreas* 2001;22(2):210–13.
55. **Chiu TY; Hu WY; Chen CY.** Revalence and severity of symptoms in terminal cancer patients: a study in Taiwan. *Supportive Care in Cancer* 2000;(4):311–3.
56. **Bruera E; Neumann CM.** Pain control. In: Cavalli F; Hansen H; Kaye SB., editors. *Textbook of Medical Oncology,* 2nd edn. London: Martin Dunitz, 2000, pp. 597–618.
57. **Ripamonti C; Zecca E; Brunelli C; Groff L; Boffi R; Caraceni A; Galeazzi G; Martini C; Panzeri C; Saita L; Viggiano V; De Conno F.** Pain experienced by patients hospitalized at the National Cancer Institute of Milan: research project 'towards a pain-free hospital'. *Tumori* 2000;86(5):412–8.
58. **Zhukovsky DS; Gorowski E; Hausdorff J; Napolitano B; Lesser M.** Unmet analgesic needs in cancer patients. *Journal of Pain and Symptom Management* 1995;10(2):113–19.
59. **Walsh D; Donnelly S; Rybicki L.** The symptoms of advanced cancer: relationship to age, gender, and performance status in 1,000 patients. *Supportive Care in Cancer* 2000;8(3):175–9.
60. **Donnelly S; Walsh D; Rybicki L.** The symptoms of advanced cancer: identification of clinical and research priorities by assessment of prevalence and severity. *Journal of Palliative Care* 1995;11(1):27–32.
61. **Portenoy RK; Thaler HT; Kornblith AB., *et al.*** The Memorial Symptom Assessment Scale: an instrument for the evaluation of symptom prevalence, characteristics and distress. *European Journal of Cancer* 1994;30A(9):1326–36.
62. **Vigano A; Bruera E; Suarez-Almazor ME.** Terminal cancer syndrome: myth or reality? *Journal of Palliative Care* 1999;15(4):32–9.
63. **Komurcu S; Nelson KA; Walsh D.** The gastrointestinal symptoms of advanced cancer. *Supportive Care in Cancer* 2001;9(1):32–9.
64. **Cunningham D; Pyrhonen S; James RD; Punt CJ; Hickish TF; Heikkila R; Johannesen TB; Starkhammar H; Topham CA; Awad L; Jacques C; Herait P.** Randomised trial of irinotecan plus supportive care versus supportive care alone after fluorouracil failure for patients with metastatic colorectal cancer. *The Lancet* 1998;352(9138):1413–8.
65. The Elderly Lung Cancer Vinorelbine Italian Study Group. Effects of vinorelbine on quality of life and survival of elderly patients with advanced non-small-cell lung cancer. *Journal of the National Cancer Institute* 1999;91(1):66–72.
66. **Vigano A; Bruera E; Jhangri GS; Newman SC; Fields AL; Suarez-Almazor ME.** Clinical survival predictors in patients with advanced cancer. *Archives of Internal Medicine* 2000;160(6):861–8.
67. **Loprinzi CL; Laurie JA; Wieand HS., *et al.*** Prospective evaluation of prognostic variables from patient-completed questionnaires. North Central Cancer Treatment Group. *Journal of Clinical Oncology* 1994;12(3):601–7.
68. **Reuben DB; Mor V; Hiris J.** Clinical symptoms and length of survival in patients with terminal cancer. *Archives of Internal Medicine* 1988;148(7):1586–91.

69. **Llobera J; Esteva M; Rifa J; Benito E; Terrasa J; Rojas C., *et al.*** Terminal cancer. Duration and prediction of survival time. *European Journal of Cancer* 2000;36(16):2036–43.

70. **Hammerlid E; Wirblad B; Sandin C; Mercke C; Edstrom S; Kaasa S; Sullivan M.** Westin. Malnutrition and food intake in relation to quality of life in head and neck cancer patients. *Head and Neck* 1998;20(6):540–8.

71. **Higginson I; Winget C.** Psychological impact of cancer cachexia on the patient and family. In: Bruera E, Higginson I., editors. *Cachexia–Anorexia in Cancer Patients.* Oxford: Oxford Medical Publications, Oxford University Press, 1996;12:172–83.

72. **Holden CM.** Anorexia in the terminally ill cancer patient: the emotional impact on the patient and the family. *Hospital Journal* 1991;7(3):73–84.

73. **Vachon M.** Emotional problems in palliative medicine: patient, family and professional. In: Doyle D; Hanks GWC; MacDonald N., editors. *The Oxford Textbook of Palliative Medicine.* Oxford: Oxford University Press, 1993;10:577–605.

74. **Dixon CE; Emery AW; Hurley RS.** Nutrition in cancer patients with a limited life expectancy. *American Journal of Hospice Care* 1985;2(3):27–33.

75. **Hockley JM; Dunlop R; Davies RJ.** Survey of distressing symptoms in dying patients and their families in hospital and the response to a symptom control team. *British Medical Journal* (*Clinical Research* Edition) 1988;296(6638):1715–17.

76. **Bruera E; Macmillan K; Kuehn N; Hanson J; MacDonald RN.** A controlled trial of megestrol acetate on appetite, caloric intake, nutritional status, and other symptoms in patients with advanced cancer. *Cancer* 1990;66(6):1279–82.

77. **Bruera E; Legris MA; Kuehn N; Miller MJ.** Hypodermoclysis for the administration of fluids and narcotic analgesics in patients with advanced cancer. *Journal of Pain and Symptom Management* 1990;5(4):218–20.

78. **Bruera E; Higginson I; Preface.** In: Bruera E, Higginson I, editors. *Cachexia–Anorexia in Cancer Patients.* Oxford: Oxford Medical Publications, Oxford University Press, 1996; v–vi.

79. **Klein S; Kinney J; Jeejeebhoy K.; *et al.*** Nutrition support in clinical practice: review of published data and recommendations for future research directions. Summary of a conference sponsored by the National Institutes of Health, American Society for Parenteral and Enteral Nutrition, and American Society for Clinical Nutrition. *American Journal of Clinical Nutrition* 1997;66(3):683–706.

80. **Laviano A; Meguid MM.** Nutritional issues in cancer management. *Nutrition* 1996;12(5):358–71.

81. **Koretz RL.** Parental nutrition: is it oncologically logical? *Review Journal of Clinical Oncology* 1984;2(5):534–8.

82. **Barber MD; Fearon KC; Delmore G; Loprinzi CL.** Should cancer patients with incurable disease receive parenteral or enteral nutritional support? *European Journal of Cancer* 1998;34(3):279–85.

83. **Klein S; Koretz RL.** Nutrition support in patients with cancer: what do the data really show? *Nutrition in Clinical Practice* 1994;9(3):91–100.

84. **Evans WK; Nixon DW; Daly JM., *et al.*** A randomized study of oral nutritional support versus ad lib nutritional intake during chemotherapy for advanced colorectal and non-small-cell lung cancer. *Journal of Clinical Oncology* 1987;5(1):113–24.

85. **Seligman PA; Fink R; Massey-Seligman EJ.** Approach to the seriously ill or terminal cancer patient who has a poor appetite. *Seminars in Oncology* 1998; 25(2 Suppl. 6):33–4.

86. **Ovesen L; Allingstrup L; Hannibal J; Mortensen EL; Hansen OP.** Effect of dietary counseling on food intake, body weight, response rate, survival, and quality of life in cancer patients undergoing chemotherapy: a prospective, randomized study. *Journal of Chemical Oncology* 1993;11(10):2043–9.

87. **Winter SM.** Terminal nutrition: framing the debate for the withdrawal of nutritional support in terminally ill patients, Review. *American Journal of Medicine* 2000;109(9):723–6.
88. **Torelli GF; Campos AC; Meguid MM.** Use of TPN in terminally ill cancer patients. *Nutrition* 1999;15(9):665–7.
89. **Tchekmedyian NS; Zahyna D; Halpert C; Heber D.** Assessment and maintenance of nutrition in older cancer patients. Review. *Oncology (Hunting)* 1992;6(Suppl. 2):105–11.
90. **Bozzetti F; Amadori D; Bruera E., *et al.*** Guidelines on artificial nutrition versus hydration in terminal cancer patients. The European Association for Palliative Care. *Nutrition* 1996;12(3):163–7.
91. **Creutzberg EC; Schols AM; Weling-Scheepers CA; Buurman WA; Wouters EF.** Characterization of nonresponse to high caloric oral nutritional therapy in depleted patients with chronic obstructive pulmonary disease. *American Journal of Respiratory and Critical Care Medicine* 2000;161(3 Pt. 1):745–52.
92. **Theologides A; Ehlert J; Kennedy BJ.** The calorie intake of patients with advanced cancer. *Minnesota Medicine* 1976;59(8):526–9.
93. **Nelson KA; Walsh D; Sheehan FA.** The cancer anorexia–cachexia syndrome. *Journal of Clinical Oncology* 1994;12(1):213–25.
94. **Body JJ.** The syndrome of anorexia–cachexia. *Current Opinion in Oncology* 1999;11(4):255–60.
95. **Bruera E.** ABC of palliative care. Anorexia, cachexia, and nutrition. *British Medical Journal* 1997;315(7117):1219–22.
96. **Brennan MF.** Uncomplicated starvation versus cancer cachexia. *Cancer Research* 1977; 37(7 Pt. 2):2359–64.
97. **Fearon KC; Preston T.** Body composition in cancer cachexia. *Infusions therapie* 1990; 17(Suppl. 3):63–6.
98. **Heymsfield SB; McManus CB.** Tissue components of weight loss in cancer patients. A new method of study and preliminary observations. *Cancer* 1985;55(Suppl. 1):238–49.
99. **Tisdale MJ.** Wasting in cancer. *Journal of Nutrition* 1999;129(Suppl. 1S):243S–246S.
100. **Jaskowiak NT; Alexander HR.** The pathophysiology of cancer cachexia. In: Doyle D; Hanks GWC; MacDonald N., editors. *The Oxford Textbook of palliative Medicine*, 2nd edn. New York: Oxford University Press, 1998, pp. 534–48.
101. **Zylicz Z; Schwantje O; Wagener DJ; Folgering HT.** Metabolic response to enteral food in different phases of cancer cachexia in rats. *Oncology* 1990;47(1):87–91.
102. **Falconer JS; Fearon KC; Plester CE; Ross JA; Carter DC.** Cytokines, the acute-phase response, and resting energy expenditure in cachectic patients with pancreatic cancer. *Annals of Surgery* 1994;219(4):325–31.
103. **Tayek JA.** A review of cancer cachexia and abnormal glucose metabolism in humans with cancer. *Journal of the American College of Nutrition* 1992;11(4):445–56.
104. **Heber D; Chlebowski RT; Ishibashi DE; Herrold JN; Block JB.** Abnormalities in glucose and protein metabolism in noncachectic lung cancer patients. *Cancer Research,* 1982;42(11):4815–19.
105. **Shaw JH; Wolfe RR.** Glucose and urea kinetics in patients with early and advanced gastrointestinal cancer: the response to glucose infusion, parenteral feeding, and surgical resection. *Surgery* 1987;101(2):181–91.
106. **Vlassara H; Spiegel RJ; San Doval D; Cerami A.** Reduced plasma lipoprotein lipase activity in patients with malignancy-associated weight loss. *Hormone and Metabolic Research* 1986;18(10):698–703.
107. **Melville S; McNurlan MA; Calder AG; Garlick PJ.** Increased protein turnover despite normal energy metabolism and responses to feeding in patients with lung cancer. *Cancer Research* 1990;50(4):1125–31.

108. **Pisters PW; Pearlstone DB.** Protein and amino acid metabolism in cancer cachexia: investigative techniques and therapeutic interventions. *Critical Review in Clinical Laboratory Sciences* 1993;30(3):223–72.

109. **Baumann H; Gauldie J.** The acute phase response. Review. *Immunology Today* 1994;15(2):74–80.

110. **Attaix D; Combaret L; Tilignac T; Taillandier D.** Adaptation of the ubiquitin–proteasome proteolytic pathway in cancer cachexia. Review. *Molecular Biology Reports* 1999;26(1–2):77–82.

111. **Williams A; Sun X; Fischer JE; Hasselgren PO.** The expression of genes in the ubiquitin–proteasome proteolytic pathway is increased in skeletal muscle from patients with cancer. *Surgery* 1999;126(4):744–9.

112. **Guttridge DC; Mayo MW; Madrid LV; Wang CY; Baldwin AS Jr.** NF–kappaB-induced loss of MyoD messenger RNA: possible role in muscle decay and cachexia. *Science* 2000;289(5488):2363–6.

113. **Mitch WE; Price SR.** Transcription factors and muscle cachexia: is there a therapeutic target? *The Lancet* 2001;357(9258):734–5.

114. **Tisdale MJ.** Biomedicine. Protein loss in cancer cachexia. *Science* 2000;289(5488):2293–4.

115. **Bozzetti F; Gavazzi C; Ferrari P; Dworzak F.** Effect of total parenteral nutrition on the protein kinetics of patients with cancer cachexia. *Tumori* 2000;86(5):408–11.

116. **Barber MD; Fearon KC; McMillan DC; Slater C; Ross JA; Preston T.** Liver export protein synthetic rates are increased by oral meal feeding in weight-losing cancer patients. *American Journal of Physiology and Endocrinology Metabolism* 2000;279(3):E707–E714.

117. **Staal-van den Brekel AJ; Schols AM; Dentener MA; ten Velde GP; Buurman WA; Wouters EF.** The effects of treatment with chemotherapy on energy metabolism and inflammatory mediators in small-cell lung carcinoma. *British Journal of Cancer* 1997;76(12):1630–5.

118. **Torelli GF; Meguid MM; Moldawer LL., *et al.*** Use of recombinant human soluble TNF receptor in anorectic tumor-bearing rats. *American Journal of Physiology* 1999;277(3 Pt 2):R850–R855.

119. **Costelli P; Carbo N; Tessitore L., *et al.*** Tumor necrosis factor-alpha mediates changes in tissue protein turnover in a rat cancer cachexia model. *Journal of Clinical Investigation* 1993;92(6):2783–9.

120. **Socher SH; Martinez D; Craig JB; Kuhn JG; Oliff A.** Tumor necrosis factor not detectable in patients with clinical cancer cachexia. *Journal of the National Cancer Institute* 1988;80(8):595–8.

121. **Maltoni M; Fabbri L; Nanni O., *et al.*** Serum levels of tumour necrosis factor alpha and other cytokines do not correlate with weight loss and anorexia in cancer patients. *Supportive Care in Cancer* 1997;5(2):130–5.

122. **Thompson MP; Cooper ST; Parry BR; Tuckey JA.** Increased expression of the mRNA for hormone-sensitive lipase in adipose tissue of cancer patients. *Biochemical and Biophysical Acta* 1993;1180(3):236–42.

123. **Scuderi P; Sterling KE; Lam KS., *et al.*** Raised serum levels of tumour necrosis factor in parasitic infections. *The Lancet* 1986;2(8520):1364–5.

124. **Kaliman P; Canicio J; Testar X; Palacin M; Zorzano A.** Insulin-like growth factor-II, phosphatidylinositol 3-kinase, nuclear factor-kappaB and inducible nitric-oxide synthase define a common myogenic signaling pathway. *Journal of Biological Chemistry* 1999;274(25):17437–44.

125. **Cahlin C; Korner A; Axelsson H; Wang W; Lundholm K; Svanberg E.** Experimental cancer cachexia: the role of host-derived cytokines interleukin (IL)-6, IL-12, interferon-gamma, and tumor necrosis factor alpha evaluated in gene knockout, tumor-bearing mice on C57 Bl background and eicosanoid-dependent cachexia. *Cancer Research* 2000;60(19):5488–93.

126. **Fujita J; Tsujinaka T; Yano M., *et al.*** Anti-interleukin-6 receptor antibody prevents muscle atrophy in colon-26 adenocarcinoma-bearing mice with modulation of lysosomal and ATP-ubiquitin-dependent proteolytic pathways. *International Journal of Cancer* 1996;68(5):637–43.

127. **Strassmann G; Fong M; Kenney JS; Jacob CO.** Evidence for the involvement of interleukin 6 in experimental cancer cachexia. *Journal of Clinical Investigation* 1992;89(5):1681–4.

128. **Espat NJ; Auffenberg T; Rosenberg JJ., *et al.*** Ciliary neurotrophic factor is catabolic and shares with IL-6 the capacity to induce an acute phase response. *American Journal of Physiology* 1996;271(1 Pt 2):R185–R190.

129. **Yasumoto K; Mukaida N; Harada A., *et al.*** Molecular analysis of the cytokine network involved in cachexia in colon 26 adenocarcinoma-bearing mice. *Cancer Research* 1995;55(4):921–7.

130. **Scott HR; McMillan DC; Crilly A; McArdle CS; Milroy R., *et al.*** The relationship between weight loss and interleukin 6 in non-small-cell lung cancer. *British Journal of Cancer* 1996;73(12):1560–2.

131. **Matthys P; Dijkmans R; Proost P., *et al.*** Severe cachexia in mice inoculated with interferon-gamma-producing tumor cells. *International Journal of Cancer* 1991;49(1):77–82.

132. **Costelli P; Llovera M; Lopez-Soriano J., *et al.*** Lack of effect of eicosapentaenoic acid in preventing cancer cachexia and inhibiting tumor growth. *Cancer Letters* 1995;97(1):25–32.

133. **Khan S; Tisdale MJ.** Catabolism of adipose tissue by a tumour-produced lipid-mobillsing factor. *International Journal of Cancer* 1999;80(3):444–7.

134. **Hussey HJ; Tisdale MJ.** Effect of a cachectic factor on carbohydrate metabolism and attenuation by eicosapentaenoic acid. *British Journal of Cancer* 1999;80(8):1231–5.

135. **Tisdale MJ.** Biology of cachexia. *Journal of the National Cancer Institute* 1997;89(23):1763–73.

136. **Tisdale MJ.** Metabolic abnormalities in cachexia and anorexia. Review. *Nutrition* 2000;16(10):1013–4.

137. **Smith KL; Tisdale MJ.** Mechanism of muscle protein degradation in cancer cachexia. *British Journal of Cancer* 1993;68(2):314–8.

138. **Smith KL; Tisdale MJ.** Increased protein degradation and decreased protein synthesis in skeletal muscle during cancer cachexia. *British Journal of Cancer* 1993;67(4):680–5.

139. **Belizario JE; Katz M; Chenker E; Raw I.** Bioactivity of skeletal muscle proteolysis-inducing factors in the plasma proteins from cancer patients with weight loss. *British Journal of Cancer* 1991;63(5):705–10.

140. **Todorov P; Cariuk P; McDevitt T; Coles B; Eearon K; Tisdale M.** Characterization of a cancer cachectic factor. *Nature* 1996;379(6567):739–42.

141. **Todorov PT; Deacon M; Tisdale MJ.** Structural analysis of a tumor-produced sulfated glycoprotein capable of initiating muscle protein degradation. *Journal of Biological Chemistry* 1997;272(19):12279–88.

142. **Cariuk P; Lorite MJ; Todorov PT; Field WN; Wigmore SJ; Tisdale MJ.** Induction of cachexia in mice by a product isolated from the urine of cachectic cancer patients. *British Journal of Cancer* 1997;6(5):606–13.

143. **Lorite MJ; Thompson MG; Drake JL; Carling G; Tisdale MJ.** Mechanism of muscle protein degradation induced by a cancer cachectic factor. *British Journal of Cancer* 1998;78(7):850–5.

144. **Lorite MJ; Cariuk P; Tisdale MJ.** Induction of muscle protein degradation by a tumour factor. *British Journal of Cancer* 1997;76(8):1035–40.

145. **Smith HJ; Lorite MJ; Tisdale MJ.** Effect of a cancer cachectic factor on protein synthesis/degradation in murine C2C12 myoblasts: modulation by eicosapentaenoic acid. *Cancer Research* 1999;59(21):5507–13.

146. **De Blaauw I; Heeneman S; Deutz NE; von Meyenfeldt MF.** Increased whole-body protein and glutamine turnover in advanced cancer is not matched by an increased muscle protein and glutamine turnover. *Journal of Surgical Research* 1997;68(1):44–55.

147. **Wigmore SJ; Todorov PT; Barber MD; Ross JA; Tisdale MJ; Fearon KC.** Characteristics of patients with pancreatic cancer expressing a novel cancer cachectic factor. *British Journal of Surgery* 2000;87(1):53–8.

148. **Rodemann HP; Goldberg Al.** Arachidonic acid, prostaglandin E2 and F2 alpha influence rates of protein turnover in skeletal and cardiac muscle. *Journal of Biological Chemistry* 1982;257(4):1632–8.

149. **Hasselgren PO; Zamir O; James JH; Fischer JE.** Prostaglandin E2 does not regulate total or myofibrillar protein breakdown in incubated skeletal muscle from normal or septic rats. *Biochemical Journal* 1990;270(1):45–50.

150. **Barrett R; Hyde SA; Scott OM; Dubowitz V.** Changes in center of gravity in boys with Duchenne muscular dystrophy. *Muscle and Nerve* 1988;11(11):1157–63.

151. **Goll DE; Thompson VF; Taylor RG; Christiansen JA.** Role of the calpain system in muscle growth. Review. *Biochimie* 1992;74(3):225–37.

152. **Baracos VE; DeVivo C; Hoyle DH; Goldberg AL.** Activation of the ATP-ubiquitinproteasome pathway in skeletal muscle of cachectic rats bearing a hepatoma. *American Journal of Physiology* 1995;268(5 Pt 1):E996–1006.

153. **Temparis S; Asensi M; Taillandier D., *et al.*** Increased ATP-ubiquitin-dependent proteolysis in skeletal muscles of tumor-bearing rats. *Cancer Research* 1994;54(21):5568–73.

154. **Kitada S; Hays EF; Mead JF.** A lipid mobilizing factor in serum of tumor-bearing mice. *Lipids* 1980;15(3):168–74.

155. **Masuno H; Yamasaki N; Okuda H.** Purification and characterization of a lipolytic factor (toxohormone-L) from cell-free fluid of ascites sarcoma 180. *Cancer Research* 1981;41(1):284–8.

156. **Beck SA; Tisdale MJ.** Production of lipolytic and proteolytic factors by a murine tumor-producing cachexia in the host. *Cancer Research* 1987;47(22):5919–23.

157. **Groundwater P; Beck SA; Barton C; Adamson C; Ferrier IN; Tisdale MJ.** Alteration of serum and urinary lipolytic activity with weight loss in cachectic cancer patients. *British Journal of Cancer* 1990;62(5):816–21.

158. **Beck SA; Groundwater P; Barton C; Tisdale MJ.** Alterations in serum lipolytic activity of cancer patients with response to therapy. *British Journal of Cancer* 1990;62(5):822–5.

159. **Bessey PQ; Watters JM; Aoki TT; Wilmore DW.** Combined hormonal infusion simulates the metabolic response to injury. *Annals of Surgery* 1984;200(3):264–81.

160. **Watters JM; Bessey PQ; Dinarello CA; Wolff SM; Wilmore DW.** Both inflammatory and endocrine mediators stimulate host responses to sepsis. *Archives of Surgery* 1986;121(2):179–90.

161. **Schaur RJ; Fellier H; Gleispach H; Fink E; Kronberger L.** Tumor host relations. I. Increased plasma cortisol in tumor-bearing humans compared with patients with benign surgical diseases. *Journal of Cancer Research and Clinical Oncology* 1979;93(3):281–5.

162. **Schaur RJ; Semmelrock HJ; Schauenstein E; Kronberger L.** Tumor host relations. II. Influence of tumor extent and tumor site on plasma cortisol of patients with malignant diseases. *Journal of Cancer Research and Clinical Oncology* 1979;93(3):287–92.

163. **Burt ME; Aoki TT; Gorschboth CM; Brennan MF.** Peripheral tissue metabolism in cancer-bearing man. *Annals of Surgery* 1983;198(6):685–91.

164. **Knapp ML; al-Sheibani S; Riches PG; Hanham IW; Phillips RH.** Hormonal factors associated with weight loss in patients with advanced breast cancer. *Annals of Clinical Biochemistry* 1991;28(Pt 5):480–6.

165. **Holroyde CP; Skutches CL; Boden G; Reichard GA.** Glucose metabolism in cachectic patients with colorectal cancer. *Cancer Research* 1984;44(12 Pt 1):5910–3.

166. **Llovera M; Garcia-Martinez C; Costelli P., *et al.*** Muscle hypercatabolism during cancer cachexia is not reversed by the glucocorticoid receptor antagaonist RU38486. *Cancer Letters* 1996;99(1):7–14.
167. **Cangiano C; Testa U; Muscaritoli M., *et al.*** Cytokines, tryptophan and anorexia in cancer patients before and after surgical tumor ablation. *Anticancer Research* 1994;14(3B):1451–5.
168. **Chance WT; Balasubramaniam A; Thompson H; Mohapatra B; Ramo J; Fischer JE.** Assessment of feeding response of tumor-bearing rats to hypothalamic injection and infusion of neuropeptide Y. *Peptides* 1996;17(5):797–801.
169. **Grunfeld C; Zhao C; Fuller J; Pollack A; Moser A; Friedman J; Feingold KR.** Endotoxin and cytokines induce expression of leptin, the ob gene product, in hamsters. *Journal of Clinical Investigation* 1996;97(9):2152–7.
170. **Sarraf P; Frederich RC; Turner EM., *et al.*** Multiple cytokines and acute inflammation raise mouse leptin levels: potential role in inflammatory anorexia. *Journal of Experimental Medicine* 1997;185(1):171–5.
171. **Simons JP; Schols AM; Campfield LA; Wouters EF; Saris WH.** Plasma concentration of total leptin and human lung-cancer-associated cachexia. *Clinical Science* (Colch) 1997;93(3):273–7.
172. **Di Marzo V; Goparaju SK; Wang L., *et al.*** Leptin-regulated endocannabinoids are involved in maintaining food intake. *Nature* 2001;410(6830):822–5.
173. **Low PA.** Autonomic neuropathies. *Current Opinion in Neurology* 1998;11(5):531–7.
174. **Lennon VA; Sas DF; Busk MF; Scheithauer B; Malagelada JR; Camilleri M; Miller LJ.** Enteric neuronal autoantibodies in pseudoobstruction with small-cell lung carcinoma. *Gastroenterology* 1991;100(1):137–42.
175. **Khawaja KI; Walker D; Hayat SA; Boulton AJ; Malik RA.** Clinico-pathological features of postural hypotension in diabetic autonomic neuropathy. *Diabetic Medicine* 2000;17(2):163–6.
176. **Bruera E; Chadwick S; Fox R; Hanson J; MacDonald N.** Study of cardiovascular autonomic insufficiency in advanced cancer patients. *Cancer Treatment Reports* 1986;70(12):1383–7.
177. **Rowe PC; Bou-Holaigah I; Kan JS; Calkinds H.** Is neurally mediated hypotension an unrecognised cause of chronic fatigue? *The Lancet* 1995;345(8950):623–4.
178. **Bruera E; Brenneis C; Michaud M., *et al.*** Association between asthenia and nutritional status, lean body mass anemia, psychological status, and tumor mass in patients with advanced breast cancer. *Journal of Pain and Symptom Management* 1989;4(2):59–63.
179. **Glaus A.** Fatigue and cachexia in cancer patients. *Support and Care for Cancer* 1998;6(2):77–8.
180. **Portenoy RK; Itri LM.** Cancer-related fatigue: guidelines for evaluation and management. *Oncologist* 1999;4(1):1–10.
181. **Meek PM; Nail LM; Barsevick A; Schewartz AL; Stephen S; Whitmer K; Beck SL; Jones LS; Walker BL.** Psychometric testing of fatigue instruments for use with cancer patients. *Nursing Research* 2000;49(4):181–90.
182. **Neuenschwander H. Bruera E.** Asthenia-cachexia. In: Bruera E; Higginson I., editors. *Cachexia-anorexia in Cancer Patients.* Oxford: Oxford Medical Publications, Oxford University Press, 1996, pp. 57–75.
183. **Theologides A.** Asthenia in cancer. *American Journal of Medicine* 1982;73:1–3.
184. **Meyers CA.** Neurocognitive dysfunction in cancer patients. *Oncology* (Huntingt) 2000;14(1):75–9.
185. **Swain MG.** Fatigue in chronic disease. *Clinical Science* (London) 2000;99(1):1–8.
186. **Patarca-Montero R; Antoni M; Fletcher MA; Klimas NG.** Cytokine and other immunologic markers in chronic fatigue syndrome and their relation to neuropsychological factors. *Applied Neuropsychology* 2001;8(1):51–64.

187. **Mendoza TR; Wang XS; Cleeland CS., *et al.*** The rapid assessment of fatigue severity in cancer patients: use of the Brief Fatigue Inventory. *Cancer* 1999;85(5):1186–96.

188. **Natelson BH.** Chronic fatigue syndrome, *Journal of the American Medical Association* 2001;285(20):2557–9.

189. **Daly E; Komaroff AL; Bloomingdale K; Wilson S; Albert MS.** Neuropsychological function in patients with chronic fatigue syndrome, multiple sclerosis, and depression. *Applied Neuropsychology* 2001;8(1):12–22.

190. **Mehler PS.** Diagnosis and care of patients with anorexia nervosa in primary care settings *Annals of Internal Medicine* 2001;134(11):1048–59.

191. **Lewinsonhn PM; Striegel-Moore RH; Seeley JR.** Epidemiology and natural course of eating disorders in young women from adolescence to young adulthood. *Journal of the American Academy of Child and Adolescent Psychiatry* 2001;39(10):1284–92.

192. **Cleeland C; Wang XS.** Measuring and understanding fatigue. NCCN Proceedings. *Oncology* 1999;13(11A):91–97.

193. **Hansen HH; Pappot H.** Primary malignant tumours of the lung and pleura. In Cavallu F; Hansen H; Kaye SB., editors. *Textbook of Medical Oncology* 2nd edn. London: Martin Dunitz 2000: pp. 253–5.

194. **Coiffier B.** Non-Hodgkin's lymphoma. In: Cavalli F; Hasen H; Kaye SB., editor. *Textbook of Medical Oncology*, 2nd edn. London: Martin Dunitz 2000: p. 422.

195. **Wessely S.** Chronic fatigue: symptom and syndrome. *Annals of Internal Medicine* 2001;134(9 Pt 2):838–43.

196. **Derogatis LR; Morrow GR; Fetting J; Penman D; Piasetsky S; Schmale AM; Henrichs M; Carnicke CL Jr.** The prevalence of psychiatric disorders among cancer patients. *Journal of the American Academy of Child and Adolescent Psychiatry* 1983;249(6):751–7.

197. **Hayes JR.** Depression and chronic fatigue in cancer patients. *Primary Care* 1991;18(2):327–39.

198. **Wilson KG; Chochinov HM; De Faye BJ; Breitbart W.** Diagnosis and management of depression in palliative care. In: Chochinov HM; Breitbart W., editors. *Handbook of Psychiatry in Palliative Medicine* New York: Oxford 2000: pp. 25–49.

199. **Gabrilove JL; Cleeland CS; Livingston RB; Sarokhan B; Winer E; Einhorn LH.** Clinical evaluation of once-weekly dosing of epoetin alfa in chemotherapy patients: improvements in hemoglobin and quality of life are similar to three-times-weekly dosing. *Journal of Clinical Oncology* 2001;19(11):2875–82.

200. **Glaspy J; Bukowski R; Steinberg D; Taylor C; Tchekmedyian S; Vadhan-Raj S.** Impact of therapy with epoetin alfa on clinical outcomes in patients with nonmyeloid malignancies during cancer chemotherapy in community oncology practice. Procrit Study Group. *Journal of Clinical Oncology* 1997;15(3):1218–34.

201. **Demetri GD; Kris M; Wade J; Degos L; Cella D.** Quality-of-life benefit in chemotherapy patients treated with epoetin alfa is independent of disease response or tumor type: results from a prospective community oncology study. Procrit Study Group. *Journal of Clinical Oncology* 1998;16(10):3412–25.

202. **Leitgeb C; Pecherstorfer M; Fritz; Ludwig H.** Quality of life in chronic anemia of cancer during treatment with recombinant human erythropoietin. *Cancer* 1994;73(10):2535–42.

203. **Ludwig H; Sundal E; Pecherstorfer M; Leitgeb C; Bauernhofer T; Beinhauer A; Samonigg H; Kappeler AW; Fritz E.** Recombinant human erythropoietin for the correction of cancer associa-ted anemia with and without concomitant cytotoxic chemotherapy. *Cancer* 1995;76(11):2319–29.

204. **Littlewood TJ; Bajetta E; Nortier JW; Vercammen E; Rapoport B.** Effects of epoetin alfa on hematologic parameters and quality of life in cancer patients receiving nonplatinum

chemotherapy: results of a randomized, double-blind, placebo-controlled trial. *Journal of Clinical Oncology* 2001;19(11):2865–74.

205. **Christensen T; Stage JG; Galbo H; Christensen NJ; Kehlet H.** Fatigue and cardiac and endocrine metabolic response to exercise after abdominal surgery. *Surgery* 1989;105(1):46–50.
206. **Zeiderman MR; Welchew EA: Clark RG.** Changes in cardiorespiratory and muscle function associated with the development of postoperative fatigue. *British Journal of Surgery* 1990;77(5):576–80.
207. **Dimeo F; Bertz H; Finke J; Fetscher S; Mertelsmann R; Keul J.** An aerobic exercise program for patients with haematological malignancies after bone marrow transplantation. *Bone Marrow Transplant* 1996;18(6):1157–60.
208. **Dimeo F; Fetscher S; Lange W; Mertelsmann R; Keul J.** Effects of aerobic exercise on the physical performance and incidence of treatment-related complications after high-dose chemotherapy. *Blood* 1997;90(9):3390–4.
209. **Dimeo FC; Tilmann MH; Bertz H; Kanz L; Mertelsmann R; Keul J.** Aerobic exercise in the rehabilitation of cancer patients after high dose chemotherapy and autologous peripheral stem cell transplantation. *Cancer* 1997;79(9):1717–22.
210. **Dimeo FC; Stieglitz RD; Novelli-Fischer U; Fetscher S; Keul J.** Effects of physical activity on the fatigue and psychologic status of cancer patients during chemotherapy. *Cancer* 1999;85(10):2273–7.
211. **Dimeo F.** Exercise as therapy for cancer fatigue: when should rehabilitation start? Cancer-Related Fatigue, 2001: March 24–25. Conference Houston: MD Anderson Cancer Center.
212. **Verweij J; Nooter K; Stoter G.** Principles of systemic therapy of cancer. In: Cavalli F; Hansen H; Kaye SB., editors. *Textbook of Medical Oncology*, 2nd edn. London: MartinDunitz Ltd., 2000, pp. 67–98.
213. Effects of vinorelbine on quality of life and survival of elderly patients with advanced non-small-cell lung cancer. The Elderly Lung Cancer Vinorelbine Italian Study Group. *Jounal of the National Cancer Institute* 1999;91(1):66–72.
214. **Cunningham D; Pyrhonen S; James RD., *et al.*** Randomised trial of irinotecan plus supportive care vesus supportive care alone after fluororacil failure for patients with metastatic colorectal cancer. *The Lancet* 1998;352(9138):1413–8.
215. **Turner JA; Deyo RA; Loeser JD; Von Korff M; Fordyce WE.** The importance of placebo effects in pain treatment and research. Review. *Journal of the American Academy of Child and Adolescent Psychiathy* 1994;271(20):1609–14.
216. **Pearce JM.** The placebo enigma. Review. *Quarterly Journal of Medicine* 1995;88(3):215–20.
217. **Korn EL; Arbuck SG; Pluda JM; Simon R; Kaplan RS; Christian MC.** Clinical trial designs for cytostatic agents: are new approaches needed? *Journal of Clinical Oncology* 2001;19(1):264–72.
218. **Mastaglia FL.** Adverse effects of drugs on muscle. *Drugs* 1982;24(4):304–21.
219. **Zuckner J.** Drug-related myopathies. *Rheumatic Disease Clinics of North America* 1994;20(4):1017–32.
220. **Cleare AJ; Heap E; Malhi GS; Wessely S; O'keane V; Miell J.** Low-dose hydrocortisone in chronic fatigue syndrome: a randomised crossover trial. *The Lancet* 1999;353(9151):455–8.
221. **Mckenzie R; O'Fallon A; Dale J; Demitrack M; Sharma G; Deloria M; Garcia-Borreguero D; Blackwelder W; Straus SE.** Low-dose hydrocortisone for treatment of chronic fatigue syndrome: a randomized controlled trial. *Journal of the American Academy of Child and Adolescent Psychiatry* 1998;280(12):1061–6.
222. **Grinspoon S; Corcoran C; Lee K., *et al.*** Loss of lean body and muscle mass correlates with androgen levels in hypogonadal men with acquired immunodeficiency syndrome and wasting. *Journal of Clinical Endocrinology and Metabolism* 1996;81(11):4051–8.

223. **Grinspoon S; Corcoran C; Miller K., *et al.*** Body composition and endocrine function in women with acquired immunodeficiency syndrome wasting *Journal of Clinical Endocrinology and Metabolism* 1997;82(5):1332–7.

224. **Morley JE.** The endocrinology of the opiates and opioid peptides. Review. *Metabolism* 1981;30(2):195–209.

225. **Abs R; Verhelst J; Maeyaert J., *et al.*** Endocrine consequences of long-term intrathecal administration of opiods. *Journal of Clinical Endocrinology and Metabolism* 2000;85(6):2215–22.

226. **Isgaard J; Bergh CH; Caidahl K; Lomsky M; Hjalmarson A; Bengtsson BA.** A Placebo-controlled study of growth hormone in patients with congestive heart failure. *European Heart Journal* 1998;19(11):1704–11.

227. **Osterziel KJ; Strohm O; Schuler J., *et al.*** Randomised, double-blind, placebo-controlled trial of human recombinant growth hormone in patients with chronic heart failure due to dilated cardiomyopathy. *The Lancet* 1998;351(9111):1233–7.

228. **Papadakis MA; Grady D; Black D., *et al.*** Growth hormone replacement in healthy older men improves body composition but not functional ability. *Annals of Internal Medicine* 1996;24(8):708–16.

229. **Burdet L;de Muralt B; Schutz Y; Pichard C; Fitting JW.** Administration of growth hormone to underweight patients with chronic obstructive pulmonary disease. A propective, randomized, controlled study. *American Journal Respiratory and Critical Care Medicine* 1997;156(6):1800–6.

230. **Schambelan M;Mulligan K: Grunfeld C., *et al.*** Recombinant human growth hormone in patients with HIV-associated wasting. A randomized, placebo-controlled trial. Serostim Study Group. *Annals of Internal Medicine* 1996;25(11):873–82.

231. **Strawford A; Barbieri T; Neese R., *et al.*** Effects of nandrolone decanoate therapy in bordeline hypogonadal men with HIV-associated weight loss. *Journal of Acquired Immune Deficiency Syndrome and Human Retrovirology* 1999;20(2):137–46.

232. **Johansen KL; Mulligan K; Schambelan M.** Anabolic effects of nandrolone decanoate in patients receiving dialysis: a randomized controlled trial. *Journal of the American Academy of Child and Adolescent Psychiatry* 1999;281(14):1275–81.

233. **Ferreira IM; Verreschi IT; Nery LE., *et al.*** The influence of 6 months of oral anabolic steroids on body mass and respiratory muscles in undernourished COPD patients. *Chest* 1998;114(1):19–28.

234. **Miller K; Corcoran C; Armstrong C., *et al.*** Transdermal testosterone administration in women with acquired immunodeficiency syndrome wasting: a pilot study. *Journal of Clinical Endocrinology and Metabolism* 1998;83(8):2717–25.

235. **Bhasin S; Storer TW; Javanbakht M., *et al.*** Testosterone replacement and resistance exercise in HIV-infected men with weight loss and low testosterone levels. *Journal of the American Academy of Child and Adolescent Psychiatry* 2000;283(6):763–70.

236. **Bhasin S; Storer TW; Asbel-Sethi N., *et al.*** Effects of testosterone replacement with a nongenital, transdermal system, Androderm, in human immunodeficiency virus-infected men with low testosterone levels. *Journal of Clinical Endocrinology and Metabolism* 1998;83(9):3155–62.

237. **DeWys WD; Walters K.** Abnormalities of taste sensation in cancer patients. *Cancer* 1975;36(5):1888–96.

238. **Davies IJ; Musa M; Dormandy TL.** Measurements of plasma zinc. II. In malignant disease. *Journal of Clinical Pathology* 1968;21(3):363–5.

239. **Mancini I; Bruera E.** Constipation in advanced cancer patients. *Supportive Care in Cancer* 1998;6(4):356–64.

240. **Rosomoff HL.** Another cause of cachexia. *Journal of Pain and Symptom Management* 1989;4(2):57.

241. **Cherel Y:Robin JP; Heitz A; Calgari C; Le Maho Y.** Relationships between lipid availability and protein utilization during prolonged fasting. *Journal of Comparative Physiology* [B] 1992;62(4):305–13.

242. **Kotler DP; Tierney AR; Wang J; Pierson RN Jr.** Magnitude of body-cell-mass depletion and the timing of death from wasting in AIDS. *American Journal of Clinical Nutrition* 1989;50(3):444–7.

243. **Jeejeebhoy KN;detsky AS; Basker JP.** Assessment of nutritional status. *Journal of Parenteral and Enteral Nutrition* 1990;Suppl. 5:193S–196S.

244. **Baker JP; Detsky AS; Wesson DE., *et al.*** Nutritional assessment: a comparison of clinical judgement and objective measurements. *New England Journal of Medicine* 1982;306(16):969–72.

245. **Dearman K; Replogle WH; Cora VL; Meeks M; Canada T.** Use of subjective global assessment to identify nutrition-associated complications and death in geriatric long-term care facility residents. *Journal of the American College of Nutrition* 2000;19(5):570–7.

246. **Lawson JA; Lazarus R; Kelly JJ.** Prevalence and prognostic significance of malnutrition in chronic renal insufficiency. *Journal of Renal Nutrition* 2001;11(1):16–22.

247. **Niyongabo T; Melchior JC; Henzel D; Bouchaud O; Larouze B.** Comparison of methods for assessing nutritional status in HIV-infected adults. *Nutrition* 1999;15(10):740–3.

248. **Figueiredo F; Dickson ER; Pasha T., *et al.*** Impact of nutritional status on outcomes after liver transplantation. *Transplantation* 2000;70(9):1347–52.

249. **Durnin JV; Womersley J.** Body fat assessed from total body density and its estimation from skinfold thickness: measurements on 481 men and women aged from 16 to 72 years. *British Journal of Nutrition* 1974;32(1):77–97.

250. **Conslisk EA; Haas JD; Martinez EJ; Flores R; Rivera JD; Martorell R.** Predicting body composition from anthropometry and bioimpedance in marginally undernourished adolescents and young adults. *American Journal of Clinical Nutrition* 1992;55(6):1051–60.

251. **Simons JP; Schools AM; Westerterp KR; ten Velde GP; Wouters EF.** The use of bioelectrical impedance analysis to predict total body water in patients with cancer cachexia. *American Journal of Clinical Nutrition* 1995;61(4):741–5.

252. **Presta E; Wang J; Harrison GG; Bjorntorp P; Harker WH; Van Itallie TB.** Measurement of total body electrical conductivity: a new method for estimation of body composition. *American Journal of Clinical Nutrition* 1983;37(5):735–9.

253. **Sarhill N; Walsh D; Nelson K; Homsi J; Komurcu S.** Bioelectrical impedance, cancer nutritional assessment, and ascites. *Supportive Care in Cancer* 2000;8(4):341–3.

254. **Loprinzi CL; Schaid DJ; Dose AM; Burnham NL.; Jensen MD.** Body-composition changes in partients who gain weight while receiving megestrol acetate. *Journal of Clinical Oncology* 1993;11(1):152-4.

255. **Mazess RB; Barden HS; Bisek JP.; Hanson J.** Dual-energy x-ray absorptiometry for total-body and regional bone-mineral and soft-tissue composition. *American Journal of Clinical Nutrition* 1990;51(6):1106–12.

256. **Roubenoff R; Kehayias JJ; Dawson-Hughes B; Heymsfield SB.** Use of dual-energy X-ray absorptiomentry in body-composition studies: not yet a 'golds standard'. Review. *American Jouran of Clinical Nutrition* 1993;58(5):589–91.

257. **Pichard C; Kyle UG.** Body composition measurements during wasting diseases. Review. *Current opinion in Clinical Nutrition and Metabolic Care* 1998;1(4):357–61.

258. **Windsor JA; Hill GL.** Grip Strength: a measure of the proportion of protein loss in surgical patients. *British Journal of Surgery* 1988;75(9):880–2.

259. **Hunt DR; Rowlands BJ; Johnston D.** Hand grip strength—a simple prognostic indicator in surgical patients. *Journal of Parenteral and Enteral Nutrition* 1985;9(6):701–4.

260. **Klidjian AM; Foster KJ; Kammerling RM; Cooper A; Karran SJ.** Relation of anthropometric and dynamometric variables to serious postoperative complications. *British Medical Journal* 1980;281(6245):899–901.

261. **Ageteresch HJ; Dagnelie PC; van der Gaast A; Stijnen T; Wilson JH.** Randomized clinical trial of adenosine 5'-triphosphate in patients with advanced non-small-cell lung cancer. *Journal of National Cancer Institute* 2000;92(4):321–8.

262. **Jatoi A; Loprinzi CL; Sloan J; Goldberg RM.** Is ATP (adenosine 5′-triphosphate), like STP, a performance-enhancing additive for the tanks of cancer patients? *Journal of the National Cancer Institute* 2000;92(4):290–1.

263. **Kaasa T; Wessel J; Darrah J; Bruera E.** Inter-rater reliability of formally trained and self-trained raters using the Edmonton Functional Assessment Tool. *Palliative Medicine* 2000;14(6):509–17.

264. **Bruera E; Kuehn N; Miller MJ; Selmser P; Macmillan K.** The Edmonton Symptom Assessment System (ESAS): a simple method for the assessment of palliative care patients. *Journal of Palliative Care* 1991;7(2):6–9.

265. **Aaronson NK; Ahmedzai S; Bergman B; Bullinger M; Cull A; Duez NJ; Filiberti A; Flechtner H; Fleishman SB; de Haes JC., *et al.*** The European Organization for Research and Treatment of Cancer QLQ-C30: a quality-of-life instrument for use in international clinical trials in oncology. *Journal of the National Cancer Institute* 1993;85(5):365–76.

266. **Schipper H; Clinch J; McMurray A; Levitt M.** Measuring the quality of life of cancer patients: The Functional Living Index-Cancer: development and validation. *Journal of Clinical Oncology* 1984;2(5):472–83.

267. **Chang VT; Hwang SS; Hulsen I; Alejandro Y; Handkinson MT; Kasimis B.** Functional Assessement of Appetite Cachexia Therapy (FAACT) in Patients with Advanced Cancer. 2000.

268. **Yellen SB; Cella DF; Webster K; Blendowski C; Kaplan E.** Measuring fatigue and other anemia-related symptoms with the Functional Assessment of Cancer Therapy (FACT) meaurement system. *Journal of Pain and Symptom Management* 1997;13(2):63–74.

269. **Piper BF; Lindsey AM; Dodd MJ; Ferketich S; Paul SM; Weller S.** The development of an instrument to measure the subjective domain of fatigue. In: Funk S; Tornquist E; Champagne M; Archer CL; Wiese R., editors. *Key aspects of Comfort: Management of Pain, Fatigue and Nauses.* New York: Springer, 1989: pp. 199–208.

270. **Schneider RA.** Reliability and validity of the Multidimensional Fatigue Inventory (MFI-20) and the Rhoten Fatigue Scale among rural cancer outpatients. *Cancer Nursing* 1998;21(5):370–3.

271. **Smets EM; Garssen B; Bonke B; De Haes JC.** The Multidimensional Fatigue Inventory (MFI) psychometric qualities of an instrument to assess fatigue. *Journal of Psychosomatic Research* 1995;39(3):315–25.

272. **Stein KD; Martin SC; Hann DM; Jacobsen PB.** A multidimensional measure of fatigue for use with cancer patients. *Cancer Practitioner* 1998;6(3):143–52.

273. **Schwartz JE; Jandorf L; Krupp LB.** The measurement of fatigue: a new instrument. *Journal of Psychosomatic Research* 1993;37(7):753–62.

274. **Hann DM; Jacobsen PB; Martin SC; Kronish LE; Azzarello LM; Fields KK.** Fatique in women treated with bone marrow transplantation for breast cancer: a comparison with women with no history of cancer. *Supportive Care in Cancer*, 1997;5(1):44–52.

275. **Kogi K; Saito Y.** Assessment criteria for mental fatique. A factor-analytic study of phase discrimination in mental fatique. *Ergonomics* 1971;14(1):119–27.

276. **Morant R; Stiefel F; Berchtold W; Radziwill A; Riesen W.** Preliminary results of a study assessing asthenia and related psychological and biological phenomena in patients with advanced cancer. *Supportive Care in Cancer* 1993;1(2):101–7.

277. **McNair DM; Lorr M; Droppleman LF.** EdlTS Manual for the Profile of Mood States. San Diego: Educational and Industrial Testing Service, 1971:8.

278. **Cella D.** Factors influencing quality of life in cancer patients: anemia and fatigue. *Seminars in Oncology* 1998;25(3 Suppl. 7):43–6.

279. **Cella D.** The functional assessment of cancer therapy-anemia (FACT-An) scale: a new tool for the assessment of outcomes in cancer anemia and fatigue. *Seminars in Hematology* 1997;34(3 Suppl 2):13–19.

280. **Cella D; Peterman A; Passik S; Jacobsen P; Breitbart W.** Progress toward guidelines for the management of fatigue. *Oncology (Huntingt)* 1998;12(11A):369–77.

281. **Burke M; Bryson EI; Kark AE.** Dietary intakes, resting metabolic rates, and body composition in benign and malignant gastrointestinal disease. *British Medical Journal* 1980;280(6209):211–5.

282. **Bruera E; Chadwick S; Cowan L; Drebit D; Hanson J; MacDonald N; van Konkelenberg Y.** Caloric intake assessment in advanced cancer patients: comparison of three methods. *Cancer Treatment Reports* 1986;70(8):981–3.

283. **Deutsch JC.** Normal digestive physiolocy and the evaluation of digestive function. Review. *Seminars in Oncology* 1998;25(2 Suppl. 6):4–11.

284. **Suarez GA; Opfer-Gehrking TL; Offord KP; Atkinson EJ; O'Brien PC; Low PA.** The Autonomic Symptom Profile: a new instrument to assess autonomic symptoms. *Neurology* 1999;52(3):523–8.

285. **Chandra RK.** Nutrition, immunity, and infection: present knowledge and future directions. *The Lancet* 1983;1(8326 Pt 1):688–91.

286. **Vigano A; Dorgan M; Bruera E; Suarez-Almazor ME.** The relative accuracy of the clinical estimation of the duration of life for patients with end of life cancer. *Cancer* 1999;86(1):170–6.

287. **Christakis NA; Lamont EB.** Extent and determinants of error in doctors' prognoses in terminally ill patients: prospective cohort study. *British Medical Journal* 2000;320(7233):469–72.

288. **Starasser F; Calder K; Tom B; Amyotte G; Willey J; Benisch-Tolley S; Palmer L; Bruera E.** A Randomized Trial of Polysaturated Fatty Acid (pufa's) in Patients with Cancer Cachexia. Copenhagen:MASCC, June 14–16, 2001 (Abstract 28).

289. **Issell BF; Valdivieso M; Zaren HA; Durdrick SJ; Freireich EJ; Copeland EW; Bodey GP.** Protection against chemotherapy toxicity by IV hyperalimentation. *Cancer Treatment Reports* 1978;62(8):1139–43.

290. **Bashir Y; Graham TR; Torrance A; Gibson GJ; Corris PA.** Nutritional state of patients with lung cancer undergoing thoracotomy. *Thorax* 1990;45(3):183–6.

291. **Clamon GH; Feld R; Evans WK; Weiner RS; Moran EM; Blum RH; Kramer BS; Makuch RW; Hoffman FA; DeWys WD.** Effect of adjuvant central iv hyperalimenatation on the survival and response to treatment of patients with small cell lung cancer: a randomized trial. *Cancer Treatment reports* 1985;69(2):167–77.

292. **Larrea J; Vega S; Martinez T; Torrrent JM; Vega V; Nunez V.** The nutritional status and immunological situation of cancer patients. *Nutrition in Hospital* 1992;7(3):178–84.

293. **Popp MB; Fisher RI; Wesley R; Aamodt R; Brennan MF.** A prospective randomized study of adjuvant parental nutrition in the treatment of advanced diffuse lymphoma: influence of survival. *Surgery* 1981;90(2):195–203.

294. **Goodwin WJ JR; Torres J.** The value of the prognostic nutritional index in the management of patients with advanced carcinoma of the head and enck. *Head and Neck Surgery* 1984;6(5):932–7.

295. **Plata-Salaman CR.** Central nervous system mechanisms contributing to the cachexia–anorexia syndrome. *Nutrition* 2000;16(10):1009–12.

296. **Turrin NP; Flynn MC; Plata-Salaman CR.** Neuropeptide Y Counteracts interferon-alpha-induced anorexia. *Neuroimmunomodulation* 1999;6(5):361–6.

Chapter 5

Oral complications of cancer

Alberto Sbanotto

Introduction

Oral cavity problems represent a major issue in advanced cancer patients. They may strongly interfere with fundamental functions, namely speaking, eating, and respiration. Moreover, they carry relevant psychosocial consequences. The treatment of these complications should often begin during the initial phases of the illness, when aggressive treatment (e.g. combined chemotherapies and radiotherapies) may produce unavoidable toxicities to normal cells. In this chapter we discuss the most frequent complications of the oral cavity, considering also cancer treatment-related problems, which may affect the oral tissues of advanced cancer patients.

Infections

The oropharyngeal region comprises many ecologically different environments, and its microflora is complex, consisting of more than 300 different bacterial species, 70% of which are anaerobes, streptococci and Gram-negative anaerobic rods. A good oral hygiene is necessary for a correct infections treatment (Tables 5.1 and 5.2).

Fungal infections: candidiasis

Candidiasis encompasses a group of mucosal and cutaneous conditions with a common etiologic agent from the *Candida* genus of fungi. It is the most common oral mycotic infection (1), although frequency rates are difficult to establish because of the prevalence of *Candida* in a large proportion of the population. Candida species are reported to be present in about

Table 5.1 Basic principles of oral hygiene

1 Check oral cavity regularly
2 Prevent, whenever possible, side-effects of anticancer and drug therapies
3 Keep lips, teeth, and oral mucosa moist, clean, soft, and intact
4 Relieve pain and maintain oral intake
5 Teach patient and relatives about good oral hygiene

Table 5.2 Oral hygiene: some symptomatic measures

Pain
◆ Systemic analgesic drugs—analgesic gargles with: Benzydamine hydrochloride 0.15%, 15 ml every 2–4 hours
◆ Xylocaine viscous 2%, 5–15 ml every 4 hours
◆ Xylocaine spray 10%, every 4 hours
◆ Aluminum hydroxide and lidocaine 2% in equal parts
◆ Dyclomine hydrochloride
◆ Benzocaine 20% solution
◆ Avoid alcohol- and lemon-containing mouthwashes
Hemorrhage
◆ Treat the basic cause
◆ Avoid using toothbrush and dental flossing
◆ Use a low-pressure dental jet and/or a gauze pad wrapped around finger or a disposable sponge moistened in a mild solution of baking soda and water
◆ Gargles with
—Saline solution
—Hexetidine 0.1%
—Sodium pernorate
—Chlorexidine gluconate 0.2%
—Povidone–iodine 1%
—Bicarbonate of soda
—Cetylpyridinium
—H_2O_2 3–6% in water (1 : 4 ratio)
◆ Gargles or use soaked gauzes with antihemorrhage drugs:
—Thrombine 1–2 g day^{-1}
—Tranexamic acid 2–4 g day^{-1}

40%–60% of the normal oral flora of population (2). Positive cultures are found in 75% of asymptomatic hospitalized people, with higher percentages if repeated cultures are obtained (3,4). In oncological wards candidiasis appears in about 25%, requiring therapy in 50% of cases (5). Oral candidiasis may complicate mucositis due to cancer therapies, especially in granulocytopenic patients, where it may be the source of systemic infections (6). Candidiasis is caused by *C. albicans* and the related species, such as *C. parapsilosis*, *C. tropicalis*, *C. glabrata* and others. Ball and colleagues examined the species of yeast present in the mouths of 30 patients with advanced cancer (7): thirty-five yeast isolates were collected from a total of 25 (83%) of the patients sampled. The two most common species were *C. albicans* (15 isolates) and *C. glabrata* (11 isolates), with smaller numbers of *C. tropicalis*, *C. parapsilosis*, *C. guilliermondii*, *C. inconspicua*, and *Saccharomyces cerevisiae*. The *Candida* organism is a unicellular yeast of the *Cryptococcaceae* family, and may exist in three different biologic and morphologic forms: the vegetative or yeasts form, the elongated cellular form (pseudohyphae), and the chlamydospore form. The pseudohyphal form is present in the commensal state. The persistence of the vegetative form intraorally (and intravaginally) is partly related to its symbiosis with *Lactobacillus acidophilus. C. albicans* is a commensal of the oral cavity of the majority of healthy persons: its transformation from a state of commensalism to pathogen relates to local and systemic factors (Table 5.3). Steroids and antibiotics are common factors involved: about 40% of patients receiving steroids, and approximately 30% of those receiving antibiotics, develop oropharyngeal candidiasis (8). Also xerostomia is an important factor (9).

Oral *candida* infection may present with different acute and chronic clinical pictures. In the acute pseudomembranous form (thrush), oral lesions are characteristically white yellowish plaques, composed of fungi, keratotic debris, bacteria, fibrin, and desquamated cell. They can be removed, leaving an erythematous, eroded surface, often tender. Favored sites comprise the buccal mucosa and mucobuccal folds, the oropharynx, and the sides of the dorsal tongue. The loss of the pseudomembrane may result in a more generalized red lesion, called acute atrophic candidiasis, also known as antibiotic stomatitis. This last form is often associated with burning, tenderness, and dysphagia, because of numerous erosions and inflammation. Chronic candidiasis, often called denture sore mouth, is a commonly seen atrophic condition, appearing in up to 65% of people wearing complete maxillary dentures. It is more common in women and in the palatal mucosa. A bright red mucosa, in the area covered by denture, is common. In individuals with accumulation of saliva due to over closure of the lips, angular cheilitis is often associated. Among chronic candidiasis, the hyperplasic form may involve the dorsum of the tongue, in a pattern referred as median rhomboid glossitis. Other forms of oral candidiasis are less important for cancer

Table 5.3 Some factors involved in *Candida* infections

1 Local factors
- Wearing dentures
- Xerostomia
- Saliva composition alterations[a]
- Oral mucosa disruption[b]
- Microbial alterations
- Reduced mechanical debridement[c]
- Previous infections
- Poor oral hygiene

2 Systemic factors
- Diabetes
- Immunosuppression
- Medical therapies (e.g. steroids)
- Nutritional status alterations

[a] Mainly proteins and electrolytes
[b] Radiotherapy, chemotherapy, surgery, and cancer
[c] Comatose patients, enterally/parenterally fed patients, trismus, etc.

patients, and often related to chronic systemic condition (e.g. mucocutaneous candidiasis in some endocrinopathies). Cytological diagnosis with wet-mounted 20% potassium hydroxide and Gram stain show typical hyphae and spore forms. Immunofluorescent techniques may be necessary in chronic atrophic forms. These laboratory tests are generally unnecessary in advanced cancer patients.

Topical or systemic treatments are available: they can be used together in more severe forms. Nystatin suspension is a classic topic treatment: it does not show prophylactic activity and results can be disappointing (10,11). Its action is limited to the time of contact with the oral mucosa. Popsicles made of water-diluted nystatin, prolonging the time of contact, are an effective alternative. Its association with chlorexidine reduces its activity (12). Clotrimazole troches show good antimycotic activity, also in nystatin-resistant patients (13,14). Also miconazole can be used, as an oral gel or lozenges four times a day. It also shows activity on some Gram-positive strains (15,16). Amphotericin B suspension or lozenges are also available, but are less active than clotrimazole or miconazole (17). Intravenous Amphotericin B is not indicated for oral infections, due to the low concentration achieved in saliva (18). Other topical treatments, such as chlorexidine rinsing or gentian violet, can be used only for minor infections (19). Systemic triazole derivatives, such as fluconazole and itraconazole, are well absorbed by the gastrointestinal route, with long half-life, allowing once daily administration. They present few side-effects. Their spectrum of action is wide, including different fungi (20,21). Their uses include oropharyngeal candidiasis and systemic infections (22–26) and present preventive properties (27,28). In advanced cancer patients resistances to this drug can be present and are usually due to non-candidal species. Results of azole antifungal agents are superior to those obtained with traditional treatments like nystatin and ketoconazole, but they are more expensive. When indicated, drugs such as steroids, tricyclic antidepressants, or antibiotics must be stopped or reduced. Lethal arrhythmias may occur with azole derivatives association with cisapride.

Non-candidal infections

An increasing number of different fungal organisms are being associated with oral infection in immunocompromised cancer patients in recent years, and includes infection by species of *Aspergillus, Mucormycosis,* and *Rhizopus* (30). The clinical presentation is not pathognomonic; lesions may appear similar to other oral toxicities. Microbiologic documentation is essential. Systemic therapy must be instituted promptly due to the high risk for morbidity and mortality. Their importance in advanced cancer patients is probably limited.

Bacterial infections

While the common oral flora is characterized by a prevalence of Gram-positive bacteria, xerostomia, radiotherapy, chemotherapy, and immunodepression cause a shift of oral flora towards Gram-negative colonization (31). This evolving epidemiology has been caused also by the use of prophylactic and therapeutic antimicrobial regimens, as well as decreased depth and duration of myelosuppression via growth factor therapy. In patients undergoing systemic anticancer therapies Gram-positive organisms, including viridans *Streptococci* and *Enterococci* species, are currently associated with systemic infection of oral origin. In addition, Gram-negative pathogens including *Pseudomonas aeruginosa, Neisseria species,* and *Escherichia coli* remain of concern. The presence of such heterogeneous flora makes bacterial cultures difficult to interpret. Previous periodontal disease is frequently linked in cancer patients to bacterial oral infections (32). Periodontal disease is very common in the normal population: about 70%–80% of adults are affected by minor periodontitis. Inflammatory signs may be masked due to the underlying myelosuppression. The treatment of bacterial infections depends first on adequate hygiene. In myelosuppressed patients neutropenic mouth care protocols that reduce microbial colonization of the dentition and periodontium are important (33). According to the National Cancer Institute, they may include: (a) oral rinses with 0.12% chlorhexidine digluconate; (b) irrigation with effervescent (peroxide) agents which may affect anaerobic bacteria colonizing the periodontal pocket; and (c) gentle mechanical plaque removal, including dental brushing and flossing. Prechemotherapy endodontic therapy should be completed at least 10 days prior to initiation of chemotherapy. Periodontal probing and scaling could possibly reduce post-chemotherapy oral complications, but the exact role of these treatments in advanced cancer patients has to be evaluated. In acute periodontal infection, broad-spectrum antibiotics therapy is usually initiated, followed by more precise therapy based on the bacterial cultures, if possible and indicated. During chemotherapy, small hemorrhages, pain, and fever may be present. Nearby structures, secondary infection can be present (34,35). Ill-fitting removable prosthetic appliances can traumatize oral mucosa and increase the risk of microbial invasion into deeper tissues. Denture soaking cups can readily become colonized with a variety of pathogens, including *Pseudomonas aeruginosa, E. coli, Enterobacter* species *Staphylococcus aureus, Klebsiella* species, and *C. albicans.* Denture cleansing solutions should be changed daily. In general, dentures should not be worn when the patient has ulcerative mucositis and is neutropenic (e.g. <500 ANC/mm^3). In a palliative care setting, pain treatment plays a major role.

Viral infections

Herpes simplex virus (HSV), cytomegalovirus (CMV), varicella zoster virus (VZV), and Epstein–Barr virus (EBV) are the main viruses involved in oral infections. In most instances HSV, VZV, and EBV infections result from the reactivation of a latent virus, while CMV infections can result from either the reactivation of a latent virus, or via a newly acquired virus. The HSV is the most common: up to 90% of the population have antibodies to HSV. Incidence of recurrent oral HSV lesions in myelosuppressed cancer patients has been considerably reduced following the introduction of prophylactic acyclovir in the mid-1980s. Reported incidence of the clinical infection in patients receiving chemotherapy is approximately 11%–65% (36–38). HSV infection is manifested by the presence of yellowish lesions, easily removed from the mucosa and extremely painful. Vesicles can also appear on the lip (cold sores), and fever, anorexia, and malaise are present. In more severe cases, pain can be so intense as to provoke dysphagia. In immunosuppressed patients early diagnosis (39) and prompt therapy remain hallmarks of management: the culture of lesions in HSV seropositive patients, including shell vial testing, are essential to accurate diagnosis. Assays, which produce more rapid results, including immunoassay for HSV antigen and/or biopsy, may also be useful. In advanced cancer patients, diagnosis is mainly clinical. Lesions have to be differentiated from aphthous ulcers: a history of vesicles preceding ulcers, a location on hard gingival and hard palate, and a crop of lesions are indicative of herpetic infection, rather than aphthous ulcers. As with other infections, risk for systemic dissemination and morbidity/mortality increases with the degree and duration of immunocompromised status. Specific treatment is provided by acyclovir. In advanced cancer patients, oral and topical routes (5% ointment) are commonly employed. chlorhexidine 0.12% twice daily rinsing can be beneficial for HSV-1 infection (40). While true resistance to antivirals may develop, clinical infection is likely due to insufficient dosing or compromised gastrointestinal absorption of oral acyclovir. In patients undergoing active therapies, the lesions typically emerge concurrently with chemotherapy-induced oral mucositis and develop into extensive, confluent mucosal ulcerations clinically similar to primary herpetic stomatitis. As such, HSV stomatitis can be confused with cancer chemotherapy-induced ulcerative mucositis; in these patients, intravenous acyclovir can be indicated. Renal function should be good and patients should be hydrated. In hematological patients lymphocytes and monocytes count recovery have been shown necessary for infection to resolve. Another viral infections is VZV; this infection classically distributes via dermatomes, although in immunocompromised patients the clinical manifestations can be altered. The lesion is typically observed several weeks after cessation of chemotherapy. This is in contrast to HSV, which often occurs within two to three weeks after chemotherapy is discontinued. Acyclovir and famcyclovir are currently the primary drugs used for treatment (40,41). Oral lesions associated with CMV have been documented in recent years (43). Appearance is not pathognomonic and is characterized by multiple mild to moderate ulcerations with irregular margins. The lesions initially present during early periods of marrow regeneration (e.g. 3 weeks after chemotherapy is discontinued). CMV-specific immunohistochemical staining of biopsy specimens remains the gold standard. Ganciclovir should be considered for treatment of acute CMV infection. Oral hairy leukoplakia has been attributed to EBV infection in immunocompromised patients, including those with acquired immune deficiency syndrome (AIDS) and renal transplant. The lesion does not appear to be clinically significant in chemotherapy recipients. Infections caused by non-herpes viruses are less common in immunocompromised chemotherapy patients. Oral lesions caused by adenovirus and oral human papilloma virus (HPV) have been described. Laser surgery or cryotherapy are typically utilized to remove oral HPV lesions; intralesional injections of alpha interferon may prove effective for recurrent lesions.

Xerostomia

Xerostomia is the subjective feeling of mouth dryness not always accompanied by a detectable decrease in salivation flow (44,45). Few data are available on the frequency of xerostomia in patients with advanced cancer. This symptom is referred by to frequent and awful in 30% of patients at the beginning of a palliative care programme (46). Oneschuk *et al.* reported mouth dryness in a group of advanced cancer patients receiving care in the community or in a hospice setting: 88% of patients reported a dry mouth at a mean intensity corresponding to 6.2 ± SD 2.21, on a 1–10 scale (47). It was a specific complaint in 40% of patients at the time of admission to a hospice, but probably 100% of patients suffer from a dry mouth at some point during the terminal stage of disease (48,49). The main causes of xerostomia are enumerated in Table 5.4. A variety of symptoms are associated with the feeling of oral dryness. In the study by Sreebny and Valdini the symptoms most frequently present in 485 or more of the xerostomic subjects were the need to do something to keep the mouth moist, the need to get out of bed at night to drink water, and difficulty with speech (45). In 13%–30% of the patients with a dry mouth it was noted that there was an association with having to keep fluids at the bedside, loss in taste acuity, difficulty with

Table 5.4 Main causes of xerostomia

1. Reduced salivary secretion caused by:
   - Radiotherapy in the head and neck region
   - Surgery in the buccal and submandibular regions
   - Drugs
   - Obstruction, infection, aplasia, and malignant destruction of salivary glands
   - Encephalitis, brain tumors, neurosurgical interventions, and autonomic pathways destruction
   - Hypothyroidism
   - Autoimmune disease
   - Sarcoidosis
2. Widespread erosion of buccal mucosa caused by:
   - Cancer
   - Chemotherapy, radiotherapy, and immunodeficiency
   - Stomatitis
   - Viral, bacterial, and fungal oral infections
3. Dehydration caused by:
   - Anorexia
   - Diarrhea
   - Fever
   - O_2 therapy
   - Breathing by mouth
   - Large bedsores and/or ulcers
   - Vomiting
   - Polyuria
   - Hemorrhage
   - Diabetes insipidus
   - Dysphagia
4. Decreased mastication
5. Depression, anxiety

chewing dry foods, burning and tingling sensations on the tongue, the presence of cracks or fissures at the corners of the lips, and difficulty in swallowing. Most of these symptoms can cause anorexia, loss of weight, and cachexia. Patients with a dental prosthesis may find poor tolerance to them due to frequent traumatic lesions; this also produces difficulty in mastication that leads to a reduced intake of food (50). Table 5.4 reports the main causes of xerostomia. Saliva is a major protector of the tissues and organs of the mouth. In its absence both the hard and soft tissues of the oral cavity may be severely damaged with an increase in ulcerations, infections such as candidiasis, and dental decay (51–54). However, numerous factors, in addition to saliva, are important in oral mucosal preservation, such as the presence of magainins, an intrinsic protective components described in frog skin (55). According to Zasloff, similar substances may have a protective role for mammalian mucosa. The volume of salivary fluid output is not the only factor in maintaining oral mucosal health. Differences in salivary composition in various states of health and disease have to be investigated. Patients treated with radiotherapy for oral or head and neck cancers suffer from xerostomia from the beginning of the treatment. Radiation directed at such areas can involve one or both parotid glands or the submandibolary salivary glands, resulting in a marked diminution of the normal salivary flow (56–59). This is a consequence of radiation-induced inflammation and degeneration of the acini and ducts, connective tissues, and vascular components of the salivary glands (57–59), even though a definitive mechanism has not been established (60). The most important factor affecting the post-irradiation salivary flow after curative dose radiotherapy seems to be the volume of the major salivary glands irradiated (61–63). A sharp decrease in the salivary flow usually occurs after the first week of radiotherapy treatment with a dose of approximately 10 Gy. This decrease in the flow rate continues throughout the treatment, resulting in almost complete xerostomia (58,61). This symptom usually persists. While one study noted a partial return of the salivary flow 8 months after the end of radiotherapy, others found minimal, if any, improvements some years after radiotherapy (64,65). After irradiation of the salivary glands, saliva become more viscous (8,58,59,64), undergoes a reduction in pH, and loses organic and inorganic components (59,66,67). The aqueous component of whole saliva is much more sharply depressed than the proteic component during the production of xerostomia: Niedermaier and colleagues took serial flow rate measurements of the parotid and palatal glands saliva over a period of approximately nine months in 13 patients who suffered from malignancies of the head and neck region (68). Twelve patients consented to take part in a second study in which salivary flow was stimulated by oral pilocarpine before and at the conclusion of radiotherapy and seven months later. After radiotherapy, the secretory performance of the parotid glands dropped off rapidly and irreversibly. Salivary secretion from the palatal glands was not totally diminished as a result of radiation. While pilocarpine produced a clinically significant increase in salivary flow from the palatal glands before and seven months after radiation, secretory performance of the parotid glands could not be sufficiently increased by stimulation with pilocarpine after radiotherapy. The authors concluded for a greater resistance and recoverability of the mucous-secreting minor palatal glands in comparison with the serous-secreting parotid glands. They also indicate the significant post-radiation ability of the mucous-secreting glands to be simulated by pilocarpine Saliva changes compromise the lubricating protective function of saliva, reducing its capacity to act as a barrier against irritating substances or remove bacterial and cellular debris. The amount of bicarbonates also diminishes (58,65,66), which further impairs the cleaning action of saliva. It is possible to observe an increase in the salivary content of Na, Cl, Mg, and protein (58,62,66). The reduction in the salivary flow rate together with these qualitative changes can alter the oral microbial flora, and results in increased growth of *Candida* organisms, Gram-negative rods, and streptococcus and *Lactobacillus* (69,70). These often-irreversible alterations can rapidly damage dental structures and increase tooth decay (71). In patients undergoing radiotherapy, the tooth decay process can be rapid and lesions can be manifest within three to six months (72). The process of decay may also provoke pain in the oral cavity, thereby adding to the suffering of the patient. Loss of already decaying teeth causes further difficulty in mastication, which, added to xerostomia, may cause difficulty in swallowing and digestion. Saving the minor oral glands may play an important role in protection against new colonization by micro-organisms (61,62, 65,73,74) or against tooth decay (75,76). In addition to the flow measurements, amylase seems to be the best indicator of salivary gland function during radiotherapy, whereas albumin and lactoferrin are good indicators of inflammatory reactions often related to irradiation (63). A large number of drugs with xerostomic side-effects are known, including antipsychotic and tricyclic antidepressants, antihistamines, anticholinergic drugs, anticonvulsants, hypnotics, beta-blockers, and diuretics (8,76–79). Drugs may directly or indirectly reduce the flow of saliva and initiate the feeling of oral dryness. Some of these drugs induce xerostomia through parasympatholytic effects. In the study by Sreebny *et al.* almost 60% of those patients with a dry mouth took xerogeneic drugs (77). The intake of xerostomia-inducing medications is positively correlated with age and with the total number of drugs taken daily, and it is highest among institutionalized patients (76,78). Xerostomia is not generally recognized as a side-effect of morphine (77), but clinical experience suggests that it is a common complaint of cancer patients treated with morphine (77–79).

Xerostomia after radiation therapy may be the most difficult to treat because of the irreversible damage to the salivary glands that may occur. A number of agents have been tested for the prevention or attenuation of xerostomia. Current therapy for chronic xerostomia includes salivary substitutes or salivary stimulants. Water, glycerin preparations, and artificial saliva are used as substitutes for saliva, while sialogogues, sugarless candies, and chewing gum are used for saliva stimulation (80). A lot of commercial products are available which patients use primarily as a gargle to relieve the symptoms of xerostomia, but they often do not provide improvement in these symptoms. Pilocarpine hydrochloride, a cholinergic agonist, was approved by the US Food and Drug Administration (FDA) after improvement was demonstrated in comfort levels in patients with post-radiotherapy xerostomia. Different studies have underlined the importance of this drug: its action seems relevant especially in stimulating residual salivary function (81). Its degranulating effects on salivary cells have also been considered to explain a possible protective action (82,83). Johnson and colleagues evaluated pilocarpine hydrochloride for the treatment of radiation-induced xerostomia, in a prospective, randomized double blind, placebo-controlled trial (84). Patients received either placebo or pilocarpine (5 mg or 10 mg orally three times a day) for 12 weeks and were evaluated at baseline and every four weeks. They enrolled 207 patients who had each received ≥ 40 Gy of radiation to the head and neck. In the patients receiving the 5-mg dose of pilocarpine, oral dryness improved in 44%, as compared with 25% of the patients receiving placebo group ($P = 0.027$). There was overall improvement in 54% of the 5-mg group as compared with 25% of the placebo group ($P = 0.003$), and 31% of the 5-mg group had improved comfort of the mouth and tongue, as compared with 10% of the placebo group ($P = 0.002$). Speaking ability improved in 33% of the 5-mg group as compared with 18% of the placebo group ($P = 0.037$). Interestingly, saliva production was improved, but it did not correlate with symptomatic relief. There were comparable improvements in the group receiving the 10-mg dose. The primary adverse effect was sweating, in addition to other minor cholinergic effects. Of the patients in the 5-mg and 10-mg groups, 6% and 29%, respectively, withdrew from the study because of adverse effects. Similar results were obtained from LeVeque *et al.* (85). In their randomized, double blind, placebo-controlled, multicenter clinical investigation, most of the enrolled 162 patients had received >60 Gy of radiation for head and neck cancers. Patients received 2.5-mg tablets for the first four weeks 5.0-mg tablets for the second four weeks, and 10.0-mg tablets for the last four weeks of the 12-weeks study; they were allowed to titrate pilocarpine or placebo for improvement in symptoms or to reduce side-effects. Patients were evaluated for symptomatic relief by questionnaires and visual analog scales (VAS), and for saliva production by sialometry. Pilocarpine produced a significant improvement ($P=0.035$) in overall global assessments compared with placebo. There was a statistically significant ($P=0.020$) decreased use of oral comfort agents such as artificial saliva, hard candy, and water. Values for symptomatic improvement in dryness approached significance ($P=0.057$). There were statistically significant post-dose improvements in whole and parotid salivary flow in pilocarpine treatment groups versus placebo. All pilocarpine dosages tested were judged to be safe. A common side-effect was mild to moderate sweating. Also, this study confirmed that best results were obtained with continuous treatment and with doses higher than 2.5 mg thrice daily. These schedules were confirmed by Rieke and colleagues (86). They evaluated pilocarpine administered in either a fixed-dose or in a dose-titration protocol three times a day for 12 weeks in two randomized, double-blind, and placebo-controlled, multicenter clinical trials. They enrolled 369 patients who had received at least 40 Gy of radiation to the head and neck with clinically significant xerostomia. In the dose–titration study 169 patients received a thrice daily regimen of 2.5 mg tablets for first four weeks, 5.0 mg tablets for the second four weeks, and 10.0 mg tablets for last four weeks of a 12-week study. In the fixed-dose study, 207 patients received placebo, 5.0 mg, or 10.0 mg tablets three times a day for 12 weeks. Patients were evaluated for symptomatic relief by responding to questionnaires using visual analog scales and categorical questions; and, for saliva production by sialometry. Evaluations were conducted at baseline, and weeks 4, 8, and 12. There were statistically significant improvements in salivary flow in pilocarpine treatment groups versus placebo. There was a significant improvement in the overall 'global' condition of xerostomia associated with the use of pilocarpine in both studies. In the fixed-dose study, there were significant improvements in oral dryness, mouth comfort, ability to speak, and reduction in the use of oral comfort agents. The dose–titration study showed improvements in dryness that approached significance and a decreased use of oral comfort agents. All pilocarpine dosages (2.5, 5.0, and 10.0 mg three times a day) were judged to be safe. Adverse effects were those expected for a cholinergic agonist, with the most common being mild to moderate sweating. The incidence of these events increased by dose. A 5.0-mg thrice-daily regimen produced the best clinical results when both efficacy and side-effects were taken into consideration. Some patients would experience some additional benefit by increasing the dose to 10 mg thrice daily (86). A recent French trial evaluated the action of pilocarpine hydrochloride versus xerostomia and the relationship of the response of dose/volume radiotherapy parameters (87). One hundred and forty-five patients with severe radiation-induced xerostomia were evaluable. They received 15 mg per day with a 5 mg optional increase at five weeks up to a daily dose of 25 mg beyond nine weeks. Treatment compliance was 75%. Thirty-eight patients (26%) stopped treatment before week 12 for acute intolerance (sweating, nausea, vomiting) or no response. No severe complication occurred. Ninety-seven patients (67%) reported a significant relief of symptoms of xerostomia at 12 weeks. Within 12 weeks, the size of the subgroup with normal food intake almost doubled (13–24 patients) while the size of the subgroup with (nearly) impossible solid food ingestion decreased by 38% (47 versus 29 patients). The impact on quality of life was considered important or very important by 77% of the responders. The authors found no difference according to dose/volume radiotherapy parameters. These results were also confirmed in long-term studies (88). Pilocarpine was also evaluated for its topical activity, trying to maximize its local action and minimize the systemic side-effects: Davies *et al.* compared a mucin-based artificial saliva and a mouthwash containing pilocarpine (5 mg three times a day). Twenty patients with radiation-induced xerostomia were entered into this prospective randomized cross-over study. Overall the patients found that the pilocarpine mouthwash was more effective than the artificial saliva in relieving their symptoms ($P=0.04$), and 47% of the patients wanted to continue with this treatment after the study had finished (89). Hamlar and colleagues evaluated pilocarpine hydrochloride suspended in a candy-like pastille as a topical treatment for radiation-induced xerostomia in head and neck cancer patients (90). They undertook a prospective, randomized, double blind, placebo-controlled trial to determine the objective and subjective efficacy in reversing the decrease in salivation. Forty previously irradiated patients received increasingly higher pilocarpine dosages in pastilles for five successive weeks. At each successive dose of pilocarpine, no significant increased salivation was noted. However, 25 (74%) of 34 patients reported that pilocarpine alleviated their subjective xerostomia. In this study topical pilocarpine administration showed similar results to previous systemic delivery methods for radiation-induced xerostomia, but with improved patient tolerance. Pilocarpine has also been tested concurrently with radiotherapy, as a preventive measure (91). In this retrospective study Zimmerman and colleagues concluded that the use of 5 mg oral pilocarpine four times a day during radiotherapy for head and neck cancer and three months thereafter was associated with significantly less subjective xerostomia than that reported by a similar cohort of patients who had not received pilocarpine.

Several recent studies show interesting radio protective action of amifostine, and its active metabolite WR-1065. These substances accumulate in many epithelial tissues, with the highest concentrations found in salivary glands and kidneys (92,93). They possibly act through scavenging radiation-induced free radicals. Brizel *et al.*, in a multicentre randomized trial, found a significative action of amifostine, 200 mg m^{-2} daily during radiotherapy, in reducing grade ≥2 acute xerostomia from 78% to 51%, and chronic grade ≥2 from 57% to 34% (94). Toxicity consisted primarily of nausea and vomiting (5%) or hypotension (5%). The production of saliva at one year following treatment was 2.5 times greater in the amifostine-treated group than in the radiation-only group. Antitumor treatment efficacy was preserved. No action was evident in reducing stomatitis, but a subset analysis showed that there was a reduction in grade 3 and 4 mucositis among 108 French and American patients receiving amifostine (22% and 39%, respectively), compared with the control group. Unfortunately patients from these groups tended to be treated with smaller radiation field sizes, potentially confounding conclusions. Additional studies are needed with a more specific focus on prevention of mucositis by amifostine. A recent economical analysis, from a randomized phase II trial, supported the use of this substance in a head and neck radiation patients setting (95).

Taste alterations

Taste alterations comprise a reduction in taste sensitivity (hypogeusia), an absence of taste sensation (ageusia), or a distortion of normal taste (dysgeusia). The incidence of these symptoms is unknown. According to Twycross and Lack (96), about 25%–50% of cancer patients have diminished taste sensation. Our clinical experience suggests that patients hardly ever report taste alterations spontaneously, but many will report it as a reason for loss of appetite if specifically questioned. Patients typically report that the food is tasteless or bitter. Taste is mediate through organs known as taste buds, which contain approximately 50 cells, continuously renewed, endowed in a network of several taste nerve fibers. They are usually specific to only one of the four primary taste stimuli (sour, bitter, sweet and salty tastes). The number of taste buds, about 3000 to 10 000 in the adult, decreases with age. Buds are found on the tongue, soft palate, pharynx, larynx, epiglottis, uvula, lips and cheeks, and in the upper third of the esophagus. The cells of the taste buds are provided with microvilli in direct communication with the oral cavity through an apical pore. A gatekeeper protein regulates the quantity of stimuli that pass through the pore per unit of time. Changes in the protein molecules are controlled by the equilibrium of metals and, consequently, a deficiency of some metals, and in particular of zinc, is associated with hypogeusia and anorexia (97,98). Taste information is sent by way of the fifth, seventh, ninth, and tenth cranial nerves to the medulla (nucleus of the solitary tract) and from there through the pons and thalamus to the cortical area subserving taste. Information in this pathway is also projected to the lateral thalamus (98). A lesion in any one of these areas can alter taste perception (99). The effects of cancer on taste are not unknown. Chemotherapy agents known to cause taste alterations include 5-FU, cylcophosphamide, methotrexate, doxorubicin, vincristine, dacarbazine. Other potential causes of taste alteration are listed in Table 5.4. Taste abnormalities in cancer patients may be correlated with the site or extent of the tumor, independent of histological type. A positive correlation exists between weight loss and the presence of an abnormal taste sensation (100). Disturbances in taste can also alter digestion because stimulation of the taste organs can increase salivary and pancreatic flow, gastric contractions, and bowel motility (99). William and Cohen demonstrated elevated thresholds for recognition of sour (HCl), but not bitter (urea), sweet (sucrose), or salt (NaCl) tastes, in a group of patients with lung cancer, who were tested prior to chemotherapy or radiotherapy (101). An elevated threshold of detection for all four basic tastes was reported in a group of patients with laryngeal cancer who had been examined before laryngectomy (102). Taste alterations have been reported as a consequence of radiotherapy for tumors in the head and neck regions. The mechanism for this effect may be due to damage to the microvilli of the taste cells and/or to reduced salivation. Taste loss was not observed until radiation doses of 20 Gy had been reached (103). Between 20 and 40 Gy taste loss increased rapidly and at the 60-Gy dose level, over 90% relative taste loss was observed (103). In most instances, taste acuity is partially restored 20–60 days after radiotherapy and is fully restored within two to four months post-radiotherapy. Three weeks after initiation of radiotherapy, the bitter and salt qualities showed the earliest and greatest impairment and the sweet quality the least (104). Drugs administered to cancer patients may also alter taste. Several drugs are considered responsible for taste alterations (105), but many of these have been reported as a cause only once. Zinc deficiency has been noted as a potential cause of anorexia, dysgeusia, or hypogeusia. Plasma zinc levels have been found to be reduced in patients with bronchial carcinoma compared the normal with healthy population, and zinc in leukemic cells appears to be lower than in normal white blood cells (106). The administration of zinc has been reported to correct abnormalities of taste in some cases (107). In uncontrolled clinical trials, the administration of oral zinc sulfate has been reported both to prevent and correct taste abnormalities in cancer patients receiving external radiotherapy to the head and neck region: Ripamonti *et al.*, in a randomized trial, observed that patients treated with placebo experienced a greater worsening of subjective perception of the four taste qualities during radiotherapy treatment compared with those treated with zinc sulfate, 45 mg daily. One month after ERT was terminated, the patients receiving zinc, 45 mg daily. One month after ERT was terminated, the patients receiving zinc sulfate had a quicker recovery of taste acuity than those receiving placebo. The authors concluded that adding oral zinc could be an effective and well-tolerated treatment for dysgeusia due to radiotherapy (108). Copper and nickel have also been used with good results in clinical trials. No patients treated prophylactically with 25 mg of oral zinc four times a day prior to radiotherapy developed as severe a hypogeusia as those who were not treated (107,109,110). Patients suffering from taste alterations need correct oral hygiene, treatment to increase salivation, and suspension of the drug that can induce or increase the symptom. Patients can usually take spicy food, with a strong smell, adding lemon or vinegar, if stomatitis or mouth ulcers are not present.

Therapies-induced stomatitis

Elimination or oral disease and implementation of oral care protocols designed to maintain maximum oral health must be a component of patient assessment and care prior to chemotherapy and radiation therapy. During and following radiation therapy, oral management will be dictated by the specific needs of the patient. Ongoing oral assessment and treatment of complications are essential, since radiation or other damage to oral tissues typically renders patients at risk for oral complications. In addition, invasive oral procedures can cause additional sequelae. Management typically needs to be altered due to underlying tissue damage (e.g. dysphagia due to stomatitis). Patients should receive a comprehensive oral evaluation several weeks prior to initiation of the treatment, especially for radiation therapy. This timing provides an appropriate interval for tissue healing in the event that invasive oral procedures including dental extractions, dental scaling/polishing, and endodontic therapy are necessary. These interventions are principally directed at reducing risk of soft tissue necrosis and osteoradionecrosis. The likelihood of these lesions occurring post-radiation increases over the patient's lifetime.

Minimizing mucosal trauma and controlling oral pain are the main principles of the pallitive treatment of mucositis. The therapeutic schedules currently used are mainly empirical and few controlled clinical studies are available. Ice chips or popsicles are soothing. Anaesthetic rinses (xylocaine viscous, benadryl, kaopectate) may allow simple oral intake, but they may impair deglutition mechanisms; analgesic treatment is usually necessary. Hydrogen peroxide rinsing appears helpful in removing debris and mucous from the teeth. Spicy or acidic food should be avoided and soft, low-salt foods should be given. Oral hygiene should be stressed: mouth care protocols, including toothbrushing, flossing, mouth rinsing, and fluoride applications, can significantly decrease the frequency or oral complications. In chemotherapy-induced stomatitis secondary infections prevention, oral hygiene, and supportive measures are most important. Spontaneous gingival bleeding appears when the platelets count falls below 10 000 cells mm^{-3}: a topical thrombin-soaked gauze held under pressure or mycrocristalline collagen may be helpful. When local measures fail, a platelets transfusion has to be considered; its role in advanced patients is limited. Severe oral pain may require systemically administered medications. Morphine or methadone can be administered orally or parenterally. In bone marrow transplanted patients, where severe mucositis is often present, intravenous continuous morphine or other strong opioids are routinely used by some groups, with good results (111,112).

Drug-induced stomatitis

Mucositis induced by chemotherapy is a common side-effect of cancer treatment: approximately 40% of patients receiving chemotherapy develop an oral problem related to treatment (113,114). Raber-Durlacher *et al.*, in a retrospective study of 185 patients treated for solid tumors with chemotherapy regimen consisting of two or more drugs, found that 31% of patients (for a total of 87 stomatitis episodes) experienced mucositis (115). Grade 2 mucositis was recorded in 16.7% of patients, and grade 3 in 4%. Patients with hematologic malignancies develop oral problems at two to three times the rate of patients with solid tumors: rates up to 76% in bone marrow transplant patients have been reported (113,114). The costs of mucositis can be high: in a recent paper Sonis and colleagues analyzed the relationships of different outcomes in a population of 92 transplanted subjects (116). Among others, mucositis with evidence of ulceration was significantly associated with $42 749 higher mean hospital charges. Patients in poor oral health have a higher risk of post-chemotherapy oral infections (117,118). Stomatotoxicity generally results from the non-specific inhibitory effect of the chemotherapeutic agents on mitoses of the rapidly dividing cells of the oral epithelium (direct toxicity). It occurs approximately five to seven days after drug administration, often a few days before the patient's hematologic nadir. Thus, the mucosal disruption provides a portal of entry for micro-organisms, at the time of maximum myelosuppression and may be accompanied by hemorrhages. A wide variety of agents may produce direct toxicity, including 5-Fluorouracil (5-FU), methotrexate, doxorubicin, bleomycin, and ifosfamide (113). In the study by Raber-Durlacher *et al.*, cited above, multivariate analysis showed that, among chemotherapy agents used, doxorubicin, paclitaxel, and etoposide presented a high risk of mucositis (115). Also the presence of fever with leucopenia is associated with a higher risk of mucositis (115). Increasing age has been cited as a possible risk factor, probably due to reduced renal clearance of chemotherapy agents, with increased toxicity (115,119). Sex differences are probably important: a recent meta-analysis of 731 patients receiving 5-FU-based chemotherapy showed a significant higher incidence (63% for female versus 52% for men, $P=0.002$) of stomatitis and its intensity (120). The precise mechanism was not evident. In general, mucositis is dose-related: divided doses, rather than a bolus, can reduce this problem; the impact of a continuing infusion regimen (e.g. 5-FU) is debatable (121,122). Specific treatment of the oral lesions induced by chemotherapy is still poor (123). In particular, 5-FU has been studied. Early pilot studies suggested that an allopurinol mouthwash could be an effective antidote to 5-FU-induced mucositis, but a controlled study did not confirm this hypothesis (124,125). Due to the very short serum half-life of 5-FU, mouth cryotherapy around the time of intravenous 5-FU bolus administration has been proposed. In randomized study, patients receiving cryotherapy presented a reduced incidence and severity of stomatitis (126). In this study also an unexpected lower incidence of stomatitis was reported among smokers than non-smokers. A further study confirmed the efficacy or cryotherapy given by a 30 minute schedule versus a 60 minute one; differences related to smoking status were evident in this other study, but not significant (127). Chamomile mouthwash, associated with cryotherapy, appeared no different from placebo in stomatitis due to 5-FU-based regimens (128). Sucralfate in association with an oral cryotherapy regimen was investigated in a placebo-randomized study in 5-FU-based chemotherapies; sucralfate was not used prophylactically, but started at the first indication of mouth soreness. No significant efficacy was evident (129). Oral glutamine has also been shown to reduce the degree of stomatitis in human subjects treated with chemotherapy (130,131). These results were not confirmed in another double blind placebo-controlled trial by Okumo and colleagues, who randomized 5-FU-based chemotherapy patients to receive oral cryotherapy with or without oral glutamine (132).

The introduction of colony-stimulating growth factors in recent years, particularly those that stimulate white blood cell production, has changed the way chemotherapy is administered and tolerated. It has been reported that granulocyte–macrophage colony-stimulating factor (GM-CSF) affects mature leukocytes, macrophages, and dendritic cells as well as fibroblasts and keratinocytes, resulting in more rapid resolution of cuts, burns, skin grafts, and leg ulcers (133–135).

The use of GM-CSF in high-dose chemotherapy and stem cell transplantation seems to be associated with a lower risk of stomatitis. The mechanism of this effect could be also related to a reduction in indirect stomatotoxicity due to the acceleration of hematopoiesis and/or an increase in the functional activation of WBC. Chi and colleagues have shown a potential reduction in both te severity and duration of stomatitis following cisplatin, 5-FU, and leucovorin among 20 patients with stage IV head and neck cancer who were randomized to receive GM-CSF or no therapy following either cycle 1 or cycle 2 of chemotherapy (136). Colony-stimulating factors were also evaluated by topical route, with disappointing results: Cartee *et al.* conducted a double blind, placebo-controlled, dose ranging study of GM-CSF mouthwash in patients with breast cancer (137). They administered a combination chemotherapy regimen which has historically produced dose-limiting (grade ≥ 3) mucositis in approximately 39% of patients. Subjects were randomized to receive either placebo mouthwash or one of four concentrations of GM-CSF mouthwash (0.01, 0.1, 1.0 or 10 $\mu g\,ml^{-1}$). Forty-five patients were evaluable for response. The primary endpoint was to evaluate the relationship between the dose of GM-CSF mouthwash received and the probability of grade ≥ 3 mucositis using a logistic model. A 42% risk (15/36) of mucositis grade ≥ 3 was evident on day 15 in patients receiving GM-CSF compared with 2 of 9 patients on the placebo arm. No evidence of dose response was found by logistic regression. A positive correlation between GM-CSF dose and leukocyte recovery was noted ($P = 0.04$). Further studies are needed, considering the high costs of these treatments.

Capsaicin applied topically to human skin produces itching, pricking, and burning sensations due to excitation of nociceptors. With repeated application, these positive sensory responses are followed by a prolonged period of hypoalgesia that is usually referred to as desensitization, or nociceptor inactivation (138). For these reasons capsaicin preparations have been proposed for controlling pain related to stomatitis (139–142). This approach to mucositis pain control is not always comfortable and convenient, and some patients are clearly not candidates for its use. Further evaluation is warranted.

The use of the low-energy helium–neon laser (LEL) appears to be a simple atraumatic technique for the prevention and treatment of mucositis of various origins, including chemotherapy-induced. Activation of epithelial healing for LEL-treated surfaces, the most commonly recognized effect, has been confirmed by *in vitro* studies. To evaluate the efficiency of LEL in the prevention of oral mucositis induced by high-dose chemoradiotherapy before autologous bone marrow transplantation (BMT), Cowen and collegues randomized 30 patients receiving BMT after high-dose chemoradiotherapy (cyclophosphamide or melphalan) to possibly receive prophylactic laser to the oral mucosa (143). Total body irradiation consisted of a 12 Gy midplane dose in six fractions (4 Gy per day for three days). LEL applications were performed daily on five anatomic sites of the oral mucosa. A daily mucositis index (DMI) and a cumulative oral mucositis score (COMS) were established.

Requirement for narcotics and parenteral nutrition was recorded. The COMS was significantly reduced among laser-treated patients ($P=0.04$). The improvement of DMI in laser-treated patients was also statistically significant ($P<0.05$). The occurrence and duration of grade III oral mucositis were reduced ($P=0.01$). LEL applications reduced oral pain as assessed by patients ($P=0.05$) and laser-treated patients required less morphine ($P=0.05$). Also, xerostomia and the ability to swallow were improved ($P=0.005$ and $P=0.01$, respectively). Requirement for parental nutrition was not reduced ($P=$NS). Similar results were obtained by Barasch and colleagues (144). They investigated LEL treatment for the prevention of conditioning-induced oral mucositis in 20 BMT patients, who received irradiation only to one side of the mouth, the others serving as control. Muscositis severity was scored independently by two modified versions of the Oral Mucositis Index Scale and the Eastern Cooperative Oncology Group Oral Toxicity Scale; pain severity was scored by subjects on a visual analog scales (VAS). Oral mucositis and pain scores were significantly lower for the treated versus the untreated side according to mucositis scales ($P<0.005$) and VAS ($P=0.027$) criteria.

Selected classes of chemotherapy, including the vinca alkaloids, vincristine, and vinblastine, can cause direct neurotoxicity. Deep-seated, throbbing mandibular pain can occur. Since this symptom is also consistent with acute dental pulpal disease, it is important that a thorough history and oral physical examination be performed when oral pain is present; radiographs and vitality testing of the dental pulp typically are necessary. Once appropriately diagnosed, management of neurotoxicity includes pain support and counseling of the patient. The symptom generally resolves within a week following cessation of the causative chemotherapy. Dental hypersensitivity may occasionally arise in patients weeks or months following discontinuation of chemotherapy. Although mechanisms are not well delineated, hot or cold thermal stimuli are typically identified. Unlike the relatively rapid resolution of symptoms associated with direct neurotoxicity as noted above, his condition may persist for several months. Topical application of fluorides and/or desensitizing toothpaste may ameliorate the discomfort.

Neutropenic ulcers

Severe neutropenia, with a neutrophil count less than 100 mm^{-3} is often complicated by mouth ulcers: up to 50% of patients admitted for acute leukemia suffer from this complication (145). In about one-third of cases neutropenic ulcers can be traced to local factors such as drug toxicity, HSV infection, leukemia infiltration, trauma, or hemorrhages; the remainder have no clear causes. Ulcers appear as one or more lesions, with few signs of inflammation, regular margins, and a yellowish appearance, not easily removed. Neutrophil count recovery is essential for healing (146).

Graft versus host disease

Patients who have received allogeneic or matched unrelated transplants are at risk for graft-versus-host disease (GVHD) (116,147). The lesion can affect oral tissues and often mimics naturally occurring autoimmune diseases such as scleroderma, erosive lichen planus, Sjogren's Syndrome, and lupus erythematosus. It may present as acute form, occurring as early as two to three weeks post-transplant, commonly with mucosal erythema and erosions/ulcerations. Chronic GVHD can occur as early as 50–60 days post-transplant, although the lesion commonly emerges three months after transplant in most patients

(148). In addition to lesions seen in acute GVHD, elevated white plaques and striae and reduced salivary function are hallmarks. Biopsy of oral mucosa or minor labial salivary glands may be of value in establishing a final diagnosis. The presence of a lymphocytic infiltrate with epithelial cell necrosis provides the diagnostic basis for oral GVHD.

Topical management of mucosal lesions may include steroids and/or oral psoralen and ultraviolet A (PUVA). However, systemic therapies (e.g. prednisone, cyclosporine, and other immunosuppressive agents) are routinely necessary primarily to treat the condition. Patients with clinically significant xerostomia may benefit from pilocarpine if salivary gland function remains partially intact (149).

Radiotherapy-induced stomatitis

Ideal management of the head/neck radiation patient is centered in prevention, based on comprehensive oral care prevaluation. The dentition, periodontium, periapices, and mucosa should be thoroughly examined in order to identify oral disease which should be eliminated prior to cancer therapy. Dentition exhibiting poor prognosis and which lie within high-dose fields should be extracted prior to radiation therapy. Ideally, at least 7 to 14 days should be allowed for healing prior to initiation of radiation, though some have suggested up to 21 days. Surgical technique should be as atraumatic as possible and utilize primary wound closure.

Virtually all patients who receive radiation therapy to the head and neck develop oral side-effects of their treatment. Radiotherapy alone, delivered in standard conventional dose fractions, has been responsible for grade 3 and 4 mucositis in approximately 25% of Radiation Therapy Oncology Group studies (150,151). Other study groups have reported grade 3 mucositis rates approaching 50% (152–154). Accelerated regimens seem to be associated with a doubled incidence of high-grade mucositis, up to 50%–60% (151,152). Aggressive schedules produce mucositis rates ranging from 66% to 86% for grade 3 and from 7% to 48% for grade 4 (154–156), necessitating treatment breaks or dose reductions. Combined chemotherapy and radiotherapy, while producing increases in disease-free and overall survival rates, produces higher rates of toxicity, with grade 3 ranging from 32% to 84% and grade 4 ranging from 0% to 30% (157–161). Radiation-induced oral mucositis is characterized by xerostomia, taste alterations, diffuse erythema, pseudomembrane formation, and ulceration. Usually a two-week interval between initiation of therapy and stomatitis onset is needed (due to the two-week renewal rate of oral mucosa). Patients may start presenting oral soreness ads little as 10 Gy into treatment. Approximately 20 Gy is usually necessary to develop diffuse erythema. Mucositis can be very painful and can strongly reduce oral intake. However, it is self-limiting: approximately three to four weeks after the end of radiation treatment are necessary for healing.

Different strategies are employed for the treatment of radiotherapy-induced stomatitis. Sucralfate, an oral non-absorbable salt of sucrose with its double action—local and systemic—on mucosal surfaces has been widely investigated for prophylactic use in radiotherapy for head and neck cancers. Different controlled studies did not show a significant advantage in the prevention of radiation-associated mucositis (162–167). Glutamine, a non-essential aminoacid, involved as an energy source in intestinal epitheoial integrity, has been tested with some results. Previous studies have shown that it reduces the extent of intestinal injury in radiotherapy and chemotherapy-treated laboratory rats (168,169). In a recent placebo-controlled trial, Huang and colleagues examined whether oral glutamine, 2 g/30 ml could also inhibit radiation-induced mucositis (170). They observed a decreased duration of grade 3 and 4 mucositis as well as decreased severity in degree of mucositis (mean, 1 grade). These early results warrant further investigation with larger patient numbers. Footie *et al.* studied the efficacy of chlorhexidine, a broad-spectrum antibiotic suspension, in a three-arm, randomized, double blind trial in which patients received chlorhexidine, placebo, or an oral non-absorbable antibiotic lozenge composed of amphotericin B, tobramycin, and polymyxin E (171). Analysis of the chlorhexidine and placebo arms among the 52 evaluable patients demonstrated a significant degree of discomfort (e.g. taste alteration and teeth staining) associated with chlorhexidine use, with no evidence of reduction or prevention of mucositis. Another widely used mouth rinse is povidone–iodine: in a small, randomized trial it has been shown to reduce the incidence, severity, and duration of chemoradiotherapy-induced stomatitis/mucositis when compared with placebo (172). A total of 40 patients with head and neck cancer, all of whom received a prophylactic suspension of nystatin, dexpanthenol, rutoside, and immunoglobulin, were treated with either povidone–iodine or water. Povidone–iodine, in contrast to chlorhexidine, was non-irritating and non-toxic. The mean grade of mucositis in the treated group was a significant 1 versus 3 in the control group. Also, the mean onset and duration of mucositis were significantly influenced in the treatment group. No cases of thyroid dysfunction were reported. After experimental work showed a protective effect of gastrointestinal mucosa exposed to radiation, prostaglandins have also been evaluated (173). In a multicenter study, Hanson and colleagues randomized subjects to receive misoprostol or placebo prior to undergoing radiotherapy for surgically resectable head and neck cancer (174). Patients were given either one tablet of misoprostol dissolved in 15 cm^3 of tap water to swish and spit 20 minutes prior to radiation on a daily basis. A modest degree of protection at weeks 4 to 5 among the 17 patients treated in one of the two institutions involved were evidenced. Azelastine, a free-radical scavenger, has shown interesting protective properties in the treatment of aphthous ulcers in Behcet's disease. These data have prompted Osaki and colleagues to evaluate this drug in combination with other antioxidants (vitamin E, vitamin C, and glutathione) for protection against radiotherapy and chemotherapy (peplomycin and 5-FU) in 63 patients, mainly affected by oral squamous cell carcinoma (175). This study demonstrated a delay in the onset to mucositis and less severe mucositis in the azelastine-treated cohort compared with placebo; the duration of mucositis was shorter in the azeslastine arm as well. No effect on tumor regression or growth was observed, and the regimen was non-toxic. Although these initial results indicated some degree of activity, azelastine has since been developed for the treatment of allergies without further investigation with regard to its usefulness in the prevention or treatment or mucositis/stomatitis. Symonds and colleagues looked at the effects of an antibiotic pastille (composed of amphotericin B, tobramycin, and polymyxin E) compared with an oral placebo among 275 patients receiving radiotherapy for head and neck cancer (176). Previously, a smaller study of 15 patients has shown excellent results in preventing higher grades of mucositis and bacterial overgrowth (177). Symonds and colleagues found no statistically significant difference in mucosal pseudomembrane thickness, which was used as a measure for the degree of mucositis; moreover, they showed confinement of the mucositis to a smaller area, a decrease in dysphagia, and a decrease in weight loss in those receiving the pastilles. They concluded that the magnitude of benefit with antibiotic pastilles was probably under-reported because of the statistical limitations of the trial design to reflect such differences (176). In a similar study of 112 patients conducted by the

North Central Cancer Treatment Group and the Mayo Clinic no objective difference in the degree or duration of mucositis was reported between the antibiotic lozenge group and the placebo group, but significantly better comfort scores and a shorter duration of symptoms were reported by the patients themselves (178). Oguchi and colleagues formulated a mucosa-adhesive, water-soluble polymer film (AD film) containing both an anesthetic (tetracaine) and antibiotics (ofloxacin, miconazole, and triacetin) for use in treating radiation-induced mucositis (179). A group of 25 head and neck cancer patients received the topical polymer; results were compared with a group of 27 patients treated for head and neck cancer two to three years earlier. This study has some methodological limitations, but some end-points were improved, including the duration of pain, which was shorter in the group using the AD film (10 days versus 15 days). Secondary bacterial or fungal infections were reported in four patients in the control group, while none was reported among AD film users. No differences in local control or overall survival rates were observed between the groups, and the AD film was associated with no toxic side-effects.

Some small, non-randomized studies indicate that subcutaneous GM-CSF given during radiation therapy reduces the severity of acute mucositis (180–182). Makkonen and colleagues recently examined the activity of GM-CSF to prevent radiation-induced mucositis (183). Forty patients were randomized to receive either sucralfate or sucralfate plus subcutaneous GM-CSF. No differences were observed between the treatment and control groups in the incidence and grade of mucositis, analgesic requirements, weight loss, or survival. A significant number of patients complained of fever, bone pain, and skin reactions at the GM-CSF injection site. In another study, Mascarin *et al.* examined the impact of granulocyte colony-stimulating factor (G-CSF) on oral mucosa in 26 patients receiving radiotherapy for head and neck cancer (184). No difference in severity or duration of mucositis was observed between the 13 patients treated with radiation alone versus the 13 patients receiving G-CSF. Treatment interruptions were significantly greater in the group receiving radiotherapy alone versus the group receiving G-CSF (69% versus 23%). This observation may be somewhat misleading, since the high rate of interruption in the radiotherapy-only goup is very different from that seen in many other studies. Candidiasis is the most common clinical infection of the oropharynx in irradiated patients. Patients receiving head and neck radiation are frequently colonized with *Candida*, as demonstrated by an increase in quantitative counts and rates for clinical infection (185). Candidiasis may exacerbate the symptoms of oropharyngeal mucositis. Treatment of oral candidiasis in the radiation patient has primarily utilized topical antifungals such as nystatin and clotrimazole. Compliance can be compromised secondary to oral mucositis, nausea and pain, and difficulty in dissolving nystatin pastilles and clotrimazole troches. The use of systemic antifungals to treat oral candidiasis has proved effective and may have advantages over topical agents for patients experiencing mucositis (28). Bacterial infections may also occur early in the course of head and neck radiation and should be treated with antibiotics appropriately targeted to culture and sensitivity data.

As noted above, use of the LEL is an interesting technique for the prevention and treatment of mucositis of various origins. In a recent double blind multicenter study, Bensadoun and colleagues randomized 30 patients with carcinoma of the oropharynx, hypopharynx, and oral cavity, treated by radiotherapy alone (65 Gy at a rate of 2 Gy per fraction, 5 fractions per week) without prior surgery or concomitant chemotherapy (186). Patients were randomized to LEL of placebo light treatment (nine application areas in the mouth, outside the tumor site), starting on the first day of radiotherapy and before each session. Grade 3 mucositis occurred with a frequency of 35.2% without LEL and of 7.6% with LEL ($P<0.01$). The frequency of 'severe pain' (grade 3) was 23.8% without LEL, falling to 1.9% with LEL ($P<0.05$). Plain relief was significantly reduced throughout the treatment period (weeks 2–7).

Limiting toxicity by reducing the amount of mucosa exposed to radiation is a logical and practical way of minimizing the damage from radiotherapy in patients with head and neck cancers. Narrow midline blocks have been used, the especially in the lower neck, since most head and neck tumors do not typically involve lower midline structures. In a retrospective review performed on 125 patients diagnosed with primary carcinoma of the head and neck who received conventional three-field post-operative definitive radiation therapy, the authors investigated weight loss, the need for nutritional support, treatment interruptions, and tumor control; the first three parameters were considered reflective of degree of mucositis (187). Among the 125 patients, 61 had a midline mucosal-sparing block (MSB). Results confirm the notion that sparing normal tissue is one of the most effective ways to reduce both short- and long-term toxicity. There was no difference in local tumor recurrence at the primary oral site whether MSBs were employed or not (25% versus 23%); three-year local control rates were equivalent as well (65% versus 64%). The local recurrence rate to the neck was similarly unaffected by the use or non-use of MSBs (22% versus 20%), with no difference seen in local control rates at three years (76% versus 75%). Intensity-modulated radiation therapy (IMRT) also seems to represent a major advance in the treatment of multiple malignancies, including head and neck cancer. With this method, the dose delivered to tumor-related targets is maintained or increased, whereas normal tissues (e.g. mucosa, salivary glands) are relatively spared. Eisbruch and colleagues have investigated 3D and IMRT techniques for parotid sparing in patients with head and neck cancer (188). Pilot results suggest significant physical tissue sparing and less symptomatic xerostomia. Submandibular salivary gland transfer at the time of surgery, prior to radiotherapy, is also under investigation in reducing the degree of acute and chronic xerostomia. Jah and colleagues, in a prospective non-randomized study including patients with head and neck cancer, transferred one submandibular gland from the side of the neck with the least risk of metastases, to the submental area during neck dissection (189). The procedure was performed after a microscopic examination of the neck dissection specimen and added about 45 minutes to the operation time. All the glands survived transfer and functioned well post-operatively as demonstrated on the salivary flow and the radioisotope studies. Post-operatively the residual gland could be easily shielded, and maintained its function.

Late oral complications of radiotherapy

Late oral complications of radiation therapy mainly result from chronic injury to vasculature, salivary glands, mucosa, connective tissue, and bone (190,191). Damage is directly related to radiation dosimetry, including total dose, fraction size, and duration of treatment. Mucosal changes include epithelial atrophy, reduced vascularization, and submucosal fibrosis, resulting in an atrophic, friable barrier. Fibrosis involving muscle, dermis, and temporomandibular joint results in compromised oral function. Loss of acinar cells, alteration in duct epithelium, fibrosis, and fatty degeneration represent the main changes in salivary tissues. Compromised vascularization and remodeling capacity of bone leads to a risk for osteoradionecrosis (ORN).

Caries

Dental caries risk increases for a number of factors including shifts to a cariogenic flora, reduced concentrations of salivary antimicrobial proteins, and loss of mineralizing components (see also Xerostomia section). Treatment strategies must be directed to each component of the caries process. Optimal oral hygiene must be maintained (192,193). Xerostomia should be managed whenever possible via salivary substitutes or replacements. Caries resistance can be enhanced via the use of topical fluorides and/or remineralizing agents. The efficacy of topical products may be enhanced by increased contact time on the teeth by application using vinyl carriers. This approach extends the contact time of the active drug with tooth structure which leads to increased uptake into the enamel. Patients not able effectively to comply with the use of fluoride trays should be instructed to use brush-on gels and rinses. Increased colonization with *Streptococcus mutans* and *Lactobacillus* species increases caries risk. Cultural data can be useful in defining the level of risk in relation to colonization patterns. Topical fluorides or chlorhexidine rinses may lead to reduced levels of *Streptococcus mutans* but not *Lactobacilli.* Due to adverse drug interactions, fluoride and chlorhexidine dosing should be separated by several hours.

Tissue necrosis

Necrosis and secondary infection of previously irradiated tissue is a serious complication for patients who have undergone radiation for head and neck tumors. Acute effects typically involve oral mucosa. Chronic changes involving bone and mucosa are a result of the process of vascular inflammation and scarring that in turn result in hypovascular, hypocellular, and hypoxic changes. Infection secondary to tissue injury and ORN confounds the process. As noted above, risk for necrosis is directly related to radiation dose and volume of tissue irradiated. The unilateral vascular supply to each half of the mandible results in ORN most frequently involving mandible versus maxilla. Presenting clinical features include pain, diminished or complete loss of sensation, fistula, and infection. Pathologic fracture can occur as the compromised bone is unable to appropriately undergo repair at the involved sites. Risk for tissue necrosis is in part related to trauma or oral infection; however, idiopathic cases can also occur. Patients who have received high-dose radiation to the head and neck are at risk for ORN for life, with an overall risk of approximately 15%. Patients who develop ORN should be comprehensively managed including elimination or trauma, avoidance of removable dental prosthesis if the denture-bearing area is within the ORN field, assuring adequate nutritional intake, and discontinuation of tobacco and alcohol use. Topical antibiotics (e.g. tetracycline) or antiseptics (e.g. chlorhexidine) may contribute to wound resolution. Wherever possible, coverage of the exposed bone with mucosa should be achieved. Analgesics for pain control are often effective. Local resection of bone sequestrae may be possible. Hyperbaric oxygen therapy (HBO) is generally recommended for the management of ORN in that it increases oxygenation of irradiated tissue, promotes angiogenesis, and enhances osteoblast repopulation and fibroblast function. HBO is usually prescribed as 20 to 30 dives at 100% oxygen and 2 to 2.5 atmospheres of pressure. If surgery is needed, 10 dives of post-surgical HBO are recommended. Unfortunately, HBO technology is not always accessible to patients who might otherwise benefit. Partial mandibulectomy may be necessary in severe cases of ORN. The mandible can be reconstructed to provide continuity for esthetics and function. A multidisciplinary cancer team including oncologists, oncology nurses, maxillofacial prosthodontists, general dentists, hygienists, and physical therapists is appropriate for management of these patients.

Mandibular dysfunction

Musculoskeletal syndromes may develop secondary ro radiation and surgery. Lesions include soft tissue fibrosis, surgically-induced mandibular discontinuity, and parafunctional habits associated with emotional stress caused by cancer and its treatment. Patients can be instructed in physical therapy interventions including mandibular stretching exercises as well as the use of prosthetic aids designed to reduce the severity of fibrosis. It is important that these approaches be instituted prior to trismus development. If clinically significant changes develop, several approaches including stabilization of occlusion, trigger point injection and other pain management strategies, muscle relaxants, and/or tricyclic medications can be considered.

Local complications of oral tumors

Facial trismus

Facial trismus is the consequence of tumor invasion of masticatory muscles, usually the pterygoids. It is common in retromolar trigone lesions, in very advanced anterior tonsillar pillar and tonsillar fossa tumors, and in soft palate lesions. It is often accompanied by local pain or by pain perceived in the external ear, in the preauricular, or in the temporal area. Occasionally, cranial nerve involvement can be present. It strongly interferes with food intake, but also respiratory function can be affected (194). It can complicate radiotherapy conducted for head and neck cancer: especially when masseter muscles lie in the radiation field, trismus can result, probably due to muscle fibrosis. Trismus frequency is especially relevant after high doses of radiotherapy (195). However, radiotherapy, when possible, is indicated for trismus secondary to tumor infiltration; also chemotherapy can be helpful (196,197). Systemic analgesics, muscle relaxants, and local anesthetic infiltrations may help when trismus depends on a painful stimulus. Oral hygiene presents many problems due to reduced access to the oral cavity. Cotton swabs soaked with antiseptics, sprays, and dental jet can help. Liquid or semisolid feeding is not always possible: whenever indicated a gastrostomy or a nasogastric line could be inserted.

Selected patients may experience spontaneous or induced pain of the temporomandibular joint, affecting mastication. This condition is not unique to cancer patients, and correlates with stress and dysfunctional habits including bruxism and clenching of the jaws. Judicious use of muscle relaxants or anxiety-reducing agents plus physical therapy (moist heat applications, massage, and gentle stretching) are standard approaches for management. For patients who have a propensity for clenching or bruxism during sleep, customized occlusal splints for use while sleeping may be of value.

Abscesses and fistulas

Infections are very common in head and neck cancer populations. They are reported to contribute to about 45% of causes of death in this population (198). Cellulitis, tumor infections, and orocutaneous fistula can contribute approximately 22% of febrile episodes in head and neck cancers (198). This group of patients is very often malnourished, with a previous history of alcoholism and chronic lung disease, and with decreased salivary flow and secretory IgA levels (58). Moreover, surgery, radiotherapy, and chemotherapy often seriously damage the head and neck structures of these patients. Gram-negative shifting of oral flora, including aerobic *Enterobacteriaceae* and *Pseudomonas aeruginosa,* is particularly important (68). Anaerobic Gram-negative bacteria also play a role in head and neck infections (199). All these aspects have to be considered when approaching the management of abscesses and orocutaneous fistulas. A simple povidone–iodine solution can be sufficient as a preventive measure in patients at risk of developing secondary bacterial infections. The same antiseptics can be used as oral medications when an abscess is already present. In the presence of signs of sepsis or of local pain or discharge, wide spectrum antibiotics, including metronidazole, should be administered (199).The patient's relatives should be taught about medication and possible emergencies (for example, massive hemorrhages).

Tumoral discharge

Many oral cavity tumors discharge, causing problems in swallowing and dysphagia and create chronic bad taste in the mouth. In some cases radiotherapy can help this symptom, reducing the tumor mass and its secretions. If not possible, local measures have to be applied. Frequent rinsing with hydrogen peroxide can help in removing tumor debris. Benzydamine hydrocloride rinse can reduce oral cavity colonization and help the patient's mouth feel cleaner (200). Prevention and treatment of other oral problems (for example, candidiasis) is important.

Conclusions

Oral complications still have a limited scientifical data strength supporting most of the everyday decisions. In particular, topical treatments and comfort measures lack convincing clinical evidence. Some of the symptoms affecting the oral cavity, e.g. taste disturbances, are poorly known and underestimated by physicians. Moreover, new cancer therapies may introduce new side-effect. Oral hygiene protocols also should be increasingly implemented. With few exceptions, costs analyses are not available and stringent efforts should be made in this field.

Some important research areas are:

- The epidemiology of oral complications
- Studies of the impact of oral problems on quality of life
- Preventive measures for the side-effects systemic therapies (e.g. radiotherapy xerostomia)
- Impact of nutritional disturbances on oral cavity problems
- Impact of new anticancer therapies and their side-effects on the oral cavity

References

1. **Bodey GP.** Candidiasis in cancer patients. *American Journal of Medicine* 1984;77D:13–19.
2. **Epstein JB; Truelove EL; Izutzu KT.** Oral candidiasis: pathogenesis and host defense. *Review of Infectious Diseases* 1984;6:96–106.
3. **Baines MJ.** Control of other symptoms. In: Baines MJ (ed.) *The Management of Terminal Disease,* 2nd edn. London: Edward Arnold, 1984.
4. **Finlay IG.** Oral symptoms and candida in the terminally ill. *British Medical Journal* 1986;293(3):592–3.

5. **Yeo E; Alvarado T; Fainstein V; Bodey GP.** Prophylaxis of oropharingeal candidiasis with clotrimazole. *Journal of Clinical Oncology* 1985;3(12):1668–71.
6. **De Gregorio MW; Lee WMF; Linker CA., *et al.*** Fungal infections in patients with acute leukemia. *American Journal of Medicine* 1984;73:543–8.
7. **Ball K; Sweeney MP; Baxter WP., *et al.*** Fluconazole sensitivities of Candida species isolated from the mouths of terminally ill cancer patients. *American Journal of Hospital Palliative Care* 1998;15(6):315–19.
8. **Dudiak LA.** Mouth care for mucositis due to radiation therapy. *Cancer Nursing* 1987;10(3):131–40.
9. **Bodey GP; Samonis G; Rolston K.** Prophylaxis of candidiasis in cancer patients. *Seminar in Oncology* 1990;17(3):24–8.
10. **Barret AP.** Evaluation of nystatin in prevention and elimination of oropharingeal Candida in immunosuppressed patients. *Oral Surgery, Oral Medicine and Oral Pathology* 1987;63:698–703.
11. **De Gregorio MW; Lee MW; Ries CA.** Candida infections in patients with acute leukemia: ineffectiviness of nystatin prophylaxis and relationship between oropharyngeal and systemic candidiasis. *Cancer* 1982;50:2780–4.
12. **Barkvoll P; Attramadal A.** Effect of nystatin and chlorexidine digluconate on Candida albicans. *Oral Surgery, Oral Medicine and Oral Pathology* 1989;67:279–81.
13. **Kirkpatrick CH; Alling DW.** Treatment of chronic oral candidiasis with clotrimazole troches: a controlled clinical trial. *New England Journal of Medicine* 1978;299:1201–3.
14. **Yeo BS; Bodey GP.** Oropharingeal candidiasis treated with a troche form of clotrimazole. *Archives of Internal Medicine* 1979;139:656–7.
15. **Roed-Petersen B.** Miconazole in the treatment of oral candidiasis. *International Journal of Oral Surgery* 1978;7:558–63.
16. **Brincker H.** Treatment of oral candidiasis in debilitated patients with miconazole—a new potent antifungal drug. *Scandinavian Journal of Infectious Diseases* 1976;8:63–5.
17. **de Vries-Hospers GH; van der Waaij D.** Salivary concentrations of amphotericin B following its use as an oral lozenge. *Infection* 1980;8:63–5.
18. **Holbrook WP.** Sensitivity of Candida albicans from patients with chronic oral candidiasis. *Postgraduate Medical Journal* 1979;55:692–4.
19. **Holmberg K.** Oral mycoses and antifungal agents. *American Dentistry Journal* 1980;4:53–61.
20. **Symoens J; Moens M; Dom J., *et al.*** An evaluation of two years of clinical experience with ketoconazole. *Review of Infectious Diseases* 1980;2:674–82.
21. **Hughes WT; Bartley DL; Patterson GG; Tufenkeji H.** Ketoconazole and candidiasis: a controlled study. *Journal of Infectious Diseases* 1983;147:1060–3.
22. **Saag MS; Dismukes WE.** Azole antifungal agents: emphasis on new triazole. *Antimicrobial Agents and Chemotherapy* 1988;32:1–8.
23. **Keykants J; Michiels M; Meuldermans W., *et al.*** The pharmacokinetics of itraconazole in animals and man: an overview. In: Fromtling RA., editor. *Recent Trends in the Discovery, Development and Evaluation of Antifungal Agents.* Barcelona: JR Prous Science Publications, 1987: pp. 223–4.
24. **Cauwenbergh G; Dedoncker P; Stoops K., *et al.*** Itraconazole in the treatment of human mycoses: review of three years of clinical experience. *Review of Infectious Diseases* 1987;**9**:S1446–S1452.
25. **De Wit S; Weerts D; Goossens H; Clumeck N.** Comparison of fluconazole and ketoconazole for oropharingeal candidiasis in AIDS. *The Lancet* 1989;1:746–8.
26. **Dupont B; Drouhet E.** Fluconazole for the treatment of fungal disease in immunosuppressed patients. *American Journal of the National Academy of Sciences* 1988;544:564–70.
27. **Allison RR; Vongtama V; Vaughan J., *et al.*** Symptomatic acute mucositis can be minimized or prophylaxed by the combination of sucralfate and fluconazole. *Cancer Investigations* 1995;13(1):16–22.

28. **Mucke R; Kaben U; Libera T., *et al.*** Fluconazole prophylaxis in patients with head and neck tumours undergoing radiation and radiochemotherapy. *Mycoses* 1998;41(9):421–3.
29. **Goodman JL; Winston DJ; Greenfield RA., *et al.*** A controlled trial of fluconazole to prevent fungal infections in patients undergoing bone marrow transplantation. *New England Journal of Medicine* 1992;326(13):845–51.
30. **Schubert MM; Peterson DE; Lloid ME.** Oral complications. In: Thomas ED; Blume KG; Forman SJ., editors. *Hematopoietic Stem Cell Transplantation.* 2nd edn., Malden: Blackwell Science, 1999: pp. 751–63.
31. **Minah GE; Rednor JL; Peterson DE., *et al.*** Oral succession of Gram negative bacilli in myelosuppressed cancer patients. *Journal of Clinical Microbiology* 1986;24:210–13.
32. **Peterson DE; Minah GE; Overholser CD., *et al.*** Microbiology of acute periodontal infection in myelosuppressed cancer patients. *Journal of Clinical Oncology* 1987;5(9):1461–8.
33. **Sonis S; Kunz A.** Impact of improved dental services on the frequency of oral complications of cancer therapy for patients with non-head and neck malignancies. *Oral Surgery, Oral Medicine and Oral Pathology* 1988;65(1):19–22.
34. **Overholsen CD; Peterson DE; Williams LT., *et al.*** Periodontal infections in patients with acute non lymphocytic leukemia: prevalence of acute exacerbations. *Archives of Internal Medicine* 1982;142:551–4.
35. **Peterson DE; Overholsen CD.** Increased morbidity associated with oral infections in patients with non acute lymphocytic leukemia. *Oral Surgery, Oral Medicine and Oral Pathology* 1981;51:390–3.
36. **Rand HR; Kramer B; Johnson AC.** Cancer chemotherapy and associated symptomatic stomatitis and the role of herpes simplex virus. *Cancer* 1986;50:1262.
37. **Barret AP.** A long term prospective clinical study of oral complications during conventional chemotherapy for acute leukemia. *Oral Surgery, Oral Medicine and Oral Pathology* 1987;63:313–16.
38. **Montgomery RT; Redding SW; Le Maistre CF.** The incidence of oral herpes simplex virus infection in patients undergoing cancer chemotherapy. *Oral Surgery, Oral Medicine and Oral Pathology* 1986;61:238–42.
39. **Barret AP; Buckley DJ; Greenberg ML., *et al.*** The value of exfoliative cytology in diagnosing of oral herpes infection in immunosuppressed patients. *Oral Surgery, Oral Medicine and Oral Pathology* 1986;62:175–8.
40. **Park JB; Park NH.** Effect of chlorexidine on the in vitro and in vivo herpes simplex virus infection. *Oral Surgery, Oral Medicine and Oral Pathology* 1989;67:149–53.
41. **Leflore S; Anderson PL; Fletcher CV.** A risk–benefit evaluation of aciclovir for the treatment and prophylaxis of herpes simplex virus infections. *Drug Safety* 2000;23(2):131–42.
42. **Snoeck R; Andrei G; Clercq ED.** Novel agents for the therapy of varicella-zoster virus infections. *Expert Opinion in the Investigation of Drugs* 2000;9(8):1743–51.
43. **Schubert MM; Epstein JB; Lloid ME., *et al.*** Oral infections due to cytomegalovirus in immunocompromised patients. *Journal of Oral Pathology and Medicine* 1993;22(6):268–73.
44. **Spielman A; Ben-Aryed H; Gutzman D; Szargel R; Deutsch E.** Xerostomia-diagnosis and treatment. *Oral Medicine* 1981;51(2):144–7.
45. **Sreebny LM; Valdini A.** Xerostomia. Part I: relationship to other oral symptoms and salivary gland hypofunction. *Oral Surgery, Oral Medicine and Oral Pathology* 1988;66:451–8.
46. **Ventafridda V; De Conno F; Ripamonti C; Gamba A; Tamburini M.** Qualità of life assessment durino a palliative care programme. *Annals of Oncology* 1990;1:415–20.
47. **Oneschuk D; Hanson J; Bruera E.** A survey of mouth pain and dryness in patients with advanced cancer. *Supportive Care in Cancer* 2000;8:372–6.

48. **Twycross RG; Lack SA.** *Control of Alimentary Symptoms in Far Advanced Cancer. The Mouth.* Edinburgh: Churchill Livingstone 1986: pp. 12–39.
49. **Sweeney MP; Bagg J; Baxter WP; Aitchinson TC.** Oral and dental disease in terminally ill cancer patients. *Oral Oncologica* 1998;34:123–6.
50. **Chen MS; Daly TE.** Xerostomia and complete denture retention. *Oral Health* 1980;70:27–9.
51. **Tapper-Jones L; Aldred M; Walker DM.** Prevalence and intraoral distribution of Candida albicans in Sjogren's syndrome. *Journal of Clinical pathology* 1980;33:282–7.
52. **Markitziu A; Gedalin I; Stabholz A; Shuval J.** Prevention of caries progress in xerostomic patients by topical fluoride applications: a study in vivo and in vitro. *Journal of Dentistry* 1982;10:248–53.
53. **Grad H; Grushka M; Yanover L.** Drug-induced xerostomia and treatment. *Canadian Dentistry Association Journal* 1985;4:296–301.
54. **Wolff A; Fox PC; Ship JA; Atkinson JC; Macynski AA; Baum BJ.** Oral mucosal status and major salivary gland function. *Oral Surgery, Oral Medicine and Oral Pathology* 1990;70:49–54.
55. **Zasloff S.** Magainins, a class of antimicrobial peptides from Xenopus skin: isolation, characterization of two active forms, and partial cDNA sequence of a precursor. *Proceedings of the National Academy of Sciences of the United States of America* 1987;84:5449–53.
56. **Makkonen TA; Nordman E.** Estimation of long term salivary gland damage induced by radiotherapy. *Acta Oncologica* 1987;26(4):307–12.
57. **Anderson MW; Izutsu KT; Rice JC.** Parotid gland pathophysiology after mixed gamma and neutron irradiation of cancer patients. *Oral Surgery* 1981;52:495–500.
58. **Brown S; Dreizen LR; Rider I.** The effect of radiation-induced xerostomia on saliva and serum lysozime and immunoglobulin levels. *Oral Surgery* 1976;41:83–92.
59. **Wescott WB; Mira JG; Starcke EN; Shannon IL; Thoruby JI.** Alterations in whole saliva flow rate induced by fractionated radiotherapy. *American Journal of Roentgenology* 1978;130:145–9.
60. **Fox PC.** Acquired salivary dysfunction. Drugs and radiation. *Annals of the New York Academy of Sciences* 1998;842:132–7.
61. **Cheng VST; Downs J; Herbert D; Aramany M.** The function of the parotid gland following radiation therapy for the head and neck cancer. *International Journal of Radiation Oncology and Biological Physics* 1986;12:401–5.
62. **Wescott WB; Starcke EN; Shannon IL.** Some factors influencing salivary function when treating with radiotherapy. *International Journal of Radiation Oncology and Biological Physics* 1981;7:535–41.
63. **Kuten A; Ben-Aryeh H; Berdicevsky I., *et al.*** Oral side-effects of head and neck irradiation: correlation between clinical manifestations and laboratory data. *International Journal of Radiation Oncology and Biological Physics* 1986;12:401–5.
64. **Liu RP; Fleming TJ; Toth BB; Keene HJ.** Salivary flow rates in patients with head and neck cancer 0.5 to 25 years after radiotherapy. *Oral Surgery, Oral Medicine and Oral Pathology* 1990;70:724–9.
65. **Mossman K; Shatzman A; Checharik J.** Long term effects of radiotherapy on taste and salivary function in man. *International Journal of Radiation Oncology and Biological Physics* 1982;8:991–7.
66. **Makkonen TA; Tenovuo J; Vilja P; Hemdahl A.** Changes in the protein composition of whole saliva during radiotherapy in patients with oral or pharyngeal cancer. *Oral Surgery* 1986;62:270–8.
67. **Dreizen S; Brown LR; Handler S; Levy BM.** Radiation-induced xerostomia in cancer patients. Effect on salivary and serum electrolytes. *Cancer* 1976;38:273–8.
68. **Niedermeier W; Matthaeus C; Meyer C., *et al.*** Radiation-induced hyposalivation and its treatment with oral pilocarpine. *Oral Surgery, Oral Medicine, Oral pathology, Oral Radiology and Endocrinology* 1998;86(5):541–9.

69. **Makkonen TA; Borthen L; Hemdahl A; Joensuu H; Lehtonen O-P; Nord CE.** Oropharyngeal colonization with fungi and Gram-negative rods in patients treated with radiotherapy of the head and neck. *British Journal of Oral Maxillofacial Surgery* 1989;27:334–40.

70. **Heimdahl A; Nord CE.** Colonization of oropharynx with pathogenic microorganisms—a potential risk factor for infection in compromized patients. *Chemioterapia* 1986;41:186–91.

71. **Beumer J; Curtis T; Harrison RE.** Radiation therapy of the oral cavity: sequelae and management. *Head and Neck Surgery* 1979;1:301–2.

72. **Carl W; Scaff NG; Chen TY.** Oral care of patients irradiated for cancer of the head and neck. *Cancer* 1972;30:448–53.

73. **Marks JE; Davis CC; Gottsman VL; Purdy JE; Lee F.** The effects of radiation on parotid salivary function. *International Journal of Radiation Oncology and Biological Physics* 1981;7:1013–19.

74. **Crawford JM; Taubman MA; Simth DJ.** Minor salivary glands as a major source of secretory immunoglobulin A in the human oral cavity. *Science* 1975;190:1206–9.

75. **Hensten-Petersen A.** Biological activities in human labial and palatine secretions. *Archives of Oral Biology* 1975;20:107–9.

76. **Handelman SL; Baric JM; Espeland MA; Berglund KL.** Prevalence of drugs causing hyposalivation in an institutionalized geriatric population. *Oral Surgery, Oral Medicine and Oral Pathology* 1986;62:26–31.

77. **Sreebny LM; Valdini A; Yu A.** Xerostomia. Part II: relationship to nonoral symptoms, drugs and diseases. *Oral Surgery, Oral Medicine and Oral Pathology* 1989;68:419–27.

78. **Sreebny LM; Scwartz SS.** Reference guide to drugs and dry mouth. *Gerodontolgy* 1986;5:75–99.

79. **White ID; Hoskin PJ; Hanks GW; Bliss JM.** Morphine and dryness of mouth. *British Medical Journal* 1989;298:1222–3.

80. **Ventafridda V; Ripamonti C; Bianchi M; Sbanotto A; De Conno F.** A randomized study on oral morphine and methadone in the treatment of cancer pain. *Journal of Pain and Symptom Management* 1986;1:203–7.

81. **Joensuu H; Bostrom P; Makkonen T.** Pilocarpine and carbacholine in treatment of radiation-induced xerostomia. *Radiotherapy and Oncology* 1993;26(1):33–7.

82. **Nagler RM; Laufer D.** Protection against irradiation-induced damage to salivary glands by adrenergic agonist administration. *International Journal of Radiation Oncology and Biological Physics* 1998;40(2):477–81.

83. **Kim KH; Kim JY; Sung MW., *et al.*** The effect of pilocarpine and atropine administration on radiation-induced injury of rat submandibular glands. *Acta Otolaryngologica* 1991;111(5):967–73.

84. **Johnson JT; Ferretti GA; Nethery WJ., *et al.*** Oral pilocarpine for post-irradiation xerostomia in patients with head and neck cancer. *New England Journal of Medicine* 1993;329(6):390–5.

85. **Le Veque FG; Montgomery M; Potter D., *et al.*** A multicenter, randomized, double-blind, placebo-controlled, dose-titration study of oral pilocarpine for treatment of radiation-induced xerostomia in head and neck cancer patients. *Journal of Clinical Oncology* 1993;11(6):1124–31.

86. **Rieke JW; Hafermann MD; Johnson JT., *et al.*** Oral pilocarpine for radiation-induced xerostomia: integrated efficacy and safety results from two prospective randomized clinical trials. *International Journal of Radiation Oncology and Biological Physics* 1995;31(3):661–9.

87. **Horiot JC; Lipinski F; Schraub S., *et al.*** Post-radiation severe xerostomia relieved by pilocarpine: a prospective French cooperative study. *Radiotherapy and Oncology* 2000;55(3):233–9.

88. **Jacobs CD; van der Pas M.** A multicenter maintenance study of oral pilocarpine tablets for radiation-induced xerostomia. *Oncology* 1996;10(3S):16–20.

89. **Davies AN; Daniels C; Pugh R; Sharma K.** A comparison of artificial saliva and pilocarpine in the management of xerostomia in patients with advanced cancer. *Palliative Medicine* 1998;12(2):105–11.

90. **Hamlar DD; Schuller DE; Gahbauer RA., *et al.*** Determination of the efficacy of topical oral pilocarpine for postirradiation xerostomia in patients with head and neck carcinoma. *Laryngoscope* 1996;106(8):972–6.
91. **Zimmerman RP; Mark RJ; Tran LM; Juillard GF.** Concomitant pilocarpine during head and neck irradiation is associated with decreased posttreatment xerostomia. *International Journal of Radiation Oncology and Biological Physics* 1997;37(3):571–5.
92. **Utley JF; Marlowe C; Waddell WJ.** Distribution of 35S-labeled WR-2721 in normal and malignant tissues of the mouse. Radiation Research 1976;68:284–91.
93. **Rasey JS; Grunbaum Z; Khron KA., *et al.*** Biodistribution of the radioprotective drug S-labeled 3-amino-2hydroxy-propyl phosphoro-thioate (WR77913). *Radiation Research* 1985;102:130–7.
94. **Brizel DM; Wasserman TH; Henke M., *et al.*** Phase III randomized trial of amifostine as a radioprotector in head and neck cancer. *Journal of Clinical Oncology* 2000;18(19):3339–45.
95. **Bennett CL; Lane D; Stinson T; Glatzel M; Buntzel J.** Economic analysis of amifostine as adjunctive support for patients with advanced head and neck cancer: preliminary results from a randomized phase II clinical trial from Germany. *Cancer Investigations* 2001;19(2):107–13.
96. **Twycross RG; Lack SA.,** editors. *Control of Alimentary Symptoms in Far Advanced Cancer. Taste Change.* Edinburgh: Churchill Livingstone, 1986: pp.57–65.
97. **Gray H.** *Anatomy, Descriptive and Surgical*, 15th edn. New York: Bounty Books, 1977.
98. **Guyton AC; Hall JA.** *Textbook of medical physiology*, 9th edn. Philadelphia: Saunders, 1996.
99. **Schiffman SS.** Taste and smell in disease. *New England Journal of Medicine* 1983;308:1275–9.
100. **De Wys WD; Walters K.** Abnormalities of taste sensation in cancer patients. *Cancer* 1975;36:1888–96.
101. **Williams LR; Cohen MH.** Altered taste thresholds in lung cancer. *American Journal of Clinical Nutrition* 1978;31:122–5.
102. **Kashima HK; Kalinowski B.** Taste impairment following laryngectomy. *Ear, Nose and Throat Journal* 1979;58:88–92.
103. **Mossman KL.** Gustatory tissue injury in man: radiation dose response relationship and mechanisms of taste loss. *British Journal of Cancer* 1986;53(7S):9–11.
104. **Mossman KL; Henkin RI.** Radiation-induced changes in taste acuity in cancer patients. *International Journal of Radiation Oncology and Biological Physics* 1978;4:663–70.
105. **Willonghby JM.** Drug-induced abnormalities of taste sensation. *Adverse Drug Reaction Bulletin* 1983;368–71.
106. **Davies IJ; Musa M; Dormandy TL.** Measurements of plasma zinc II. In malignant disease. *Journal of Clinical Pathology* 1968;21(3):363–5.
107. **Henkin RI; Brandley DF.** Hypogeusia corrected by Hi++ and Zn++. *Life Sciences* 1970;9:701–9.
108. **Ripamonti C; Zecca E; Bruelli C., *et al.*** A randomized, controlled clinical trial to evaluate the effects of zinc sulfate on cancer patients with taste alterations caused by head and neck irradiation. *Cancer* 1998;82:1938–45.
109. **Henkin RI; Schecter PJ; Hoye R; Mattern C.** Idiopathic hypogeusia with dysgeusia, hyposmia and dysosmia: a new syndrome. *Journal of the American Medical Association* 1971;217:434–40.
110. **Henkin RI.** Prevention and treatment of hypogeusia due to head and neck irradiation. *Journal of the American Medical Association* 1972;220:870–1.
111. **Pillitteri LC; Clarck RE.** Comparison of a patient-controlled analgesia system with continuous infusion for administration of diamorphine for mucositis. *Bone Marrow Transplantation* 1998;22(5):495–8.
112. **Strupp C; Sudhoff T; Germing U., *et al.*** Transdermal fentanyl during high-dose chemotherapy and autologous stem cell support. *Oncology Reports* 2000;7(3):659–61.

113. **Sonis ST.** Oral complications of cancer therapy. In: De Vita Jr; Hellman S; Rosenberg SA., editors. *Cancer—Principles and Practice of Oncology*. Philadelphia: Lippincott-Raven, 1989, pp. 2144–52.

114. **Sonis ST.** Mucositis as a biological process: a new hypothesis for the development of chemotherapy-induced stomatotoxicity. *Oral Oncology* 1998;34:39–43.

115. **Raber-Durlacher JE; Weijl NI; Abu Saris M; de Koning B; Zwinderman AH; Osanto S.** Oral mucositis in patients treated with chemotherapy for solid tumors: a retrospective analysis of 150 cases. *Supportive Care in Cancer* 2000;8(5):366–71.

116. **Sonis ST; Oster G; Fucks H., *et al.*** Oral mucositis and the clinical and economic outcomes of hematopoietic stem-cell transplantation. *Journal of Clinical Oncology* 2001;19(8):2201–5.

117. **Beck S.** Impact of a systematic oral care protocol on stomatitis after chemotherapy. *Cancer News* 1979;2:185–99.

118. **Greenberg MS; Cohen SG; Mckifrick JC., *et al.*** The oral flora as a source of septicemia in patients with acute leukemia. *Oral Surgery, Oral Medicine and Oral Pathology* 1982;53:32–6.

119. **McCarthy GM; Awde JD; Ghandi H; Vincent M; Kocha WI.** Risk factors associated with mucositis in cancer patients receiving 5-fluorouracil. *Oral Oncology* 1998;34(6):484–90.

120. **Sloan JA; Loprinzi CL; Novotny PJ; Okuno S; Nair S; Barton DL.** Sex differences in fluorouracil-induced stomatitis. *Journal of Clinical Oncology* 2000;18(2):412–20.

121. **Feld R.** The role of surveillance cultures in patients likely to develop chemotherapy-induced mucositis. *Supportive Care in Cancer* 1997;5(5):371–5.

122. **Loprinzi CL; Dose AM.** Studies on the prevention of 5-fluorouracil-induced oral mucositis. *Oral Oncology* 1996;34:484–90.

123. **Poland JM.** Stomatitis and specific oral infections of the oncologic patients. *American Journal of Hospice Care* 1987;4:30–2.

124. **Clark PI; Slevin ML.** Allopurinol mouthwash and 5-fluorouracil-induced oral toxicity. *European Journal of Surgical Oncology* 1985;11:267–8.

125. **Dose AM; Loprinzi CL; Cianflone S., *et al.*** A controlled evaluation of an allopurinol mouthwash as prophylaxis against 5-fluorouracil-induced stomatitis: a North Central Treatment Group and Mayo Clinic Study. *Proceedings of American Society of Clinical Oncology* 1989;2:55–9.

126. **Mahood DJ; Dose AM; Loprinzi CL., *et al.*** Inhibition of fluorouracil-induced stomatitis by oral cryotherapy. *Journal of Clinical Oncology* 1991;9:449–52.

127. **Rocke LK; Loprinzi CL; Lee JK., *et al.*** A randomized clinical trial of two different durations of oral cryotherapy for prevention of 5-fluorouracil-related stomatitis. *Cancer* 1993;72(7):2234–8.

128. **Fidler P; Loprinzi CL; O'Fallon JR., *et al.*** Prospective evaluation of a chamomile mouthwash for prevention of 5-FU-induced oral mucositis. *Cancer* 1996;77(3):522–5.

129. **Loprinzi CL; Ghosh C; Camoriano J., *et al.*** Phase III controlled evaluation of sucralfate to alleviate stomatitis in patients receiving fluorouracil-based chemotherapy. *Journal of Clinical Oncology* 1997;15(3):1235–8.

130. **Skubitz KM; Anderson PM.** Oral glutamine to prevent chemotherapy induced stomatitis: a pilot study. *Journal of Laboratory and Clinical Medicine* 1996;127:223–8.

131. **Anderson PM; Schroeder G; Skubitz KM.** Oral glutamine reduces the duration and severity of stomatitis after cytotoxic cancer chemotherapy. *Cancer* 1998;83:1433–9.

132. **Okuno SH; Woodhouse CO; Loprinzi CL., *et al.*** Phase III controlled evaluation of glutamine for decreasing stomatitis in patients receiving fluorouracil (5-FU)-based chemotherapy. *American Journal of Clinical Oncology* 1999;22(3):258–61.

133. **Lieschke GJ; Burgess AW.** Granulocyte colony-stimulating factor and granulocyte–macrophage colony-stimulating factor (2). *New England Journal of Medicine* 1992;327:99–106.

134. **Schuchter LM; Luginbuhl WE; Meropol NH.** The current status of toxicity protectants in cancer therapy. *Seminars in Oncology* 1992;19:742–51.

135. **Masucci G.** New clinical applications of granulocyte–macrophage colony-stimulating factor. *Medical Oncology* 1996;13:149–54.

136. **Chi KH; Chen CH; Chan WK., *et al.*** Effect of granulocyte–macrophage colony-stimulating factor on oral mucositis in head and neck cancer patients after cisplatin, fluorouracil, and leucovorin chemotherapy. *Journal of Clinical Oncology* 1995;13:2620–8.

137. **Cartee L; Petros WP; Rosner GL., *et al.*** Evaluation of GM-CSF mouthwash for prevention of chemotherapy-induced mucositis: a randomized, double-blind, dose-ranging study. *Cytokine* 1995;7(5):471–7.

138. **Nolano M; Simone DA; Wendelschafer-Crabb G., *et al.*** Topical capsaicin in humans: parallel loss of epidermal nerve fibers and pain sensation. *Pain* 1999;81(1–2):135–45.

139. **Dray A.** Mechanism of action of capsaicin-like molecules on sensory neurons. *Life Sciences* 1992;51(23):759–65.

140. **Green BG.** Evidence that removal of capsaicin accelerates desensitization on the tongue. *Neuroscience Letters* 1993;150(1):44–8.

141. **Green BG; Rentmeister-Bryant H.** Temporal characteristics of capsaicin desensitization and stimulus-induced recovery in the oral cavity. *Physiological Behavior* 1998;65(1):141–9.

142. **Berger A; Henderson M; Nadoolman W., *et al.*** Oral capsaicin provides temporary relief for oral mucositis pain secondary to chemotherapy/radiation therapy. *Journal of Pain and Symptom Management* 1995;10(3):243–8.

143. **Cowen D; Tardieu C; Schubert M., *et al.*** Low energy Helium-Neon laser in the prevention of oral mucositis in patients undergoing bone marrow transplant: results of a double blind randomized trial. *International Journal of Radiation Oncology and Biological Physics* 1997;38(4):697–703.

144. **Barasch A; Peterson DE; Tanzer JM., *et al.*** Helium-neon laser effects on conditioning –induced oral mucositis in bone marrow transplantation patients. *Cancer* 1995;76(12):2550–6.

145. **Barret AP.** Long term prospective clinical study of neutropenic ulceration in acute leukemia. *Journal of Oral Medicine* 1987;42(2):102–5.

146. **Lockhart PB; Sonis ST.** Relationship of oral complications to peripheral blood leukocyte and platelets count in patients receiving cancer chemotherapy. *Oral Surgery, Oral Medicine and Oral Pathology* 1979;48:21–8.

147. **Schubert MM; Sullivan KM.** Recognition, incidence, and management of oral graft-versus-host disease. *National Cancer Institute, Monograph* 1990;(9):135–43.

148. **Loughran TP Jr; Sullivan K; Morton T., *et al.*** Value of day 100 screening studies for predicting the development of chronic graft-versus-host disease after allogeneic bone marrow transplantation. *Blood* 1990;76(1):228–34.

149. **Schubert MM; Peterson DE; Lloid ME.** Oral complications. In: Thomas ED; Blume KG; Forman SJ, editors. *Hematopietic Cell Transplantation,* 2nd edn. Malden: Blackwell Science, 1999;751–63.

150. **Lee DJ; Cosmatos D; Marcial VA., *et al.*** Results of an RTOG phase III trial (RTOG 85-27) comparing radiotherapy plus etanidazole with radiotherapy alone for locally advanced head and neck carcinomas. *International Journal of Radiation Oncology and Biological Physics* 1995;32:567–76.

151. **Fu KK.** RTOG (90–03): a phase III randomized study to compare twice daily hyperfractionation, accelerated hyperfractionation with concomitant boost to standard fractionation radiotherapy for squamous cell carcinomas of the head and neck. Data on file. Radiation Treatment Oncology Group, Philadelphia, 1993.

152. **Horiot K; Le Fur R; N'Guyen T., *et al.*** Hyperfractionation versus conventional fractionation in oropharyngeal carcinoma: final analysis of a randomized trial of the EORTC cooperative group of radiotherapy. *Radiotherapy in Oncology* 1992;25:231–41.

153. **Dische S; Saunders M; Barrett A., *et al.*** A randomised multicentre trial of CHART versus conventional radiotherapy in head and neck cancer. *Radiotherapy in Oncology* 1997;44:123–36.

154. **Horiot JC; Bontemps P; van den Bogaert W., *et al.*** Accelerated fractionation (AF) compared to conventional fractionation (CF) improves loco-regional control in the radiotherapy of advanced head and neck cancers: results of the EORTC 22851 trial. *Radiotherapy in Oncology* 1997;44:111–21.

155. **Maciejewski B; Skladowski K; Pilecki B., *et al.*** Randomized clinical trial on accelerated 7 days per week fractionation in radiotherapy for head and neck cancer: preliminary report on acute toxicity. *Radiotherapy in Oncology* 1996;40:137–45.

156. **Jackson SM; Weir LM; Hay JH., *et al.*** A randomised trial of accelerated versus conventional radiotherapy in head and neck cancer. *Radiotherapy in Oncology* 1997;43:39–46.

157. **Brownman GP; Cripps C; Hodson DI., *et al.*** Placebo-controlled randomized trial of infusional fluorouracil during standard radiotherapy in locally advanced head and neck cancer. *Journal of Clinical Oncology* 1994;12:2648–53.

158. **Al-Sarraf M; LeBlanc M; Giri PG., *et al.*** Chemoradiotherapy versus radiotherapy in patients with advanced nasopharyngeal cancer: phase III randomized Intergroup study 0099. *Journal of Clinical Oncology* 1998;16:1310–17.

159. **Adelstein DJ; Kalish LA; Adams GL., *et al.*** Concurrent radiation therapy and chemotherapy for locally unresectable squamous cell head and neck cancer: an Eastern Cooperative Oncology Group pilot study. *Journal of Clinical Oncology* 1993;11:2136–42.

160. **Adelstein DJ; Saxton JP; Lavertu P., *et al.*** A phase III randomized trial comparing concurrent chemotherapy and radiotherapy with radiotherapy alone in resectable stage III and IV squamous cell head and neck cancer: preliminary results. *Head and Neck* 1997;19:567–75.

161. **Brizel DM; Albers ME; Fisher SR., *et al.*** Hyperfractionated irradiation with or without concurrent chemotherapy for locally advanced head and neck cancer. *New England Journal of Medicine* 1998;338:1798–804.

162. **Epstein JB; Wong FL.** The efficacy of sucralfate suspension in the prevention of oral mucositis due to radiation therapy. *International Journal of Radiation Oncology and Biological Physics* 1994;28:693–8.

163. **Makkonen TA; Bostrom P; Vilja P; Joensuu H.** Sucralfate mouth washing in the prevention of radiation-induced mucositis: a placebo-controlled double-blind randomized study. *International Journal of Radiation Oncology and Biological Physics* 1994;30:177–182.

164. **Franzen L; Henriksson R; Littbrand B; Zackrisson B.** Effects of sucralfate on mucositis during and following radiotherapy of malignancies in the head and neck region: a double-blind placebo-controlled study. *Acta Oncologica* 1995;34:219–23.

165. **Lievens Y; Haustermans K., *et al.*** Does sucralfate reduce the acute side-effects in head and neck cancer treated with radiotherapy? A double-blind randomized trial. *Radiotherapy in Oncology* 1998;47:149–53.

166. **Carter DL; Hebert ME; Smink K., *et al.*** Double-blind randomized trial of sucralfate vs placebo during radical radiotherapy for head and neck cancers. *Head and Neck* 1999;21:760–6.

167. **Etiz D; Erkal HS; Serin M., *et al.*** Clinical and histopathological evaluation of sucralfate in prevention of oral mucositis induced by radiation therapy in patients with head and neck malignancies. *Oral Oncology* 2000;36:116–20.

168. **Klimberg VS; Souba WW; Dolson DJ., *et al.*** Prophylactic glutamine protects the intestinal mucosa from radiation injury. *Cancer* 1990;66:62–8.

169. **Souba WW; Klimberg VS; Copeland EM.** Glutamine nutrition in the management of radiation enteritis. *Journal of Parenteral and Enteral Nutrition* 1990;14(4S):106S–108S.

170. **Huang EY; Leung SW; Wang CJ., *et al.*** Oral glutamine to alleviate radiation-induced oral mucositis: a pilot randomized trial. *International Journal of Radiation Oncology and Biological Physics* 2000;46(3):535–9.

171. **Foote RL; Loprinzi CL; Frank AR., *et al.*** Randomized trial of a chlorhexidine mouthwash for alleviation of radiation-induced mucositis. *Journal of Clinical Oncology* 1994;12:2630–3.

172. **Adamietz IA; Rahn R; Bottcher HD., *et al.*** Prophylaxis with povidone–iodine against induction of oral mucositis by radiochemotherapy. *Supportive Care in Cancer* 1998;6(4):373–7.

173. **Hanson WR; Houseman KA; Collins PW.** Radiation protection in vivo by prostaglandins and related compounds of the arachidonic acid cascade. *Pharmacology and Therapeutics* 1988;39(1–3):347–56.

174. **Hanson WR; Marks JE; Reddy SP; Simon S; Mihalo WE; Tova Y.** Protection from radiation-induced oral mucositis by a mouth rinse containing the prostaglandin E1 analog, misoprostol: a placebo controlled double blind clinical trial. *Advances in Experimental Medicine and Biology* 1997;400B:811–8.

175. **Osaki T; Ueta E; Yoneda K; Hirota J; Yamamoto T.** Prophylaxis of oral mucositis associated with chemoradiotherapy for oral carcinoma by azelastine hydrochloride (azelastine) with other antioxidants. *Head and Neck* 1994;16:331–9.

176. **Symonds RP; McIlroy P; Khorrami J., *et al.*** The reduction of radiation mucositis by selective decontamination antibiotic pastilles: a placebo-controlled double-blind trial. *British Journal of Cancer* 1996;74:312–17.

177. **Spijkervet KL; Van Saene HK; Van Saene JJ., *et al.*** Effect of selective elimination of the oral flora on mucositis in irradiated head and neck cancer patients. *Journal of Surgical Oncology* 1991;46:167–73.

178. **Okuno SH; Foote RL; Loprinzi CL., *et al.*** A randomized trial of a non-absorbable antibiotic lozenge given to alleviate radiation-induced mucositis. *Cancer* 1997;79:2193–9.

179. **Oguchi M; Shikama N; Sasaki S., *et al.*** Mucosa-adhesive water-soluble polymer film for treatment of acute radiation-induced oral mucositis. *International Journal of Radiation Oncology and Biological Physics* 1998;40:1033–7.

180. **Kannan V; Bapsy PP; Anantha N., *et al.*** Efficacy and safety of granulocyte—macrophage colony-stimulating factor (GM-CSF) on the frequency and severity of radiation mucositis in patients with head and neck carcinoma. *International Journal of Radiation Oncology and Biological Physics* 1997;37:1005–10.

181. **Throuvales N; Antonadou D; Pullizi M., *et al.*** Evaluation of efficacy and safety of GM-CSF in the prophylaxis of mucositis in patients with head and neck cancer treated with radiation therapy. *European Journal of Cancer* 1997;41A(S7):431.

182. **Nicolatou O; Sotiropoulou-Lontou A; Skarlatos J., *et al.*** A pilot study of the effect of granulocyte–macrophage colony-stimulating factor on oral mucositis in head and neck cancer patients during X-radiation therapy: a preliminary report. *International Journal of Radiation Oncology and Biological Physics* 1998;42:551–6.

183. **Makkonen TA; Minn H; Jekunen A., *et al.*** Granulocyte–macrophage colony-stimulating factor (GM-CSF) and sucralfate in prevention of radiation-induced mucositis: a prospective randomized study. *International Journal of Radiation Oncology and Biological Physics* 2000;46:525–34.

184. **Mascarin M; Franchin G; Minatel E., *et al.*** The effect of granulocyte colony-stimulating factor on oral mucositis in head and neck cancer patients treated with hyperfractionated radiotherapy. *Oral Oncology* 1999;35:203–8.

185. **Epstein JB; Freilich MM; Le ND.** Risk factors for oropharyngeal candidiasis in patients who receive radiation therapy for malignant conditions of the head and neck. *Oral Surgery, Oral Medicine and Oral Pathology* 1993;76(2):169–74.

186. **Bensadoun RJ; Franquin JC; Ciais G., *et al.*** Low-energy He/Ne laser in the prevention of radiation-induced mucositis. A multicenter phase III randomized study in patients with head and neck cancer. *Supportive Care in Cancer* 1999;7(4):244–52.

187. **Perch SJ; Machtay M; Markiewicz DA; Kligerman MM.** Decreased acute toxicity by using midline mucosa-sparing blocks during radiation therapy for carcinoma of the oral cavity, oropharynx, and nasopharynx. *Radiology* 1995;197:863–6.

188. **Eisbruch A; Dawson LA; Kim HM., *et al.*** Conformal and intensity modulated irradiation of head and neck cancer: the potential for improved target irradiation, salivary gland function, and quality of life. *Oto-Rhino-Laryngology (Belgian)* 1999;53:271–5.

189. **Seikaly H; Jha N; McGaw T., *et al.*** Submandibular gland transfer: a new method of preventing radiation-induced xerostomia. *Laryngoscope* 2001;111(2):347–52.

190. **Myers RA; Marx RE.** Use of hyperbaric oxygen in postradiation head and neck surgery. *National Cancer Institute, Monograph* 1990;(9):151–7.

191. **Epstein JB; Wong FL; Stevenson-Moore P.** Osteoradionecrosis: clinical experience and a proposal for classification. *Journal of Oral Maxillofacial Surgery* 1987;45(2):104–10.

192. **Jansma J; Vissink A; Spijkervet FK., *et al.*** Protocol for the prevention and treatment of oral sequelae resulting from head and neck radiation therapy. *Cancer* 1992;70(8):2171–80.

193. **Dose AM.** The symptom experience of mucositis, stomatitis, and xerostomia. *Seminars in Oncology Nursing* 1995;11(4):248–55.

194. **Krennmair G; Ulm CW; Lenglinger F.** Effects of reduced mouth opening capacity (trismus) on pulmonary function. *International Journal of Oral Maxillofacial Surgery* 2000;29(5):351–4.

195. **De Crevoisier R; Bourhis J; Domenge C; Wibault P; Koscielny S; Lusinchi A., *et al.*** Full-dose reirradiation for unresectable head and neck carcinoma: experience at the Gustave-Roussy Institute in a series of 169 patients. *Journal of Clinical Oncology* 1999;16(11):3556–62.

196. **Goldstein M; Maxymiw WG; Cummings BJ; Wood RE.** The effects of antitumor irradiation on mandibular opening and mobility: a prospective study of 58 patients. *Oral Surgery, Oral Medicine, Oral Pathology, Oral Radiology and Endocrinology* 1999 Sep;88(3):365–73.

197. **MacKenzie R; Balogh J; Choo R; Franssen E.** Accelerated radiotherapy with delayed concomitant boost in locally advanced squamous cell carcinoma of the head and neck. *International Journal of Radiation Oncology and Biological Physics* 1999;45(3):589–95.

198. **Hussain M; Kish JA; Crane L., *et al.*** The role of infection in the morbidity and mortalità of patients with head and neck cancer undergoing multimodality therapy. *Cancer* 1991;67:716–21.

199. **Barret AP.** Metronidazole in the management of anaerobic neck infection on acute leukemia. *Oral Surgery, Oral Medicine and Oral Pathology* 1988;66:287–9.

200. **Epstein JG; Stevenson-Moore P.** Benzydamine hydrocloride in prevention and management of pain in oral mucositis associated with radiation therapy. *Oral Surgery, Oral Medicine and Oral Pathology* 1988;62:145–8.

Chapter 6

Hiccup

Paul Walker

Introduction

Every person has experienced hiccups of a transient nature. These short spells are commonly experienced by healthy individuals and disappear spontaneously or with simple measures. Fortunately, prolonged episodes of hiccup are rare, but when they do occur, cause significant distress to the patient and caregiver. It has been reported to cause significant discomfort, fatigue, sleep deprivation, weight loss, and depression (1–3).

The known record for prolonged hiccup is held by an individual who hiccupped every $1^1/2$ seconds for 69 years and 5 months (4). There is a paucity of scientific information related to this phenomenon with much of the literature consisting of case reports outlining specific etiologies or treatments. Launois *et al.* have written the most recent comprehensive review of this topic (1).

Definition

The terms hiccup, hiccough, or singultus have been used to describe this phenomenon in the current literature. Hiccup is defined as an involuntary, synchronous, clonic spasm of the intercostal muscles and diaphragm causing sudden inspiration followed by abrupt glottic closure resulting in a characteristic sound (1,5,6). This sound has interestingly been mimicked by the term used for hiccup in most languages which represents an onomatopoeia (1).

Pathophysiology

Electrophysiologic studies were performed on three male patients who suffered from persistent hiccups, by Newsom Davis in 1970 (5). Measurements were performed on these individuals documenting electromyography, arterial blood gases, chest excursion, air flow, and expired CO_2. It was determined that glottic closure occurred 35 msec after diaphragmatic discharge and persisted until discharged had ceased. Because of this early glottic closure, it was determined that hiccups had only a minimal effect on ventilation in these subjects. Each hiccup was found to exhibit synchronous activity of the diaphragm and inspiratory intercostal muscles with coincident inhibition of expiratory intercostal muscle activity. It was initiated by a supraspinal mechanism separate from the normal breathing center. Interaction of the hiccup drive occurred with other respiratory motor neuron stimuli at the spinal level. The characteristics suggested that a hiccup was closer to a gastrointestinal reflex such as vomiting, than a respiratory reflex such as coughing or sneezing. Breath-holding, which increased the PCO_2, was found to reduce the frequency but not amplitude of the hiccup, whereas decreasing the PCO_2 resulted in a significant increase in the amplitude but no alteration in the frequency of the hiccup.

Hiccup may vary in frequency from two to 60 per minute (5,6). It occurs much more frequently in males than females (5) with one source suggesting a 20:1 ratio (7). The complete pathophysiology of this reflex remains poorly understood but the current model favors initiation involving stimulation of the vagus nerve, phrenic nerves, or thoracic sympathetic afferent fibers T6–T12 (5,8). A coordinating hiccup center has been postulated in the brain stem or the cervical spinal cord between C3 and C5 (5). The efferent limb of the reflex is mediated through the phrenic nerve (5,7). A recent case report involving hiccups produced by demyelination secondary to multiple sclerosis at the C5–C6 level confirms that the cervical spinal cord may be involved in this process (9). This is not unexpected as this region innervates the phrenic nerve. Previous reports of intractable hiccups occurring in multiple sclerosis have all been due to lesions located in the medulla (9).

The functional significance of hiccup is unknown. After the eighth week of gestation it is often present in the fetus (10–13). It is frequently observed in young children, becoming less frequent with age. A number of theories have been postulated to ascribe a significance to the hiccup reflex (see Table 6.1).

Hiccup episodes may be transient or prolonged and can occur in healthy individuals or in association with a wide variety of conditions (1,6). Chronic hiccup has been defined as episodes lasting 48 hours or recurring attacks (1,2). Although not particularly helpful, in some articles the term intractable hiccups has been reserved for episodes lasting greater than one month (7). Chronic hiccup that affects multiple members of the same family has been described (14). An autosomal dominant pattern of transmission is suspected (14). This author has presented a schema for the classification of hiccup (Table 6.2).

The incidence and prevalence of this symptom have not been studied extensively (1,15). Cases of hiccup in the terminally ill population are not unusual and have been reported particularly in cases of acquired immune deficiency syndrome (AIDS) and cancer (1,3,15). One group has studied the prevalence of symptoms in the palliative care setting and has found a prevalence of 19 cases among 942 patients studied (16). Approximately 4000 hospital admissions for hiccup each year are reported based on 300 million computerized admissions assembled by the Columbia-Presbyterian Medical Center in New York City (17).

Table 6.1 Postulated theories to explain the function of the hiccup reflex

Persistence of a primitive reflex
Prepares respiratory muscles for breathing after birth
A digestive reflex preventing amniotic fluid aspiration (or caused by gastric distention following amniotic fluid ingestion)
Protects the respiratory tract from esophageal reflux

From ref. (25). Reproduced with permission.

Table 6.2 Classification of hiccup

Acute (transient, occurs commonly)	
Chronic (lasting 48 h or recurring attacks)	
	Associated with disease
	Iatrogenic (medication-induced)
	Idiopathic
	Familial

From ref. (25). Reproduced with permission.

Etiology

A large number of conditions are known to cause or be associated with chronic hiccup. The exact relationship and mechanism of provoking hiccup by these varied conditions is not known. Launois *et al.* chose to classify these etiologies anatomically (Table 6.3)(1). It is surmised that conditions effecting the thorax, abdomen, and ear, nose and throat may cause irritation of the afferent fibers of the hiccup reflex. Diseases of the central nervous system as well as metabolic and psychiatric disorders may influence the higher centers where hiccup is coordinated. Conditions involving the efferent limb of the reflex, namely the phrenic nerves, may also play a role. In all, the number of conditions that have been attributed to inciting chronic hiccup remain extensive and do not aid greatly in the understanding of this phenomenon.

Among hiccup reports gastrointestinal causes rank highly, especially gastroesophageal reflux disease (GERD). This condition is believed to be the most frequent cause of chronic hiccup and treatment of the reflux may result in abolishing the hiccups (18–20). Conversely, one report suggests that esophageal reflux was a direct consequence of the hiccup episode (21). Investigating for esophageal disease or evidence of reflux, or alternatively empiric treatment of such, is commonly suggested to manage hiccup. Esophageal candidiasis is believed to be a common cause of hiccups in AIDS (22,23).

In the setting of advanced cancer, tumors and complications in the abdomen, the thorax, and central nervous system all may play a role in inciting hiccup. Metabolic conditions such as diabetes, hyponatrenia, hyperuracemia, and hypocalcemia, as well as renal failure, may contribute to the development of hiccup in the cancer patient (1). Hiccup may be induced by medication. Common culprits in this regard include corticosteroids such dexamethasone as well as benzodiazapines such as midazolam (22). These drugs are commonly used in the palliative setting to improve symptom control or provide palliative sedation and have been described in the literature as inciting chronic hiccup (1,22). Attributing this condition to a psychogenic cause has been described in multiple cases. However, one authority cautions that with more intensive investigation, an organic factor can usually be found (1). In many advanced cancer patients, with extensive metastatic disease and complications related to cancer, it may not be unusual to have a number of possible causes for prolonged hiccup.

Investigation

Considerations in the medical history include the duration of the hiccup episode, distressing symptoms attributed to them, persistence of hiccup in sleep, or disruption of sleep by

Table 6.3 Etiology of chronic hiccup

Central nervous system

- Craniocerebral injury
- Neoplastic disease:
  - Intracranial neoplasms
  - Brainstem neoplasms
- Demyelinating disease:
  - Multiple sclerosis
- Spinal cord:
  - Syringomyelia
  - Tables dorsalis
  - Cervical hydromyelia
- Cerebrovascular diseases:
  - Ischemic disease
  - Intracranial hemorrhage
  - Arteriovenous malformation
  - Temporal arteritis
- Infectious disease:
  - Meningitis
  - Encephalitis
  - Neurosyphilis
  - Brain abscess
  - Tuberculomas
- Miscellaneous:
  - Epilepsy
  - Hydrocephalus
  - Ventriculo-peritoneal shunt
  - CNS sarcoidosis

Psychiatric causes

- Reaction to grief or shock
- Hysteria
- Personality disorders
- Anorexia nervosa
- Enuresis
- Malingering

Metabolic, infectious, and toxic causes

- Renal failure
- Diabetes
- Metabolic disorders:
  - Hyponatremia
  - Hypocalcemia
  - Hypocapina
  - Hyperuricemia
  - Combination of metabolic disorders
- Fever, septic shock
- Insulin shock therapy
- Alcohol
- Drugs:
  - Alpha methyldopa
  - Dexamethasone
  - Methylprednisolone
  - Sulphonomides
  - Diazepam
  - Midazolam
  - Chlordiazepoxide
  - Barbiturates
  - Methsuximide
  - Heroin addiction
  - Nicotine
  - Etoposide
- Malaria
- Herpes zoster
- Typhoid fever
- Acute rheumatic fever
- Influenza

Ear, nose, and throat

- Pharyngitis, laryngitis
- Goiter
- Neck tumor or lymphadenopathy
- Glaucoma
- Hair or insect in external auditory canal

Thorax

- Lung and bronchi:
  - Pneumonia, bronchitis
  - Tuberculosis
  - Lung cancer
  - Asthma
- Pleura:
  - Pleuritis
  - Emphysema
- Mediastinum:
  - Mediastinitis
  - Tumor
  - Pericarditis
  - Abscess
- Cardiovascular
  - Myocardial infarction
  - Angina pectoris
  - Thoracic aortic aneurysm
  - Irritation caused by foreign body
  - Corpulmonale
- Esophagus:
  - Esophageal cancer or obstruction
  - Esophagitis, esophageal ulcers
  - Hiatus hernia and esophageal reflux
- Diaphragm:
  - Diaphragmatic hernia
  - Diaphragmatic tumors
  - Neurofibroma of phrenic nerve
  - Irritation of foreign body

(Continued)

Table 6.3 (continued) Etiology of chronic hiccup

Abdomen	Peritoneum:
Gastric disorders:	Subphrenic abscess
Gastric cancer, or ulcer	Intra-abdominal abscess
Gastritis	Appendicitis
Gastric distention	Parasitic infection
Foreign body	Peritonitis
Gastrointestinal bleeding	Post-operative
Pancreatic disorders	Cardiovascular disorders:
Pancreatic cancer	Abdominal aortic aneurysm
Pancreatitis	Aortorenal graft
Hepatobiliary disorders:	Irritation caused by wiring of abdominal aorta
Hepato- or splenomegaly	Kidney and urinary tract:
Hepatitis, perihepatitis	Hydronephrosis
Cholecystitis	Prostatic infection and cancer
Cholelithiasis	Prostatic and urinary tract interventions
Cirrhosis	
Intestinal disorders:	
Crohn's disease, ulcerative colitis	
Bowel obstruction	

Note: It is unclear whether conditions reported to cause hiccup are true etiologies or only associations. CNS, central nervous systems.
From ref. (1). Reproduced with permission.

hiccup (1). Situations or conditions that may provoke hiccup, previous alcohol or drug use, surgeries, and medical conditions, as well as previous maneuvers and pharmacological treatments attempted to treat the episodes, should be documented. A complete physical examination should be undertaken with attention to the head and neck, thorax, abdomen, and central nervous system. Laboratory investigations such as complete blood count, electrolytes, glucose, creatinine, BUN, uric acid, and calcium carry little burden and may reveal potential etiologies that are remediable. In some situations an electrocardiogram may be helpful to rule out an atypical myocardial infarction that can provoke a hiccup episode (1). Consideration of the benefits to the individual patient of investigating for esophageal disease or reflux with upper gastrointestinal (GI) endoscopy, esophageal pH monitoring and manometry needs to be considered, as well as imaging of the brain (CT, MRI), thorax (CXR, CT) and abdomen (U/S, CT)(1). This approach is recommended for healthy indi-viduals with chronic hiccup but may not be appropriate for the advanced cancer patient. The patient's ability to tolerate the procedure and the likelihood of positive findings, as well as the potential therapies available should pathology be found, must be considered. It is useful to give forethought to changes in management that would be appropriate, based on scenarios of positive or negative investigations, to most intelligently and compassionately investigate the patient.

Treatment

If possible, treatment of a recognized cause such as GERD or esophageal candidiasis may be possible and may result in resolving the hiccups (1,22). Empiric treatment may be warranted when these conditions are expected. If possible, discontinuing medications, which may have provoked the hiccups, is warranted. Medications that have been linked to causing hiccup are listed in Table 6.3. The patient's medication list should be carefully checked for these potentially troublesome agents. Dexamethasone may commonly contribute to this problem in the oncology setting. A large variety of folk remedies and maneuvers have been suggested (Table 6.4). However, it is unusual in the setting of chronic hiccup for these techniques to be effective. Moreover, caution must be exercised as over-zealous administration of non-drug maneuvers and phrenic nerve disruption have resulted in serious consequences for patients (1).

Drug treatment relies heavily on the case literature reporting anecdotal evidence of medications that have helped resolve or reduce troublesome hiccups. To date, a large number of medications have been reported, including most medications that are thought to have an effect on the GI or nervous systems (24). Most agents cited would usually have less than five reported cases (1). A list of the most common drug treatments is presented

Table 6.4 Non-pharmacological treatment of hiccup (from case reports)

Common remedies

1. Respiratory maneuvers
   - Breathholding associated with: neck extension, quickly drinking a large glass of water, steady inspiratory effort against closed airway, application of 20–40 cm H_2O CPAP
   - Coughing, valsalva maneuvers, hyperventilation
   - Rebreathing in a bag, or breathing a 5% CO_2 mixture
   - Compression of the diaphragm by drawing legs up or leaning forward, compression of thyroid cartilage
   - Application of ice or mustard plaster on epigastrum
2. Nasal and pharyngeal stimulation
   - Pressure on the bridge of nose, sneezing, pressure on the upper lip
   - Inhalation or instillation of irritants (smelling salts, ether, ammonia)
   - Gargling with water
   - Firm traction of the tongue
   - Drinking: from the far side of a glass, from a glass covered with a piece of fabric, one can of lemonade quickly then lie down, carbonated beverages, ice water, alcohol, tea, vinegar, sweet pickle juice
   - Swallowing: granulated sugar, crushed ice or stale bread, crushed pepper, sugar lump dipped in vinegar, lemon wedge, and Angostura bitter
   - Touch soft palate with tip of the tongue then swallow, posterior pharyngeal wall stimulation, massage of hard/soft palate junction
3. Miscellaneous vagal stimulation
   - Ocular compression, carotid massage, digital rectal massage
4. Psychiatric treatment
   - Behavioral therapy, hypnosis
5. Gastric distension relief
   - Fasting for 24 h, gastric aspiration or lavage, vomiting

Other remedies

Bilateral compression of radial arteries while gazing into the subject's eyes, rest in bed, fright, acupuncture, prayers, wrap patients in wet cold sheets, hydrotherapy, relaxation, concentration, bilateral pressure on external auditory meatus, homeopathy, mesotherapy, pinching the external side of the wrist

Phrenic nerve disruption

Transient disruptions:
- Cooling
- Local anesthetic injection
- Compression of phrenic nerve at the neck

Phrenic nerve stimulation

Phrenic crush or section
- Bilateral
- Unilateral

From ref. (1). Reproduced with permission.

in Table 6.5. Chlorpromazine is mentioned in many textbooks and is commonly considered by many practitioners as the agent they would consider first. However, the literature has recently been replete with cases of Baclofen's effectiveness in the setting of chronic hiccup unresponsive to multiple agents including chlorpromazine. Baclofen was first suggested by Burke in 1988. Since that time case reports of its effectiveness have outnumbered other drugs, and it is now widely regarded as the most effective agent for this condition (Table 6.6)(1,14,25–30). An oral preparation of Baclofen is available and intrathecal administration is used in severe cases of spasticity due to multiple sclerosis and spinal cord injury. Little information is available regarding subcutaneous or intravenous routes of administration (25). The limited experience of this author with Baclofen tablets administered rectally was unsuccessful.

Only one controlled trial has been published. Ramirez and Graham performed a double-blind, randomized, placebo-controlled, crossover trial using Baclofen in four men with idiopathic hiccup of at least six month duration, unresponsive to medical therapy (31). All four subjects had not responded to cholorpromazine or metaclopramide. A statistically significant improvement in the severity of hiccup was seen with baclofen. This was reported by the patient subjectively and by hiccup-free periods as assessed by a blinded observer. Hiccup frequency was not effected, however. In these four subjects hiccup was not eliminated, in contrast to what is reported in the case literature. This may be related to the modest dosages that were administered in the trial (15 and 30 mg day^{-1}). Benefit persisted for the duration of treatment with Baclofen but relapsed with discontinuation of the drug. During the study no side-effects were reported. Following the protocol some patients

Table 6.5 Drug treatment of hiccup

Drug	Dosage
Baclofen	5–60 mg daily PO
Chlorpromazine	25–50 mg IV in 30–60 min then 50–60 mg daily PO
Metoclopramide	10 mg IV then 10–40 mg daily PO
Haloperidol	2 mg IM, 5–10 mg daily PO
Amitriptyline	25–90 mg daily PO
Gabapentin	400 mg PO thrice daily
Carbamazepine	600–1200 mg daily PO
Diphenylhydantoin	200 mg IV then 300–400 mg daily
Valproic acid	5 mg kg^{-1} daily PO then increase by 250 mg per week until hiccup stops
	500 mg × three PO
Nifedipine	10–80 mg daily PO
Nefopam	10 mg IV
Mephensin	1000 mg PO
Orphenadrine	400 mg PO or 60 mg IM

Divided dosing schedules required for most daily does noted.
PO, oral; IM, intramuscular; IV, intravenous.
Adapted from refs. (1) and (25).

Table 6.6 Baclofen

GABA analog, oral route provides rapid absorption, half-life of 3–4 h, renal excretion
Mechanism of action uncertain, possibly as an agonist at GABA-B receptor
Acts at the level of the spinal cord by inducing presynaptic motor neuron inhibition (centrally active antispasticity effect) Commonly used in multiple sclerosis and spinal cord injury patients
Dosage: start with 5 mg orally every 8 h increasing each dose by 5 mg every three days until effective
Some references report the maximum dose to be 80 mg day^{-1}; however, oral doses up to 300 mg day^{-1} have been used to treat spasticity
Sedation: commonest side-effect. Alcohol and other centrally acting depressants have an additive effect
Other side-effects: insomnia, dizziness, weakness, ataxia, mental confusion
May be poorly tolerated by the elderly
Interactions with tricyclic antidepressants can increase Baclofen's effect
Should not be discontinued suddenly; gradual tapering is recommended to avoid withdrawal symptoms such as anxiety, seizure, tachycardia, auditory and visual hallucinations

From ref. (25). Reproduced with permission.

tried to increase the dose of Baclofen to improve symptom control further. They experienced sedation at a dose of 20 mg four times daily; this resolved when the dose was decreased.

Guelaud *et al.* a multidisciplinary group established in Paris in 1991 to study the pathophysiology and treatment of chronic hiccup, performed an open trial on 72 male patients with chronic hiccup (32). Fifty-five patients with evidence of GERD were treated with full doses of omeprazole and cisapride; 35 patients responded completely to this treatment. Of the remaining 20 patients who did not respond, Baclofen was added to the regimen starting at 5 mg three times daily and increasing by 15 mg per day every three days, until the hiccups were controlled; a maximum dose of 75 mg per day was reached, or adverse events occurred. Seventeen patients from the original group who did not have empiric treatment for GERD also received Baclofen treatment. Of these 37 patients with chronic hiccup (average duration of 4.6 years) the addition of Baclofen resulted in complete resolution (18 cases) or considerable decrease of hiccups (10 cases) in 28 of the 37 patients. Treatments failure was reported in six patients and three patients were lost to follow-up. Overall, substantial improvement or complete resolution was reported in 82% of cases (76%, if patients lost to follow-ups are counted as failures). Adverse events were not encountered except for nausea and somnolence reported in a few patients requiring more than 45 mg per day. This resolved when the doses were decreased. This was an open study and the authors commented that questions may arise on whether the effect was purely by coincidence or due to the placebo effect. They believe this was very unlikely as the great majority of the cases had persistent hiccups for many years which were not improved by a variety of mechanical, psychological, alternative medical, or standard pharmaceutical therapies. During the treatment hiccups were found to stop rapidly after Baclofen treatment or, alternatively, to progressively decrease in frequency and amplitude over a number of days. Withdrawal of medications was suggested following successful hiccup treatment, as hiccups may not relapse. In the case of relapse, the authors of the study have found that reapplication of the drug had always been efficacious. This study suggests that a large portion of idiopathic chronic hiccup may be due to silent gastroesophageal reflux. It was the first to suggest an algorithm utilizing cisapride and omeprazole as initial therapy followed by the addition of baclofen.

Petroianu *et al.* utilized this combination approach in an open trial of 15 male patients with various medical disorders and chronic hiccup of mean duration 100 months (7). The regimen consisted of cisapride 10 mg three times daily, omeprazole 20 mg daily, and baclofen 15 mg three times daily. These patients had tried an average of five medications to alleviate hiccup prior to the study. Hiccups disappeared completely in six patients while three experienced substantial relief. The remaining six patients had no hiccup relief. This combination therapy was stated to produce significant relief of hiccup in 60% (9 of 15) of patients treated.

These same researchers reported four cases of chronic hiccup associated with a variety of medical conditions (33). In two of the cases the combination of cisapride, omeprazole and gabapentin required the addition of baclofen, with improvement resulting. In one patient the combination of cisapride, omeprazole, and gabapentin resolved the hiccups while in another cisapride, omeprazole, and baclofen required the addition of gabapentin before hiccups resolved. These authors stated that they believed gabapentin is a useful agent for this condition and speculated that unlike baclofen, which is a GABA agonist, acting by depressing synaptic transmission at the spinal level, gabapentin may increase endogenous GABA release and thus modulate CNS excitability. They propose an algorithm where cisapride and omeprazole are used initially and then stepwise, baclofen and then gabapentin are added as required until successful hiccup treatment occurs. Their approach is to maintain the successful therapy for six months and then slowly withdraw the regimen over three to six months.

Gregory *et al.* performed a controlled trial in 51 anesthesized patients with hiccup but that did not stop spontaneously. No difference was found between treatment with methylphenidate or treatment with the saline solution (34).

Bilotta reports three cases where an infusion of 10 mg of nefopam IV resulted in hiccups being abolished within one minute (35). These patients had limited duration hiccup which had failed to respond to vagal maneuvers in one case, vagal maneuvers and bolus lidocaine infusion in the second case, and vagel maneuvers, chlorpromazine, and lidocaine infusion in the third case. These patients had not been administered baclofen or treatment for GERD. These patients had troublesome, severe hiccups of a short duration which would not be termed intractable. Nefopam is a non-opioid analgesic available in Europe and Israel but only available in the United States on an investigational basis. These cases provide interesting data that require further support.

Based on the above findings a rational approach to the advanced cancer patient with chronic hiccup can be extrapolated (Fig. 6.1). Clinical judgment is required regarding the extent of investigations that would be appropriate in each individual case. The limited evidence to date supports empiric trials of medications for GERD. Since cisapride has been discontinued in some countries, including the United States and Canada, because of the concerns that it may produce fatal ventricular arrhythmia, it may be necessary to substitute metaclopramide or domperidone for cisapride, in combination with omeprazole.

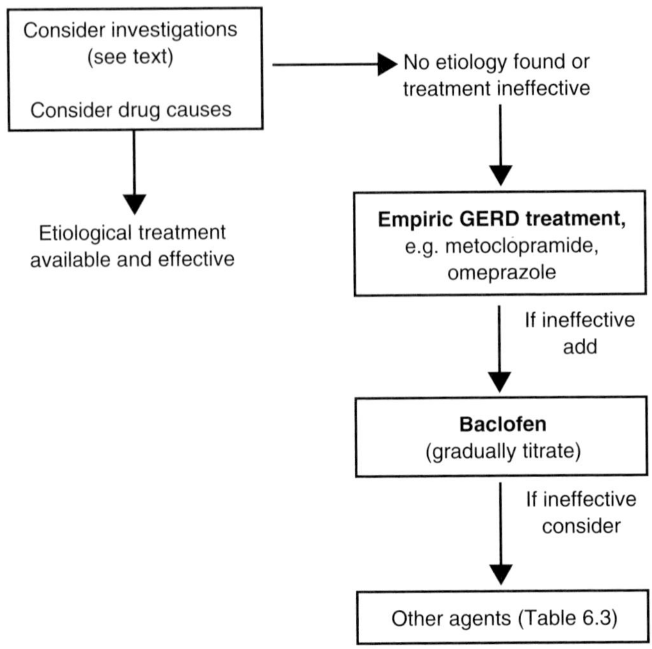

Figure 6.1 Management of chronic hiccup in advanced cancer.

If this is not effective, baclofen may then be added starting at a dose of 5 mg three times daily and increasing each dose by 5 mg every three days until improvement or side-effects occur. If this is not effective, then a further agent such as gabapentin may be considered for addition to the regimen. Following regular use of baclofen abrupt discontinuation can lead to serious withdrawal symptoms such as seizures, and therefore gradual discontinuation is recommended.

Treatments that disrupt the phrenic nerve have been reported in situations where all else fails. Phrenic nerve crush or section techniques used unilaterally or bilaterally have resulted in severe consequences. Dobelle reports a selected series of seven patients who underwent implantation of breathing pacemakers which electronically stimulate the phrenic nerve in a continuous fashion (17). One patient is reported to be hiccup-free for five years and no known systemic effects are reported. This data appear preliminary and further study is required.

Summary

While transient hiccup may be trifling, chronic hiccup can be a severe problem. This peculiar symptom has eluded more intensive study due to its rarity. Its function remains unknown and much remains to be learned about the hiccup reflex. Treatment is based largely on case reports and a few clinical studies. Investigating for reversible causes and empiric treatment for GERD may be considered as first approaches to management. Baclofen has emerged as the agent with the strongest pedigree for managing chronic hiccup.

References

1. **Launois S; Bizec JL; Whitelaw WA; Cabane J; Derenne J.** Hiccup in adults: an overview. *European Respiratory Journal* 1993;6:563–75.
2. **Souadjian JV; Cain JC.** Intractable hiccup. *Postgraduate Me*dicine 1968;43: 72–7.
3. **Howard RS.** Persistent hiccups. *British Medical Journal* 1992;305:1237–8.
4. **Young MC.**, editor. Hiccuping. *The Guinness Book of Records.* New York: Bantam Dell Doubleday, 1997: p. 28.
5. **Newsom Davis J.** An experimental study of hiccup. *Brain* 1970;93:851–72.
6. **Samuels L.** Hiccup. *Canadian Medical Association* 1952;67:315–22.
7. **Petroianu G; Hein G; Petroianu A; Bergler W; Rufer R.** Idiopathic chronic hiccup: combination therapy with Cisapride, Omeprazole, and Baclofen. *Clinical Therapeutics* 1997;19:1031–8.
8. **Salem M; Baraka A; Rattenborg C; Holaday DA.** Treatment of hiccups by pharyngeal stimulation in anesthetized and conscious subjects. *Journal of the American Medical Associatio*n 1967;202:32–6.
9. **Funakawa I; Terao A.** Intractable hiccups and syncope in multiple sclerosis. *Acta Neurologica Scandinavica* 1998;98:136–9.
10. **Norman HN.** Fetal hiccups. *Journal of Comparative and Physiological Psychology* 1942;34:65–73.
11. **Lewis PJ; Trudinger B.** Fetal hiccups. *The Lancet* 1988;2:355.
12. **Brouillettte TR; Thatch BT; Abu-Osba YK; Wilson SL.** Hiccups in infants: Characteristics and Effects on Ventilation. *Journal of Pediatrics* 1980;96:219–25.
13. **Pillai M; James D.** Hiccups and breathing in human fetuses. *Archives of Disease in Childhood* 1990;65:1072–5.
14. **Lance JW; Bassil GT.** Familial intractable hiccup relieved by baclofen. *The Lancet* 1989;2:76–277.
15. **Twycross RG.** Dysphagia depression and hiccup. In: Doyle D; Hanks GWC; Macdonald N. editors. *The Oxford Textbook of Palliative Medicine.* London: Oxford Medical Publications, Oxford University Press, 1992: pp. 291–9.
16. **Donnelly S; Walsh D.** The symptoms of advanced cancer. *Seminars in Oncology* 1995;2:67–72.
17. **Dobelle W.** Use of breathing pacemakers to suppress intractable hiccups of up to thirteen years duration. *ASAIO Journal* 1999;45:524–5.
18. **Cabane J; Desmet V; Detrenne JP., *et al.*** Le hoquet chronique. *Revue de Medicine Interne* 1992;13:454–9.
19. **Seibert D; Al-Kawas F.** Trimethoprimsulfamethoxazole, hiccups, and esophageal ulcers. *Annals of Internal Medicine* 1986;105:976.
20. **Gluck M.** Chronic hiccups and gastroesophageal disease: the acid perfusion test as a provocative maneuver. *Annals of Internal Medicine* 1986;105:219–20.
21. **Triadafilopoulos G.** Hiccups and esophageal dysfunction. *American Journal of Gastroenterology* 1989;84:164–9.
22. **Gilson I; Busalacchi M.** Marijuana for intractable hiccups. *The Lancet* 1998;351:267.
23. **Albrecht H; Stellbrink HJ.** Hiccups in people with AIDS. *Journal of Acquired Immune Deficiency Syndrome* 1994;7:735.
24. **Williamson BWA; MacIntyre IMC.** Management of intractable hiccup. *British Medical Journal* 1977;20:501–3.
25. **Walker P; Watanabe S; Bruera E.** Baclofen, a treatment for chronic hiccup. *Journal of Pain and Symptom Management* 1998;16:125–32.
26. **Burke AM; White AB; Brill N.** Baclofen for intractable hiccup. *New England Journal of Medicine* 1998;319:1354.

27. **Yaqoob M; Prabhu P; Ahmad R.** Baclofen for intractable hiccups. *The Lancet* 1989;2:562–3.
28. **Haas C; Lowenstein W; Fadlallah JP; Durand H.** Traiement du hoquet rebelle par—le baclofen. *Presse Medicale* 1991; 20–658.
29. **Bhaloatra R.** Baclofen therapy for intractable hiccoughs. Letter. *Journal of Clinical Gastroenterology* 1990;12:122.
30. **Grant JA; Steiner EM; Johnson RH.** Treatment of persistent hiccups. Letter, *Journal of Neurology, Neurosurgery and Psychiatry* 1991;54:468.
31. **Ramirez F; Graham D.** Treatment of intractable hiccup with Baclofen: results of a double-blind randomized, controlled, cross-over study. *American Journal of Gastroenterology* 1992;87:1789–91.
32. **Guelaud C; Similowski T; Bizec J-L; Cabane J; Whitelaw WA; Derenne JP.** Baclofen therapy for chronic hiccup. *European Respiratory Journal* 1995;8:235–7.
33. **Petroianu G; Stegmeier-Petroianu A; Bergler W.** Gabapentin 'Add-on Therapy' for Idiopathic Chronic Hiccup (ICH). *Journal of Clinical Gastroenterology* 2000;30(3):321–35.
34. **Gregory GA; Way WL.** Methylphenidate for the treatment of hiccups during anesthesia. *Anesthesiology* 1969;31:89–90.
35. **Bilotta F; Giovanni R.** Nefopam for severe hiccups. Letter. *New England Journal of Medicine* 2000;343:1973–4.

Chapter 7

Gastrointestinal motility disorders

Mellar P. Davis and Declan Walsh

Symptoms of dysmotility in the normal population

A three-month prevalence survey from 10 international sites using 5581 face-to-face interviews revealed that 46% of subjects experienced one or more of 14 different gastrointestinal symptoms (217). Upper gastrointestinal symptoms were experienced in 28%, reflux symptoms by 7.7%, ulcer-like dyspepsia in 4.1%, and dysmotility-like dyspepsia (nausea, bloating, and satiety) in 15.5% (217). Women experienced more reflux and dysmotility than men. Reflux symptoms increased and dysmotility decreased with age (217).

In a second study of 1036 Canadian adults closely matched to the normal population, 28% reported substantial gastrointestinal symptoms occurring within three months of interview with most experiencing symptoms for over one year (233). Only 34% never experienced gastrointestinal symptoms. Dysmotility-like symptoms were experienced in nearly 55% of those with chronic symptoms, ulcer-like symptoms in 12%, and reflux symptoms in 42% (233). Chronic intestinal symptoms significantly reduced psychological well-being.

Gastrointestinal symptoms in advanced cancer

A survey of patients in the Cleveland Clinic Palliative Medicine Program included age, gender, diagnosis, current treatment, gastrointestinal symptoms, changes in weight, and food intake (196). This survey included 353 consecutive admissions to an acute palliative medicine unit, 180 of whom were men (196). The median age was 61 years (range 20–94 years). The most common diagnosis was lung cancer. Metastatic disease was present in 81%, and 42% had intra-abdominal metastases. Weight loss had occurred in the past six months in 85% (196). There was anorexia in 80%, early satiety in 69%, constipation in 58%, nausea in 48%, bloating in 43%, vomiting in 38%, and abdominal pain in 37% (162,196). Both belching and indigestion were found in 35%. Symptoms of dyspepsia, including early satiety, nausea, bloating and abdominal pain, were found in up to two-thirds of individuals (162,196).

Normal anatomy and gastrointestinal motility

The absorptive, motility, and secretory functions must be coordinated to digest nutrients (250). Bowel motility is governed by muscle cells; predominantly smooth muscle, which has intrinsic depolarization (29,34). An extrinsic nervous system of parasympathetics from the vagus and sacral nerve roots, and sympathetics in prevertebral ganglia along the thoracic and lumbar spine coordinate complex gastrointestinal reflexes (29,34,78,250). Both post-ganglionic parasympathetics and sympathetic fibers innervate the enteric nervous system (29,250). The gastroileal and gastrocolic reflexes exert 'positive forward' control of intestinal transport and the inhibitory reflex caused by rectal distention (delaying ileal and gastric emptying) is governed by the extrinsic parasympathetic and sympathetic pathways (53,78,250). Vagus innervation extends from the esophagus to the transverse colon (34,78). The sacral parasympathetic plexus innervates the descending colon, sigmoid, and rectum (29). Parasympathetic ganglia are within the walls of the gastrointestinal tract, whereas the sympathetics are prevertebral (63). Sympathetic fibers inhibit motility, whereas parasympathetics are prokinetic (29,78,252).

Four levels of motility control exist. The enteric nervous system is a 'minibrain' with interconnected ganglia to integrate, coordinate, and process information from the brain and spinal cord (53,122,231,252). This system divides into the myenteric and submucosal plexus which controls muscle contraction, mucosal transport, and intramural blood flow (78,252). The enteric system is responsible for specialized behaviors such as (a) post-prandial fundic relaxation, (b) triturabation of the stomach, (c) migratory motor complexes (MMC) of the small bowel and stomach, (d) giant migratory contractions (GMC) of the distal small bowel, through the proximal colon, and (e) retropulsive behavior of the upper small bowel, stomach, and sphincter relaxation (34,78,122,230). A system of ganglion and interganglionic fibers are located circumferentially and longitudially along the gastrointestinal tract (34,78,189,230,245,252). Enteric nerve fibers are unmyelinated C-fibers. The dominant myenteric plexus is closely applied to the longitudinal muscle between the circular and longitudinal muscle layers (143,250). The lesser submucosal plexus is between the circular muscle and the mucosa (78,230). Interconnections exist so as to function as a unified system (34,189). Neural elements consist of sensory, motor, and interneurons (78,143,189). Like the brain, there are multiple synapses and interconnections (34,53,122, 230,252). The primary sensory receptors respond to mechanical and chemical sensory stimuli (37,252). Nociceptive equivalents to C-fibers and A-delta fibers ascend as sensory afferent fibers within the vagus and when stimulated elicit nausea and vomiting (34,37,250,251). The stimulation of afferents traveling with the sympathetic fibers to the dorsal root via the splanchnic nerves evoke pain (37,78,250,251).

The second level within the prevertebral sympathetic ganglia acts as a gastrointestinal 'brake' mediated by norephinephrine (34,78,250,251). The parasympathetics in the medulla and sacral cord release acetylcholine and are prokinetic (250,251,252). The third and fourth levels include the higher brain centers, which integrate sympathetic and parasympathetic output (37,73,250,252). They receive afferent information by dorsal horn sympathetics and the nucleus tractus solitarius by the vagus ascending through the thalamus and cingulate gyrus and other cortical centers resulting in the sensory experience of gastrointestinal symptoms (37,73,78,250,252).

The enteric nervous system has both excitatory and inhibitory neurons (78,79,189). Acetylcholine and substance P are the main excitatory neurotransmitters evoking muscular contraction (34,78,189,250). Inhibitory motor neurons release adenosine triphosphate, vasoactive intestinal peptide (VIP), and nitric oxide, which suppress contractile activity (34,78,189,250). Interstitial cells of Cajal act as pacemakers to the smooth muscle which uniquely have an electrical syncytium (53,79,95,123,252). Inhibitory neurons to circular muscle discharge continuously; action potentials leading to contraction within the syncytium occur only when these inhibitory neurons are switched off by input from interneurons (34,78,189,252). In sphincters the opposite is true. The inhibitory neurons are normally inactive but are switched on when appropriate to coordinate sphincter opening with peristalsis. Inhibitory neurons govern the length of contraction by controlling the distant spread of action potentials within the syncythium.

Neuropeptide and effectors of gastrointestinal motility and their receptors

The enteric nervous system uses more than 25 neurotransmitters, many are colocalized with other transmitters and similar to those within the central nervous system (78,250). These include acetylcholine (ACh), serotonin (5HT), vasoactive intestinal peptide (VIP), nitric oxide (NOS), and somatostatin (164,189). Norephinephrine is in the post-ganglionic efferent sympathetic nerves (78). Norephinephrine action on alpha$_2$-adrenoceptors through enteric colon neurons inhibits proximal motility when the distant colon is distended, i.e. the colocolonic inhibitory reflex (34,78,94). Tachykinins delay gastric emptying and mediate giant migrating contractions of the colon and small bowel (89,182,197). The right colon contains fewer VIP and nitric oxide containing fibers than the left (34,78,144,164,190). Both VIP and nitric oxide positive neurons are differently distributed in the inner and outer portions of circular muscle (34,78,144,164,190). Glutamate, a major excitatory neurotransmitter in the central nervous system, is also an excitatory neurotransmitter in the enteric nervous systems (113). A subset of enteric neurons express *N*-methyl-D-asparate (NMDA) receptors (113). Opioid receptors, found on intestinal smooth muscle, nerves, and mucosal surfaces decrease in density from proximal to distal small bowel (50).

Serotonin is a secretagogue in the small and large intestine and modulates motility (80,85). It mediates secretion via epithelial 5HT2 and neuronal 5HT3 and 5HT4 receptors in the submucosal plexus (27,80,85). Serotonin alters motility both through cholinergic and non-cholinergic pathways (85,224). Many 5HT3 receptors are in the vagus primary afferent neurons which initiate the vomit reflex (78,85,224). The three enteric serotonin excitatory neuron receptor subtypes are 5HT1P, 5HT3, and 5HT7 (9,27,85,100,149,175,224,228, 229,231). The receptor 5HT2B mediates a contractile response in the longitudinal muscle of the small bowel (23). The receptor 5HT1A is an inhibitory motor receptor.

Gastrin induces fundic relaxation and increases gastric wall compliance (102,151). Motilin, a prokinetic intestinal peptide, stimulates contraction of smooth muscle and has its highest concentration in the antrum of the stomach (102,158,222). Cholecystokinin delays gastric emptying (182). Motilin, gastrin, cholecystokinin, and insulin stimulate small bowel contraction (78,102,157,222). Secretin and glucagon inhibit small bowel motility (102). Morphine and thyrotropin releasing hormone (TRH) inhibit transit (19,21).

Gastrointestinal motility physiology

The enteric nervous system coordinates reflex behavior and repetitive cyclic patterns. Reflex behavior requires sensory input such as bowel distension, whereas repetitive patterns do not. Reflex behaviors like peristalsis occur as a result of relaxation of the circular muscle and contraction of the longitudinal muscle ahead of the distending bolus, and relaxation of the longitudinal muscle with contraction of the circular muscle behind (250). Vomiting, as occurs with intestinal obstruction, reverses normal peristalsis.

Recurring intestinal myoelectric activity produces a slow oscillating wave pattern (97). Slow waves do not lead to contractions but action potentials on the crest of the slow wave do (179,249). Slow waves occur at 3 cycles per minute in the stomach, 11–12 cycles per minute in the duodenum, and 9 per minute in the distal ileum (179). In the fasting state migratory motor complexes (MMCs) occur in three phases (97,143,191,208,249). Phase I is motor quiescent, phase II is random irregular contractions, and phase III is an uninterrupted phasic migratory contraction (179). Phases I and III are enterically mediated, whereas phase II depends upon the extrinsic nervous system and diminishes with sleep (97,208). True rhythmic activity in the stomach occurs only in the distal antrum (179). As phase III approaches, antropylorodudenal coordination increases with high amplitude contractions from antrum to duodenum (97,179,208,249). In the proximal small bowel, phase III contractions occur at 1 to 2 hours, slowing as the contraction moves distally towards the ileum (97,179).

If food is ingested, the MMC pattern is replaced by random contractions called 'the fed pattern' lasting 2.5 to 8 hours (208). A specialized function called trituration occurs within the proximal antrum and propagates to the pylorus (179). As propagation proceeds to the mid-antrum the pylorus opens and duodenal contractions are inhibited allowing small particles and liquid to pass (179). When the contraction reaches the distal antrum the pylorus contracts causing retropulsion of large food particles (179). Larger particles are prevented from exiting and are moved about the antrum, grinding until small enough to exit (179).

Feeding also abolishes small bowel MMCs and sets up nearly continuous contractions of varying amplitude (97,208). Gastrin and cholecystokinin (CCK) mediate this change. The flow from the small bowel is impeded by the ileocecal sphincter mechanism. Pressures within this sphincter are higher than proximal ileal and cecal pressures (97). Periodic sphincter relaxation combined with proximal ileal contraction propels the contents into the colon.

Colonic contractions during the fed state are mostly segmental, mixing intestinal contents and exposing them to mucosal surfaces for absorption. Segmental contractions cause haustra (164,190). An occasional aboral organized segmental contraction produces propulsion (190). One to three times daily a generalized migratory contraction (GMC) occurs (139). As the GMC develops, haustra cease and a long extended contraction sweeps the contents towards the rectum (139,190,193). When the rectum is filled with fecal material the internal anal sphincter relaxes as part of the rectosphincteric reflex (190,193). A defecation response is signaled. Restoration of the internal anal sphincter tone is transient until defecation (193). Defecation is accomplished by contraction of the descending colon, sigmoid colon, and rectum with relaxation of the internal and external anal sphincters (139,190,193). Intra-abdominal pressure increases and the pelvic floor relaxes (193). Gastrointestinal hormones influence colon motility. Both gastrin and CCK increase colonic motility (164). Prostaglandins decrease segmental contractions and increases propulsion (190). Epinephrine inhibits both activities. Serotonin will either increase or decrease colonic motility based upon receptor subtype.

Aging, gender, and motility

Aging does not significantly alter small bowel motility (98,133,185). Colonic transit time is longer in women and smokers (153). The menstrual cycle does not alter transit time (153).

Gastrointestinal motility studies

Gastrointestinal dysmotility produces symptoms from localized or generalized distention of intestinal segments without involvement of the entire bowel. Radiographic studies outline mucosal lesions or obstruction but are poor tests to evaluate motility (1,36). Radiographs detect ileus but not mild to moderate dysmotility. Radioactive breath hydrogen studies (after ingestion of substrates metabolized by cecal bacteria) do not separate gastric from small bowel dysmotility (200). These studies reflect oral to colonic transit and do not locate the site of dysmotility (36). Bacterial overgrowth in the small bowel will produce a falsely normal study despite severe upper gastrointestinal dysmotility (36). Endoscopy will detect the effects but not the cause of dysmotility, such as occurs with GERD, and hence is also of limited value.

Scintigraphic gastric emptying studies

Indications for gastric emptying studies include:

- unexplained nausea and vomiting which fails to respond to prokinetics;
- motility-like dyspepsia, i.e. bloating, nausea, satiety;
- diabetes with poor glycemic control and gastroparesis;
- post-gastrectomy dumping, stasis, or nausea;
- reflux esophagitis unresponsive to proton pump inhibitors (PPI) and high-dose histamine (H_2) receptor antagonist (H_2RA) (35,43,111,177–179,208);
- chronic intestinal pseudo-obstruction.

Gastric emptying of solids is clinically more meaningful than liquids except in the 'dumping syndrome' (35,36,153,208). Gastric emptying is altered by small bowel or colonic dysfunction, constipation, and rectal distention (56,94,106). A positive study may preclude manometry or electrogastrography (EGG). Ultrasound studies of gastric emptying are not as sensitive as scintigraphy (14,35,147,173,178,200). Gastric emptying abnormalities may not correlate with symptoms. It is controversial whether gastric emptying studies are useful in predicting response to therapy.

Small bowel transit studies by scintography

Symptoms of small bowel dysmotility can mimic gastroparesis (37). Transit times widely vary (16). In contrast to gastric emptying time, small bowel transit for liquids and solids does not differ nor are there gender differences (16). Small bowel transit studies are indicated when gastric transit is normal but symptoms of gastroparesis persist (35,45,111,146, 147,167,178, 200,208,234).

Intraluminal gastroduodenal pressure recordings (manometry)

Indications include:

- unexplained nausea and vomiting with normal scintography;
- document etiology of gastric or small bowel stasis, i.e. neuropathic or myopathic etiology;
- generalized dysmotility where limited dysmotility is clinically apparent as in slow transit constipation, and gastroesophageal reflux disease (GERD);
- suspected chronic intestinal pseudo-obstruction (CIP);
- unexplained abdominal pain without obstruction or mucosal lesions;
- medication effects;

- preoperative evaluation for intestinal transplant in CIP (35,136,142,178,208,210, 234,239).

Occult intestinal obstruction is suspected by manometry when clustered or sustained contractions are recorded (177,178). Myopathic disorders produce low amplitude contractions with otherwise normal motility patterns, whereas neuropathic disorders produce abnormal MMC waves, discoordinated hypercontractions, and failure to elicit a 'fed response' with meals (35,177,178). Manometry and histological correlates are not well documented (35,178). Stationary recordings of reduced antral motility correspond to impaired gastric emptying caused by disease or medication (50). In the post-vagotomy syndrome duodenal frequencies of MMCs increase and phase III MMCs are absent when monitored by antral recordings (29,208). Post-prandial antral hypomotility also occurs after vagotomy. In the Roux Syndrome, the jejunal limb shows sustained uncoordinated pressure activity (35,50,125,191,208). Normal manometry suggests dysmotility is not the cause of patients' gastrointestinal symptoms (143). The absence of MMCs and a myopathic recording are predictors of a poor response to prokinetics. Forty per cent of patients with nausea and vomiting associated with unexplained abdominal pain will have abnormal manometry (181,182,210).

Cutaneous electrogastrography (EGG)

The surface EGG is a non-invasive test to evaluate nausea, vomiting, and post-prandial abdominal pain and bloating (35,178,208). It is a tool which can assess gastroparesis and abnormal gastric motor function (35,178,208). The EGG measures myoelectric frequency and amplitude. Recordings are not diagnostic of a particular disease but may help define a gastric motility disorder in a different subset than those studied by scintography emptying studies or manometry (35,178). Post-prandial dysrhythmia and lack of post-prandial crescendo amplitudes may reliably indicate delayed gastric emptying (168). However, EGG will be abnormal in motion sickness, eating disorders, and pregnancy (35). Dysrhythmia, which includes tachygastria, bradygastria, and mixed arrhythmia occur with idiopathic or diabetic gastroparesis (35,168,178). The EGG may be abnormal and correlate with symptoms even when gastric emptying studies are normal (12,168,178). Gastric dysrhythmia may better predict symptoms such as nausea and satiety than gastric emptying (35,168).

Radiopaque markers

Radiopaque markers or capsules have been used to detect abnormal gastric emptying. The number of markers retained in the stomach at 30–120 minutes post-prandial or the percentage of residual marker retained at 2 hours is significantly greater with dysmotility.

Assessment of colonic motility

A plain abdominal radiograph will demonstrate luminal distention, gas patterns, and fecal material, which indirectly reflects colonic compliance and transit (209). Contrast studies with fluoscopy illuminate segmental contractions and peristalsis. Stool consistency directly reflects transit through the gastrointestinal tract. Stool consistency correlates poorly with colorectal transit and more closely relates to whole gut transit (2,106,142,164). Ingested radiographic marker excretion time can be quantified as a measure of total intestinal transit (2,106,154, 164,167,209).

Colonic transit time is 75% of entire gastrointestinal transit. Scintigraphy using indium labeled radioisotope pellets encased with a pH-sensitive polymer coated capsule will isolate colon transit (50,106,164). Manometry of the colon is difficult (35,214). Accurate placement is difficult (164,214). Colonic lavage is necessary and the large diameter of the colon precludes accurate occlusive pressure measurements (164,214). Movement artifact is common. Electromyography requires either surgical placement of electrodes on serosal surfaces or intraluminal electrodes, which are also subject to motion artifact (35,164,214).

Upper gastrointestinal symptoms

The prevalence of dyspepsia in the United States is reported to be 26%. Dyspepsia is a symptom complex rather than a diagnosis (6,11,179,227). Symptoms include abdominal pain, anorexia, belching, bloating, early satiety, heartburn, nausea, post-prandial fullness, and regurgitation (1,6,42,48,227). There is a considerable overlap between epigastric discomfort and heartburn symptoms and the predictability of pattern to pathology is poor (6,11,48,88,227). Investigations by barium contrast radiograph or endoscopy will detect structural dyspepsia by outlining mucosal lesions in patients who have alarming symptoms or signs. Non-ulcerative dyspepsia is not well defined; the diagnosis is almost exclusively symptomatic (178,179). Functional dyspepsia excludes an organic etiology and is divided into ulcer-like, dysmotility-like, and reflux-like dyspepsia (6,45,48,88,179,227). Most consider dyspepsia to be a constellation of symptoms arising from the gastroduodenal region rather than a single disease entity (6,48,88). Either delayed esophageal or gastric transit is found in two-thirds to one-half with dysmotility-like dyspepsia (45,110). Two main groups can be identified. Males who have predominantly epigastric pain, and normal gastric emptying studies make up 61%. Females with non-painful symptoms and delayed gastric emptying are the other large subset (88). A high frequency of associated irritable bowel syndrome (30%) is found with the second group (88). Abnormal proximal stomach relaxation with meals is a cause of dyspepsia in some (88). Gastric emptying is normal with abnormal fundic relaxation in this group (88,256).

In a study of 340 patients with dyspepsia, 43% had upper abdominal pain, 42% had dysmotility-like symptoms, 35% reflux symptoms, and 22% mixed symptoms (22,88,219). Approximately 12% had alarming symptoms, particularly weight loss. Non-steroidal anti-inflammatory drug use occurred in 18%. Using guidelines established by the British Society for Gastroenterology, 1% of previously unstudied dyspeptic patients should undergo endoscopy with initial presentation due to certain alarming symptoms. Endoscopy is also indicated for dyspepsia and (a) age of 45 or older, (b) complicated refractory symptoms, and (c) patients on NSAIDs (Figure 7.1) (22). Patients who have both an abnormal EGG and gastric emptying studies have more severe symptoms than those with either an abnormal EGG and normal manometry or an abnormal manometry and normal EGG.

Dysphagia

Dysphagia as opposed to dyspepsia describes disability with associated swallowing and may be accompanied by pain. Impaired transport of a bolus from mouth to stomach occurs as a result of an uncoordinated or weakened esophageal peristalsis or from a failure of relaxation of the lower esophageal sphincter. Dysphagia and non-cardiac chest pain are due to (a) structural abnormalities, (b) a hypercontractile esophagus (nutcracker esophagus), or

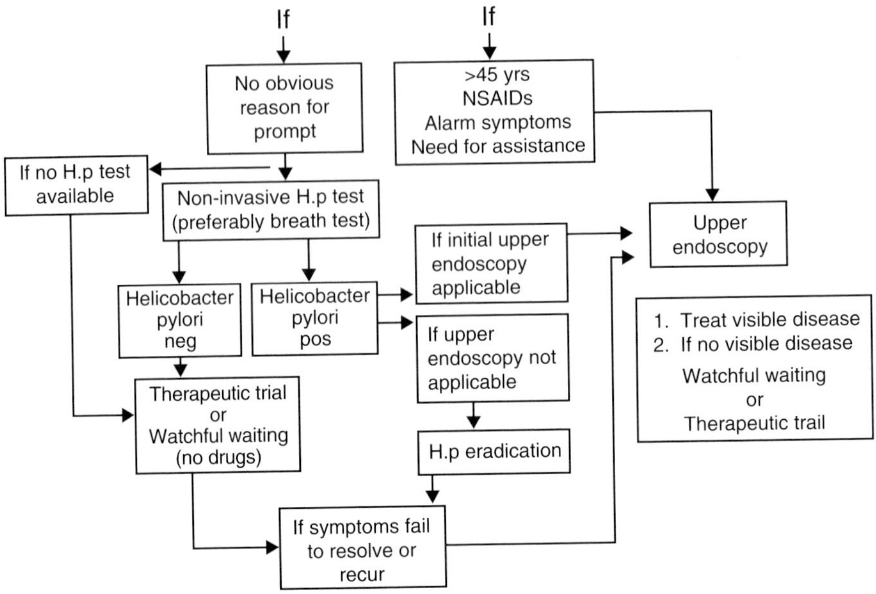

Figure 7.1 New dyspepsia. Reprinted from Agreus, L. and Talley, N. Dyspepsia: current understanding and management (1997) *Annual Review of Medicine* 49:475–93, by permission of Annual Reviews.

(c) gastroesophageal reflux (GERD) (11,42,142). Endoscopy is initially performed and, if normal, then a 24 hour esophageal pH monitoring study (220). The two major esophageal dysmotility disorders are achalasia and diffuse esophageal spasm (11,122,142). The cause of achalasia is failure of LES relaxation from a loss of inhibitory enteric motor neuron function (78,82,221). Reflux is caused by transient LES relaxation leading to the reflux of acid gastric contents into the stomach (110). Esophageal spasm is associated with either GERD or peristaltic incoordination. A close relationship exists between hypercontractile esophageal disorders and GERD. Respiratory problems can arise as a result of GERD, gastroparesis, or achalasia (78,82,201). Reflux is a cause of asthma, laryngitis or chronic cough (78,82,201). Gastroparesis is associated with cough and aspiration, and achalasia with aspiration (201).

Tumor-associated dysphagia

Carcinoma associated achalasia accounts for 4% of achalasia. Adenocarcinoma of the gastric cardia is most closely related. Achalasia is either due to direct tumor invasion of the myenteric plexus, invasion of the vagus nerve or the dorsal motor neuron in the brain stem (34). In addition, paraneoplastic degeneration may destroy the sphincter controlling neurons of the myenteric plexus (59,250). The age of onset is usually after the age of 60 and symptoms are present less than one year and weight loss is greater than 9 kg. Diffuse esophageal spasm (DES) like achalasia has been reported with cancer. Both neurofibromatosis and multiple endocrine neoplasia (MEN) type IIB produce overgrowth of neural tissue in the intestinal wall (59). No systematic study of symptoms or motility have been done with neurofibromatosis or MEN type IIB; however, achalasia-like syndromes have been reported with both. Amyloid, either primary or secondary, can be found throughout the intestinal tract (30,59) and infiltrates both muscle and myenteric plexus (59,230). Esophageal involvement with amyloid is usually asymptomatic. Manometry studies in amyloid patients do demonstrate some enteric neural involvement which produces incomplete fundic relaxation and diminished peristalsis. Achalasia and DES have been reported with amyloid resulting in pyrosis and dysphagia (30,59).

Dermatomyositis in the elderly may be a paraneoplastic disorder, which also affects the esophagus (50). Striated esophageal muscle is more often involved than distal smooth muscle. Muscle cell degeneration, destruction, and inflammation results in fibrosis (59). Dysphagia is predominantly oropharyngeal due to the destruction of striated muscle in the upper esophagus resulting in nasal regurgitation and aspiration pneumonitis (50,59). Manometry demonstrates a lack of coordination of cricopharyngeal relaxation with pharyngeal peristalsis (50). Diminished esophageal peristalsis is classically myopathic (50). A hypotensive LES has also been described with dermatomyositis as a result of smooth muscle dysfunction.

Paraneoplastic visceral neuropathy is caused by an IgG antienteric neuron antibodies (Anna-1) binding to gastrointestinal neurons (59,78). This is predominantly associated with small cell carcinomas. An inflammatory process destroys the myenteric plexus thereby destroying motor neuron function (50,78). Dysmotility occurs with manometry consistent with either achalasia or DES.

Brain stem tumors in the region of the posterior pons or near the dorsal motor nucleus of the vagus result in oropharyngeal dysphagia (30,59). Spinal cord injury or spinal tumors rarely produce dysphagia but cause profound dysfunction of the anal sphincter (30,50,59).

Esophageal involvement with Epstern–Barr virus or varicella-zoster infections in immunosuppressed individuals leads to enteric ganglionitis (30,50,59,78). Gastrointestinal involvement may precede other symptoms producing dysphagia as initial presentation. Fortunately, dysmotility is usually temporary.

Both corticosteroids and vinca alkaloids are associated with dysphagia (59). Steroids induce myopathy and vinca alkaloids are associated with neurotoxic to the myenteric plexus (59). Morphine decreases LES pressures (59). A severe form of esophageal spasm has been reported with hypomagnesemia (99).

Acute radiation induces submucosal edema and subacutely increases granulation tissue (52,59). Large irregular fibroblasts are eventually found within the esophagus, which are the hallmark of radiation therapy. Late effects include endothelial fibrosis with scar and stricture (52,59). Early dysphagia is the result of dysmotility and late dysphagia to stricture (52,59).

The division of esophageal musculature into two parts, striated muscle and smooth muscle, are affected differently by disease processes. Striated pharyngeal and proximal esophageal musculature are affected by polymyositis and dermatomyositis, which usually spares more distal smooth muscle (40,59). The pharmacology of the two muscle systems differ. Both benzodiazepines and muscle relaxants selectively affect striated muscle. Vagal motor neurons directly innervate striated muscle, whereas smooth muscle innervation is indirect by the vagus via the enteric myenteric nervous system.

Treatment of esophageal disorders (Figure 7.2)

Achalasia

Achalasia is associated with an imbalance of excitatory and inhibitory motor neurotransmission (252). The loss of inhibitory motor neurons results in failure of LES relaxation. Peristalsis may also be abnormal. Chagas disease causes achalasia, as can a degenerative disease of the myenteric plexus or as a final result of an autoimmune process (78,250,251). The standard treatment is balloon dilatation (221). Medical management includes nitrates, calcium channel blockers (nefedipine and verapamil), beta-2 adrenergic agonist, and loperamide (122,221,246). Botulinum toxin decreases the release of acetylcholine from presynaptic neurons, and can be injected repeatedly at 7- to 12-month intervals without systemic side-effects and with gratifying benefit (78,221). A transcutaneous nerve stimulator which increases VIP release and benefits some (207). Drug therapy is less beneficial than balloon dilatation, myotomy, or botulinum toxin injections (221). Nefidipine or other medical therapies are added in patients partially responding to usual measures. The outcome for balloon dilitation and botulinum toxin is poorer when patients are less than 50 years of age. These patients usually require myotomy (221).

Diffuse esophageal spasm (DES)

There is overlap clinically and manometrically between DES and achalasia (11). A subset of patients with DES have reflux and respond to antireflux measures (4,11). A 24-hour esophageal pH monitoring study is helpful in discovering this subset of patients (110,221).

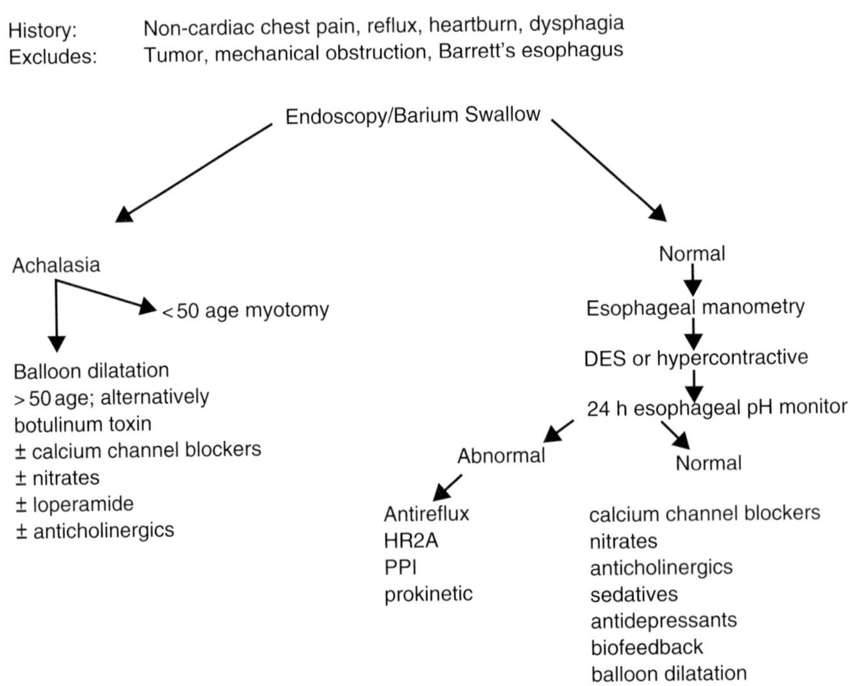

Fig. 7.2 Esophageal dysmotility.

Evidence of symptom benefit from anticholinergics, calcium channel blockers, and nitrate are not compelling, but do not exclude a trial of medical management (91,122,246). Botulinum toxin is beneficial in a few patients. However, it is important to rule out GERD before botulinum toxin injection (221).

Hypercontractile (nutcracker esophagus)

Normal propulsion and transit but muscular hypertrophy characterize nutcracker esophagus. Like DES, nutcracker esophagus may be associated with GERD and 24-hour esophageal pH monitoring is an important diagnostic tool (110,221). Calcium channel blockers are therapeutically disappointing (221). In addition, little experience exists for combining calcium channel blockers with anticholinergics or nitrates (221). Dilatation is helpful in some. Occasional responses have been recorded with weak sedatives, antidepressants, behavioral therapy, and biofeedback (221).

Mechanical obstruction of the esophagus

Progressive dysphagia in advanced esophageal cancer is due to intrinsic tumor or extrinsic paraesophageal spread. In advanced intrathoracic cancers, commonly lung cancer, dysphagia occurs when mediastinal structures or nodes are invaded and the esophagus is extrinsically compressed. Malignant esophageal obstruction complicated by esophago-respiratory fistula leads to dysphagia and recurrent aspiration pneumonia.

Chemoradiation therapy for thoracic cancers causes odynaphagia and dysphagia, which fortunately in most circumstances is temporary, but in a few leads to permanent esophageal stenosis and chronic dysphagia. Post-surgical anastomotic stenosis mimics locally recurrent esophageal cancer. Esophagoscopy differentiates the two.

Patients with an intrathoracic cancer and dysphagia will frequently require both upper endoscopy and computer tomography of the chest to differentiate intrinsic tumor from extrinsic and benign from malignant causes of dysphagia.

Treatment of mechanical obstructions

The treatment of a mechanical obstruction will depend upon the etiology (intrinsic tumor, extrinsic compression, or benign). Treatment will also depend upon the prognosis and performance status of the patient.

Intrinsic tumor

Dilatation is the oldest technique for palliating obstructing intrinsic primary esophageal carcinomas (26). Newer techniques include neodymium–yttrium–aluminum–garnet (Nd: YAG) laser, photodynamic therapy, BICAP tumor probe, intracavitary radiation (selectron therapy), and absolute alcohol injection (26,69,87,160,165,188,204,247). Both plastic and expandable metal stents palliate dysphagia (58,204). Metal stents are more costly but have fewer early complications compared to plastic prosthesis (18,188,204). The late morbidity may differ depending upon the type of stent but is not less with metal stents (58,204). Stents are particularly helpful when palliating esophago-respiratory fistulas (204). A plastic prosthesis is more cost effective if the patient's life expectancy is short (less than 3 months). Tumor ablation procedures should be done without stenting if survival is a month or less since regrowth of the tumor is not a major concern. Tumor ablation therapy (i.e. laser or photodynamic therapy) can be combined with prosthesis placement.

Palliative (non-curative) resections of obstructing esophageal cancer may significantly improve the patient's quality of life (40). Surgical bypass is a lessor option compared with endoluminal tumor ablation and/or stenting (40). Patients must be able to tolerate surgery and understand the potential complications and mortality associated with a surgical procedure. The goals of palliative surgery should be clearly outlined to the patient.

Esophageal obstruction from extrinsic compression

Endoluminal laser therapy, photodynamic therapy, and brachytherapy are not appropriate to palliate dysphagia from extrinsic tumor compression. Endoprosthesis with either a plastic or expandable metal stent are options depending upon the patient's prognosis and symptoms. The palliative response is less than when an endoprosthesis is used for intrinsic tumor (18). A clear and cogent discussion of the goals of prosthesis placement and complications as well as risks should precede placement of a stent.

Percutaneous endoscopic gastrostomy (PEG)

Patients hospitalized with acute illnesses for which a PEG tube is being considered as part of management are at high risk for serious adverse events after a PEG insertion (3). Additional care burdens accompany PEG tube placement and limited evidence exists for the improvement of function, nutrition, and subjective health particularly in the advanced cancer population (28,68,108). Nearly 25% die during hospitalization in which a PEG tube is placed (28,184,205). Thirty-day survival with a PEG tube correlates directly with serum albumin and inversely with creatinine and may be used in the decision-making process for tube placement (71,108).

Adverse events associated with a PEG tube occur in 35%. Complications include peristomal wound infections and aspiration (195). Antibiotic prophylaxis significantly reduces the risk of peristomal infections (77). PEG tubes do not eliminate the risk of pulmonary aspiration of gastric contents and a percutaneous endoscopic jejunostomy tube also does not reduce the risk of aspiration compared with a PEG tube (68,103,130). The cost of PEG-associated aspiration pneumonitis is $808 million per year in the United States (205). Tube dysfunction is a third complication. A mushroom-retained gastrostomy catheter is more durable, secure, and less prone to dysfunction compared with a pigtail-retained catheter (72).

PEG tube-feeding to reverse cancer associated anorexia and cachexia is clearly futile. The only indication for PEG placement in these patients is for medication administration (183). Patients with dysphagia unassociated with other symptoms and with good quality of life benefit from PEG tube placement and nutrition (183). Nutrition can be started safely 3 hours after PEG tube placement (51). Patients with dysphagia and reduced quality of life due to multiple symptoms should have other alternatives recommended before PEG tube placement. An explanation of complications as previously outlined is necessary if this option is considered (183). The PEG tube placement may be presented to the patient as a 'trial of management' in which the patient and physician periodically re-evaluate the burden and benefits of the PEG tube (183).

Aspiration pneumonia

Aspiration pneumonia is common with dysphagia either as a result of neuromuscular dysfunction, mechanical obstruction, or esophageal intubation. Approximately 10% of aspiration pneumonias occur with a PEG or involve PEG placement. Aspiration pneumonias most frequently involve the posterior segments of the upper lobes and superior segments of the lower lobes and are best visualized by chest computer tomography (70,141). Esophagoscopy and computer tomography are particularly useful when esophago-respiratory fistula is suspected (70). Mortality is high (24%) even more so when associated with *Pseudomonas* and *Acinetobacter* (35%–75%) (44). Metoclopramide delays nosocomial pneumonia in intubated ICU patients but does not decrease frequency or mortality (253).

Managing secretions in patients with esophageal obstruction

Difficulty swallowing, retained secretions, and sialorrhea are common problems associated with dysphagia from esophageal cancer. Sialorrhea results in drooling which produces considerable discomfort, inconvenience, social embarrassment, and leads to aspiration pneumonia. Glycopyrrolate, a quaternary antimuscarinic medication, decreases secretions within 24–48 hours (156,186). Glycopyrrolate is virtually without central nervous system (CNS) side-effects since it penetrates the blood–brain barrier poorly (186). Approximately 20% of children on glycopyrrolate experience side affects severe enough to require discontinuation (156). Alternatives are nebulized hyoscine hydrobromide, sublingual hyoscyamine, or transdermal scopolamine for patients unable to swallow and for whom parenteral glycopyrrolate is not feasible (15). A prospective comparative audit of hyoscine (scopolamine) hydrobromide, hyoscine butylbromide (not available in the United States), and glycopyrrolate in patients with retained secretions demonstrated better responses from glycopyrrolate and hysocine butylbromide than with hyoscine hydrobromide (15,93). Overall 54%–65% of patients had their secretions reduced (93). Antimuscarinics will not eliminate secretions already present and are less effective for bronchial secretions (93). Postural drainage and suctioning may be necessary at the start of antimuscarinic therapy to mobilize secretions.

Gastroduodenal-related dyspepsia

The discomfort of dyspepsia when mild produces bloating, nausea, early satiety, and when dyspepsia is severe, pain (6,50). Fifty per cent of assessments fail to uncover a structural or biochemical cause for dyspepsia. Structural lesions may be the end result of dysmotility rather than the cause and thus can be misleading (110). Some with organic upper gastrointestinal disease will not have dyspepsia. Patients with GERD are frequently misdiagnosed with functional dyspepsia since nearly half have normal endoscopy (110). Esophageal hypersensitivity to acid is an underlying cause for their dyspepsia. Overlap between esophageal and gastroduodenal symptoms clearly exists, and both may appear simultaneously (50,88,216,219). Certainly with the complaint of heartburn, reflux needs to be considered (88). Dyspeptic subgroups fail to accurately predict manometric or endoscopic findings (50,124,219). When manometry, 24-hour esophageal pH monitoring, lactose tolerance tests, and scinitigraphic evaluation of the esophagus, stomach, and biliary transit are done, approximately 50% will have abnormal findings not predicted based upon symptom cluster, i.e. reflux-like, dysmotility-like, and unspecified symptoms (88). Patients experiencing dyspepsia-associated dysmotility have large fasting and post-prandial gastric dimensions measured by ultrasound (62). Dysmotility does correlate with severe nausea, vomiting, abdominal pain, early satiety, post-prandial fullness, and weight loss. Neither symptoms nor motility findings correlate with *Helicobacter pylori* infections (6,140,208,216).

Endoscopy and dyspeptic patients

Endoscopic findings in dyspeptic patients are normal in 43%. Endoscopically detected pathologies include esophagitis in 15%, GERD in 12%, duodenal erosions in 9%, gastric ulcers in 4%. Erosive duodenitis occurs in 2% (238). Lactose intolerance occurs in 9%, biliary disease in only 2%, and malignancy in 2% (238). Patients with cancer are usually over the age of 45 and have weight loss or anemia which are considered alarming findings. Patients on NSAIDs also should undergo endoscopy.

Manometry and dyspepsia

Twenty-four-hour ambulatory manometry in significant dyspepsia will uncover antral or jejunal dysmotility in 71% during the interdigestive period, and 79% during the postprandial state (239). The most prevalent findings is prolonged phase II and phase III MMC configurations during fasting, or antral, and jejunal hypomotility or hypermotility in the fed state. Minute fasting rhythms occur in 21% and during the fed state in 29%. No positive correlation exists between symptom score and gastric emptying times determined by scintigraphy or manometric motility scores (249).

Gastric dysmotility associated with neoplastic conditions

Causes of gastric dysmotility are divided into myopathic, enteric neuropathic, extrinsic neuropathic, and unknown (8). Gastroparesis is the commonest abnormality of gastrointestinal motor function due in part to the availability of radionuclide studies. Dysmotility may be related to altered gastric relaxation, antropyloroduodenal dysmotility, and abnormal visceral sensation. Cancer-associated dyspeptic syndrome (CADS) refers to anorexia, early satiety, nausea, vomiting, and bloating unassociated with mechanical obstruction or tumor invasion (162). Early satiety predicts dysmotility and gastroparesis. CADS has been attributed to autonomic dysfunction. However, recent evidence suggests that interleukin-1 reduces gastric motility via its influence on the hypothalamus which disrupts the MMCs (61). Interleukin-1 also directly suppresses acetylcholine release within the myenteric plexus (61). Improvement of CADS frequently occurs with metoclopramide. Amyloid, dermatomyositis, paraneoplastic visceral neuropathy, and central nervous tumors delay gastric emptying (39,50,134). Spinal cord tumors rarely impair gastric emptying (34,50,107). Viral infections with cytomegalovirus (CMV), Epstein–Barr virus, varicella, and human immunodeficiency virus (HIV) temporarily or permanently delay gastric emptying (29,34,50,117,162,163). Delayed gastric emptying is associated with morphine analgesia (10,50) (Table 7.4). Cannabinoids delay gastric emptying and slow small bowel transit. Vinca alkaloids do the same by a neuropathic mechanism. Chemotherapy otherwise does not have a direct effect on gastric myoelectric activity or motility (46). Acute radiation injury of the stomach impedes gastric emptying, as determined by scintigraphy (52). This is usually temporary. Hypothyroidism, either primary or iatrogenic, causes gastroparesis and impairs small bowel motility through reduced slow wave frequency within gastric smooth muscle (50). Renal failure causes dysmotility and delays gastric emptying and is associated with abnormal myoelectric activity on EGG (131). Gastroparesis also occurs from constipation and inflammation or distention of the proximal, distal colon and small bowel (55,94,106). Vagal injury by tumor causes gastroparesis (34,208). Progesterone, tricyclic antidepressants, and anticholinergics delay gastric emptying (75,78,107,142) (Table 7.4).

Gastroparesis in the normal population

One-third of individuals presenting with gastroparesis have no obvious underlying disease to account for gastroparesis (107). Diabetes mellitus is a factor in 24%, post-gastrectomy surgery in 19%, Parkinson's Disease 5%, collagen vascular disease 5%, and anorexia nervosa 5% (78,107,182). Pseudo obstruction is a factor in 3% (107).

Treatment of dyspepsia (Figure 7.2)

Patients with dyspepsia and either associated reflux symptoms or ulcer-like pain derive benefit from proton pump inhibitors (PPIs) to a greater percentage then to H_2RA and antacids (57,122,211,225). Approximately 40% improve with H_2RA and antacids with an additional 20% improvement with PPIs (57,122,211,225,238). Painless dyspepsia and dysmotility-like symptoms do not respond any better to PPIs than to placebo (211,238). Prokinetic agents are better with nausea and early satiety than when heartburn is the major symptom (91,122,211,238). Early endoscopy is deferred with a negative *H. pylori* test unless alarming signs or symptoms are present. If *H. pylori* is present by laboratory tests, the infection is appropriately treated and symptoms readdressed afterwards. Endoscopy is recommended for refractory symptoms, age >45 years at symptom onset, history of NSAIDs, weight loss, and anemia.

Management of gastroparesis (Figure 7.3)

Gastroduodenal manometry is helpful when gastroparesis is detected by gastric and small bowel transit studies (Figure 7.2). Patients should also have a normal endoscopic examination.

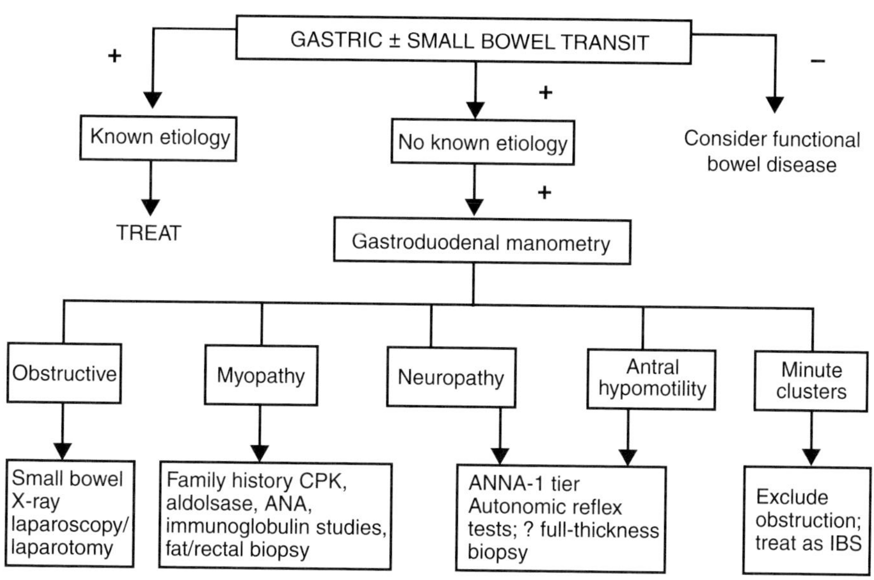

Figure 7.3 Approach to upper gastrointestinal dysmotility. Reprinted from Camilleri, M. Hasler, W. *et al*. Measurements of gastrointestinal motility in the GI laboratory (1998) *Gastroenterology* (118) 747–62 by permission of W.B. Saunders Company.

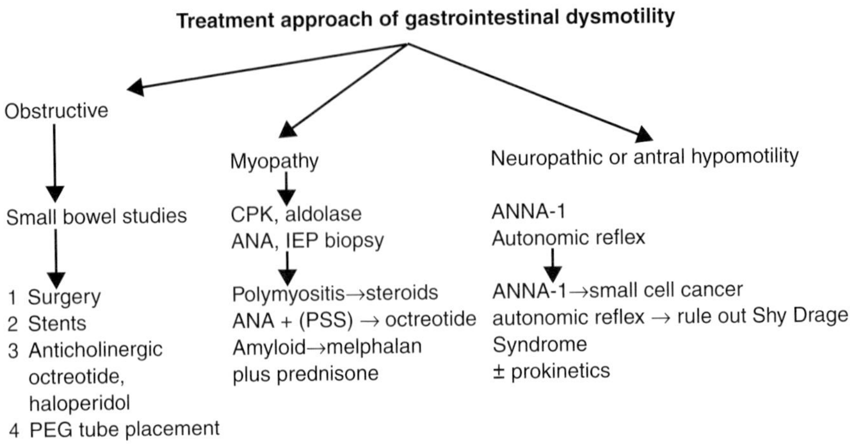

Figure 7.4 Treatment approach of gastrointestinal dysmotility.

If clustering or sustained contractions are detected by manometry, obstruction of the small bowel is suspected and small bowel radiographs should follow. If low amplitude but regular contractions, a smooth muscle myopathy is present and a CPK, aldolase, ANA and immunoglobulin studies as well as a fat or rectal biopsy performed. With neuropathic abnormalities, an ANNA-1 and autonomic study (i.e. orthostatic pressures as well as additional studies) (20,182) as well as gastric biopsy are indicated. The mainstay of treatment is nutritional support, antiemetics, prokinetic medications and rarely surgery (Figure 7.4) (31,32,66). Nutritional support is best by a laparoscopy-placed jejunal tube (66). Percutaneous endoscopic gastrostomy (PEG) is usually not helpful due to gastroparesis. Before adding prokinetics, medications that delay gastric emptying are discontinued (66). These include aluminium hydroxide, calcium channel blockers, dopamine, isoproterenol, opioids, phenothiazines, potassium, synthetic estrogens, sulcafate, and tricyclic antidepressants (30–32,50,75,91). 5HT3 antagonists do not delay gastric emptying (31,114,182) (Table 7.4).

If nausea is prevalent, metoclopramide is a reasonable first choice (83,132,185). Metoclopramide has central D2 dopaminergic antagonism and peripheral prokinetic action through facilitating acetylcholine release from enteric nerves (34,50,83,91,232). The majority of prokinesis occurs in proximal gut (83,91,109). Metoclopramide increases esophageal peristalsis, accelerates gastric emptying, increases antral contractions, and relaxes the pylorus and duodenal bulb (66,83,91,109,232). Subcutaneous and intravenous dosing are preferred if highly symptomatic (83,109). Subcutaneous metoclopramide provides drug levels 80% of equivalent intravenous doses and 300% greater than equivalent oral doses (83). Domperidone, unavailable in the United States, is a benzimidazole derivative with prokinetic activity through blockade of dopaminergic receptors (13,109,132). Domperidone increases LES pressure, accelerates gastric emptying (by inhibiting receptive fundic relaxation), and improves gastrointestinal peristalsis (13,109,132,232). Cisapride, an active agent in the treatment of dysmotility dyspepsia and a benzamide derivative, has recently been placed on limited availability due to its multiple drug interactions (81,91,109,189). Prokinesis by cisapride is induced by acetylcholine release from the myenteric plexus and 5HT4 agonism (33,66,81). Erythromycin, a macrolide antibiotic, acts on motilin receptors concentrated in the antroduodenal junction (31,32,66,132). Motilin elicits phase III MMC

Table 7.1 Evaluation of extrinsic neurologic disease in gastrointestinal motor dysfunction

Component	Specific features
History	Postural dizziness, control of blood pressure Disturbances of vision Sweating Urinary disturbances or infections Sensory or motor deficits
Medications	Calcium channel blockers, anticholinergic agents, antiarrhythmic drugs, antipsychotic agents, antihypertensive agents
Past history	Diabetes mellitus, spinal cord injury
Family history	Amyloidosis, other neuropathy
Examination	Blood pressure and pulse (with patient supine and standing) Pupils (size, reaction to light) Cranial nerves Sensation Motor function
Studies	Gastrointestinal manometry (±) RR interval (electrocardiographic) responses to valsalva maneuver and pulse rate variation (oscillation) with deep breathing Pupillary responses to 0.1% epinephrine, 0.125% pilocarpine, 5% cocaine drops Thermoregulatory sweat test Quantitative sudomotor axon reflex test (to iontophoresed acetylcholine) Blood pressure and plasma norephinephrine (with patient supine and standing) Screen for peripheral neuropathy Magnetic resonance imaging of the brain

Reproduced from Camilleri, M., Disorders of Gastrointestinal Motility in Neurologic Disease (1996) *Mayo Clinic Proceedings* 65: p. 838, by permission of *Mayo Clinic Proceedings*.

in the antroduodenal region. Tachyphylaxis occurs after a month of therapy. Experimental agents, which have prokinetic properties, are leuprolide and cholecystokinin receptor antagonists (66,109,189,232). Opioid receptor antagonists, by blocking the gastrointestinal mu and kappa opioid receptors, are prokinetic when patients are on opioids (92,105,254,255).

The response to prokinetics is poor with vagal dysfunction or with generalized autonomic failure as manifested by orthostatic hypotension (29,31,32) (Table 7.1). Myopathic dysmotility also responds poorly to prokinetics (29–32). Lack of response with vagal dysfunction suggests that an intact vagus nerve is an important effector of overall motor function. Failure of prokinetics to elicit a response in myopathic dysmotility is anticipated since neither 5HT4 stimulation nor acetylcholine release from the myenteric nerves will initiate prokinesis if smooth muscle function is diminished or absent.

Small bowel motility

The MMC of the small bowel requires an intact enteric nervous system and modulation from the extrinsic nervous system (30,98,143,176). Intestinal microflora significantly stimulate phase III activity (96). Diminished phase III MMC activity leads to Gram-negative bacterial overgrowth within the small bowel (29,30,96). The diminished velocity of phase III contractions is a second factor predicting bacterial overgrowth. Vagal activity controls phase II activity (97). Abdominal surgery inhibits phase II MMC and decreases the amplitude of phase II MMC (17). Small bowel transit is therefore delayed post-operatively despite a rapid recovery of phase III MMC response (usually within 3 hours of surgery) (17). The major determinant of small bowel dysmotility associated with surgery is absent phase II MMC (17). Somatostatin, opioids, sumatripan, and paroxetine initiate a phase III MMC response but diminish phase II activity (Table 7.4). Small bowel transit is therefore delayed overall by somatostatin and opioids despite initiation of phase III MMC (97). Small bowel MMC frequency is a marker of enteric neuromuscular functional integrity and the absence of phase III indicates severe dysfunction (30,179,207,208). Enteral feeding is likely to fail in cases of myopathy or absence of a phase III MMC (30,31,208). However, recordings to detect the absence of MMC should be over an extended period of time since wide interindividual differences exist and some normal individuals do not have phase III MMC during a usual three to four hours daytime recording (97,142,178,179).

After the post-prandial period, initial phase III recovery occurs in the mid-jejunal region. This is usually three to 10 hours after eating (79). Extrinsic innervations control the fed state motility pattern via the vagus which, when stimulated, abolishes usual MMC activity(208). Regulatory peptides, released by feeding, include secretin, gastrin, CCK, and insulin (97). Gastrin, secretin, and neural function induce post-prandial small bowel motility thus interrupting gastric MMC. Absorption is enhanced by the slow transit and inhibition of phase III MMC (97).

During the fasting state, 50% of aboral intestinal flow transpires during phase III MMC, whereas phase II accounts for 30%–40% of intestinal flow (97). Aboral transport must be sufficient during fasting to prevent bacterial overgrowth as shown by the inverse relationship between the presence of fasting phase III MMC and small bowel bacterial overgrowth (30,96,97,178,191,207,208). Distal ileal resections, if it includes the ileal cecal valve, produce greater dysmotility than proximal ileal or jejunal resections (97). Celiac sprue produces rapid transit by preserving phase II activity and increasing phase III MMC activity (97). High-frequency phase III MMC also occurs in the short bowel syndrome (30,36,178,179). Low-amplitude wave manometric recordings characterize myopathic disorders (scleroderma and amyloid). These disorders respond to octreotide, particularly scleroderma (34,36,84,143,207,212). Gastrointestinal neuropathies produce intense uncoordinated contraction, with bursts, an important feature of chronic intestinal pseudo-obstruction (30,84,97,178,190, 206,208). The absence or marked reduction in the fed motility response characterizes neuropathic dysfunction (97,178,179,180,181). Such irregular bursts also occur late as a result of radiation-induced enteropathy. Late radiation effects on the small bowel damage enteric neurons. Dysmotility in the proximal small bowel from pelvic radiation is caused by colonic reflex inhibition of small bowel motility. Giant migrating contracting waves which last 15–20 seconds and generate pressures greater than 33 mm Hg within the proximal small bowel are associated with dysmotility (97,208). Non-propagating prolonged contractions located in the upper small bowel which last greater than 20 seconds are known to occur with small bowel obstruction (36,97,178,179,208).

Patients with irritable bowel syndrome will have small bowel transit times shorter than normal when diarrhea is present and prolonged transit with constipation or when there is bloating and pain (106,178,179). Patients with IBS and constipation or bloating have delayed gastroduodenal ileal reflex and delayed ileal cecal valve opening (97,106,178,179). Patients with diarrhea associated with IBS have an unusually rapid recurrence of MMC post-prandially (178,179). Despite varying transit rates, all patients will have transit times within the range of healthy controls (178,179). Stress reduces the recurrence of phase III MMC and increases phase II activity leading to diarrhea (97).

Chronic intestinal pseudo-obstruction (CIP)

Patients with CIP present have signs and symptoms of intestinal obstruction without mechanical obstruction (30,54,56,126,218,252). Some have non-ulcer dyspepsia symptoms, and most have nausea with vomiting, abdominal distention with pain, bloating, and altered bowel movements (138,143,218). Weight loss and occasionally malabsorption accompany these symptoms (34,56,126,143,218,240). Malnutrition is common (66,138). Extra intestinal smooth muscle (particularly within the urinary bladder) is affected in some, resulting in associated bladder symptoms (56). Physical examination reveals a distended abdomen and high-pitched bowel sounds. Plain abdominal radiographs will have air fluid levels but small bowel contrast studies will appear normal (34).

Either the extrinsic autonomic neurons, the myenteric neurons, or smooth muscle are principally involved resulting in the same signs and symptoms (Table 7.2) (34,38,54,78,121, 218,240,252). If regions circular muscle are replaced with collagen, the bowel will appear segmentally distended and without peristalsis in the affected segment (207). Manometry of myopathic CIP will have low-amplitude but coordinated contractions (Figure 7.3) (30,34,36, 136, 178,191). Neuropathic pseudo-obstruction results from either interruption of the extrinsic nerve supply by retroperitoneal tumor, brainstem tumor, pandysautonomia, or through destruction of the enteric nervous system (Figure 7.3) (30,38,106,136,178,182, 191,218,252). Manometry will record excessive or uncoordinated contractions (36,56,136, 178,240). The extrinsic nerve supply is assessed by computerized tomography (CT) or magnetic resonance imaging (MRI) of the brain and by non-invasive autonomic function testing (Table 7.1) (34). If either MRI or CT are normal and non-invasive autonomic testing is normal yet neuropathic findings are discovered on manometry, an intrinsic neuropathic disorder is present (34,106,112,134). Antinuclear neuronal antibody type 1 (ANNA-1) test is obtained with a suspected paraneoplastic disorder or with small cell carcinoma (30,106,207). If a myopathic process is demonstrated by manometry, then rectal biopsy for amyloid, and serology for scleroderma, is performed (30,106,207). The patient should be questioned about the use of anticholinergic drugs, phenothiazines, clonidine, tricyclic antidepressants, and opioids (30,31,34,78,143) (Table 7.4). The diagnosis of an underlying disease such as scleroderma or diabetes precludes gut dysmotility testing (34,106,181, 182,207). Some patients with diabetes will have decreased fasting gastric phase III MMC with clinically apparent CIP (56). Paradoxically, these patients may have normal numbers and configuration in small bowel MMC (30,34,56). This accounts for increased bezoar formation in diabetics (182,185). A recent finding suggests that a post-prandial somatostatin response is suboptimal in patients with chronic idiopathic intestinal pseudo-obstruction resulting in discoordinated motor function (171).

Treatment of chronic idiopathic pseudo-obstruction (Figure 7.5)

Patients with mild vagal dysfunction or normal function will have decreased symptoms when treated with prokinetics (33). Octreotide generates phase III MMC complexes and

Table 7.2 Causes of chronic intestinal pseudo-obstruction

AIDS enteropathy	***Neurologic disorders***
Drug intake	Amytrophic lateral sclerosis
Alpha-adrenergic agonist	Burn-injury sequelea
Vasopressors (e.g. ephendrine, phenylephrine HCl [Carapres])	Cathartic colon (from long-term laxative use or abuse)
Antiparkinson agents	***Chagas' disease***
Designer drugs (e.g. MPTP)	Ganglioneuroma of intestine
Opiates	Hirschsprung's disease
Phenothiazine derivatives	Multiple sclerosis
Tricyclic antidepressants	Parkinson's disease
	Porphyria
Endocrine disorders	Radiation enteritis
Diabetes mellitus	Virally acquired hollow visceral neuropathy
Hyperglycemia	
Hyperosmolar non–ketotic coma	***Organ transplantation***
Hypoparathyroidism	Cytomegalovirus
Ketoacidosis	Epstein–Barr virus
Myxedema	*Herpes simplex* virus
Pheochromocytoma	
	Other
Intestinal smooth-muscle disease	Eosinphilic gastroenteritis
Amyloidosis	Jejunal diverticulosis
Collagen vascular disease	Jejunoileal bypass
◆ CREST syndrome	Non-tropical sprue
◆ Dermatomyositis	Paraneoplastic syndromes
◆ Raynaud's disease	(e.g. oat cell carcinoma, carcinoid syndrome)
◆ Rheumatoid arthritis	Psychosis
◆ Sceleroderma	
◆ Sjogren's syndrome	
◆ Systemic lupus erythematosus	
Hollow visceral myopathy	
Muscular dystrophy	
◆ Duchenne–Aran muscular atrophy	
◆ Myotonic dystrophy	

Reproduced from Mathias, J. and Clench, M. Neuromuscular Diseases of the Gastrointestinal Tract (1995) *Postgraduate Medicine* 97(3):p. 102 by permission of *Postgraduate Medicine*.

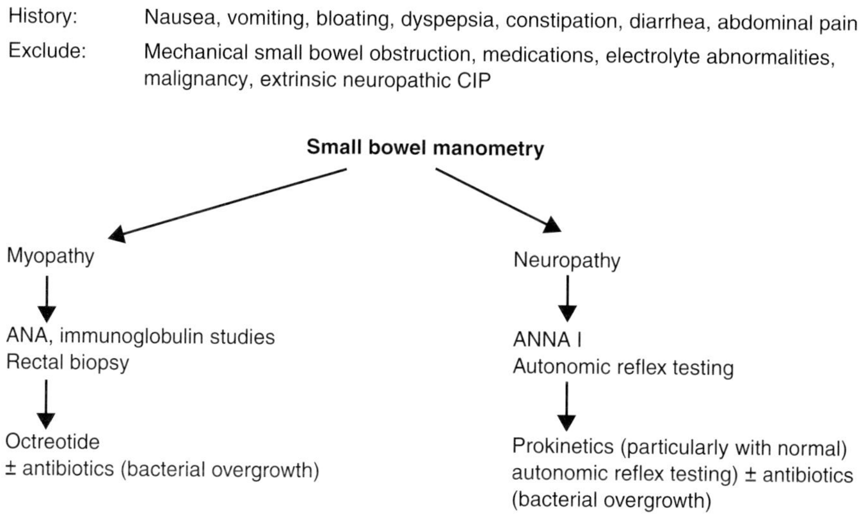

Figure 7.5 Treatment of CIP.

decreases bacterial overgrowth in small bowel limiting malabsorption and diarrhea in myopathic CIP (particularly scleroderma) (30,31,56,63,84,126,166). Metoclopramide is therapeutically disappointing in myopathic CIP (31,32,56,232). Macrolide antibiotics may reduce diabetic gastroparesis but are usually ineffective in CIP (56,182,232). Macrolide antibiotics will lose prokinetc activity in a matter of weeks due to the down regulation of motilin receptors (30,31,232). Anecdotal benefits are reported with domperidone, leuprolide, naloxone, cholecystokinin, and trimebutine (31,56,66,232). Bacterial overgrowth is only reliably confirmed by small bowel aspirate culture, but if steatorrhea is present, then a trial of one week of antibiotics (trimethoprim-sulfa, amoxicillin, cirprofloxin and metronidazole) out of two to four weeks may benefit some CIP patients (30,31,56,66,126,182,192).

Nutritional support includes a low-lactose, low-fiber, polypeptide hydrolized protein diet supplemented with multivitamins, iron, folate, calcium and vitamins D, K, and B_{12} (30,31,54, 66,138). Liquids are better tolerated due to associated gastroparesis (66). A therapeutic trial of nasogastric feeding should be done prior to jejunal tube placement (30,31). Sixty milliliters per hour of an isoosmolar solution should be tolerated if jejunal feeding is to successfully nourish the patient. Myopathic pseudo-obstruction is a relative contraindication to jejunal feeding (30,31,66). Selected patients will benefit from surgical bypass or resection of the affected segment of intestine (31,32,56,126,127). However, most patients have a generalized process, for which surgery is pointless (106,107).

Liver disease and small bowel motility

Cirrhosis impedes small bowel motility. Even though prolonged phase II like patterns occur during fasting, the MMC frequency is less than normal and MMC velocity is slower particularly in patients who develop spontaneous bacterial peritonitis (47,49). Bacterial overgrowth of the small bowel in cirrhotic patients is a risk factor for spontaneous bacterial peritonitis (47,49). The influence of cirrhosis on small bowel motility is an indirect effect since small bowel motility returns to normal after orthotopic liver transplantation (135).

Acute intestinal and colonic pseudo-obstruction

Acute pseudo-obstruction (Ogilvie's Syndrome) is most frequently encountered as an isolated colonic disturbance but can extend to affect the entire gastrointestinal tract (including acute gastroparesis) (59). Excessive sympathetic stimulation from the spinal cord occurs and decreased parasympathetic tone is diminished (78,107). Clinical features resemble CIP. The causes are protean (Table 7.3) (59). However, it most commonly occurs as a

Table 7.3 Factors associated with acute intestinal pseudo-obstruction with neoplastic conditions

Systemic infections
◆ Sepsis syndrome
◆ Varicella–Zoster virus
◆ Epstein–Barr virus
Gastrointestinal infections
◆ *Clistridium difficile*
Post-transplant lymphoproliferative disease
Central nervous system tumors
◆ Brain stem
◆ Spinal cord
Retroperitoneal abnormalities
◆ Tumor
◆ Hematoma
Graft-versus-host disease
Neutropenic entercolitis
Medications
◆ Opiates
◆ Anticholinergics
◆ Antineoplastic agents
◆ Octreotide
Miscellaneous
◆ Pelvic irradiation
◆ Electrolyte disturbances
◆ Pancreatitis
◆ Pulmonary emboli
◆ Intra-abdominal inflammatory conditions
◆ Multisystem organ failure

Reproduced from DiBaise, J. and Quigley, E. Tumor-related Dysmotility Gastrointestinal Dysmotility Syndromes Associated with Tumors (1998) *Digestive Diseases and Science* 43(7) p. 1387, by permission of Kluwer Academic Publishers.

physiological response to surgery (107). Ogilvie's Syndrome does not normally produce permanent impairment of control mechanisms or permanent structural damage (107). Diagnosis is frequently delayed resulting in increased morbidity and mortality. Plain films demonstrate proximal colonic distention with preserved haustra and mucosal patterns which distinguishes it from toxic meglacolon and inflammatory bowel disease, respectively (59). The worst complications are cecal perforation and ischemia, which is rare if the cecal diameter is less than 12 cm. Contrast enemas are used to rule out mechanical obstruction.

Treatment of acute pseudo-obstruction

The initial treatment of acute pseudo-obstruction includes hydration, minimal oral fluid intake, nasogastric suctioning, correction of electrolyte abnormalities, and elimination of offending drugs (59,107). Colonic decompression is necessary to avoid cecal ischemia and perforation. Chemical decompression of the distended colon involves acetylcholine-estrase inhibitors (59). Failing chemical decompression, colonoscopy decompression will be successful in 75%–90% (107). Recurrence after colonoscopy decompression occurs in 15% and requires a repeat procedure. Rarely cecostomy is necessary. Mortality in the appropriately treated is 15% but is 36%–44% if perforation or ischemia develop (59).

Colonic dysmotility

Constipation and disordered defecation are symptoms of underlying colonic disease (1). Dysmotility may not be associated with structural abnormalities. Constipation arises from impaired colonic motility (inertia coli), increased and frequent haustrating colonic contractions, or paradoxical strain on the pelvic floor musculature during defecation (anismus) (190,209). The initial approach excludes structural disorders and is followed by motility studies with radiopaque markers and sequentially timed plain abdominal radiographs (164,209). Defaecography is indicated for anismus (200,209). Ano-rectal manometry assesses intestinal neuronal disorders such as aganglionesis (Hirschsbrung's Disease) and intestinal neuronal dysplasia associated with structural ganglia (7,56,78,159,209,237,243,244).

Slow transit constipation

Slow transit constipation is a severe condition of colonic motor function affecting predominantly women (115,164,170). Medical management, which frequently includes prokinetics, is often ineffective (128,232). The outcome from surgery is unpredictable (115,116,164). Slow transit constipation is associated with low substance P in mucosal and submucosa of the colon (235). Oral–cecal transit is delayed but antroduodenal motility is well preserved (115,170). A panenteric neurological deficit can be present dispite the limited extent of symptoms (213,220).

Irritable bowel syndrome

Irritable bowel syndrome affects 12%–14% of individuals in the United States (190,214). The most consistent symptoms are abdominal pain relieved by defecation, loose stools at the onset of colicky pain, frequent stools with pain, and post-prandial bloating or discomfort (8,86,92). It is unclear whether these symptoms are a normal perception of abnormal motility or an abnormal perception of normal motility (90,92,137,178,199). Radiopaque marker studies for dysmotility are helpful in this regard (90). The mid and lower gut are

Table 7.4 Drugs and motility

Drug	Esophageal	Gastric	Small bowel (SB)	Colon
Ranitidine (23,169)		↑Antral MMC phase III; post-prandial delayed gastric emptying; increased EEG power; increased antral manometric motility index		
Famotidine				
Omeprazole (187)				
Cimetidine	No effect on emptying rates Reduced spikes			
Morphine (4,109,129,248)		Delays gastric emptying; prolongs orocecal transit time	Increases SB contraction followed by distention; increases phase III MMC; reduces phase II MMC	Increases defecation urge threshold; prolongs right colon transit time by segmental contraction
Tramadol, codeine (148,248)				
Cholinergic agonists (23) [bethanecol (122), neostigmine (232)]	Increases LES; increase amplitude and velocity of esophageal contraction		Increases amplitude of contraction throughout gastrointestinal tract which are not coordinated nor accelerate transit	
Metoclopramide (66,83,232)	Raises LES	Stimulates gastric motility and coordinates gastric pyloric and duodenal motility		
Domperidone (13,122,232)	Raises LES pressure (high doses)	Stimulates gastric motility and improves emptying of solids and liquids		
Cisapride (66,118,120, 122,198)	Increases LES pressure, improves peristalsis	Improves gastric emptying (via motilin receptor)	Stimulates contactility	Decreases substance P; stimulates contactility; accelerates proximal colonic transit

Octreotide (60,63–66, 84, 122,166,212,223,241)	Increases LES pressure and esophageal contraction	Delays emptying; inhibits antral contraction by inhibition of motilin release	Low doses ↑ MMC; high doses ↑ phases III MMC and decreases phase II MMC; delays transit	↓ Rectal sensation ↓ Post-prandial tone ↑ Phasic pressure activity
(Macrolides) (60,67,122,232)		Decreases gastric transit initiation of phase III MMC		
Erythromycin (152,202,222,236)	Increases LES pressure	Increases antral contraction; abolishes lag phase for solids; reduces pyloric tone	Suppresses SB activity; reduces frequency of propagated contractions and amplitude of contraction; initiates phase III MMC	Normal transit to accelaration transit
Ondansetron Tropisetron Cilansetron (76,85,114,161, 215,226) (5HT3 antagonist)	No effect	Increases gastric emptying of solids		No effect on transit time or slow colonic transit through left colon
Midazolam (41)			Increases phase III MMC in proximal duodenum; increases median motility index	
Magnesium sulfate (242)		Delays the reappearance of phase III MMC in fasting state and antroduodenal motility in fasting state	Accelerates duodenal transit	
Antidepressants 1. Tricyclic (74,75,128) 2. Paroxetine (74)		1. Delays orocecal transit; slows phase III MMC	1. Increases SB transit (decreases SB transit time) 2. Diminished phase II activity	1. Markedly reduces GMC

(Continued)

Table 7.4 (Continued) Drugs and motility

Drug	Esophageal	Gastric	Small bowel (SB)	Colon
Peppermint oil and caraway oil (155)		Reduces number and amplitude of contraction of gastroduodenal smooth muscle; occurs during various phases of MMC		
Tegaserod (25,122,172,174)		Unaltered gastric emptying	Accelerates orocecal transit	
Prucalopride (5HT4 agonist)				Increases proximal colon emptying (reducing transit) with no change in mean colonic transit time
Isosorbide dinitrate (145)	Lowers LES pressures	No delay in gastric emptying		
Methylnaltexone (254,255)		Reverses delayed orocecal transit caused by morphine		
Dopamine	Decreases tone and motility	Decreases tone and motility	Decreases tone and motility	Dose dependence increase in sigmoid contractility
Verapamil (119)	Reduces LES and peristalsis	Normal gastric emptying	Normal transit	Delays colonic transit
Bran (150)		Delays gastric emptying	Accelerates SB	
Pramlintide (194)		Delays gastric emptying	Normal	Normal
Cox (2) Inhibitors (104)			Improves post-operative dysmotility	

primarily affected. Females are more commonly afflicted with a female to male ratio of 1 to 2 (86,214). Stool weight is usually normal (214). Lactose intolerance, which occurs in 25%, is of uncertain significance (214). Those with bloating and alternating diarrhea and constipation have faster small bowel transit (90,164). Exaggerated post-prandial giant migratory complexes (GMCs) occur upon wakening, resulting in several bowel movements in the morning (214). GMC frequency is diminished in those with constipation. Abnormal central processing of intestinal afferents, and increased rectal sensitivity, leads to either symptoms without abnormal motility or rectal urgency and normal motor and sphincter function (92,164,178,182,214). The patient may have exaggerated colonic responses to stress, perhaps mediated by corticotropin releasing factor (78). Finally, an imbalance exists between sympathetic and parasympathetic input which leads to diarrhea or constipation, respectively (78,180,182). Post-dysentery irritable bowel syndrome is related to post-infectious enteroendocrine hyperplasia and release of either 5HT, and substance P (inducing diarrhea) or somatostatin (producing constipation) (55,78,214). Activated mast cells increase in post-campylobacter dysentery leading to continuous diarrhea, which responds to sodium cromoglycate (214).

Treatment of irritable bowel syndrome (Figure 7.6)

Smooth muscle relaxants are given for abdominal colic (101). Dicyclomine is used, although evidence is supported by only one trial. Cimetropium, pinaverium, and trimebutine are other agents that may benefit the patient. Hyoscyamine is an alternative (101). Bulking agents are not usually helpful (101). Tricyclic antidepressants for psychiatric disturbances and irritable bowel syndrome will have both a neuromodulatory effect on bowel sensitivity (producing analgesia) and an antidepressant effect (74,75,101). SSRIs have not been reported as a treatment for IBS. Cisapride is also not helpful (101). Loperamide decreases diarrhea but does not reduce abdominal pain. Peppermint oil is an antispasmodic which reduces diarrhea and cramps (101). Dietary modification and a trial of a lactose-free diet is reasonable (101). Patient education, reassurance, and a good physician–patient relationship may be as valuable as any medication.

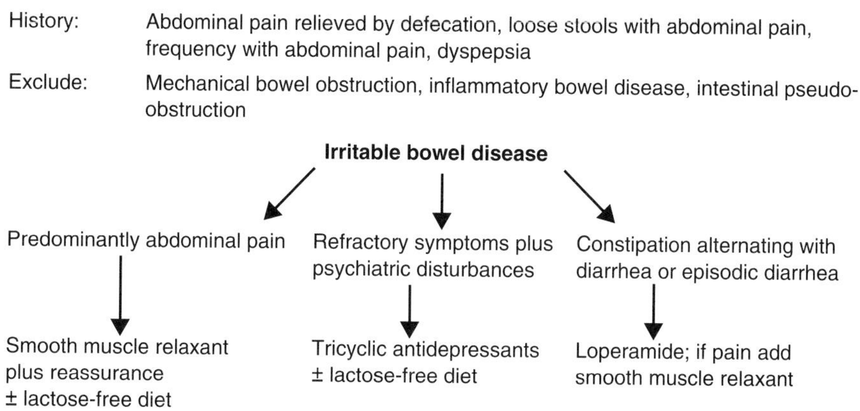

Figure 7.6 Irritable bowel syndrome.

Toxic megacolon

Toxic megacolon is an acute colonic dilatation (total or segmental, ascending or transverse) of 6 cm or more associated with sepsis or systemic toxicity (203). It is most common with inflammatory bowel disease but may occur with pseudo-membranous colitis, salmonella, shigella, campylobactor, or amoebic colitis, CMV colitis, ischemic colitis, diverticulitis, volvulus, or with an obstructing cancer. Lifetime risk for toxic megacolon in inflammatory bowel disease is 1%–5% and usually occurs early in the course of the illness (203). Toxic megacolon is the end result of an acute inflammatory cell infiltration which extends into smooth muscle layers leading to smooth muscle paralysis. The myenteric plexus is uninvolved. Nitric oxide released from nitric oxide synthetase in macrophages and smooth muscle inhibits motility (78,203). Toxic megacolon is a common complication of pancolitis. Precipitating factors, with colitis, are hypokalemia, opioids, anticholinergics, loperamide and antidepressants, as well as psyllium seed (203). Anemia and electrolyte disturbances, particularly hypokalemia, complicate toxic megacolon. Dehydration and metabolic alkalosis are poor prognostic factors (203). Plain abdomen radiographs demonstrate a dilated right and/or transverse colon, air fluid levels, and an absent haustral pattern. Limited endoscopy may help differentiate the colitis of inflammatory bowel disease from pseudo-membranous colitis (203). Limited sigmoidoscopy may miss a CMV infection. Full colonoscopy is risky and contraindicated.

Treatment of toxic megacolon (Figure 7.7)

Medical management will circumvent surgery in 50% (203). The main goal is to reduce colitis, restore motility, and prevent ischemia and perforation. Initial steps are to correct dehydration and electrolyte disturbances, and decompress the bowel by nasogastric suctioning placing the bowel at rest (203). Anti-motility agents are stopped. Prophylaxis for gastric stress ulcers and venous thrombosis is started. In inflammatory bowel disease, hydrocortisone 100 mg every 6–8 hours is given with broad-spectrum antibiotics in order to reduce the risk of sepsis (203). In pseudo-membranous colitis intravenous metronidazole plus oral vancomycin is indicated. Subtotal colectomy and end-ileostomy is done in those whose colitis fails to respond in 48–72 hours or who show evidence of colonic perforation (203). Early surgery is associated with reduced mortality. Mortality is 2%–8% if done before perforation. Overall mortality associated with toxic megacolon from pseudo-membranous colitis is 18% and 42% for medically and surgically managed patients, respectively (203). The high mortality in the surgical patients may be related to patient selection rather than treatment modality. Toxic megacolon associated with HIV and CMV responds poorly to medical management and colectomy is frequently necessary (203).

Summary

Dysmotility syndromes produce many symptoms, which overlap. The discovery of dysmotility by scintigraphy, manometry, and EGG signifies either a structural or functional disease but is not diagnostic of a single disease. Dysmotility studies may help guide therapy. There are few data which correlate histopathology with abnormal motility. Dysmotility studies frequently does not correlate with symptoms. Further research is needed to understand the pathophysiology of dysmotility disorders associated with cancer and chronic

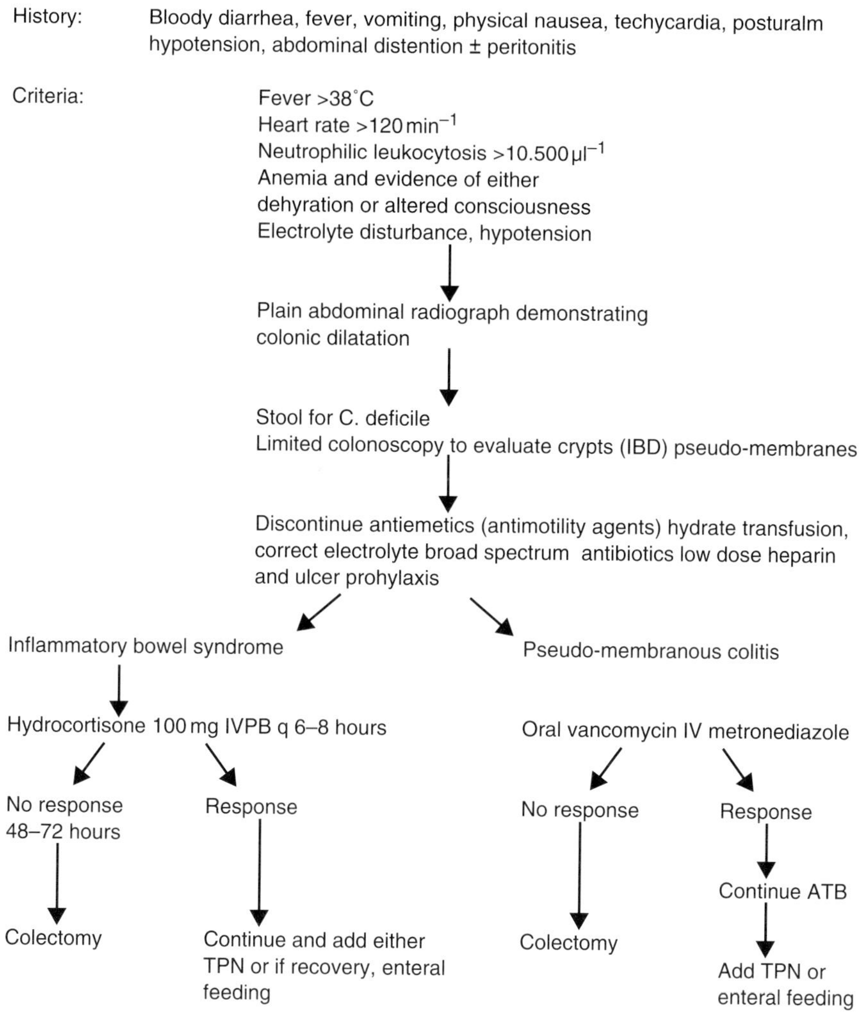

Figure 7.7 Toxic megacolon.

intestinal pseudo-obstruction. Newer agents with fewer extra-intestinal side-effects and drug interactions would be helpful. Further research into leuprolide analogs and CCK antagonists would be fruitful and hopefully provide a new class of agents that are beneficial in the palliation of dysmotility disorders.

References

1. **Abell TL; Werkman RF.** Gastrointestinal motility disorders. *American Family Physician* 1996;53(3):895–902.
2. **Abrahamsson H; Antov S; Bosaeus I.** Gastrointestinal and colonic segmental transit time evaluated by a single abdominal X-ray in healthy subjects and constipated patients. *Scandinavian Journal of Gastroenterology*. Supplement. 1988;152:72–80.

3. **Abukis G; Mor M; Negba S; Shemesh I; Plout S; Sulkes J; Fraser GM; Niv Y.** Percutaneous endoscopic gastrostomy: high mortality rates in hospitalized patients. *The American Journal of Gastroenterology* 2000;95(1):128–32.
4. **Achem SR; Robinson M.** A prokinetic approach to treatment of gastroesophageal reflux disease. *Digestive Diseases* 1998;16(1):38–46.
5. **Adams HA; Pohlemann T.** Effect of anesthetics on the function of the gastrointestinal tract. *Anaesthesiologie und Reanimation* 1999;24(4):88–94.
6. **Agreus L; Talley NJ.** Dyspepsia: current understanding and management. *Annual Review of Medicine* 1997;49:475–93.
7. **Ammann K; Stoss F; Meier-Ruge W.** Intestinal neuronal dysplasia in adults as a cause of chronic constipation: morphmetric characterization of colon innervation. *Chirurg.* 1999;70(7):771–7.
8. **Anuras S.** Classification of neuromuscular disease of the gastrointestinal tract and the spectrum of clinical manifestation. In: Anuras S, editor. *Motility Disorders of the Gastrointestinal Tract.* New York: Raven Press, 1992: pp. 157–164.
9. **Appel S; Kumle A; Hubert M; Duvauchelle T.** First pharmacokinetic–pharmacodynamic study in humans with a selective 5-hydroxytryptamine4 receptor agonist. *Journal of Clinical Pharmacology* 1997;37(3):229–37.
10. **Asai T.** Effects of morphine, nalbuphine and pentazocine on gastric emptying of indigestible solids. *Arzneimittelforschung* 1998;48(8):802–5.
11. **Bak YT; Lorang M; Evans PR; Kellow JE; Jones MP; Smith RC.** Predictive value of symptom profiles in patients with suspected esophageal dysmotility. *Scandinavian Journal of Gastroenterology* 1994;29(5):392–7.
12. **Barbar M; Steffen R; Wyllie R; Goske M.** Electrogastrography versus gastric emptying scintography in children with symptoms suggestive of gastric motility disorders. *Journal of Pediatric Gastroenterology and Nutrition* 2000;30(2):134–6.
13. **Barone JA.** Domperidone: a peripherally acting dopamine2-receptor antagonist. *Annals of Pharmacotherapy* 1999;33(4):429–40.
14. **Benini L; Sembenini C; Heading RC; Giorgetti PG; Montemezzi S; Zamboni M; Di Benedetto P; Brighenti F; Vantini I.** Simultaneous measurement of gastric emptying of a solid meal by ultrasound and by scintigraphy. *American Journal of Gastroenterology* 1999;94(10):2861–5.
15. **Bennett MI.** Death rattle: an audit of hyoscine (scopolamine) use and review of management. *Journal of Pain and Symptom Management* 1996;12(4):229–33.
16. **Bennink R; Peeters M; Van den Maegdenbergh V; Geypens B; De Roo M; Mortelmans L.** Evaluation of small-bowel transit for solid and liquid test meal in healthy men and women. *European Journal of Nuclear Medicine* 1999;26(12):1560–6.
17. **Benson MJ; Roberts JP; Wingate DL; Rogers J; Deeks JJ; Castillo FD; Williams NS.** Small bowel motility following major intra-abdominal surgery: the effects of opiates and rectal cisapride. *Gastroenterology* 1994;106:924–36.
18. **Bethge N; Sommer A; Vakil N.** Palliation of malignant esophageal obstruction due to intrinsic and extrinsic lesions with expandable metal stents. *The American Journal of Gastroenterology* 1998;93(10):1829–32.
19. **Bhargava HN; Pillai NP.** Stereospecific opiate receptors in the actions of thyrotropin releasing hormone and morphine on gastrointestinal transit. *Life Sciences* 1985;36(1):83–8.
20. **Bharucha AE; Camilleri M; Low PA; Zinsmeister AR.** Autonomic dysfunction in gastrointestinal motility orders. *Gut* 1993;34(3):397–401.
21. **Bhounsule SA; D'Sa S; Fernandes N; D'Souza RD; Dhume VG.** Gastrointestinal actions of buprenorphine: are different receptors involved? *European Journal of Pharmacology* 1996;316(2–3):253–6.

22. **Bodger K; Eastwood PG; Manning SI; Daly MJ; Heatley RV.** Dyspepsia workload in urban general practice and implications of the British Society of Gastroenterology Dyspepsia Guidelines (1996). *Alimentary Pharmacology and Therapeutics* 2000;14(4):413–20.
23. **Bortolotti M; Cucchiara S; Sarti P; Brunelli F; Mazza M; Bagnato F; Barbara L.** Comparison between the effects of neostigmine and ranitidine on interdigestive gastroduodenal motility of patients with gastroparesis. *Digestion* 1995;56(2):96–9.
24. **Borman RA; Burleigh DE.** Functional evidence for a 5-HT2B receptor mediating contraction of longitudinal muscle in human small intestine. *British Journal of Pharmacology* 1995;114(8):1525–7.
25. **Bouras EP; Camilleri M; Burton DD; McKinzie S.** Selective stimulation of colon transit by the benzofuran 5HT4 agonist, prucalopride, in healthy humans. *Gut* 1999;44(5):682–6.
26. **Boyce GA.** Palliation of malignant esophageal obstruction. *Dysphagia* 1990;5(4):220–6.
27. **Burleigh DE.** Evidence for more than one type of 5-hydroxytryptamine receptor in the human colon. Journal of Pharmacy and Pharmacology 1977;29(9):538–41.
28. **Callahan CM; Haag KM; Weinberger M; Tierney WM; Buchanan NN; Stump TE; Nisi R.** Outcomes of percutaneous endoscopic gastrostomy among older adults in a community setting. *Journal of American Geriatrics Society* 2000;48:1048–54.
29. **Camilleri M.** Disorders of gastrointestinal motility in neurologic diseases. *Mayo Clinic Proceedings* 1990;65:825–46.
30. **Camilleri M.** Small bowel motility disorders. *Review of Gastroenterology Mexico* 1994;59(2):120–6.
31. **Camilleri M.** Appraisal of medium- and long-term treatment of gastroparesis and chronic intestinal dysmotility. *The American Journal of Gastroenterology* 1994a;89(10):1769–74.
32. **Camilleri M; Balm RK; Zinsmeister AR.** Determinants of response to a prokinetic agent in neuropathic chronic intestinal motility disorder. *Gastroenterology* 1994b;106:916–23.
33. **Camilleri M; Balm RK; Zinsmeister AR.** Symptomatic improvement with one-year cisapride treatment in neuropathic chronic intestinal dysmotility. *Alimentary Pharmacology and Therapeutics* 1996;10(3):403–9.
34. **Camilleri M; Bharucha AE.** Gastrointestinal dysfunction in neurologic disease. *Seminars in Neurology* 1996;16(3):203–16.
35. **Camilleri M; Hasler WL; Parkman HP; Quigley EMM; Soffer E.** Measurements of gastrointestinal motility in the GI laboratory. *Gastroenterology* 1998;115:747–62.
36. **Camilleri M; Phillips SF.** Disorders of small intestinal motility. *Gastroenterology Clinics of North America* 1989;18(2):405–24.
37. **Camilleri M; Saslow SB; Bharucha AE.** Gastrointestinal sensation: mechanisms and relation to functional gastrointestinal disorders. *Gasteroenterology* 1996;25(1):247–59.
38. **Camilleri M; Vassallo M.** Small intestinal motility and transit in disease. *Baillieres Clinics of Gastroenterology* 1991;5(2):431–51.
39. **Caras S; Laurie S; Cronk W; Tompkins W; Brashear R; McCallum RW.** Pancreatic cancer presenting with paraneoplastic gastroparesis. *American Journal of the Medical Sciences* 1996;312(1):34–6.
40. **Carlini S; Grauso F; Perri P; Pasquali Lasagni R; Piarulli L; Cavallari A; Bruno P; Benaglia A; Cerasoli V; Campioni N.** Role of surgery in the treatment of recurrent esophageal cancer. *Hepatogastroenterology* 1997;44(13):187–91.
41. **Castedal M; Bjornsson E; Abrahamsson H.** Effects of midazolam on small bowel motility in humans. *Alimentary Pharmacology and Therapeutics* 2000;14(5):571–7.
42. **Champion MC.** Prokinetic therapy in gastroesophageal reflux disease. *Canadian Journal of Gastroenterology*. Suppl. B 1997;55B–65B.

43. **Charles F; Camilleri M; Phillips SF; Thomforde GM; Forstrom LA.** Scintigraphy of the whole gut: clinical evaluation of transit disorders. *Mayo Clin Proceedings* 1995;70(2):113–8.
44. **Chastre J; Trouillet JL.** Problem pathogens (Pseudomonas aeruginosa and Acinetobactor). *Seminars in Respiratory Infections* 2000;15(4):287–98.
45. **Chauduri S; Santra A; Dobe PB; Das AS; Dasgupta J; Roy A; Mazumder DN.** Esophageal and gastric dysmotility in non-ulcer dyspepsia. *Indian Journal of Gastroenterology* 2000;19(3):109–11.
46. **Cheng W; Chan CG; Tam PK.** Cytotoxic chemotherapy has minimal direct effect on gastric myoelectric activity in children with 5HT(3) antagonist prophylaxis. *Medical and Pediatric Oncology* 2000;34(6):421–3.
47. **Chesta J; Defilippi C; Defilippi C.** Abnormalities in proximal small bowel motility in patients with cirrhosis. *Heptology* 1993;17(5):829–32.
48. **Chiba N.** Definitions of dyspepsia: time for a reappraisal. *European Journal of Surgery.* Suppl. 1998;583:14–23.
49. **Chang CS; Chen GH; Lien HC; Yeh HZ.** Small intestine dysmotility and bacterial overgrowth in cirrhotic patients with spontaneous bacterial peritonitis. *Hepatology* 1998;28:1187–90.
50. **Chokhavatia S; Anuras S.** Neuromuscular disease of the gastrointestinal tract. *American Journal of Medical Science* 1991;301(3):201–14.
51. **Choudhry U; Barde CJ; Markert R; Gopalswamy N.** Percutaneous endoscopic gastrostomy: a randomized prospective comparison of early and delayed feeding. *Gastrointestinal Endoscopy* 1996;44:164–7.
52. **Coia LR; Myerson RJ; Tepper JE.** Late effects of radiation therapy on the gastrointestinal tract. *International Journal of Radiation Oncology and Biological Physics* 1995;31(5):1213–36.
53. **Cole SJ; Duncan HD; Silk DBA.** Intestinal motility. *Current Opinion in Clinical Nutrition and Metabolic Care* 1998;1:415–17.
54. **Colemont LJ; Camilleri M.** Chronic intestinal pseudo-obstruction: diagnosis and treatment. *Mayo Clinic Proceedings* 1989;64(1):60–70.
55. **Collins SM.** The immunomodulation of enteric neuromuscular function: implications for motility and inflammatory disorders. *Gastroenterology* 1996;111:1683–99.
56. **Coulie B; Camilleri M.** Intestinal pseudo-obstruction. *Annual Review of Medicine* 1999;50:37–55.
57. **Delaney BC; Innes MA; Deeks J; Wilson S; Oakes R; Moayyedi P; Hobbs FDR; Forman D.** Initial management strategies for dyspepsia. *The Cochran Library* 2000;3.
58. **De Palma GD; di Matteo E; Romano G; Fimmano A; Rondinone G; Catanzano C.** Plastic prosthesis versus expandable metal stents for palliation of inoperable esophageal thoracic carcinoma: a controlled prospective study. *Gastrointestinal Endoscopy* 1996;43:478–82.
59. **DiBase JK; Quigley EMM.** Tumor-related dysmotility: gastrointestinal dysmotility syndromes associated with tumors. *Digestive Diseases and Sciences* 1998;43(7):1369–1401.
60. **Di Lorenzo C; Lucanto C; Flores AF; Idries S; Hyman PE.** Effect of sequential erythromycin and octreotide on antroduodenal manometry. *Journal of Pediatric Gastroenterology and Nutrition* 1999;29(3):293–6.
61. **Dunlop RJ; Campbell CW.** Cytokines and advanced cancer. *Journal of Pain and Symptom Management* 2000;20(3):214–32.
62. **Eberl T; Barnert J; Dumitrascu DL; Fischer J; Weinbeck M.** The effect of cisapride on dysmotility-like functional dyspepsia: reduction of the fasting and postprandial area, but not of the postprandial antral expansion. *European Journal of Gastroenterology and Hepatology* 1998;10(12):991–5.
63. **Edmunds MC; Chen JD; Soykan I; Lin Z; McCallum RW.** Effect of octreotide on gastric and small bowel motility in patients with gastroparesis. *Alimentary Pharmacology and Therapeutics* 1998;12(2):167–74.

64. **Farthing MJG.** Octreotide in dumping and short bowel syndromes. *Digestion* 1993;54:47–52.
65. **Farthing MJG.** Octreotide in the treatment of refractory diarrhoea and intestinal fistulae. *Gut* 1994;35:5–10.
66. **Farrugia G; Camilleri M; Whitehead WE.** Medications, nutrition, biofeedback, and hypnotherapy. *Gastroenterology Clinics of North America* 1996;25(1):225–47.
67. **Faure C; Wolff VP; Navarro J.** Effect of mean and intravenous erythromycin on manometric and electrogastrographic measurements of gastric motor and electrical activity. *Digestive Diseases and Sciences* 2000;45(3):525–8.
68. **Fay DE; Poplausky M; Gruber M; Lance P.** Long-term enteral feeding: a retrospective comparison of delivery via percutaneous endoscopic gastrostomy and nasoenteric tubes. *The American Journal of Gastroenterology* 1991;86(11):1604–9.
69. **Ferraro P; Beauchamp G; Aumais G.** Endoscopic Nd: YAG laser therapy of malignant esophageal obstruction on an outpatient basis. *Canadian Journal of Surgery* 1990;33(6):479–82.
70. **Franquet T; Gimenez A; Roson N; Torrubia S; Sabate JM; Perez C.** Aspiration diseases: findings, pitfalls, and differential diagnosis. *Radiographics* 2000;20(3):673–85.
71. **Friedenberg F; Jensen G; Gurjal N; Braitman LE; Levine GM.** Serum albumin is predictive of 30-day survival after percutaneous endoscopic gastrostomy. *Journal of Parenteral and Enteral Nutrition* 1997;21:72–4.
72. **Funaki B; Zaleski GX; Lorenz J; Menocci PB; Funaki AN; Rosenblum JD; Straus C; Leef JA.** Radiologic gastrostomy placement: pigtailversus mushroom-retained catheters. *American Journal of R* 2000;175:375–9.
73. **Furness JB; Kunze WA; Bertrand PP; Clerc N; Bornstein JC.** Intrinsic primary afferent neurons of the intestine. *Progress in Neurobiology* 1998;54(1):1–18.
74. **Gorand DA.** Libby GW; Farthing MJG. Essence of antidepressants on whole gut and orocaecal transit times in health and irritable bowel syndrome. *Alimentary Pharmacology and Therapeutics* 1994;8:159–66.
75. **Gorand DA; Libby GW; Farthing MJG.** Effect of a tricyclic antidepressant on small intestinal motility in health and diarrhea-predominant irritable bowel syndrome. *Digestive Diseases and Sciences* 1995;40(1):86–95.
76. **Gore S; Gilmore IT; Haigh CG; Brownless SM; Stockdale H; Morris AI.** Colonic transit in man is slowed by ondansetron (GR38032F), a selective 5-hydroxytriptamine receptor (type 3) antagonist. *Alimentary Pharmacology and Therapeutics* 1990;4(2):139–44.
77. **Gossner L; Keymling J; Hahn EG; Ell C.** Antibiotic prophylaxis in percutaneous endoscopic gastrostomy (PEG): a prospective randomized clinical trial. *Endoscopy* 1999;31(2):119–24.
78. **Goyal RK; Hirano I.** Mechanisms of disease: the enteric nervous system. *The New England Journal of Medicine* 1996;334(1):1106–15.
79. **Hagger R; Finlayson C; Jeffrey I; Kumar D.** Role of intestinal cells of Cajal in the control of gut motility. *British Journal of Surgery* 1997;84(4):445–50.
80. **Hansen MB; Skadhauge E.** Signal transduction pathways for serotonin as an intestinal secretogue. *Comparative Biochemistry and Physiology, Part A Physiology* 1997;118(2):283–90.
81. **Hansen JM; Bytzer P; Schaffalitzky de Mukadell OB.** Placebo-controlled trial of cisapride and nizatidine in unselected patients with functional dyspepsia. *American Journal of Gastroenterology* 1998;93(3):368–74.
82. **Harding SM.** Nocturnal asthma: role of noctural gastroesophageal reflux. *Chronobio International* 1999;16(5):641–62.
83. **Harrington RA; Hamilton CW; Brogden RN; Linkewich JA; Romankiewicz JA; Heel RC.** Metoclopramide: an updated review of its pharmacological properties and clinical use. *Drugs* 1983;25:451–94.

84. **Haruma K; Wiste JA; Camilleri M.** Effect of octreotide on gastrointestinal pressure profiles in health and in functional and organic gastrointestinal disorders. *Gut* 1994;35:1064–9.
85. **Hasler WL.** Serotonin receptor physiology: relation to emesis. *Digestive Diseases and Sciences* 1999;44(8):108s–113s.
86. **Heaton KW.** Diagnosis of acute non-specific abdominal pain. *The Lancet* 2000;355(9215):1644.
87. **Heier SK; Rothman KA; Heier LM; Rosenthal WS.** Photodynamic therapy for obstructing esophageal cancer: light dosimetry and randomized camparison with Nd: YAG laser therapy. *Gastroenterology* 1995;109:63–72.
88. **Holtmann G; Stanghellini V; Talley NJ.** Nomenclature of dyspepsia, dyspepsia subgroups and functional dyspepsia: clarifying the concepts. *Bailliere's Clinical Gastroenterology* 1998;12(3):417–33.
89. **Holzer P; Holzer-Petsche U.** Tachykinins in the gut. Part I Expression, release and motor function. *Pharmacology and Therapeutics* 1997;73(3):173–217.
90. **Horikawa Y; Mieno H; Inoue M; Kajiyama G.** Gastrointestinal motility in patients with irritable bowel syndrome studies by using radiopaque markers. *Scandinavian Journal of Gastroenterology* 1999;34(12):1190–5.
91. **Horn JR.** Use of prokinetic agents in special population. *American Journal of Health System Pharmacy* 1996;53(Suppl.3):S27–S29.
92. **Houghton LA.** Sensory dysfunction and the irritable bowel syndrome. *Best Practice and Research in Clinical Gastroenterology* 1999;13(3):415–27.
93. **Hughes A; Wilcock A; Corcoran R; Lucas V; King A.** Audit of three antimuscarinic drugs for managing retained secretions. *Palliative Medicine* 2000;14:221–2.
94. **Hughes SF; Scott SM; Pilot MA; Williams NS.** Adrenoreceptors and colocolonic inhibitory reflex. *Digestive Diseases and Sciences* 1999;44(12):2462–8.
95. **Huizinga JD.** Gastrointestinal peristalsis: joint action of enteric nerves, smooth muscle, and interstitial cells of Cajal. *Microscopy Research and Technique* 1999;47(4):239–47.
96. **Husebye E.** Gastrointestinal motility disorders and bacterial overgrowth. *Journal of Internal Medicine* 1995;237(4):419–27.
97. **Husebye E.** The patterns of small bowel motility: physiology and implications in organic disease and functional disorders. *Neurogastroenterology and Motility* 1999;11:141–61.
98. **Husebye E; Engedal K.** The patterns of motility are maintained in the human small intestine throughout the process of aging. *Scandinavian Journal of Gastroenterology* 1992;27(5):397–404.
99. **Iannello S; Spina M; Leotta P; Prestipino M; Spina S; Ricciardi N; Belfiore F.** Hypomagnesemia and smooth muscle contractility: diffuse esophageal spasm in an old female patient. *Mineral and Electrolyte Metabolism* 1998;24(5):348–56.
100. **Itoh K; Kanzaki K; Ikebe T; Kuroita T; Tomozane H; Sonda S; Sato N; Haga K; Kawakita T.** Synthesis and pharmacological evaluation of carboxmide derivatives as selective serotoninergic 5-Ht(4) receptor agonists. *European Journal of Medicinal Chemistry* 1999;34(11):977–89.
101. **Jailwala J; Imperiale TF; Kroenke K.** Pharmacologic treatment of the irritable bowel syndrome: a systematic review of randomized, controlled trials. *Annals of Internal Medicine* 2000;133(2):136–47.
102. **Johnson LR.** Peptides of the gastrointestinal tract. In: Johnson LR., editor. *Gastrointestinal Physiology.* 5th edn.: Mosby, St. Louis, MO. 1997; pp. 1–58.
103. **Jorgensen F; Elsborg L.** Sucralfate versus cimetidine in reflux oseophagitis. The effect on oesophageal pH and motility. *Scandinavian Journal of Gastroenterology* 1991;26(3):263–3.
104. **Josephs MD; Cheng G; Ksontini R; Moldawer LL; Hocking MP.** Products of cyclooxygenase–2 catalysis regulate postoperative bowel motility. *Journal of Surgical Research* 1999;86(1):50–4.

105. **Kamei J; Ohsawa M; Misawa M; Nagase H; Kasuya Y.** Effect of diabetes on the morphine-induced inhibition of gastrointestinal transit. *Nihon Shinkei Seishin Yakurigaku Zasshi* 1995;15(2):165–9.

106. **Kamm MA.** The small intestine and colon: scintigraphic quantitation of motility in health and disease. *European Journal of Nuclear Medicine* 1992;19:902–12.

107. **Kamm MA.** Primary and secondary disorders to gut muscle and nerve. *Scandinavian Journal of Gastroenterology* 1996;220:91–3.

108. **Kaw M; Sekas G.** Long-term follow-up of consequences of percutaneous endoscopic gastrostomy (PEG) tubes in nursing home patients. *Digestive Diseases and Sciences* 1994;39(4):738–43.

109. **Kendall BJ; McCallum RW.** Gastroparesis and the current use of prokinetic drugs. *The Gastroenterologist* 1993;1(2):107–14.

110. **Karzka DA.** Motility abnormalities in gastroesophageal reflux disease. *Gastroenterology Clinics of North America* 1999;28(4):905–15.

111. **Kikuchi K; Kusano M; Kawamura O; Mori M; Sekiguchi T.** Measurement and evaluation of gastric emptying using radiopaque barium markers. *Digestive Diseases and Science* 2000;45(2):242–7.

112. **King PH; Redden D; Palmgren JS; Nabors LB; Lennon VA.** Hu antigen specificities of ANNA-1 autoantibodies in paraneoplastic neurological disease. *Journal of Autoimmunity* 1999;13(4):435–43.

113. **Kirchgessner AL; Liu MT; Alcantara F.** Excitotoxicity in the enteric nervous system. *Journal of Neuroscience* 1997;17(22):8804–16.

114. **Klatt S; Bock W; Rentschler J; Beckh K; Adler G.** Effects of tropisetron receptor, a 5-HT_3 receptor antagonist, on proximal gastric motor and sensory function in nonulcer dyspepsia. *Digestion* 1999;60:147–52.

115. **Knowles CH; Martin JE.** Slow transit constipation: a model of human gut dysmotility. Review of possible aetiologies. *Neurogastroenterology and Motility* 2000;12(2):181–96.

116. **Knowles CH; Scott M; Lunniss PJ.** Outcome of colectomy for slow transit constipation. *Annals of Surgery* 1999;230(5):627.

117. **Konturek JW; Fischer H; van der Voort IR; Domschke W.** Disturbed gastric motor activity in patients with human immunodeficiency virus infection. *Scandinavian Journal of Gastroenterology* 1997;32(3):221–5.

118. **Krevsaky B; Maurer AH; Malmud LS; Fisher RS.** Cisapride accelerates colonic transit in constipated patients with colonic inertia. *American Journal of Gastroenterology* 1989;84(8):882–7.

119. **Krevsky B; Maurer AH; Niewiarowski T; Cohen S.** Effect of verapamil on human intestinal transit. *Digestive Diseases and Science* 1992;37(6):919–24.

120. **Krevsky B; Malmud LS; Maurer AH; Somers MB; Siegel JA; Fisher RS.** The effect of oral cisapride on colonic transit. *Alimentary Pharmacology and Therapeutics* 1987;1(4):293–304.

121. **Krishnamurthy S; Schuffler MD.** Pathology of neuromuscular disorders of the small intestine and colon. *Gastroenterology* 1987;93(3):610–39.

122. **Kuemmerle JF.** Therapy of gastrointestinal motility disorders: moving in the right decision. *The Gastroenterologist* 1994;2:166–73.

123. **Kunze WA; Furness JB.** The enteric nervous system and regulation of intestinal motility. *Annual Review of Physiology* 1999;61:117–42.

124. **Kusano M; Sekiguchi T; Kawamura O; Kikuchi K; Miyazaki M; Tsunoda T; Hirikoshi T; Mori M.** Furthering the classification of dysmotility-like dyspepsia by interdigestive gastroduodenal manometry and plasma motilin level. *American Journal of Gastroenterology* 1997;92(3):481–4.

125. **Le Blanc-Louvry J; Ducrotte P; Peillon C; Michel P; Chiron A; Denis P.** Roux-en-Y limb motility after total or distal gastrectomy in symptomatic and asymptomatic patients. *Journal of the American College of Surgeons* 2000;190(4):408–17.

126. **Lecomte T; Cavicchi M; Delchier JC.** Small bowel pseudo-obstruction revealing an early scleroderma. *Gastrointestinal Clinical Biology* 2000;24(3):361–3.

127. **LePort J; Larvol L; Zeitoun E; Cerf M.** Chronic small intestine obstructions. *Review Pratique* 1993;43(6):684–90.

128. **Leroi AM; Lalaude O; Antonietti M; Touchais JY; Ducrotte P; Menard JF; Denis P.** Prolonged stationary colonic motility recording in seven patients with severe constipation secondary to antidepressants. *Neurogastroenterology and Motility* 2000;12(2):113–15.

129. **Lewis TD.** Morphine and gastroduodenal motility. *Digestive Diseases and Sciences* 1999;44(11):2178–86.

130. **Lien HC; Chang CS; Chen GH.** Can percutaneous endoscopic jejunostomy prevent gastro-esophageal reflux in patients with preexisting esophagitis? *The American Journal of Gastroenterology* 2000;95(12):3441–3.

131. **Lin X; Mellow MH; Southmayd L; Pan J; Chen JD.** Impaired gastric myoelectrical activity in patients with chronic renal failure. *Digestive Diseases and Science* 1997;42(5):898–906.

132. **Longo WE; Vernava AM.** Prokinetic agents for lower gastrointestinal motility disorders. *Diseases of the Colon and Rectum* 1993;36(7):696–708.

133. **Lovat LB.** Age related changes in gut physiology and nutritional status. *Gut* 1996;38(3):306–9.

134. **Lucchinetti CF; Kimmel DW; Lennon VA.** Paraneoplastic and oncologic profiles of patients seropositive for type 1 antineuronal nuclear autoantibodies. *Neurology* 1998;50(3):652–7.

135. **Madrid AM; Brahm J; Buckel E; Silvia G; Defilippi C.** Orthotopic liver transplantation improves small bowel motility disorders in cirrhotic patients. *American Journal of Gastroenterology* 1997;92(6):1044–5.

136. **Madrid AM; Quera R; Defilippi C.** Value of intestinal manometry in gastrointestinal pathology. *Revista Medica de Chile* 1999;127(10):1176–82.

137. **Malagelada JR.** Conscious perception of gut activity. *Digestive Diseases and Science* 1994;39(Suppl. 12):51s–53s.

138. **Maladelada JR; Distrutti E.** Management of gastrointestinal motility disorders. A practical guide to drug selection and appropriate ancillary measures. *Drugs* 1996;52(4):494–506.

139. **Malcolm A; Camilleri M.** Coloanal motor coordination in association with high-amplitude colonic contractions after pharmacological stimulation. *American Journal of Gastroenterology* 2000;95(3):715–19.

140. **Manes G; Mafertheiner P.** Relationship of helicobacter pylori infection with gastrointestinal motility. *Italian Journal of Gastroenterology and Hepatology* 1999;31(8):705–12.

141. **Marom EM; McAdams P; Erasmus JJ; Goodman PC.** The many faces of pulmonary aspiration. *American Journal of Roentgenology* 172:121–8.

142. **Marshall JB.** Diagnosis of esophageal motility disorders. *Postgraduate Medicine* 1990;87(7):81–4.

143. **Mathias JR; Clench MH.** Neuromuscular diseases of the gastrointestinal tract. *Postgraduate Medicine* 1995;97(3):95–8.

144. **Matini P; Faussone-Pellegrini MS; Cortesini C; Mayer B.** Vasoactive intestinal polypeptide and nitric oxide synthase distribution in the enteric plexuses of the human colon: an histochemical study and quantitative analysis. *Histochemistry and Cell Biology* 1995;103(6):415–23.

145. **Matsuda NM; Oliveira RB; Dantas RO; Iazigi N.** Effect of isosorbide dinitrate on gastroesophageal reflux in health volunteers and patients with Chagas' disease. *Digestive Diseases and Science* 1995;40(1):177–82.

146. **Maurer AH; Fisher RS.** Current applicability of scintigraphic methods in gastroenterology. *Bailliere's Clinical Gastroenterology* 1995;9(1):71–95.

147. **Maurer AH; Krevsky B.** Whole-gut transit scintigraphy in the evaluation of small-bowel and colon transit disorders. *Seminars in Nuclear Medicine* 1995;25(4):326–38.

148. **Maurer AH; Krevsky B; Knight LC; Brown K.** Opioid and opioid-like drug effects on whole-gut transit measured by scintigraphy. *Journal of Nuclear Medicine* 1996; 37(5):818–22.

149. **McLean PG; Coupar IM.** Further investigation into the signal transduction mechanism of the 5-HT4-like receptor in the circular smooth muscle of human colon. *British Journal of Pharmacology* 1996;118(4):1058–1164.

150. **McIntyre A; Vincent RM; Perkins AC; Spiller RC.** Effect of bran, ispaghula, and inert plastic particles on gastric emptying and small bowel transit in humans: the role of physical factors. *Gut* 1997;40(2):223–7.

151. **Mearadji B; Straathof JW; Lamers CB; Masclee AA.** Effect of gastrin on proximal gastric motor function in humans. *Neurogastroenterology and Motility* 1999;116(6):449–55.

152. **Medhus AW; Bondi J; Gaustad P; Husebye E.** Low-dose intravenous erythromycin: effects on postprandial and fasting motility of the small bowel. *Alimentary Pharmacology and Therapeutics* 2000;14(2):233–40.

153. **Meir R; Belinger C; Dederding JP; Meyer-Wyss B; Fumagalli M; Rowedder A; Turberg J; Brignoli R.** Age- and sex-specific standard values of colonic transit time in healthy subjects. *Schweizerische Medizinische Wochenschrift* 1992;122(24):940–3.

154. **Metcalf AM; Phillips SF; Zinsmeister AR; MacCarty RL; Beart RW; Wolff BG.** Simplified assessment of segmental colonic transit. *Gastroenterology* 1987;92(1):40–7.

155. **Micklefield GH; Greving I; May B.** Effects of peppermint oil and caraway oil on gastroduodenal motility. *Phytotherapy Research* 2000;14(1):20–3.

156. **Mier RJ; Bachrach SJ; Lakin RC; Barker T; Childs J; Moran M.** Treatment of sialorrhea with glycopyrrolate: a double-blind, dose-ranging study. *Archives of Pediatric and Adolescent Medicine* 2000;154:1214–18.

157. **Milenoy K; Kalfin R; Todoroy S; Raichey P.** Neuropeptides of the cholcystokinin group: effects and mechanisms of action on the gastro-intestinal and gall bladder motility. *Acta Physiologica et Pharmalogica Bulgarica* 1998;23(3–4):85–91.

158. **Miller P; Roy A; St-Pierre S; Dagenais M; Lapointe R; Poitras P.** Motilin receptors in the human antrum. *American Journal of Physiology - Gastrointestinal and Liver Physiology* 2000;278(1):18–23.

159. **Molenaar JC; Tibboel D; van der Kamp AW; Meijers JH.** Diagnosis of innervation-related motility disorders of the gut and basic aspects of enteric nervous system development. *Progress in Pediatric Surgery* 1989;24:173–85.

160. **Murray FE; Bowers GJ; Birkett DH; Cave DR.** Palliative laser therapy of advanced esophageal carcinoma: an alternative perspective. *The American Journal of Gastroenterology* 1988;83(8):816–19.

161. **Nagukura Y; Naitoh Y; Kamato T; Yamano M; Miyata K.** Compounds possessing 5-HT3 receptor antagonistic activity inhibit intestinal propulsion in mice. *European Journal of Pharmacology* 1996;311(1):67–72.

162. **Nelson KA; Walsh D; Sheehan FG; O'Donovan PB.** Assessment of upper gastrointestinal motility in the cancer associated dyspepsia syndrome. *Journal of Palliative Care* 1993;9(1):27–31.

163. **Nowak TV; Goddard M; Batteiger B; Cummings OW.** Evolution of acute cytomegalovirus gastritis to chronic gastrointestinal dysmotility in the nonimmunocompromised adult. *Gastroenterology* 1999;116(4):953–8.

164. **O'Brien MD; Phillips SF.** Colonic motility in health and disease. *Gastroenterology Clinics of North America* 1996;25(1):147–67.

165. **O'Sullivan G; Grundy A.** Palliation of malignant dysphagia with expanding metallic stents. *Journal of Vascular and Interventional Radiology* 1999;10:346–51.

166. **Owyang C.** Octreotide in gastrointestinal motility disorders. *Gut* Supplement 3. 1994;S11–S14.

167. **Parkman HP; Miller MA; Fisher RS.** Role of nuclear medicine in evaluating patients with suspected gastrointestinal motility disorders. *Seminars in Nuclear Medicine* 1995;25(4):289–305.

168. **Parkman HP; Miller MA; Trate D; Knight LC; Urbain JL; Maurer AH; Fisher RS.** Electrogastrography and gastric emptying scintigraphy are complementary for assessment of dyspepsia. *Journal of Clinical Gastroenterology* 1997;24(4):214–19.

169. **Parkman HP; Urbain JLC; Knight LC; Brown KL; Trate DM; Miller MA; Maurer AH; Fisher RS.** Effect of gastric acid suppressants on human gastric motility. *Gut* 1998;42:243–50.

170. **Penning C; Gielkens HA; Hemelaar JB; Bemelman WA; Lamers CB; Masclee AA.** Prolonged ambulatory recording of antroduodenal motility in slow-transit constipation. *British Journal of Surgery* 2000;87(2):211–17.

171. **Peracchi M; Basilisco G; Bareggi B; Quatrini M; Velio P; Bianchi PA.** Plasma somatostatin levels in patients with chronic idiopathic intestinal pseudo-obstruction. *American Journal of Gastroenterology* 1997;92(10):1884–6.

172. **Poen AC; Felt-Bersma RJ; Van Dongen PA; Meuwissen SG.** Effect of prucalopride, a new enterokinetic agent, on gastrointestinal transit and anorectal function in health volunteers. *Alimentary Pharmacology and Therapeutics* 1999;13(11):1493–7.

173. **Portincasa P; Colecchia A; Di Ciaula A; Larocca A; Muraca M; Palsciano G; Roda E; Festi D.** Standards for diagnosis of gastrointestinal motility disorders. Section: ultrasonography. A position statement from the Gruppo Italiano di Studio Montilita Apparato Digerente. *Digestive and Liver Diseases* 2000;32(2):160–72.

174. **Prather CM; Camilleri M; Zinsmeister AR; McKinzie S; Thomforde G.** Tegaserod accelerates orocecal transit in patients with constipation-predominant irritable bowel syndrome. *Gastroenterology* 2000;118(3):463–8.

175. **Prins NH; Shankley NP; Welsh NJ; Briejer MR; Lefebvre RA; Akkermans LM; Schuurkes JA.** An improved in vitro bioassay for the study of 5-HT(4) receptors in the human isolated large intestinal circular muscle. *British Journal of Pharmacology* 2000;129(8):1601–8.

176. **Quigley EM.** Small intestinal motor activity—its role in gut homostasis and disease. *Quarterly Journal of Medicine* 1987;65(246):799–810.

177. **Quigley EM.** Intestinal manometry in man: a historical and clinical perspective. *Digestive Diseases* 1994;12(4):199–209.

178. **Quigley EM.** Gastrointestinal motility testing—a personal perspective. *Irish Medical Journal* 1995;88(6):210–12.

179. **Quigley EM.** Gastric and small intestinal motility in health and disease. *Gastroenterology Clinics of North America* 1996;25(1):113–44.

180. **Quigley EM.** Enteric neuropathology: recent advances and implications for clinical practice. *Gastroenterologist* 1997;5(3):233–41.

181. **Quigley MM.** Disturbances in small bowel motility. *Best Practice and Research in Clinical Gastroenterology* 1999;13(3):385–95:481–91.

182. **Quigley EMM.** Gastrointestinal motility. Current Opinion in Gastroenterology 1999;15:481–91.

183. **Rabeneck L; McCullough LB; Wray NP.** Ethically justified, clinically comprehensive guidelines for percutaneous endoscopic gastrostomy tube placement. *The Lancet* 1997;349(9050):496–8.

184. **Rabeneck L; Wray NP; Petersen NJ.** Long-term outcomes of patients receiving percutaneous endoscopic gastrostomy tubes. *Journal of General Internal Medicine* 1996;11:287–93.

185. **Raiha I; Sourander L.** GI motility disorders: diagnostic workup and use of prokinetic therapy. *Geriatrics* 1993;48(11):57–66.

186. **Rashid H; Long JD; Wadleigh RG.** Management of secretions in esophageal cancer patients with glycopyrrolate. *Annals of Oncology* 1997;8:198–9.

187. **Rasmussen L; Oster-Jorgensen E; Qvist N; Pedersen SA.** The effects of omeprazole on intragastric pH, intestinal motility, and gastric emptying rate. *Scandinavian Journal of Gastroenterology* 1999;34(7):671–5.

188. **Reed CE.** Pitfalls and complications of esophageal prothesis, laser therapy, and dilation. *Chest Surgery Clinics of North America* 1997;7(3):623–36.

189. **Reiche D; Pfannkuche H; Michel K; Schemann M.** Structural and functional organization of the enteric nervous system in the stomach. *Deutsche Tieraerztliche Wochenschrift* 1998;105(12):461–5.

190. **Reynolds JC.** Challenges in the treatment of colonic motility disorders. *American Journal of Health System Pharmacy* 1996;53:S17–S26.

191. **Richards W; Parish K; Williams LF.** The usefulness of small-bowel manometry in the diagnosis of gastrointestinal motility disorders. *American Surgeon* 1990;56(4):238–44.

192. **Riordan SM; Mclver CJ; Wakefield D; Bolin TD; Duncombe VM.** Small intestinal bacterial overgrowth in the symptomatic elderly. *American Journal of Gastroenterology* 1997;92(1):47–51.

193. **Sagar PM; Pemberton JH.** Anorectal and pelvic floor function: relevance to continence, incontinence, and constipation. *Gastroenterology Clinics of North America* 1996:163–82.

194. **Samson M; Szarka LA; Camilleri M; Vella A; Zinsmeister AR; Rizza RA.** Pramlintide, an amylin analog, selectively delays gastric emptying: potential role of vagal inhibition. *American H Physiol Gastrointestinal Liver Physiology* 2000;278(6):G946–G951.

195. **Santos PM; McDonald J.** Percutaneous endoscopic gastrostomy: avoiding complications. *Otolaryngology and Head and Neck Surgery* 1999;120:195–9.

196. **Sarhill N; Nelson K; Walsh D; Komurcu S; Homsi J; Davis M; LeGrand SB.** Gastrointestinal symptoms (GI) of advanced cancer patients in a palliative medicine unit. *Twelth International Symposium on Supportive Care in Cancer.* Abstract.

197. **Sarna SK.** Tachykinins and in vivo gut motility. *Digestive Diseases and Science* 1999;44(8):114–18.

198. **Satake K; Hongo M; Ujiie H; Okuno Y; Goto Y.** The effect of cisapride on intestinal transit. *Nippon Heikatsukin Gakkai Zasshi* 1988;24(1):55–60.

199. **Scarpignato C; Pelosini I.** Management of irritable bowel syndrome: novel approaches to the pharmacology of gut motility. *Canadian Journal of Gastroenterology.* Suppl.A 1999;50A–65A.

200. **Schiefer B; Stange EF.** Motility diagnosis in chronic constipation. *Zentralblatt fuer Chirurgie* 1999;124(9):775–83.

201. **Schiller LR.** Upper gastrointestinal motility disorders and respiratory symptoms. *American Journal of Health System Pharmacy* 1996;53(Suppl. 3):S13–S16.

202. **Sharma SS; Bhargava N; Mathur SC.** Effect of oral erythromycin on colonic transit in patients with idiopathic constipation. A pilot study. *Digestive Diseases and Sciences* 1995;40(11):2446–9.

203. **Sheth S; LaMont JT.** Toxic megacolon. *The Lancet* 1998;351(9101):509–13.

204. **Shimi SM.** Self-expanding metallic stents in the management of advanced esophageal cancer: a review. *Seminars in Laparoscopy Surgery* 2000;7(1):9–21.

205. **Siddique R; Neslusan CA; Crown WH; Crystal-Peters J; Sloan S; Farup C.** A national inpatient cost estimate of percutaneous endoscopic gastrostomy (PEG)-associated aspiration pneumonia. *American Journal of Managing Care* 2000;6:490–6.

206. **Sinha SK; Kochhar R; Rana S; Bupuraj R; Singh K.** Intestinal pseudo-obstruction due to neurofibromatosis responding to cisapride. *Indian Journal of Gastroenterology* 2000;19(2):83–4.

207. **Sjogren RW.** Gastrointestinal motility disorders in scleroderma. *Arthritis and Rheumatism* 1994;1265–82.

208. **Snape WJ.** Role of motility measurements in managing upper gastrointestinal dysfunction. *The Gastroenterologist* 1998;6(1):44–58.
209. **Smout AJ; Brummer RJ.** Gastrointestinal surgery and gastroenterology. Obstipation: etiology and diagnosis. *Nederlandsch Tijdschrift voor Geneeskunde* 2000;144(19):878–84.
210. **Soffer E; Thongsawat S.** Clinical value of dudeojejunal manometry. Its usefulness in diagnosis and management of patients with gastrointestinal symptoms. *Digestive Diseases and Science* 1996;41(5):859–63.
211. **Soo S; Moayyedi P; Deeks J; Delaney B; Innes M; Forman D.** Pharmacological interventions for non-ulcer dyspepsia. *The Cochran Library* 2000;3:1–33.
212. **Soudah HC; Hasler WL; Owyang C.** Effect of octreotide on intestinal motility and bacterial overgrowth in scleroderma. *New England Journal of Medicine* 1991;325(21):1461–7.
213. **Spiller RC.** Upper gut dysmotility in slow-transit constipation: is it evidence for a pan-enteric neurological deficit in severe slow transit constipation? *European Journal of Gastroenterology and Hepatology* 1999;11(7):693–6.
214. **Spiller RC.** Disturbances in large bowel motility. *Bailliere's Clinical Gastroenterology* 1999;13(3):397–413.
215. **Stacher G; Weber U; Stacher-Janotta G; Bauer P; Huber K; Holzapfel A; Krause G; Steinborn C.** Effects of the 5-HT3 antagonist cilansetron vs placebo phasic sigmoid colonic motility in healthy man: a double-blind crossover trial. *British Journal of Clinical Pharmacology* 2000;49(5):429–36.
216. **Stanghellini V.** Treatment of dyspepsia. *Clinical Therapy* 1998;Suppl. D1–D12.
217. **Stanghellini V.** Three-month prevalence rates of gastrointestinal symptoms and the influence of demographic factors: results from the Domestic/International Gastroenterology Surveillance study. *Scandinavian Journal of Gastroenterology.* Supplement 1999;231:20–8.
218. **Stanghellini V; Corinaldesi R; Barbara L.** Pseudo-obstruction syndromes. *Bailliere's Clinical Gastroenterology* 1988;2(1):225–54.
219. **Stanghellini V; Tosetti C; Paternico A; De Giorgio R; Barbara G; Salvioli B; Corinadesi R.** Predominant symptoms identify different subgroups in functional dyspepsia. *American Journal of Gastroenterology* 1999;94(8):2080–5.
220. **Stivland T; Camilleri M; Vassallo M; Proano M; Rath D; Brown M; Thomforde G; Pemberton J; Phillips S.** Scintigraphic measurement of regional gut transit in idiopathic constipation. *Gastroenterology* 1991;101(1):107–15.
221. **Storr M; Allescher HD.** Esophageal pharmacology and treatment of primary motility disorders. *Disease of the Esophagus* 1999;12:241–67.
222. **Tack J.** Georges Brohee Prize 1994. Motilin and the enteric nervous system in the control of interdigestive and postprandial gastric motility. *Acta Gastroenterologica Belgica* 1995;58(1):21–30.
223. **Takeda T; Taniyama K; Baba S; Tanaka C.** Putative mechanisms involved in excitatory and inhibitory effects of somatostatin on intestinal motility. *American Journal of Physiology* 1989;257:532–8.
224. **Talley NJ.** Review article: 5-hydroxytryptamine agonists and antagonists in the modulation of gastrointestinal motility and sensation: clinical complications. *Alimentary Pharmacology and Therapeutics* 1992;6(3):273–89.
225. **Talley NJ; Meineche-Schmidt V; Pare P; Duckworth M; Raisanen P; Pap A; Kordecki H; Schmid V.** Efficacy of omprazole in functional dyspepsia: double-blind, randomised, placebo-controlled trials (the Bond and Opera studies). *Alimentary Pharmacology and Therapeutics* 1998;12(11):1055–65.

226. **Talley NJ; Phillips SF; Haddad A; Miller LJ; Twomey C; Zinsmeister AR; MacCarty RL; Ciociola A.** GR 38032F (ondansetron), a selective 5HT3 receptor antagonist, slows colonic transit in healthy man. *Digestive Diseases and Science* 1990;35(4):477–80.

227. **Talley NJ; Stanghellini V; Heading RC; Koch KL; Malagelada JR; Tytgat GN.** Functional gastroduodenal disorders. *Gut* 1999;45(Suppl. 2):37–42.

228. **Tam FS; Hillier K; Bunce KT.** Characterization of the 5-hydroxytryptamine receptor type involved in inhibition of spontaneous activity of human isolated colonic circular muscle. *British Journal of Pharmacology* 1994;113(1):143–50.

229. **Tam FS; Hillier K; Bunce KT; Grossman C.** Differences in response to 5-HT4 receptor agonists and antagonists of the 5-HT4-like receptor in human colon circular smooth muscle. *British Journal of Pharmacology* 1995;115(1):172–6.

230. **Taraviras S; Pachnis V.** Development of the mammalian enteric. *Current Opinion in Genetics and Development* 1999;9(3):321–7.

231. **Thomas DR; Atkinson PJ; Ho M; Bromidge SM; Lovell PJ; Villani AJ; Hagan JJ; Middlemiss DN; Price GW.** [(3) H]—SB-2669970—A selective antagonist radioligand for 5-HT-(7) receptors. *British Journal of Pharmacology* 2000;130(2):409–17.

232. **Thompson JS; Quigley EMM.** Prokinetic agents in the surgical patient. *The American Journal of Surgery* 1999;177(6):508–14.

233. **Tougas G; Chen Y; Hwang P; Liu MM; Eggleston A.** Prevalence and impact of upper gastrointestinal symptoms in the Canadian population: findings from the DIGEST study. Domestic/International Gastroenterology Surveillance Study. *American Journal of Gastroenterology* 1999: 2845–54.

234. **Turberg Y; Dederding JP.** Evaluation of small intestinal motility. *Schweizerische Medizinische Wochenschrift.* Suppl. 1993;54:26–31.

235. **Tzavella K; Riepl RL; Klauser AG; Voderholzer WA; Schindlbeck NE; Muller-Lissner SA.** Decreased substance P levels in rectal biopsies from patients with slow transit constipation. *European Journal of Gastroenterology and Hepatology* 1996;8(12):1207–11.

236. **Ueberschaer B; Ewe K; Alles U; Schmidtmann I.** Effect of 4×250 mg erythromycin on human gastrointestinal tract. *Zeitschrift fuer Gastroenterologie* 1995;33(6):340–4.

237. **Ure BM; Holschneider AM; Schulten D; Meier-Ruge W.** Clinical impact of intestinal neuronal malformations: a prospective study in 141 patients. *Pediatric Surgery International* 1997;12(5–6):377–82.

238. **van Pinxteren B; Numans ME; Bonis PA; Lau L.** Short-term treatment with proton pump inhibitors, H2-receptor antagonists and prokinetics for gastro-esophageal reflux disease-like symptoms and endoscopy negative reflux disease. *The Cochrane Library* 2000;3:1–25.

239. **Verhagen MA; Samsom M; Jebbink RJ; Smout AJ.** Clinical relevance of antroduodenal manometry. *European Journal of Gastroenterology and Hepatology* 1999;11(5):523–8.

240. **Verne GN; Sninsky CA.** Chronic intestinal pseudo-obstruction. *Digestive Disease* 1995;13(3):163–81.

241. **von der Ohe MR; Camilleri M; Thomforde GM; Klee GG.** Differential regional effects of octreotide on human gastrointestinal motor function. *Gut* 1995;36(5):743–8.

242. **Vu MK; Nouwens MA; Biemond I; Lamers CB; Maselee AA.** The osmotic laxative magnesium sulphate activates the ileal brake, *Alimentary Pharmacology and Therapeutics* 2000;14(5):587–95.

243. **Wendel T; Gleiss J; Schiedeck T; Herold A; Bruch HP.** Megacolon in adults—the spectrum of underlying intestinal innervation disorders. *Langenbecks Archiv fuer Chirurgie—Supplement—Kongressband* 1998;115:979–81.

244. **Wendel T; Roblick U; Gleiss J; Ott V; Eggers R; Kuhnel W; Krammer HJ.** Disorders of intestinal innervation as a possible cause for chronic constipation. *Zentralblatt fuer Chirurgie* 1999;124(9):796–803.

245. **Wendel T; Roblick U; Gleiss J; Schiedeck T; Bruch HP; Kuhnel W; Krammer HJ.** Organization of the enteric nervous system in the human colon demonstrated by wholemount immunohistochemistry with special reference to the submucous plexus. *Anatomischer Anzeiger* 1999;181(4):327–37.

246. **Wen A; Wang Y.** Nitrates for achalasia. *The Cochran Library* 2000;(3):1–4.

247. **Wetstein L; Brenner A.** Management of unresectable malignant esophageal obstruction. *Military Medicine* 1990;155(7):324–6.

248. **Wilder-Smith CH; Hill L; Wilkins JB; Denny L.** Effects of morphine and tramadol on somatic and visceral sensory function and gastrointestinal motility after abdominal surgery. *Anesthesiology* 1999;91(3):639–42.

249. **Wilmer A; Van Cutsem E; Andrioli A; Tack J; Coremans G; Janssens J.** Ambulatory gastrojejunal manometry in severe motility-like dyspepsia: lack of correlation between dysmotility, symptoms, and gastric emptying. *Gut* 1998;42:235–42.

250. **Wood JD.** Enteric nervous control of motility in the upper gastrointestinal tract in defensive states. *Digestive Diseases and Science* 1999;44(8):44–52.

251. **Wood JD.** Neuropathy in the brain-in-the gut. *European Journal of Gastroenterology and Hepatology* 2000;12(6):597–600.

252. **Wood JD; Alpers DH; Andrews PLR.** Fundamentals of neurogastroenterology. *Gut* 1999;45(11):II-6–II-16.

253. **Yavagal DR; Karnad DR; Oak JL.** Metoclopramide for preventing pneumonia in critically ill patients receiving enteral tube feeding: a randomized control trial. *Critical Care in Medicine* 2000;28(5):1408–11.

254. **Yuan CS; Foss JF; O'Connor M; Osinski J; Roizen MF; Moss J.** Effects of intravenous methylnaltrexone on opioid-induced gut motility and transit time changes in subjects receiving chronic methadone therapy: a pilot study. *Pain* 1999;83(3):631–5.

255. **Yuan CS; Foss JF; O'Connor M; Karrison T; Osinski J; Roizen MF; Moss J.** Effects of enteric-coated methylnaltrexone in preventing opioid-induced delay in oral-cecal transit time. *Clinical Pharmacology and Therapeutics* 2000;67(4):398–404.

256. **Zerbib F; des Varannes SB; Ropert A; Lamouliatte H; Quinton A; Galmiche JP.** Proximal gastric tone in gastro-oesophageal reflux disease. *European Journal of Gastroenterology and Hepatology* 1999;11(5):511–15.

Chapter 8

Chronic nausea and vomiting

Carla Ripamonti and Eduardo Bruera

How frequent is the problem?

There is no standard definition of chronic nausea in terms of duration in advanced cancer patients. According to Pereira *et al.* (1) the presence of nausea for more than one week in the absence of a well-identified and self-limiting cause, such as chemotherapy or radiation therapy, may be defined as chronic nausea. In advanced cancer patients, the frequency of nausea is higher than vomiting and varies from 6% to 98% (Table 8.1) (1–19). However, no study reports how long nausea is present. Nausea occurs both at an early stage of the unresectable disease (11,12), in advanced disease (1,2,4,6,7,9,11–14,20) as well as during the last weeks and days of life (5,16,18,20). Nausea is reported to be distressing for 33%–75% of patients (12,13,19). Bruera *et al.* (17) found a frequency of greater than 90% among patients admitted to a tertiary Palliative Care Unit. Although the frequency was extremely high, in this patient population managed with metoclopramide-based protocol the intensity was lower than other symptoms such as pain or asthenia.

In some surveys it is among the 10 most frequent symptoms of advanced cancer patients upon referral to the Palliative Care Service (7,14) and/or admission to hospital, hospice, or home care programs (3,8,10,15,17,19). Advanced cancer patients are polysymptomatic. Walsh *et al.* (7) found the median number of symptoms was 11 (range 1–27) and the median number of gastrointestinal (GI) symptoms was 4 (range 0–11).

The differences found by various authors in the frequency and the severity of the symptom are probably due to the non-homogeneous characteristics of the patients (different sites and stage of the disease and different survival), evaluated at different points in time (on admission and/or at certain intervals before death), using a different study design (retrospective, cross-sectional study or prospective), and different evaluations and assessment tools (self-reports, interviews with patients, and/or primary care-givers, team-based evaluation, structured questionnaire or sets of shuffled cards, visual analogue scale, numerical or verbal scales) in various settings of care (hospice/home care/palliative care unit, conventional care) and treated with a different approach (Table 8.2). Various authors report that nausea, vomiting, as well as other GI symptoms occur more frequently in females (4,5,7,8,11,14,19,21–23). This fact can be due to cancer type and increased sensitivity to opioids and other drugs. Nausea and vomiting have been commonly associated with cancers of the GI tract (4,5), breast (4), genitourinary system (3–5,8), and lymphatic–hematopoietic system (4). Vainio *et al.* (3) showed that nausea was most prevalent in gynecological cancer (42%) and stomach cancer (36%), and occurred less frequently in head and neck cancer

Table 8.1 Frequency of GI symptoms in advanced cancer patients

Number of patients	6677	1840	1635	1592	1103	1000	1000	352	275	254	243	115	100	100	100	100	90	50
(References)	(2)	(3)	(4)	(5)	(6)	(7)	(8)	(9)	(10)	(11)	(12)	(13)	(14)	(15)	(16)	(17)	(18)	(19)
Anorexia (%)	67	30	48	79	31	66	46	73	85	–	44	30	55	75	–	–	8	58
Dysphagia (%)	23	–	22	43	22	18	8	–	–	24	–	9	9	43	–	–	3	–
Nausea (%)	40	21	27	44	19	36 42% F 31% M	16 80%[a]	24	68	39	44	6	32	30	71	32 98%[b]	12	42
Vomiting (%)	–	–	20	–	–	23 28% F 18% M	10	13	–	27	21	4	25	22	–	–	–	32
Constipation (%)	47	23	33	54	–	52	31	36	65	41	35	23	40	35	–	–	4	36
Diarrhea (%)	4	–	6	25	–	8	–	–	–	–	11	5	–	–	–	–	<5	4

F: female; M: male and associated with age.

[a]16% in all populations up to 80% in cervix–vagina cancers.

[b]32% admission→98% during hospitalization in Palliative Care Unit.

(–) Not reported.

(6%) and lung cancer (14%). Donnelly and Walsh (8) found that the prevalence of moderate to severe nausea in 1000 patients was 16%; this increased to 80% in cervix–vagina cancers. A comprehensive prospective analysis of symptoms carried out in 1000 patients on initial referral to a Palliative Medicine Program (7) showed that gender was associated with different symptoms: males had more dysphagia, hoarseness, >10% weight loss, and sleep problems; females had more early satiety, nausea, vomiting, and anxiety. Younger age was associated with at least four GI symptoms such as nausea, vomiting, bloating, and constipation.

Mechanisms

Figure 8.1 shows the most frequent causes of nausea and vomiting (24–29). Figure 8.2 shows the emetic pathways and neurotransmitters (1).

Chronic nausea and vomiting are usually described as a multicausal syndrome. GI motility disorders (24), opioid treatment (4,27–30), metabolic abnormalities, brain metastases, and autonomic failure (31–39) have been associated with chronic nausea and vomiting in advanced cancer. In general, GI symptoms resulting from motility disorders are caused by delayed or accelerated transit, non-peristaltic contractions, or alterations of the motility patterns at GI sphincter sites. Early satiety, nausea, vomiting, bloating, and post-prandial fullness may all be, at least partially, the results of gastroparesis due to autonomic dysfunction. Cardiovascular alterations such as postural hypotension, tachycardia, syncopal episodes, painless myocardial infarction as well as low performance status and malnutrition may be associated (31–39).

The incidence of nausea and vomiting in patients treated with oral morphine is about 70% (40). Morphine (as do other opioids) stimulates nausea and vomiting by action on the chemoreceptor trigger zone in the area postrema by increasing vestibular sensitivity and delaying gastric emptying, and consequently adds to the accumulation of morphine-6-glucuronide in patients with renal insufficiency. Nausea and vomiting are frequent complications of early exposure to morphine and usually disappear spontaneously within the first 3 to 4 days of treatment. In some patients, nausea may persist or develop for the first time in those receiving long-term opioid therapy. In the study of Ventafridda *et al.* (40) nausea and vomiting diminished when dosages greater than 270 mg/day were achieved. Also, in animals low doses of morphine were more emetogenic than high (41).

There is increasing evidence to suggest that nausea may be a component of the cancer anorexia–cachexia syndrome (42,43). Cancer-associated dyspepsia syndrome (CADS) appears to be associated with the cancer anorexia–cachexia syndrome (44,45). The causes of this syndrome may be due to central abnormalities (metabolic, biochemical, or humoral) or peripheral abnormalities (direct tumor invasion or esophagus and stomach motility disorders) or both. Some causes of functional dyspepsia are specific to the cancer population. These include delayed gastric emptying due to the administration of opioids, anticholinergics, or chemotherapeutics; gastritis due to irritant drugs such as iron, metronidazole, non-steroidal anti-inflammatory drugs (NSAIDs), and corticosteroids; direct effects of gastric cancer; gastroparesis due to autonomic dysfunction; small stomach syndrome; and reflux esophagitis following surgery and/or radiotherapy. Patients with CADS show radiographic evidence of reduced upper GI motility (44). On the other hand, nausea may predispose to the above-mentioned syndromes or increase their severity. It is of interest that drugs such as megestrol, metoclopramide, dexamethasone, and cannabinoids, which are used in the treatment of anorexia–cachexia syndrome, are also antiemetics (43–46).

Table 8.2 Data collection/assessment on GI symptoms in advanced cancer patients

Authors (Ref.)	Time of assessment	Setting of care	Data collection	Assessment	Type of study
Vainio *et al.* (3)	Referrral–admission First contact	Home, hospice, hospital	Patient interview by physician or nurse using a structured questionnaire	Pain = 4 grade scale. Other symptoms: dichotomous indicator for none/mild or moderate/severe	Multicenter 7 PC centers Prospective
Grond *et al.* (4)	Admission	Pain clinic	Patient questionnaire	Pain = VRS (verbal rating scale) Other symptoms: presence/absence	Prospective
Reuben *et al.* (5)	Admission and every two weeks until death	Hospice and conventional terminal care	Patient and/or primary care person interview	Patient self-report of presence and intensity Primary care person report of presence/absence	Retrospective
Brescia *et al.* (6)	Admission	Calvary Hospital	Presence or absence of symptoms from the patient's medical record and not from direct clinical assessment	Pain = severe, mild, none Other symptoms: presence/absence	Retrospective
Donnelly *et al.* (8)	Initial referral	In-patients–out-patients	Patient interview by physician or nurse using a structured questionnaire	Graded moderate/severe	Prospective
Edmonds *et al.* (9)	Initial referral and twice weekly	St George's Hospital	Team-based evaluation tool	E-STAS (extended version of support team assessment schedule)	Prospective
Bruera *et al.* (10)	Admission	Palliative Care Unit	Patient questionnaire	(ESAS) Edmonton Symptom Assessment System	Retrospective
Grosvenor *et al.* (11)	Admission	Clinical Research Centre	Patient interview	Symptoms: presence/absence	Prospective
Portenoy *et al.* (12)		In-patient units and out-patient clinic, Memorial Sloan-Kettering Cancer Centre	Questionnaire to the patients with breast, colon, prostate or ovary cancer	(MSAS) Memorial System Assessment Scale	Prospective

Ventafridda *et al.* (13)	A sample week	Palliative Care Unit (in- and out-patients) Home care patients	Patient questionnaire	TIQ (Therapy Impact Questionnaire) 4 point scale: not at all, slight, a lot, awful	Cross-sectional study
Curtis *et al.* (14)	Admission	Palliative Care Unit	Patient interview by personnel	Symptom severity = mild, moderate, severe	Prospective
Ng, K., *et al.* (15)	Admission	Hospice, Palliative Care Unit	Patient or primary care interview	Survey instrument presence/absence of symptom + to describe their main complaint in their own words	Prospective
Faisinger *et al.* (16)	Admission and every day	Palliative Care Unit; in-patient	Patient or nurse rated symptoms	VAS (Visual Analogue Scale)	Retrospective
Bruera *et al.* (17)	Admission	Palliative Care Unit	Patient questionnaire	(ESAS) Edmonton Symptom Assessment System	Retrospective
Coyle *et al.* (18)	From admission until death	Supportive Care Program Memorial Sloan-Kettering Cancer Centre	Symptoms reported spontaneously by the patients	Pain = categorical scale Other symptoms = presence	
Dunlop (19)	Not defined	Hospices and hospitals with terminal care support team	Patients presented with a set of shuffled cards; the patients select the cards which describe symptoms that they experienced over the last three days	Symptoms: presence/absence + most to least distressing	Prospective

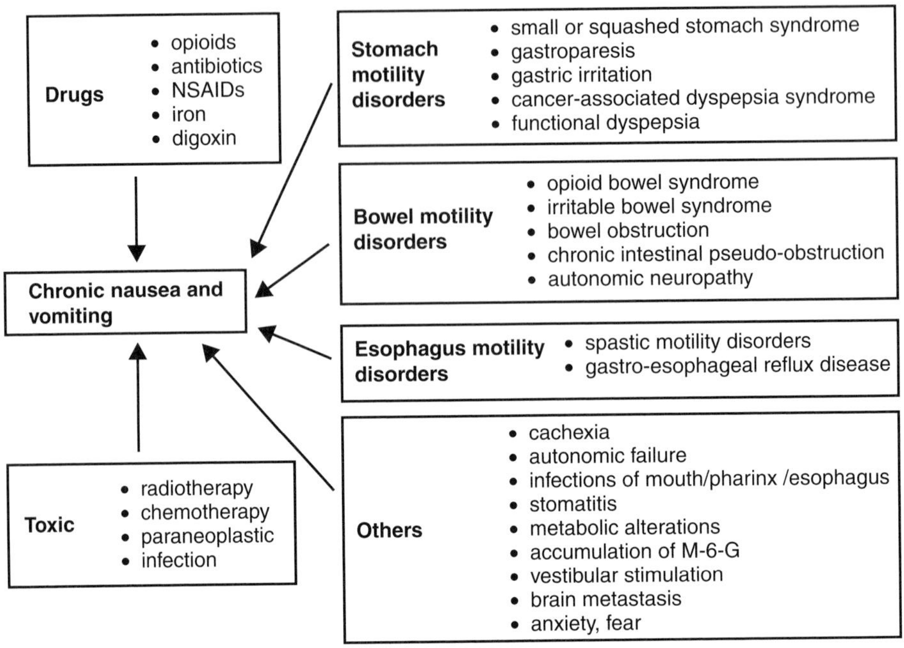

Figure 8.1 Most frequent causes of chronic nausea and vomiting.

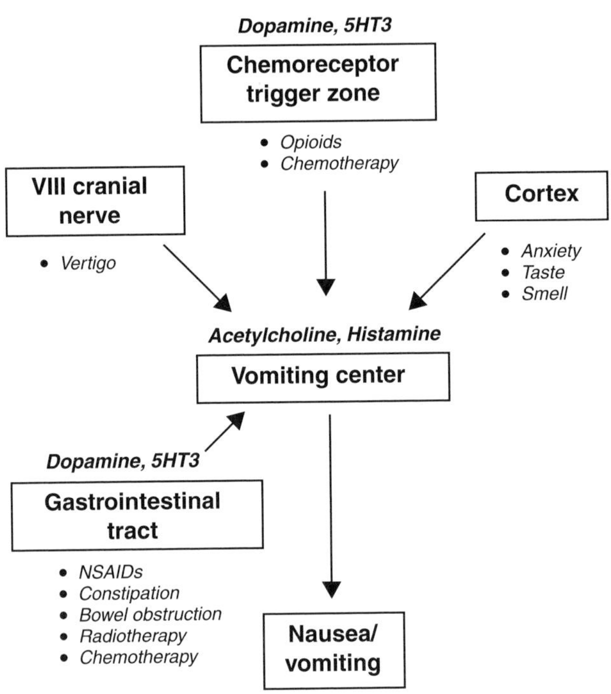

Figure 8.2 Emetic pathways and neurotransmitter.

While much research has been, and is being carried out on the cause and treatment, and the impact on quality of life of chemotheraphy-induced emesis, chronic nausea in advanced cancer has received minimal attention, despite its high prevalence and the patient's discomfort (47).

The most frequent causes of bowel dismotility are reported in Figure 8.1 and discussed in detail in Chapter 7 by Davis and Walsh. Narcotic bowel syndrome (NBS) appeared in 4% of advanced cancer patients treated with oral opioids (48). This syndrome is characterized by nausea and vomiting, mild abdominal discomfort, constipation, gaseous abdominal distension, features of intestinal pseudo-obstruction, and weight loss. Rapid resolution of symptoms and signs of NBS can occur within days of complete withdrawal of opioids (49). The treatment with parenteral opioids in association with continuous subcutaneous infusion of metoclopramide significantly improved the symptoms (48,50). Bowel obstruction is a distressing outcome especially in patients with abdominal and pelvic cancer who are in the advanced and terminal stages of the disease (see Chapter 12 by Ripamonti). As a consequence of the partial or complete occlusion of the lumen, the accumulation of unabsorbed secretions produces nausea, vomiting, and pain. When patients are unfit for surgery, medical measures such as antisecretory drugs and/or antiemetics should be considered to relieve nausea and vomiting. Moreover, the intensity of nausea decreases when patients are treated with more than 1 litre per day of parenteral fluids (51,52). Constipation can also result in chronic nausea in cancer patients. This is a frequent and undiagnosed problem (see Chapter 9 by Mancini and Bruera) with multiple causes including opioids, immobility, decreased oral intake, and other drugs. Psychological distress, including depression and anxiety, frequently result in GI symptoms. Mood problems can result in increased symptom awareness and expression. Autonomic failure is a frequent complication in patients with advanced cancer (1,35–39,53–55). These patients have evidence of cardiovascular autonomic failure such as postural hypotension and lack of change in heart rate or blood pressure during positional changes or Valsalva maneuvers. In addition, they have GI symptoms such as chronic nausea, anorexia, and early satiety. The causes are unclear, but cachexia, autonomic effects of drugs such as opioids, anticholinergics, autonomic neuropathy from chemotherapy (56) paraneoplastic effect (1,57) and hypocalcemia are all likely causes.

Autonomic neuronopathy (AN) is a rare syndrome usually associated with small-cell lung cancer (SCLC) and may occur with other cancers (pancreas, breast, pulmonary carcinoid). Patients present a subacute onset of intestinal dysmotility characterized by chronic nausea and anorexia secondary to gastroparesis with delayed gastric emptying, marked small and large intestinal dilatation, and poor propulsive activity. Antinuclear neuronal antibody I was found in serum of patients with SCLC, myenteric plexopathy, and AN (58,59). Anti-Hu antibody is a polyclonal complement-fixing IgG that reacts strongly with the nuclei of virtually all neurons in the peripheral nervous system and CNS, sparing the nucleoli (34).

From a clinical stand-point, serological testing offers a simple way to determine which patients with gut dysmotility syndromes may have associated small-cell carcinoma, thereby enabling earlier diagnosis and treatment of the tumor. Treatment of AN, using steroids, plasmapheresis, or immunosuppressants does not appear to improve the paraneoplastic symptoms (24).

Chronic intestinal pseudo-obstruction is a clinical syndrome characterized by recurrent symptoms of gastroparesis and intestinal obstruction in the absence of mechanical obstruction. The causes of intestinal pseudo-obstruction include diabetes mellitus, hypothyroidism, hypoparathyroidism, sclerodermia amyloidosis as well as medications with opioid, dopaminergic, and anticholinergic properties. Gastroparesis has also been reported after viral illness, including cytomegalovirus and *Herpes zoster*. Less common abnormal GI motility has been associated with thyrotoxicosis, abdominal radiation, traumatic brain injury, brainstem tumors, ischemic brain lesions, as well as familial forms of pseudo-obstruction (24).

Autonomic neuropathy and intestinal pseudo-obstruction are increasingly recognized in clinical practice, particularly with the introduction of antroduodenojejunal manometry, scintigraphic transit, electrophysiological studies, and autonomic function tests (24). Early recognition of such a syndrome might permit successful treatment of the underlying malignancy, with improved prognosis as well as symptomatic improvement or resolution of the pseudo-obstruction.

The differential diagnosis of this is like any intestinal motility disorders: mechanical obstruction, pseudo-obstruction or dysmotility due to visceral myopathy, familial pseudo-obstruction, connective tissue diseases, endocrine disorders, treatment with anticholinergics or other neurologic diseases that affect the autonomic nervous system.

Most studies have reported no reversal of intestinal pseudo-obstruction after treatment of the underlying neoplasm with symptomatic improvement after chemotherapy or radiotherapy noted in only few cases.

Assessment

The most effective way to take care of these patients in daily clinical practice is to let them guide us, and to assess and regularly reassess the presence and the intensity of their symptoms and the impact they have on physical and emotional well-being, activities, social, and spiritual life. One of the main priorities in palliative care education is to make the physicians and nursing staff aware of the importance of a systematic assessment of the patient's symptomatology by means of validated assessment tools that can be chosen according to experience, the human resources available, and the care settings. Patients must be informed and instructed on the importance and usefulness of a systematic assessment. This must not be a substitute for a good patient/doctor/nurse empathetic relationship, and this assessment must be obtained with the patient's full consent.

The information on symptoms has to be obtained by physicians and nurses using structured questionnaires at referral and throughout the course of the disease. To give a definition of chronic nausea, the duration of the symptom has to be reported at the first evaluation and at every assessment if the symptom is not assessed daily.

One of the crucial points in research is that of characterizing the population under consideration in terms of age, gender, type of cancer and site of metastases, stage of the disease, prognostic parameters, performance status, care setting, metabolic and cognitive condition, ability to self-rate the presence, severity and distress caused by the physical and emotional symptoms, awareness of the disease and prognosis, type of treatment including oncological therapy (chemo-, radio- and hormone therapy) carried out with curative and/or palliative intent. Whilst oncological treatment is not administered in patients cared for at home or in hospice, this treatment is frequent for patients attending out-patient departments for pain therapy and palliative care, especially in oncological research centers. Unfortunately, it may be difficult to characterize the population that receives palliative care due to a dynamic process in which the presence, nature and intensity of symptoms and the clinical features of the illness can change from day to day.

The second issue is the multidimensional assessment of nausea. Knowing that nausea is present does not give any indication regarding treatment unless the causes (tumor and/or metastases, drugs, metabolic alterations, GI dysmotility, etc.), exacerbating and alleviating factors (body position/movement, food/drug administration) onset and duration, and diurnal variation are taken into consideration. If there is co-existing vomiting, then the nature of the vomiting and how long nausea lasts after vomiting should also be reviewed. The presence of cardiovascular signs and symptoms such as syncopal episodes, tachycardia, and early satiety, which may indicate autonomic failure, should also be investigated.

Nausea may be present and not produce any discomfort to the patient, so additional information regarding the symptom is required, such as the intensity and the impact of the symptom on the patient's well-being.

A detailed and thorough description on how to measure symptoms has been given by Ingham and Portenoy (60,61). The same indications can be applied to nausea and other GI symptoms provoked by bowel dysmotility. Chronic nausea is a subjective symptom and must be evaluated separately from vomiting and retching and systematically together with all the other physical and emotional symptoms. The fact that nausea and vomiting can occur independently points to the validity of their assessment as separate behaviors. It is also important to note that their severity and duration are separate phenomena. These symptoms are subjective and therefore are referred by the patient himself.

Neither the medical/nursing staff nor the care-giver can evaluate the presence and intensity of nausea in relation to the vomiting episodes without noting that these two events need not be associated. The patient can best describe the distress caused by nausea, which is the main target for the treatment.

In terminal and/or confused patients the symptoms are often referred by the nurses or the care-givers. However, this method cannot be considered reliable for research as it has been shown that the severity of the symptoms referred by the care-givers not always agree with patients' ratings (62–65).

The intensity of nausea is easily measured by simple tools such as a visual analogue scale, a numerical scale, or verbal descriptors. There are specific tools for measuring nausea and/or vomiting, particularly for patients on chemotherapy, such as the Rhodex Index (66), the Overall Nausea Index (67), and the Morrow Assessment of Nausea and Emesis (68). These tools have a particular role when nausea and/or vomiting are the only symptoms present in the population under study to evaluate both drug-induced nausea and vomiting as well as the efficacy of a pharmacological therapy.

In advanced cancer patients presenting more than one symptom, the intensity of nausea alone might not give us enough information if we do not know the degree of the distress that nausea causes; the possible interaction between nausea and other physical and emotional symptoms such as pain, anorexia, dyspepsia, asthenia, anxiety, sense of well-being; and the impact of nausea on performance status and the social life of the patient. These are the reasons why a multidimensional assessment is required. Different multidimensional assessment tools have been devised (69). Among these there is the Edmonton Symptom Assessment System (ESAS) based on visual analogue scales (VAS) looking not only at nausea but also pain, anxiety, depression, appetite, shortness of breath, and also the feeling of well-being (70). This is used twice a day in patients admitted to the palliative care unit and is completed either by the patient alone, by the patient with a nurse's assistance, or by the nurses or relatives, depending on the physical and cognitive condition of the patient. The information is then transferred to a graph, allowing staff to visualize patterns of symptom control over time. It is a simple and easy test to use. Further testing of this measure's validity and reliability are required, particularly with reference to the potential bias introduced by a change in the person recording the answers on the VAS as care continues (69).

The Therapy Impact Questionnaire is a validated tool used to evaluate the quality of life of advanced cancer patients. It includes 36 items to assess the degree of discomfort experienced and evaluated subjectively by the cancer patient through a verbal Likert scale with four possible answers (not at all, slight, a lot, very much) (71). This tool allows us to evaluate five areas:

1 physical symptoms resulting from disease or therapies,

2 functional conditions,

3 psychological conditions,

4 family and social relationships, and

5 global judgment of not feeling well.

The period of reference is the previous week.

Nausea and/or other GI symptoms may be present but not distressing to the patient (12). The expression 'symptom distress' refers to the degree of discomfort caused by a specific symptom as it is perceived by the patient.

One of the most widely tested instruments for the evaluation of symptom distress is the Symptom Distress Scale (SDS) by McCorkle and Young (72). The most recent version of SDS comprises 13 symptoms that are considered to be of most concern to patients and among these the intensity and frequency of nausea and bowel pattern are reported. This instrument is self-rated and has been described for several potential applications:

1 to measure the variations in the degree of symptom distress linked to the course of the disease (73–76),

2 to correlate the trend of some symptoms over time (72),

3 to measure the variance of a specific symptom or group of symptoms in correlation with specific therapeutic or home care programs (76),

4 to compare the symptom distress scores for different kinds of chronic diseases (73), and

5 to assess the efficacy of treatment provided by a Palliative Care Division (77).

Peruselli *et al.* (78) used the Italian version of the SDS to assess the quality of life in advanced cancer patients cared for at home. The scores showed a reduction in symptom distress, which was primarily due to an improvement in pain, nausea, and bowel pattern.

The Memorial Symptom Assessment Scale (MSAS) (79) provides a method for the comprehensive evaluation of physical and psychological symptomatology in patient care, epidemiological surveys, and clinical trials. By means of separate four- or five-point Likert scales, three dimensions are considered: severity of the symptom, frequency with which it occurs, and the distress it produces. The study carried out to evaluate the reliability and validity of the MSAS (79) shows that the use of a distress scale gives significant information on the relationship between symptoms and quality of life, but that the combination of a distress measurement with either a frequency or severity measurement provides significantly more information than the distress measurement alone. Moreover, it was found that the frequency of the symptom was a more remarkable complement to distress than the severity.

The Rotterdam Symptom Checklist (RSC) (80) is a validated, patient-rated measure that evaluates a spectrum of common symptoms in terms of patient-rated distress. Thirty physical and psychological symptoms are described plus eight other items that specifically attempt to define the impact of symptoms on physical activity and function. The intensity of distress is evaluated by means of a four-point Likert scale. The RSC assessment tool gives quantitative information on physical and psychological symptom distress.

Other questionnaires on the quality of life often used in oncology (The Functional Living Index for Cancer, the EORTC QLQ-C30, The Functional Assessment of Cancer Therapy) (81–83) contain evaluation methods on nausea and vomiting representing a relatively simple system of data collection using descriptive or visual analogue scales. Other multidimensional assessment tools used in palliative care are available and have been recently reviewed (69).

Management

Various antiemetics acting on the central nervous system and/or on the GI tract proved to be effective in reducing nausea and vomiting in advanced cancer patients in uncontrolled (10,26,84–87) and controlled clinical trials (45,88–92).

However, there are no controlled clinical trials comparing the efficacy and tolerability of the different antiemetics in the treatment of morphine-induced nausea and vomiting.

Prokinetic drugs such as metoclopramide, domperidone, and cisapride have been proposed as a rational treatment, particularly for patients with dysmotility-like symptoms. Prokinetic agents rarely alleviate the symptoms of paraneoplastic pseudo-obstruction, probably because of widespread neuronal degeneration. There is no evidence that metoclopramide is efficacious in myopathic or neuropathic intestinal pseudo-obstruction (93). In advanced cancer patients chronic nausea and vomiting have been shown to improve after the administration of metoclopramide in uncontrolled (17,86,87) and controlled studies (89–92). Metoclopramide is also effective in reversing tumor-related gastroparesis (94,95), nausea, and anorexia in advanced cancer patients (86,87).

Sustained plasma metoclopramide concentrations are required to suppress nausea, vomiting, and other GI symptoms associated with cancer, resulting in the need for frequent administration of short-acting formulations of metoclopramide.

In a double-blind, cross-over study, controlled release metoclopramide was able to reduce the intensity of nausea significantly more than immediate release metoclopramide in advanced cancer patients (89). Recently Bruera *et al.* (45) carried out a double-blind, cross-over study of controlled release metoclopramide and placebo for mild to moderate chronic nausea lasting for an average of 19 weeks and dyspepsia of advanced cancer. Nausea was significantly lower in the controlled release metoclopramide group compared with placebo.

Preliminary data suggest that continuous subcutaneous infusion of metoclopramide is superior to intermittent administration for the management of chronic nausea in advanced cancer (87,96). Domperidone (not available in the United States) 10 or 20 mg three to four times daily has been shown to be more effective than, or comparable with, an equal dose of metoclopramide in patients with symptoms of dyspepsia caused mainly by gastritis (97).

In comparison with metoclopramide, cisapride showed similar or superior efficacy in reducing the time of gastric emptying in healthy volunteers as well as in patients with idiopathic or diabetic gastroparesis (98–100). In patients with functional dyspepsia the superiority of cisapride in comparison with standard doses of metoclopramide or domperidone is still controversial. Cisapride was more effective than metoclopramide in reversing delayed gastric emptying due to the intramuscular administration of morphine (101). In a double-blind, cross-over study (102) carried out on patients suffering from constipation, the time of emptying of the caecum and ascending colon was significantly reduced after cisapride administration. Furthermore, cisapride (20 mg twice daily) was found to significantly increase spontaneous stool frequency and consistency and to reduce the laxative intake in 126 patients with idiopathic constipation (103).

Unfortunately, because of the potential for serious drug interactions, cisapride has been withdrawn from the market in the United States and other countries.

The treatment of nausea is also successfully carried out in most cases using drugs such as haloperidol (88), prochlorperazine, dimenhydrinate, and phenothiazine (26,85) which are also potent antiemetics but may also produce sedation.

A number of novel pro-motility agents are currently under development but they are not available for clinical use yet.

Corticosteroids are among the most potent antiemetics. These agents are synergistic with metoclopramide and 5HT3 antagonist against chemotherapy-induced emesis and chronic nausea (17). These drugs can be given orally, subcutaneously, or intravenously. In addition to nausea, corticosteroids are capable of impacting appetite, pain, and asthenia (104–107). Their main drawback is potentially serious toxicity with prolonged used. The ideal dose is not known, but higher dosages are usually tolerated well for a short period of time. After an initial response it is important to descrease the dose to the minimally effective as soon as possible. Response is usually observed within 24 to 48 hours of therapy.

No clinical trials have been carried out on the role of selective 5HT3 antagonists in the treatment of chronic nausea. Recently, some case reports and retrospective analyses have showed the efficacy of one of these drugs—ondansetron—in the management of intractable nausea in advanced cancer patients (108–112) and in AIDS patients (112). All the patients reported had no benefit from standard or combination antiemetics. In these patients ondansetron was used as a third- or fourth-line therapy. Treatment with ondansetron was well tolerated, and response rates were rapid, high, and sustained over time. There is limited evidence from animal models suggesting that 5HT3 antagonists are efficacious in the suppression of opioid-induced vomiting (113).

Switching the opioid and/or its route of administration to manage GI symptoms

According to the data in the literature, opioids can act on different receptors or subtype receptors, and individual receptor profiles may influence analgesia as well as the side-effects. The genetic makeup of the individual also plays an important role. An important role may also be related to differences in the profile of active metabolites between various opioids (114–116).

In view of this data, which opioid produces less nausea and fewer GI symptoms? Is opioid or route switching beneficial in the management of GI symptoms?

Table 8.3 shows the results of comparative studies between different opioids (117–120). In a controlled clinical trial, controlled release morphine and controlled release oxycodone showed comparable efficacy and tolerability (117). However, preliminary results from controlled clinical trials show that morphine can cause more nausea, vomiting, hallucinations, and delirium in comparison with oxycodone (118,119). In a prospective randomized study, 16 patients were treated with dextropropoxyphene and 16 patients with morphin sulphate slow release. The patients on morphine reported significantly more intensity and severity of drowsiness, nausea, vomiting, and xerostomia (120).

Table 8.3 Comparative studies between different opioids

Authors (Ref.)	Study design	Number of patients	Opioid	Opioid	Results
Mercadante *et al.* (120)	Prospective Randomized	32 Opioid naives	16 pts DPP 120–240 mg/day	16 pts CR morphine 20 mg/day	Pts on morphine had significant more frequency and severity of drowsiness, vomiting, dry mouth 11 pts on DPP switched to CR morphine to increase analgesia 3 pts on morphine switched to DPP due to intolerable vomiting and drowsiness and had pain relief until death
Bruera *et al.* (117)	Prospective Double-blind Cross-over	32 23 completed the study	CR morphine for 7 days	CR oxycodone for 7 days	Comparable efficacy and tolerability
Kalso *et al.* (118)	Double-blind Cross-over	20	Oral oxycodone every 4 h 2.7 mg/ml after IV PCA for titration	Oral morphine every 4 h; 4.0 mg/ml after IV PCA for titration	Comparable pain relief Morphine caused more nausea hallucinations occurred only during morphine treatment Both drugs produced sedation
Heiskanen *et al.* (119)	Double-blind Randomized Cross-over	27	CR oxycodone	CR morphine[a]	Comparable analgesia Significantly more vomiting with morphine Constipation more common with oxycodone Nightmares only with morphine (n.s.)

Notes: pts: patients; DPP: dextropropoxyphene; CR: controlled release; IV: intravenous; PCA: patient-controlled analgesia

[a]Opioid consumption ratio of oxycodone: morphine was 2:3 when oxycodone was administered first and 3:4 when oxycodone was administered after morphine

Table 8.4 shows the results of studies on different routes of opioid administration (121,126). Drexel *et al.* (121) found that the incidence of constipation, drowsiness, and nausea was significantly lower in patients treated with low doses of a continuous subcutaneous morphine infusion compared with conventional intermittent oral or subcutaneous boluses of morphine. The incidence of nausea and its severity were significantly higher when oxycodone was administered intravenously as compared with oral administration (122).

In a double-blind, cross-over study, 27 patients with cancer pain were randomized to receive controlled release morphine suppositories versus controlled release morphine tablets every 12 hours for 7 days each. There was a small but significant difference particularly in the nausea VAS score in favor of rectal morphine (123).

Pre-clinical (127) and clinical data (128) support the relatively low incidence of constipation observed with transdermal fentanyl in comparison with morphine. However, no difference in nausea was found between the two drugs (128).

There is some clinical evidence showing that switching the route of opioid administration may improve the opioid tolerability (Table 8.5) (129,130).

Switching from oral morphine to epidural or subcutaneous morphine produces improvement of pain as well as a reduction in adverse effects, including nausea and vomiting (129). Moreover, no significant benefits, either in efficacy or in adverse effects, were achieved by administering morphine epidurally compared with continuous subcutaneous infusion(CSI).

MacDonald *et al.* (130) prospectively studied the analgesia and toxicity of regular four-hourly subcutaneous bolus morphine in 164 patients with cancer-related pain previously treated with oral morphine. Subcutaneous morphine was associated with significant improvement in pain relief and significant less nausea and vomiting compared with aqueous solution.

In a recent prospective study (131) a switch from oral morphine to oral methadone was performed in 50 cancer patients with poor pain control and/or moderate to severe opioid adverse effects not responsive to adjuvant medications during oral morphine therapy. Significant improvement was found also in GI symptoms such as nausea, vomiting, and constipation. Future research is necessary to evaluate the duration of this benefit over time.

Which opioid/opioids should be considered for switching (116)? The selection of an alternative opioid is largely empirical. A pure opiod agonist such as oxycodone, methadone, hydromorphone, and fentanyl is recommended. Theoretically there may be some benefit in opioid switching in any situation where there are unacceptable adverse effects with the initial opioid.

Short- and long-term goals of clinical research

Clinical research in the field of the prevention and treatment of nausea and vomiting are equally important as for other GI symptoms.

1 First of all, it is important to define the terms used in clinical practice. What is the definition of chronic nausea in advanced cancer patients? That is to say, how long should nausea be present before defining it as chronic?

2 The high incidence of GI symptoms in women has implications for future research in the area of drug development, clinical attention to complaints of these symptoms, symptom management, and the relationship between the symptom and cancer site.

Table 8.4 Comparative studies between different routes of morphine administration

Authors (Ref.)	Study design	Number of patients	Route	Route	Results
Drexel *et al*. (121)	Prospective	36	Morphine 10–90 mg/day intermittent oral or SC	Morphine 5–48 mg/day CSI conversion rate 2:1	Significant lower incidence of constipation, nausea, and drowsiness with CSI
Leow *et al*. (122)	Open, cross-over, single dose	12	Oral oxycodone 9.1 mg	IV oxycodone 4.6–9.1 mg	IV oxycodone had a faster onset of pain relief than oxycodone tablets but the duration of analgesia was the same (4 h) IV oxycodone had a significantly higher incidence and severity of nausea, drowsiness; and light-headedness than oral oxycodone
Bruera *et al*. (123)	Double-blind, cross-over	23	CR morphine sulfate suppository every 12 h	SC morphine rect/parent ratio 2.5:1	Comparable analgesia and side-effects
Babul *et al*. (124)	Double-blind, cross-over	27	CR morphine suppository every 12 h	CR morphine tablets every 12 h conversion rate 1:1	No difference in pain and sedation small but significant difference in nausea in favor of rectal administration
De Conno *et al*. (125)	Double-blind, double-dummy, cross-over, single dose study	34 opioid naives	Rectal morphine conversion rate 1:1	Oral morphine	Rectal morphine had a faster onset of action and longer duration of analgesia than an acute dose of oral morphine. No significant difference in intensity of sedation, nausea, or number of vomiting episodes between the two routes
Bruera et al. (126)	Randomized, double-blind, cross-over	12 6 evaluable	CR morphine sulfate suppository every 12h	CR morphine sulfate suppository every 24h	There was no significant difference between the q12h and q24h treatment groups in symptom (pain, nausea, sedation) intensity, adverse effects, patient choice

SC: subcutaneous; CSI: continuous subcutaneous infusion; CR: controlled release; IV: intravenous

Table 8.5 Switching the route of opioid administration

Authors (Ref.)	Study design	Number of patients	Route	Route	Results
Kalso *et al.* (129)	Randomized, double-blind, cross-over	10	Oral morphine every 4 h median dose 225 mg/day	CSI morphine median dose 327 mg/day	Pain at rest significantly less during CSI compared with oral morphine
			Switch to CSI or CEI	CEI morphine median dose 106 mg/day	Pain when moving significantly less during both CSI and CEI compared with oral morphine No significant difference in pain relief between CSI and CEI Total amount of adverse effects (sum of VAS values) significantly higher during oral compared with CSI Median of the sum of adverse effects during CEI did not differ significantly from oral or CSI
MacDonald et al. (130)	Prospective	164 switched due to drowsiness, nausea, vomiting, not controlled pain, difficulty in swallowing	Oral morphine	Bolus SC morphine every 4h Conversion rate 2:1	Significant improvement in pain relief and significant less nausea and vomiting but not drowsiness with SC

CSI: continuous subcutaneous infusion; CEI: continuous epidural infusion; SC: subcutaneous; CR: controlled release; IV: intravenous

3 Do physical and/or psychological symptoms such as constipation, taste adversions, oral mouth infections, depression, anxiety, and fear have any influence on the onset or worsening of nausea? It is important to study the interactions among the symptoms with the aim of prioritizing the treatment of those symptoms that cause the most distress to the patient and that trigger other symptoms so that we can reduce to the minimum drug administration by avoiding drug interaction and further side-effects.

4 Staging systems are very important in the development of clinical research. In pain assessment, certain clinical descriptors, such as those associated with neuropathic and/or incident pain, have therapeutic and prognostic implications. Do specific characteristics of nausea, vomiting and/or other GI symptoms have similar meaning?

5 Specific drugs have to be targeted at specific syndromes of chronic nausea in cancer. Prospective clinical trials of different prokinetics and antiemetics should be conducted. As far as prokinetics are concerned it would be interesting to study drugs that have a propulsive action on the large bowel too. Among antiemetics the role of 5HT3 antagonists in palliative care should be investigated together with their administration routes. In particular, the possible worsening of constipation in advanced cancer patients taking opioids and these drugs should be examined.

6 Parenteral hydration use in the care of terminal cancer patients is still a controversial topic (see Chapter 22 by Fainsinger and Chapter 23 by MacDonald). What is the role of parenteral hydration in the management of nausea and vomiting?

7 Many other questions need to be answered: What is the cost of treating nausea and other GI symptoms? How often is it possible to find the cause of nausea and how often is it possible to manage the symptom? How many times do patients have to be admitted to hospital for adequate evaluation and treatment of nausea and other GI symptoms? Could intractable nausea be considered as a poor prognostic indicator of survival for the patient and/or for the doctor? Is there a circadian rhythm for nausea as there is for pain? How often is nausea present without vomiting and are antiemetic drugs always able to control nausea in this case?

Conclusions

The presence and intensity of nausea and vomiting as well as the impact on quality of life are dynamic events which can change in respect to both physical and psychological factors. To obtain an adequate follow-up on symptom control, assessment should be held frequently during the course of the illness.

The assessment tools can be used to document the intensity of the nausea, initially as a baseline assessment, and then on a regular basis thereafter aiding doctors and nurses in clinical decision-making and in research.

The therapeutic intervention for managing nausea and/or other GI symptoms foresees careful research on causes and triggering factors in order to act adequately. Since some symptoms are caused by multiple factors, it is necessary to identify the different factors involved, and then to seek to correct those that are reversible. Treatment for the same symptom may vary considerably from patient to patient.

Before administration of symptomatic antiemetics to manage nausea and vomiting, the patient's drug regimen should be checked for substances that can trigger the symptom through different mechanisms and eventually stop or substitute the drug.

Secondly, it is necessary to optimize the therapy that the patient is taking to control other symptoms. As already mentioned, prospective studies should be carried out to evaluate the effects of different opioids and the different routes of their administration on the GI tract. Prospective studies are necessary to evaluate the efficacy of opioid switching as well as hydration on GI symptoms and/or side-effects.

The treatment of nausea and GI symptoms should not be limited to the use of drugs alone.

It is advisable to administer antiemetic drugs only after all possible causes of nausea have been investigated and the therapy that the patient is receiving has been optimized. Patients should be evaluated for drowsiness due to antiemetics acting at the central level and for confusion due to anticholinergic side-effects.

In the pharmacological research field, a space should be dedicated to prospectively studying the role of 5HT3 antagonist in chronic nausea in advanced cancer patients and to compare the efficacy and tolerability of such drugs with those commonly used such as metoclopramide and haloperidol. In some studies, large numbers of patients are required to evaluate the effects of different drugs. This is not always possible in one center alone; the solution would be to undertake these studies in collaboration with other centers around the world (multicenter studies). Unfortunately, the major problem is the need to use the same validated assessment tools in all centers. Whereas this is possible for studies on pain control, this is not yet the case for studies on other symptoms. A common effort must be made in order to solve the problem. This would be a stepping stone in the field of research for palliative care.

References

1. **Pereira J; Bruera E.** Chronic nausea. In: Bruera E; Higginson I., editors. *Cachexia–anorexia in Cancer Patients.* Oxford: Oxford Medical Publications, Oxford University Press, 1996; 2: pp. 23–37.
2. **Twycross RG; Lack SA.** *Control of Alimentary Symptoms in Far Advanced Cancer.* Edinburgh: Churchill Livingston, 1986.
3. **Vainio A; Auvinen A.** with Members of the Symptom Prevalence Group. Prevalence of symptoms among patients with advanced cancer: an International Collaborative Study. *Journal of Pain and Symptom Management* 1996;12:3–10.
4. **Grond S; Zech D; Diefenbach C; Bischoff A.** Prevalence and pattern of symptoms in patients with cancer pain: a prospective evaluation of 1635 patients referred to a pain clinic. *Journal of Pain and Symptom Management* 1994;9:372–82.
5. **Reuben DB; Mor V; Hiris J.** Clinical symptoms and length of survival in patients with terminal cancer. *Archives of Internal Medicine* 1988;148:1586–91.
6. **Brescia FJ; Adler D; Gray G; Ryan MA; Cimino J; Mamtani R.** Hospitalized advanced cancer patients: a profile. *Journal of Pain and Symptom Management* 1990;5:221–7.
7. **Walsh D; Donnelly S; Rybicki L.** The symptoms of advanced cancer: relationship to age, gender, and performance status in 1,000 patients. *Supportive Care in Cancer* 2000;8:175–9.
8. **Donnelly S; Walsh D.** The symptoms of advanced cancer: identification of clinical and research priorities by assessment of prevalence and severity. *Journal of Palliative Care* 1995;11(1):27–32.
9. **Edmonds PM; Stuttaford JM; Penny J; Lynch AM; Chamberlain J.** Do hospital palliative care teams improve symptom control? Use of a modified STAS as an evaluation tool. *Palliative Medicine* 1998;12:345–51.
10. **Bruera E.** Clinical management of anorexia and cachexia in patients with advanced cancer. *Oncology* 1992;49:35–42.

11. **Grosvenor M; Bulcavage L; Chlebowski RT.** Symptoms potentially influencing weight loss in a cancer population. Correlations with primary site, nutritional status, and chemotherapy administration. *Cancer* 1989;63(2):330–4.

12. **Portenoy RK; Thaler HT; Kornblith AB., *et al.*** Symptom prevalence, characteristics and distress in a cancer population. *Quality of Life Research* 1994;3:183–9.

13. **Ventafridda V; De Conno F; Ripamonti C; Gamba A; Tamburini M.** Quality-of-life assessment during palliative care programme. *Annuals of Oncology* 1990;1:415–20.

14. **Curtis EB; Krech R; Walsh TD.** Common symptoms in patients with advanced cancer. *Journal of Palliative Care* 1991;7(2):25–9.

15. **Ng K; von Gunten CF.** Symptoms and attitudes of 100 consecutive patients admitted to an acute hospice/palliative care unit. *Journal of Pain and Symptom Management* 1998;16:307–16.

16. **Fainsinger R; Miller MJ; Bruera E; Hanson J; MacEachern T.** Symptom control during the last week of life on a palliative care unit. *Journal of Palliative Care* 1991;7(1):5–11.

17. **Bruera E; Seifert L; Watanabe S; Babul N; Darke A; Harsanyi Z; Suarez-Almazor M.** Chronic nausea in advanced cancer patients: a retrospective assessment of a metoclopramide-based antiemetic regimen. *Journal of Pain and Symptom Management* 1996;11:147–53.

18. **Coyle N; Adelhardt J; Portenoy RK; Foley KM.** Character of terminal illness in the advanced cancer patient: pain and other symptoms during the last four weeks of life. *Journal of Pain and Symptom Management* 1990;5:83–93.

19. **Dunlop GM.** A study of the relative frequency and importance of gastrointestinal symptoms and weakness in patients with far advanced cancer. *Palliative Medicine* 1989;4:37–43.

20. **Mercadante S; Casuccio A; Fulfaro F.** The course of symptom frequency and intensity in advanced cancer patients followed at home. *Journal of Pain and Symptom Management* 2000;20:104–12.

21. **Wachtel T; Allen-Masterson S; Reuben D; Goldberg R; Mor V.** The end-stage cancer patient: terminal common pathway. *Hospice Journal* 1988;4:43–80.

22. **Baines M.** Nausea and vomiting in the patient with advanced cancer. *Journal of Pain and Symptom Management* 1988;3:81–5.

23. **Saunders DC.** Pain and impending death. In: Wall PD; Melzack R. editors. *Textbook of Pain.* Edinburgh: Churchill Livingstone, 1989: pp. 624–31.

24. **Ripamonti C; Rodriguez C.** Gastrointestinal motility disorders in patients with advanced cancer. In: Portenoy RK; Bruera E., editors. *Topics in Palliative Care, Vol. 1.* Oxford: Oxford University Press, 1997;4: pp. 61–93.

25. **Hagen NA; Foley KM; Cerbone DJ; Portenoy RK; Inturrisi CE.** Chronic nausea and morphine-6-glucuronide. *Journal of Pain and Symptom Management* 1991;6:125–8.

26. **Twycross R; Back I., *et al.*** Nausea and vomiting in advanced cancer. *European Journal of Palliative Care* 1998;5(2):39–45.

27. **Campora E; Merlini L; Pace M; Bruzzone M; Luzzani M; Gottlieb A; Rosso R.** The incidence of narcotic-induced emesis. *Journal of Pain and Symptom Management* 1991;6:428–30.

28. **McIllmurray MB; Warren MR.** Evaluation of a new hospice: the relief of symptoms in cancer patients in the first year. *Palliative Medicine* 1989;3:135–40.

29. **Schug SA; Zech D; Grond S; Jung H; Meuser T; Stobbe B.** A long term survey of morphine in cancer pain patients. *Journal of Pain and Symptom Management* 1992;7:259–66.

30. **Manara L; Bianchetti A.** The central and peripheral influence of opioids on gastrointestinal propulsion. *Annual Review of Pharmacology and Toxicology* 1985;25:249–73.

31. **Lautenbach E; Lichtenstein GR.** Retroperitoneal leiomyosarcoma and gastroparesis: a new association and review of tumor-associated intestinal pseudo-obstruction. *The American Journal of Gastroenterology* 1995;90(8):1338–41.

32. **Gould GA; Ashworth M; Lewis GT.** Are cardiovascular reflexes more commonly impaired in patients with bronchial carcinoma? *Thorax* 1986;41:372–5.
33. **Liang B; Albers J; Sima A., *et al.*** Paraneoplastic pseudo-obstruction, mononeuropathy multiplex, and sensory neuropathy. *Muscle and Nerve* 1994;17:91–6.
34. **Posner J.** Paraneoplastic syndromes. In: Reinhardt R; Wissler B; Massey R; Forgione L., editors. *Neurologic Complications of Cancer.* New York: F.A. Davis Company Press, 1995; pp. 353–84.
35. **Bruera E; Catz Z; Hooper R; Lentle B; MacDonald N.** Chronic nausea and anorexia in advanced cancer patients: a possible role for autonomic dysfunction. *Journal of Pain and Symptom Management* 1987;2:19–21.
36. **Kvale G; Psychol C; Hugdahl K.** Cardiovascular conditioning and anticipatory nausea and vomiting in cancer patients. *Behavioral Medicine* 1994;20(2):78–83.
37. **Martin R; Delgado JM; Molto JM; Vincent JM; Manzanares R; Insa R; Matias-Guiu J.** Cardiovascular reflexes in patients with malignant disease. *Italian Journal of Neurological Sciences* 1992;13(2):125–9.
38. **Bruera E; Chadwick S; Fox R; Hanson J; MacDonald N.** Study of cardiovascular autonomic insufficiency in advanced cancer patients. *Cancer Treatment Reports* 1986;70:1383–7.
39. **Bruera E.** Autonomic failure in patients with advanced cancer. *Journal of Pain and Symptom Management* 1989;4(3):163–6.
40. **Ventafridda V; Oliveri E; Caraceni A; Spoldi E; De Conno F; Saita L; Ripamonti C.** A retrospective study on the use of oral morphine in cancer pain. *Journal of Pain and Symptom Management* 1987;2:77–81.
41. **Blancquaert JP; LeFebvre RA; Willems JL.** Emetic and antiemetic effects of opioids in the dog. *European Journal of Rheumatology* 1986;128:143–50.
42. **MacDonald N; Alexander R; Bruera E.** Cachexia–anorexia–asthenia. *Journal of Pain and Symptom Management* 1995;10:151–5.
43. **Nelson KA; Walsh D; Sheehan FG.** The cancer anorexia–cachexia syndrome. *Journal of Clinical Oncology* 1994;12:213–25.
44. **Nelson KA; Walsh D; Sheehan FG; O'Donovan PB; Falk GW.** Assessment of upper gastrointestinal motility in the cancer associated dyspepsia syndrome (CADS). *Journal of Palliative Care* 1993;9(1):27–31.
45. **Bruera E; Belzile M; Neumann C; Harsanyi Z; Babul N; Darke A.** A double-blind, crossover study of controlled-release metoclopramide and placebo for the chronic nausea and dyspepsia of advanced cancer. *Journal of Pain and Symptom Management* 2000;19:427–35.
46. **Loprinzi CL.** Controlled trial of megestrol acetate for the treatment of cancer, anorexia and cachexia. *Journal of the National Cancer Institute* 1990;12:1127–32.
47. **Tamburini M.** *Quality of Life Assessment in Medicine.* CD ROM for Windows and companion report. Milano: Glamm Interactive Srl., 1997 and 1998.
48. **Bruera E; Brenneis C; Michand M; MacDonald N.** Continuous Subcutaneous infusion of metoclopramide for treatment of narcotic bowel syndrome. *Cancer Treatment Reports* 1987;71:1121–2.
49. **Sandgren J; McPhee M; Grenberger N.** Narcotic bowel syndrome treated with Clonidine. *Annals of Internal Medicine* 1984;101:331–4.
50. **Bruera E; Brenneis C; MacDonald RN., *et al.*** Continuous subcutaneous infusion of metoclopramide using a disposable portable pump. *Annals of Internal Medicine* 1986;104:896–7.
51. **Ripamonti C; Mercadante S; Groff L; Zecca E; De Conno F; Casuccio A.** Role of octreotide, scopolamine butylbromide and hydration in symptom control of patients with inoperable bowel obstruction having a nasogastric tube. A prospective trial. *Journal of Pain and Symptom Management* 2000;19:23–34.

52. **Mercadante S; Ripamonti C; Casuccio A; Zecca E; Groff L.** Comparison of octreotide and hyoscine butylbromide in controlling gastrointestinal symptoms due to malignant inoperable bowel abstruction. *Supportive Care in Cancer* 2000;3:133–91.

53. **Kris MG; Yeh SDJ; Gralla RJ., *et al.*** Symptomatic gastroparesis in cancer patients. A possible cause of cancer-associated anorexia that can be improved with oral metoclopramide. *Proceedings of the American Society for Clinical Oncology* 1985;4:1038A (Abstract).

54. **Thomas J; Shields R.** Associated autonomic dysfunction and carcinoma of the pancreas. *British Medical Journal* 1970;4:32.

55. **Gilbert HA; Kagan AR.** *Radiation Damage to the Nervous System, a Delayed Therapeutic Hazard,* 1st edn. New York: Raven Press, 1980: pp. 94–5.

56. **Roca E; Bruera E; Politi P., *et al.*** Vinca alkaloids-induced cardiovascular autonomic neuropathy. *Cancer Treatment Reports* 1985;69(2):149–51.

57. **Schuffer M; Wallace H; Fleming C., *et al.*** Intestinal pseudo-obstruction as the presenting manifestation of small cell carcinoma of the lung: paraneoplastic neuropathy of the gastrointestinal tract. *Annals of Internal Medicine* 1983;98:129–34.

58. **Anderson E; Rosenblum EK; Gravs F., *et al.*** Auto antibodies in paraneoplastic syndromes associated with small-cell lung cancer. *Neurology* 1988;38:1391–8.

59. **Lennon V; Sas D; Busk M., *et al.*** Enteric neuronal autoantibodies in pseudo-obstruction with small-cell lung carcinoma. *Gastroenterology* 1991;100:137–42.

60. **Ingham J; Portenoy RK.** Cachexia in context: the interactions among anorexia, pain, and other symptoms. In: Bruera E; Higginson I., editors. *Cachexia-anorexia in Cancer Patients.* Oxford Medical Publications, Oxford University Press, 1996;11:158–71.

61. **Ingham J; Portenoy RK.** The measurement of pain and other symptoms. In: Doyle D; Hanks GWC; MacDonald N., editors. *The Oxford Textbook of Palliative Medicine.* Oxford: Oxford University Press, 2nd edn, 1998; 6: pp. 203–19.

62. **Grossman SA; Sheidler VR; Sweedeen K; Mucenski J; Piantadosi S.** Correlation of patients and caregiver ratings of cancer pain. *Journal of Pain and Symptom Management* 1991;6:53–7.

63. **Clipp EC; George LK.** Patients with cancer and their spouse caregivers. Perceptions of the illness experience. *Cancer* 1992;69:1074–9.

64. **Higginson I; Priest P; McCarthy M.** Are bereaved family members a valid proxy for a patient's assessment of dying? *Social Science and Medicine* 1994;38:553–7.

65. **Khan SB; Houts PS; Harding SP.** Quality of life and patients with cancer: a comparative study of patient versus physician perceptions and its implications for cancer education. *Journal of Cancer Education* 1992;7:241–4.

66. **Rhodes VA; Watson PM; Johnson MH.** Development of reliable and valid measures of nausea and vomiting. *Cancer Nursing* 1984;7(1):33–41.

67. **Melzack R.** Measurement of nausea. *Journal of Pain and Symptom Management* 1989;4:157–60.

68. **Morrow G.** The assessment of nausea and vomiting. Past problems, current issues, and suggestions for future research. *Cancer* 1984;53:2267–78.

69. **Hearn J; Higginson IJ.** Outcome measures in palliative care for advanced cancer patients: a review. *Journal of Public Health Medicine* 1997;19(2):193–9.

70. **Bruera E; Kuehn N; Miller MJ; Selmser P; Macmillan K.** The Edmonton Symptom Assessment System (ESAS): a simple method for the assessment of palliative care patients. *Journal of Palliative Care* 1991;7(2):6–9.

71. **Tamburini M; Rosso S; Gamba A; Mencaglia E; De Conno F; Ventafridda V.** A therapy impact questionnaire for quality-of-life assessment in advanced cancer research. *Annals of Oncology* 1992;3:565–70.

72. **McCorkle R; Young K.** Development of a symptom distress scale. *Cancer Nursing* 1978;1:373–8.
73. **McCorkle R; Benoliel JQ.** Symptom distress, current concerns and mood disturbance after diagnosis of life-threatening disease. *Society of Scientific Medicine* 1983;17:431–8.
74. **Young KJ; Longman AJ.** Quality of life and person with melanoma. *Cancer Nursing* 1983;6:219–25.
75. **Monipur C; Feigl P; Metch B; Hayden KA; Meyskens FL; Crowley J.** Quality of life end points in cancer clinical trials: review and recommendations. *Journal of the National Cancer Institute* 1989;81:485–95.
76. **McCorkle R; Benoliel JQ; Donaldson G; Georgiadou P; Monipur C; Goodell B.** A randomized clinical trial of home nursing care for lung cancer patients. *Cancer* 1989;64:1375–82.
77. **Degner LF; Henteleff PD; Ringer C.** The relationship between theory and measurement in evaluations of palliative care services. *Palliative Care* 1987;3(2):8–13.
78. **Peruselli C; Camporesi E; Colombo AM; Cucci M; Mazzoni G; Paci E.** Quality-of-life assessment in a home care program for advanced cancer patients: a study using the Symptom Distress Scale. *Journal of Pain and Symptom Management* 1993;8:306–11.
79. **Portenoy RK; Thaler HT; Kornblith AB; McCarthyLepore J; Friedlander-Klar H; Kiyasu E; Sobel K; Coyle N; Kemeny N; Norton L; Scher H.** The Memorial Symptom Assessment Scale: an instrument for the evaluation of symptom prevalence, characteristics and distress. *European Journal of Cancer* 1994;30A(9):1326–36.
80. **de Haes J; van Knippenberg F; Neijt J.** Measuring psychological and physical distress in cancer patients: structure and application of the Rotterdam Symptom Checklist. *British Journal of Cancer* 1990;62:1034–8.
81. **Schipper H; Clinch J; McMurray A., *et al.*** Measuring the quality of life of cancer patients: The Functional Living Index—Cancer: development and validation. *Journal of Clinical Oncology* 1984;2:472–83.
82. **Cella DF; Tulsky DS; Gray G., *et al.*** The functional assessment of cancer therapy scale : development and validation of the general measure. *Journal of Clinical Oncology* 1993;11:570–9.
83. **Aaronson NK; Ahmedzai S; Bergman B., *et al.*** The European Organization for Research and Treatment of Cancer QLQ-C30: a quality-of-life instrument for use in international clinical trials in oncology. *Journal of the National Cancer Institute* 1993;85:365–76.
84. **Pisters KMW; Kris MG.** Treatment-related nausea and vomiting. In: Berger A., *et al.*, editor. *Principles and Practice of Supportive Oncology.* Philadelphia: Lippincott-Raven, 1998;11:165–77.
85. **Lichter I.** Which antiemetic? *Journal of Palliative Care* 1993;9(1):42–50.
86. **Nelson KA; Walsh D.** Metoclopramide in anorexia caused by cancer-associated dyspepsia syndrome (CADS). *Journal of Palliative Care* 1993;9(2):14–18.
87. **Bruera E; Brenneis C; MacDonald N; Simpson I; LeGatt D.** Metoclopramide infusion with a disposable portable pump (letter). *Annals of Internal Medicine* 1986;104:896.
88. **Cole DR; Duffy DF.** Haloperidol for radiation sickness: control of associated nausea, vomiting, and anorexia. *New York State Journal of Medicine* 1974;74:1558–62.
89. **Bruera E; MacEachern TJ; Spachynski KA; LeGatt DF; MacDonald RN; Babul N; Harsanyi Z; Darke AC.** Comparison of the efficacy, safety, and pharmacokinetics of controlled release and immediate release metoclopramide for the management of chronic nausea in patients with advanced cancer. *Cancer* 1994;74:3204–11.
90. **Perkel MS; Moore C; Hersh T; Davidson ED.** Metoclopramide therapy in patients with delayed gastric emptying: a randomized, double-blind study. *Digestive Disease Science* 1979;24:662–6.
91. **Snape WJ; Battle WM; Schwartz SS., *et al.*** Metoclopramide to treat gastroparesis due to diabetes mellitus. *Annals of Internal Medicine* 1982;96:444–6.
92. **McCallum RW; Ricci DA; Rakatansky H., *et al.*** A multicentre placebo controlled clinical trial of oral metoclopramide in diabetic gastroparesis. *Diabetes Care* 1983;6:463–7.

93. **Schuffler MD; Rohrmann CA; Chaffee RG., *et al.*** Chronic intestinal pseudo-obstruction. *Medicine* 1981;60:173–96.
94. **Shivshanker K; Bennett RW; Haynne TP.** Tumor-associated gastroparesis: correction with metoclopramide. *American Journal of Surgery* 1983;145:221–5.
95. **Stewart JJ; Weisbraodt NW; Burko TF.** Intestinal reverse peristalsis associated with morphine-induced vomiting. In: Kosterlitz HW., editor. *Opiates and Endogenous Opioid Peptides.* Amsterdan: Elsevier, 1976: pp. 46–58.
96. **Bruera E; Brenneis C; Michand M; MacDonald N.** Continuous subcutaneous infusion of metoclopramide for treatment of narcotic bowel syndrome. *Cancer Treatment Reports* 1987;71:1121–2.
97. **O'Shea M.** A double-blind comparison of domperidone and metoclopramide in the treatment of the postprandial dyspepsia. *Current Therapeutic Research* 1980;26:367.
98. **Corinaldesi R; Raiti C; Stanghellini V., *et al.*** Comparative effects of oral cisapride and metoclopramide on gastric emptying of solids and symptoms in patients with functional dyspepsia and gastroparesis. *Current Therapeutic Research* 1987;42:428–35.
99. **McHugh S; Lico S; Diamant N.** Cisapride vs. metoclopramide: an acute study in diabetic gastroparesis. *Digestive Disease Science* 1992;37:997–1001.
100. **De Caestecker JS; Ewing DJ; Tothill P; Clarke BF; Heading RC.** Evaluation of oral cisapride and metoclopramide in diabetic autonic neuropathy: an eight-week double-blind crossover study. *Alimentary Pharmacology and Therapeutics* 1989;3:69–81.
101. **Rowbotham DJ; Bamber PA; Nimmo WS.** Comparison of the effect of cisapride and metoclopramide on morphine-induced delay in gastric emptying. *British Journal of Clinical Pharmacology* 1988;26:741–6.
102. **Krevsky B; Maurer AH; Malmud LS; Fisher RS.** Cisapride accelerates colonic transit in constipated patients with colonic inertia. *American Journal of Gastroenterology* 1989;84:882–7.
103. **Muller-Lissner SA, and The Bavarian Constipation Study Group.** Treatment of chronic constipation with cisapride and placebo. *Gut* 1987;28:1033–8.
104. **Moertel C; Shutte A; Reitemeir R., *et al.*** Corticosteroid therapy in pre-terminal gastro-intestinal cancer. *Cancer* 1974;33:1607–9.
105. **Bruera E; Roca E; Cedaro L., *et al.*** Action of oral methylprednisolone in terminal cancer patients: a prospective randomized double-blind study. *Cancer Treatment Reports* 1985;69:751–4.
106. **Della Cuna GR; Pellegrini A; Piazzi M.** Effect of methylprednisolone sodium succinate on quality of life in preterminal cancer patients. A placebo-controlled, multicenter study. *European Journal Cancer and Clinical Oncology* 1989;25:1817–20.
107. **Popiela T; Lucchi R; Giongo F.** Methylprednisolone as palliative therapy for female terminal cancer patients. *European Journal of Cancer and Clinical Oncology* 1989;25:1823–6.
108. **Pereira J; Bruera E.** Successful management of intractable nausea with ondansetron: a case study. *Journal of Palliative Care* 1996;12(2):47–50.
109. **Cole R; Robinson F; Harvey L; Trethowank; Murdoch V.** Successful control of intractable nausea and vomiting requiring combined ondansetron and haloperidol in a patient with advanced cancer. *Journal of Pain and Symptom Management* 1998;16:259–62.
110. **Mercadante S; Sapio M; Serretta R.** Ondansetron in nausea and vomiting induced by spinal morphine. *Journal of Pain and Symptom Management* 1998;16:259–62.
111. **Kock KL; Xu L; Bingman J; Summy-Long J; Seaton J; Stern RM; Joslyn A; William M.** Effects of ondansetron on morphine-induced nausea, vasopressin and gastric myoelectrical activity. *Gastroenterology* 1993;104(Suppl):A535.
112. **Currow DC; Coughlan M; Fardell B; Cooney NJ.** Use of ondansetron in palliative medicine. *Journal of Pain and Symptom Management* 1997;13:302–7.

113. **Wynn R; Essien E; Thut P.** The effects of different antiemetic agents on morphine-induced emesis in ferrets. *European Journal of Pharmacology* 1993;159:125–7.

114. **de Stoutz ND; Bruera E; Suarez-Almazor M.** Opioid rotation for toxicity reduction in terminal cancer patients. *Journal of Pain and Symptom Management* 1995;10:378–84.

115. **Watanabe S.** Intraindividual variability in opioid response: a role for sequential opioid trials in patient care. In: Portenoy RK; Bruera E., editors. *Topics in Palliative Care, Vol. 1.* New York: Oxford University Press, 1997; 10: pp. 195–203.

116. **Cherny N; Ripamonti C; Pereira J., *et al.*** Strategies to manage the adverse effects of oral morphine. *Journal of Clinical Oncology* 2001;19:2542–54.

117. **Bruera E; Belzile M; Pituskin E; Fainsinger R; Darke A., *et al.*** Randomized, double blind, cross-over trial comparing safety and efficacy of oral controlled-release oxycodone with controlled-release morphine in patients with cancer. *Journal of Clinical Oncology* 1998;16:3222–9.

118. **Kalso E; Vainio A.** Morphine and oxycodone hydrochloride in the management of cancer pain. *Clinical Pharmacology and Therapeutics* 1990;47:639–46.

119. **Heiskanen T; Kalso E.** Controlled-release oxycodone and morphine in cancer related pain. *Pain* 1997;73:37–45.

120. **Mercadante S; Salvaggio L; Dardanoni G; Agnello A; Garofalo S.** Dextropropoxyphene vs morphine in opioid-naive cancer patients with pain. *Journal of Pain and Symptom Management* 1998;15:76–81.

121. **Drexel H; Dzien A; Spiegel RW; Lang AH; Breier C; Abbrederis K., *et al.*** Treatment of severe cancer pain by low-dose continuous subcutaneous morphine. *Pain* 1989;36:169–76.

122. **Leow KP; Smith MT; Williams B; Cramond T.** Single-dose and steady-state pharmacokinetics and pharmacodynamics of oxycodone in patients with cancer. *Clinical Pharmacology and Therapeutics* 1992;52:487–95.

123. **Bruera E; Fainsinger R; Spachinsky K; Suarez-Almazor M; Inturrisi C.** Clinical efficacy and safety of a novel controlled-release morphine suppository and subcutaneous morphine in cancer pain: a randomized evaluation. *Journal of Clinical Oncology* 1995;13:1520–7.

124. **Babul N; Provencher L; Laberge F; Harsanyi Z; Moulin D.** Comparative efficacy and safety of controlled-release morphine suppositories and tablets in cancer pain. *Journal of Clinical Pharmacology* 1998;38:74–81.

125. **De Conno F; Ripamonti C; Saita L; MacEachern T; Hanson J; Bruera E.** Role of rectal route in treating cancer pain: a randomized cross-over clinical trial of oral vs rectal morphine administration in opioid-naive cancer patients with pain. *Journal of Clinical Oncology* 1995;13:1004–8.

126. **Bruera E; Belzile M; Neumann CM; Ford I; Harsanyi Z; Darke A.** Twice-daily versus once-daily morphine sulphate controlled-release suppositories for the treatment of cancer pain. A randomized controlled trial. *Supportive Care in Cancer* 1999;7:280–3.

127. **Megens A; Artois K., *et al.*** Comparison of the analgesic and intestinal effects of fentanyl and morphine in rats. *Journal of Pain and Symptom Management* 1998;15:253–8.

128. **Hunt R; Fazekas B; Thorne D; Brooksbank M.** A comparison of subcutaneous morphine and fentanyl in hospice cancer patients. *Journal of Pain and Symptom Management* 1999;18:111–9.

129. **Kalso E; Heiskanen T; Rantio M; Rosenberg PH; Vainio A.** Epidural and subcutaneous morphine in the management of cancer pain: a double-blind cross-over study. *Pain* 1996;67:443–9.

130. **MacDonald P; Graham P; Clayton M; Buhagiar A; Stuart-Harris R.** Regular subcutaneous bolus morphine via an indwelling cannula for pain from advanced cancer. *Palliative Medicine* 1991;5:323–9.

131. **Mercadante S; Casuccio A; Groff L; Boffi R; Villari P; Gebbia V; Ripamonti C.** Switching from morphine to methadone to improve analgesia and tolerability in cancer patients. A prospective study. *Journal of Clinical Oncology* 2001;19:2898–904.

Chapter 9

Constipation

Isabelle Mancini and Eduardo Bruera

Introduction

Constipation is a common and distressing symptom in patients with advanced cancer. The term refers to infrequent or difficult defaecation with reduced number of bowel movement, which may or may not be abnormally hard, with increased difficulty or discomfort (1). Constipation occurs in approximately 40% of patients referred to a palliative care service and 90% of patients treated by opioids (2). Terminally ill cancer patients have many risk factors, but the routine assessment of constipation in this population is insufficient (3).

Pathophysiology

Normal bowel function requires the coordination of motility, mucosal transport, and defaecation reflexes. Motility depends on central nervous system mechanisms (Figure 9.1), on the activity of the peripheral or autonomic nervous system (both parasympathetic and sympathetic), and on a variety of gastrointestinal hormones (4). The ascending colon and proximal half of the transverse colon receive their parasympathetic input from the vagus nerve, while the remainder of the colon is supplied by parasympathetic fibres from the second, third, and fourth sacral segments. These fibres pass through the pelvis as the nervi erigentes, enter the bowel wall in the low rectum, and then travel as six major nerve trunks for 50% or more of the distance around the colon (5). Sympathetic fibres innervate the proximal part of the large intestine via the superior mesenteric plexus, the distal part of the large intestine via the inferior mesenteric, and superior hypogastric plexus. Stimulation of the sympathetic nerves stops colonic movements (6); however, sympathectomy either has no effect on bowel function or may unmask colonic propulsion (5). Colonic propulsion and defaecation appear to be coordinated by a spinal centre that is modulated by excitatory and inhibitory influences from the brain. Patients with neurological lesions involving the cauda equina or low spinal cord have all the abnormalities observed after section of the pelvic nerves, but in addition, the external anal sphincter contractions are weak or absent and may not occur in response to rectal distension, increases in intra-abdominal pressure, and anal stimulation (5). Patients with lesions involving the high spinal cord may also be constipated, probably because they are unable to perceive the presence of faeces in the rectum. However, colonic reflexes are intact, and sphincter pressure is often normal (5). Colonic motility can also be abnormal in patients with pontine, hypothalamic, or cortical lesions (5). The nerve cells in the intestines include the submucosal plexus and myenteric plexus.

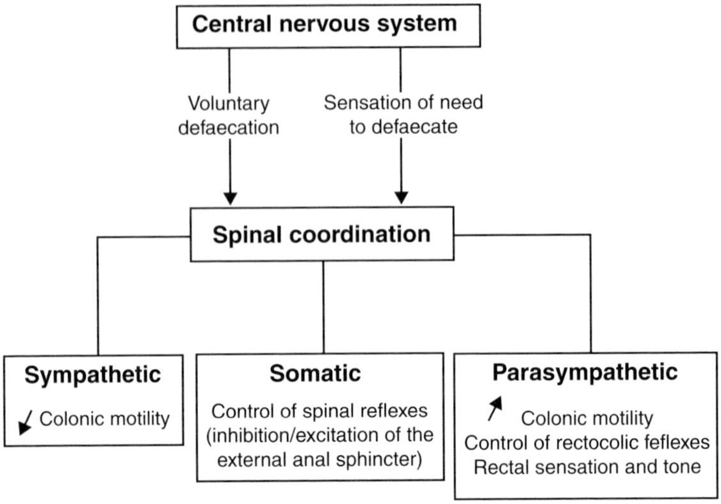

Figure 9.1 Central nervous control of bowel motility (↙ = decrease; ↗ = increase).

These two groups of nerve cells are the major components of the enteric nervous system and integrate the motor and secretory activities of the gastrointestinal tract (6). The intrinsic electrical and mechanical properties of gut smooth muscle are modulated by transmitters released from neurons of the myenteric plexus. The two principal neurotransmitters involved in the control of peristalsis appear to be acetylcholine and vasoactive intestinal peptide (VIP) (7). The autonomic nervous system can influence both motor and secretory activities, but gut motility ultimately depends on the presence on an intact enteric nervous system (6). Activation of the enteric plexus and release of acetylcholine inhibit contraction of the circular layer and stimulate contraction of the longitudinal layer. When the circular layer contracts it makes the gut longer; when the longitudinal layer contracts the gut is shortened. This coordinated action results in the movements of the content of the intestinal lumen. Anticholinergic drugs tend to produce constipation because they inhibit control of these two parts of the peristaltic complex. Three types of motility have been distinguished: segmental (non-propulsive), short segment propulsive, and long segment propulsive. Segmental movements of the colon churn and mix the content, and propulsive movements, or peristalsis, drive the content forward. Increases in segmental non-propulsive motility of the bowel are associated with the development of constipation (8).

Electrolyte and water transports are under neuronal control (7). The basic secretory condition of intestinal epithelium is cholinergic and is mediated through changes in intracellular calcium concentrations. Anticholinergic agents and hypercalcaemia tend to produce constipation, and hypocalcaemia tends to cause diarrhoea. Increased absorption of fluids could potentially cause constipation, but it is more likely that desiccation of bowel content is due to prolonged transit time rather than mucosal processes. Finally, interference in defaecation reflexes can cause constipation (see above) (4): normal defaecation depends on the ability of the upper anal canal receptors to detect the presence of stool and on the relaxation of the involuntary internal sphincter and the puborectalis muscle, which also exerts a sphincter function. These actions are abolished by lower motor neuron lesions, producing low of rectal sensation, decreased rectal tone, and inability to defaecate.

Opioid effects on the gastrointestinal tract

Opioids affect the intestines by one of three mechanisms: reduction in motility (propulsive peristalsis); secretions (pancreatic, biliary, electrolytes and fluid); and increases in intestinal fluid absorption and blood flow (9–12). Opioids augment the tope and non-propulsive motility of both the ileum and the colon, thereby increasing transit time. The dominant effect of morphine on the gut is due partly to its ability to accumulate in intestinal tissue (13). Morphine appears in the intestinal lumen of rats approximately 10–20 minutes after IV administration, and it persists there for a long period of time (14). A local effect can be demonstrated by the efficacy of poorly absorbed opioid antagonist in the treatment of opioid-related constipation (15,16), by the response of the bowel to oral administration of non-absorbable opioids (9,17), and by the persistence of the gastrointestinal effects of systemic opioids even after extirpation of the neural supply to the bowel (18). Opiod receptors are present on gut smooth muscle and at all levels of nervous input to the intestine (9–11). μ-Receptors and δ-receptors are apparently the most important for motility, the first predominating in the myenteric plexus and the second in the submucous plexus.

Several classes of endogenous opioids and their receptors have been identified in the intestine and also suggest that there is a local effect of opioid drugs (10,11). Changes in the gut motility observed during experimental administration of opioid drugs into the cerebral ventricles in animals suggest that there are also central opioid effects (11,19–21). However, at present, the precise areas of the central nervous system that control the above effects remain unknown.

Exogenous opioid administration extends the transit time and desiccates the intraluminal content. There is some evidence that morphine stimulates mucosal sensory receptors, which, in turn, activate a reflex arc to increase fluid absorption further (22). The mechanism of the antisecretory affect of opioids has been shown to be indirect. A series of events is initiated within the intestine that requires at least two neurotransmitters and three classes of receptors: morphine may act locally through μ-opioid receptors probably located on neurons of the myenteric plexus, submucosa, villus core, and crypt regions. This is followed by the release of 5HT, possibly from tryptaminergic neurons with cell bodies located in the myenteric plexus. 5HT-receptors are then activated, and this results in the release of noradrenaline, which acts on α-adrenoceptors to antagonize the secretary mechanism of the enterocytes (9,22). The action of opioid on secretion results in decreased biliary, pancreatic and intestinal secretions, further delayed food digestion and, finally, increased fluid absorption owing to longer exposure of the intestinal contents to the mucosal surface (6).

Causes of constipation in advanced cancer patients

In the cancer population, constipation may develop from general disturbances that may or may not be cancer related (Table 9.1). Mechanical obstruction (intra- or extraluminal), metabolic disturbances, neurological disorders, the use of constipating drugs such as opioids, advanced age, confusion, sedation, reduced physical activity, diminished fluid intake, low-fibre diet intake, inconvenient bathroom availability, and depression are all frequent aetiologies in patients with advanced cancer (1,10). A survey conducted by Twycross suggests the importance of these multiple factors: in a hospice population, 50% of patients receiving no opioids required regular doses of laxatives (23). A recent retrospective study (24) found a significant correlation between laxative dose and abdominal involvement,

Table 9.1 Causes of constipation in advanced cancer patients

1 Structural abnormalities
Obstruction
Pelvic tumour mass
Radiation fibrosis
Painful anorectal conditions (anal fissure, haemorroids, perianal abscess)
2 Drugs
Opioids
Drugs with anticholinergic actions (anticholinergics, antispasmodics, antidepressants, phenothiazines, haloperidol, antacids)
Antiemetics (ondansetron)
Diuretics
Anticonvulsants
Iron
Antihypertensive drugs
Anticancer agents (vinca alkaloids)
3 Metabolic disturbances
Dehydration (fever, vomiting, polyuria, poor fluid intake, diuretics)
Hypercalcaemia
Hypokalaemia
Uraemia
Hypothyroidism
4 Neurological disorders
Cerebral tumours
Spinal cord involvement
Sacral nerve infiltration
Autonomic failure
5 General
Advanced age
Inactivity
Depression
Sedation
Decreased intake
Low-fibre diet
Poor fluid intake
Physical or social impediments

older age, female gender, and treatment by opioids other than methadone. There were no significant correlations between laxative doses and food intake, cognitive status and functional status, in opposition with Fallon who found a highly significant correlation between persistent constipation and deteriorating performance status (25).

Structural disorders include both intracolonic and extracolonic mass lesions, either primary or metastatic, radiation fibrosis, and painful anorectal conditions caused, for example, by the presence of anal fissures, haemorrhoids, or perianal abscess.

A large variety of metabolic disorders predispose to constipation. Of particular relevance to cancer patients are dehydration (due to vomiting, fever, polyuria, poor fluid intake, or diuretics), hypercalcaemia, hypokalaemia, and uraemia. Some patients may also present with other diseases that have compounding constipating effects, such as diabetes and hypothyroidism (1,10).

Diseases affecting every level of the nervous system can potentially disturb bowel function. Constipation frequently accompanies compression of the spinal cord, conus medullaris, or cauda equina by epidural metastases. Other common neurological lesions producing this effect include peripheral neuropathy and local sacral plexus disease, which is usually due to tumor infiltration (10). In addition, patients with advanced cancer frequently develop autonomic failure. This abnormality is more frequent in patients with anorexia–cachexia syndrome and is associated with abnormal gastrointestinal motility and symptoms such as anorexia, chronic nausea, and constipation (26).

Many drugs induce constipation: in cancer patients, opioid analgesics are the most notable offenders. A large retrospective study conducted by Sykes concluded that opioids accounted for about a quarter of the constipation found in terminally ill cancer patients in a hospice (27). Clinical observation suggests that the constipation caused by these medications is a dose-related phenomenon with wide interindividual variability (28), but the form of the relationship between laxative dose and opioid dose is probably more hyperbolic than linear (27). Tolerance to the effect develops very slowly, and many patients require laxative therapy for as long as they take the drugs. Little research has been done to elucidate the effects of different opioids on the bowel. Recent clinical researches have found that laxative doses may be lower in patients using methadone (29) or transdermal fentanyl (30) as analgesic. Other drugs commonly used in the treatment of cancer have prominent constipating effects, including those with anticholinergic action (antispasmodics, antidepressants, phenothiazines, haloperidol, antacid), some anticonvulsants or antihypertensive drugs, antiemetics (ondansetron), and diuretics (1). Chemotherapeutic agents can produce the same effects, mediated by the development of autonomic neuropathy.

Clinical manifestations

Constipation can cause a number of significant symptoms (Table 9.2). Severely constipated patients can present complaining of diarrhoea and continue to pass faecal material. Faecal impaction or rectal obstruction causes increased production of mucus, which may present as a rectal discharge or diarrhoea (31). Similarly, bacterial liquefaction of faecal material proximal to an obstruction can also lead to the frequent passage of small watery faeces or the continuous seepage of moist stool and mucus. As the condition progresses there is variable rectal pain, abdominal fullness and distension, usually with some colics. Untreated constipation may progress to obstipation, which can lead to life-threatening complications associated with bowel obstruction. Some patients rapidly develop nausea with or without vomiting in the presence of intestinal blockage. Unexplained nausea or vomiting should prompt inquiry and examination for constipation (32). Faecal impaction is well recognized as a factor in urinary incontinence in the elderly (33). Abdominal and rectal examination should be performed in all patients with urinary incontinence of recent onset. Rectal tearing, haemorrhoids, and rectal fissures caused by passing hard, dry stool are a frequent complication of constipation. Faecal impaction will cause pressure on the bowel wall and may lead to ischaemic necrosis of the mucosa, with increased pain and bleeding and, occasionally, perforation. Constipation has also been determined to be a risk factor for intestinal perforation in patients receiving corticosteroids for intracranial lesions (34).

Table 9.2 Clinical manifestations and complications of constipation

Clinical manifestations
- Abdominal pain
- Increase of liver or retroperitoneal pain
- Distension
- Anorexia
- Nausea and vomiting
- Urinary retention
- Confusion
- Diarrhoea

Complications when untreated
- Inadequate absorption of oral drugs
- Faecal impaction
- Rectal tearing, fissures, and haemorrhoids
- Bowel obstruction
- Intestinal perforation

In addition, constipation can also cause confusion (35), increase retroperitoneal or liver pain, and lead to inadequate absorption of oral drugs (29,36,37).

Assessment

Terminally ill cancer patients have many risk factors for severe constipation and should, therefore, be carefully assessed for this complication. The assessment of the patient with constipation includes at least the history of the frequency and difficulty of defaecation and of symptoms attributed to constipation, and physical and rectal examination. When the diagnosis of constipation is unclear, an abdominal X-ray may be required (Table 9.3) (38–40). Examination of the abdomen may reveal faecal masses in the left iliac fossa all along the wall of the colon. Faecal masses are usually not tender, are relatively mobile and can be indented with pressure. Rectal examination will reveal any painful rectal condition or local tumour infiltration, whether or not there are faeces in the rectum and whether they are hard or soft. Patients with spinal cord lesions may have reduced sensation, but the anal tone and reflex are preserved. Patients with sacral nerve root infiltration will have reduced or absent anal tone and reflex as well as sensory loss of the sacral dermatomes. Routine assessment of constipation is unusual, and clinicians must be encouraged to maintain a high level of vigilance. In a retrospective review in a palliative care unit, 72 of 122 patients (59%) did not undergo a rectal examination on admission and there was minimal documentation in the charts by either physician or nurse that had any bearing on symptoms of constipation, even in patients who were symptomatic (3). This same study also showed that simple bedside questions and clinical manoeuvres may be insufficient for the diagnosis of, or assessment of, the degree of constipation in this population at high risk of severe constipation. The assessment of a radiological constipation score may be necessary for adequate diagnosis in some patients (for example, patients who have cognitive failure). The constipation score is determined by the assessment of the amount of stool in each of the four abdominal quadrants using the following score: 0 = no stool, 1 = stool occupying <50% of lumen, 2 = stool occupying >50% of the lumen, and 3 = stool completely occupying the whole of the lumen of the colon. The total score would, therefore, range from 0 to 12.

Table 9.3 Assessment of constipation

Information required
- Pattern of patient's recent bowel movements
- Pattern of patient's pre-illness bowel movements, any previous long-term use of laxatives
- Use of potentially constipating drugs (cf. Table 9.1)
- Use of laxatives and their effects
- Patient's food and fluid intake
- Concomitant disease (diabetes, hypothyroidism)

Physical examination
- Palpation of faecal masses
- Presence or absence of faeces in the rectum—consistency
- Presence of anal tone and reflex
- Sacral nerve root sensation

Abdominal X-ray
- Rule out bowel obstruction
- Assessment of a constipation score
- Amount of stool in each quadrant (ascending colon, transverse colon, descending colon, and rectum) assessed:
  - 0 = no stool
  - 1 = stool < 50%
  - 2 = stool occupying > 50%
  - 3 = stool occupying whole of lumen
- Score ≥ 7/12 indicates severe constipation and requires immediate intervention

Others
- Determination of electrolytes, renal and hepatic function, and level of thyroid hormones
- Imaging procedures: ultrasound and/or CT scan of the abdomen and pelvis if extraluminal processes suspected; barium enema or colonoscopy for evaluation of intraluminal pathology

A constipation score greater than 7/12 indicates the presence of severe constipation and requires immediate treatment (3,38–40).

The need to pursue further clinical evaluation depends on the course and the medical setting. Many patients develop constipation after the initiation of opioid therapy. In this case, further evaluation is not needed unless there is reason to suspect a previously unidentified contributing cause that may be amenable to treatment. In contrast, the patient who develops progressive constipation in the absence of any clear precipitating cause should be considered for an evaluation that may include determination of electrolytes, renal and hepatic function tests, levels of thyroid hormones, and more sophisticated imaging procedures.

Treatment of constipation in advanced cancer patients

The management of constipation can be divided into general interventions and therapeutic measures. The general interventions involve elimination of medical factors that may be contributing to constipation (for example, treatment of electrolyte abnormalities or discontinuation of all non-essential constipating drugs), the increase of fluid intake and fibre consumption, if possible, and the availability of comfort, privacy, and convenience during defaecation.

Therapeutic interventions for the routine management of constipation may be administered orally or rectally (1,4,7,10,37). Oral laxatives include bulk agents, osmotic (saline) agents, contact cathartics, agents for colonic lavage, lubricants, prokinetic drugs, and opioid antagonists (Table 9.4).

Bulk agents (cellulose or psyllium seeds) are used to supplement the use of fibre in the food. These are usually safe, although some experience suggests that they may worsen symptoms, causing distension, bloating, or abdominal pain. These agents increase stool bulk and correct its consistency by increasing the mass and water content of the stool. Transit time through the colon is decreased. These products are typically effective after 2–4 days of daily use. Bulk laxatives are unsuitable for advanced cancer patients: they require the patient to drink extra fluids as otherwise a viscous mass may form and aggravate a partial bowel obstruction. In addition, significant allergy to these substances has been reported, and their effectiveness in severe constipation is doubtful.

Saline laxatives, including magnesium salt (magnesium hydroxide and magnesium citrate) and sodium salts (sodium phosphate), are osmotically active particles and act by drawing fluid into the intestinal lumen. The transit time of the resulting semi-liquid stools is decreased. With dose-related variation in latency, magnesium and sodium salts usually produce results in 3–6 hours. The action is not physiological, and long-term use should be avoided. In addition, in patients with cardiac failure or renal insufficiency the use of these agents should be carefully monitored. Lactulose and sorbitol are not broken down or absorbed in the small gut, where, as a result, they exert an osmotic influence, causing water retention in the lumen. In addition, bacterial degradation in the colon produces short-chain organic acids, which lower the intestinal pH and possibly stimulate peristalsis. The use of these substances may cause flatulence in about 20% of patients, and their sweet taste is sickly to some.

The contact cathartics are the most commonly administered laxatives for opioid-induced constipation. This group comprises the anthraquinone derivatives (cascara, senna, and danthron), the diphenylmethan derivatives (phenophthalein, bisacodyl, and oxyphenisatin), the docusates, and castor oil. Although there are some differences in actions between the different classes, all of these drugs act by increasing peristalsis by way of a direct stimulating effect on the myenteric plexus and reducing net absorption of water and electrolytes from the intraluminal contents (41,42). Short-term use of contact cathartics is safe; however, overuse can cause dehydration and long-term ingestion may result in dependence on laxatives for bowel function. This 'laxative bowel' is the result of drug-induced damage to the myenteric plexus but is certainly not a contraindication to therapy for advanced cancer patients. The anthraquinone derivatives (cascara, senna, and danthron) affect mucosal electrolyte transport and motility. They act primarily in the colon, and colonic electromyography following oral administration of senna in man shows an increase in myoelectrical activity of the type seen in diarrhoea. Net absorption of water and electrolytes in the colon is reduced, partly through the inhibition of Na, K-ATPase and also probably by stimulation of cAMP, prostaglandin E2 and, perhaps, serotonin synthesis (43). These laxatives are generally effective within 12–24 hours. The diphenylmethan derivatives (phenophthalein, bisacodyl, and oxyphenisatin) also act primarily on the colon and produce effects similar to those of the anthraquinone derivatives. Allergy to these substances has been reported. They are usually effective within 12–24 hours. Although the docusates act *in vitro* as a contact cathartics, causing changes in gut secretions and motility, the relatively low doses used clinically

Table 9.4 Classification and pharmacological properties of laxatives [adapted from ref. (4)]

Laxative	Onset of action (h)	Site of action*	Mechanism of action	Comments
Bulk agents				
Methylcellulose Psyllium Polycarbophil	12–24	SLI	Hold water in stool, mechanical distension	Require to drink extra fluid
Saline laxatives				
Magnesium hydroxide Magnesium citrate Magnesium sulphate	0.5–3	SLI	Osmotically active particles draw fluid into the intestinal lumen	May alter fluid and electrolyte balance To be avoided in patients with heart failure or renal insufficiency
Sodium phosphate	0.03–0.25	Colon		
Lactulose and Sorbitol	24–48	Colon	Deliver osmotic active molecules to the colon	
Contact cathartics				
Anthraquinones (cascara, senna, danthron) Diphenylmethan (phenophthalein, bisacodyl)	6–10	Colon	↑ Peristalsis by ↓ stimulating effect on the myenteric plexus and net absorption of water and electrolytes	
Castor oil	2–6	SI		
Docusate	24–72	SLI	Detergent activity; facilitates admixture of fat and water to soften stool	Highly beneficial when faeces are hard or dry or in anorectal conditions where passage of a firm stool is painful
Mineral oil	6–8	Colon	Acts both as a lubricant and as a faecal softener	May ↓ absorption of fat-soluble vitamins Risk of lipoid pneumonia in debilitated patients
Prokinetic agents				
Domperidone		SLI	Dopamine antagonist	The use of these drugs may be considered for constipation that has not responded to conventional measures
Metoclopramide		O, G, SI	Dopamine antagonist/ cholinergic agonist, ↓ transit time	May be a useful adjunctive measure for treatment of constipation in patients with spinal cord involvement and colonic inertia
Oral Naloxone		SLI	Opioid antagonist	Occurrence of withdrawal reaction; high cost
Methylnaltrexone		SLI	Opioid antagonist	Does not cross the blood–brain barrier—no withdrawal reaction

*SLI: small and large intestine, SI: small intestine, O: oesophagus, G: gastric antrum, ↑: increased, ↓: decreased.

produce only a detergent effect, allowing water and fats to mix with the faeces (41,44). Docusate also promotes water, sodium, and chloride secretion in the jejenum and colon. This drug is often added to other contact cathartics as a stool softener. This is reasonable, although there are no controlled studies establishing the added efficacy of such a combination. However, an increased risk of hepatotoxicity from the combination of this drug and others is likely (45), and periodic evaluation of liver function tests is indicated if other medications are added. These laxatives are usually effective within 1–3 days. Castor oil is hydrolysed by gut microflora to ricinoleic acid. This compound, in turn, acts on the small intestine, producing abundant mucosal secretion. Castor oil may have a very rapid onset of action and cause considerable cramping. With chronic use, malabsorption of nutrients may occur. This drug is seldom needed. It should be considered only for the management of acute constipation.

Lubricant laxatives (mineral oil) lubricate the stool surface and soften the stools, allowing easier passage. These may be useful in the management of transient acute constipation or faecal impaction, but are not recommended for chronic laxation in the cancer population. Their long-term use is limited by perianal irritation, poor absorption of fat-soluble vitamins, and the potential risk of lipoid pneumonia, especially in debilitated patients. These drugs are usually effective within 1–3 days.

It has been shown that the μ-opioid antagonist naloxone can reverse certain cases of idiopathic constipation or opioid-induced constipation when given by mouth (15,46,47). Presumably this is because gut opioid receptors are involved in normal control of gut motility (48,49) and because the extensive first-pass hepatic and possibly intestinal mucosal glucuronidation of oral naloxone at the 3-hydroxy position results in its much greater bioavailability at the enteric wall than in the systemic circulation (50). In a recent study, Sykes shows that the oral administration of naloxone at a daily dose of 20% or more of the prevailing 24-hour morphine dose is capable of providing a clinical laxative effect without antagonizing opioid analgesia (16). However, opioid withdrawal was observed, and it is suggested that initial individual naloxone doses should not exceed 5 mg. Further research is needed to clarify the risks of causing withdrawal and the relationship between serum naloxone levels and adverse effects. Methylnaltrexone is a quaternary ammonium opioid receptor antagonist which, in opposition to naloxone, does not cross the blood–brain barrier in humans. Intravenous or orally methylnaltrexone has been showed to reverse chronic opioid-induced constipation in patients in methadone maintenance programmes without causing adverse effects such as withdrawal or abdominal cramps (51,52). The dose of methylnaltrexone ranged from $0.3\,mg\,kg^{-1}$ to $3\,mg\,kg^{-1}$ with an effect which is significantly dose-dependant.

The use of prokinetic agents such as bethanechol, metoclopramide, or domperidone could be considered for constipation that has not responded to conventional measures (53). These agents may enhance intestinal function through one of two distinct pathways: either by promoting the effect of an agonist, such as acetylcholine, or by inhibiting the effect of an inhibitory transmitter, such as dopamine (54). Bethanechol is the most commonly prescribed agonist. It enhances the amplitude of contractions throughout the gastrointestinal tract, including the lower oesophageal sphincter. However, recent studies show that bethanechol has little effect in coordinating contraction or accelerating gastric or small bowel transit (53) and should no longer be considered a prokinetic agent. In addition, the side-effects of this drug, which include abdominal cramps, diarrhoea, salivation, flushing, bradycardia, and blurred vision, limit its use. The effects of metoclopramide on the gastrointestinal tract are mediated by three mechanism: central antidopamine effect, a peripheral antidopamine effect, and both direct and indirect stimulation of cholinergic receptors (55). Despite basic studies showing dose-related effects of metoclopramide on the colon (56,57) and the demonstration of a colonic effect by dopaminergic agonists and antagonists (54,58), metoclopramide has not been shown to be effective in the treatment of colonic motility disorders. Domperidone is a benzimidazole derivative that acts as a specific antagonist to the inhibitory effects of dopamine on the upper intestinal tract (59) and causes a dose-dependent stimulation of antroduodenal coordination (60). It has no cholinergic activity and diffuses poorly into the central nervous system, rarely causing any of the dystonic or extrapyramidal symptoms that occur commonly with metoclopramide.

For most cancer patients, the use of enemas and rectal suppositories is limited to the acute short-term management of more severe episodes of constipation. Occasional patients who cannot tolerate oral laxatives may be able to use long-term rectal laxatives or enemas effectively. These are usually administered two to three times per week. Rectal suppositories may be inert or inactive. Inert suppositories are usually fashioned from glycerin alone. They draw fluid into the rectum and act as a stimulus to defaecation. Active suppositories contain a cathartic. Enemas are use to relieve constipation where suppositories are ineffective. Various commercially prepared formulations are available, based on a variety of laxative substances. Microenemas such as Microlax are particularly useful in patients with cancer, as their small volume makes them less distressing for the patient. Docusate and bisacodyl are also available as ready-to-use enemas. Sodium phosphate enemas, which are commercially available, may cause fluid and electrolyte imbalance, particularly in a dehydrated patient. Soap and water enemas may be irritant to the mucosa and there is a risk of fluid overload if a significant amount of water is absorbed.

There have been no adequate comparative studies of long-term management of opioid-induced constipation, and therefore the therapy must be based on a comprehensive assessment of the patient's medical needs, capabilities, and expectations. Combination therapy is often used. One limitation of the traditional oral laxatives is the need to take a large number of pills or capsules or a large volume of liquid. Most of the time, laxatives account for the majority of oral medications taken by advanced cancer patients. This makes compliance difficult because of the high prevalence of chronic nausea, anorexia, and dysphagia in this population.

Patients with severe refractory constipation should be considered for opioid rotation, especially for opioids that are likely to cause less constipation than morphine. One randomized control trial thus found that fentanyl causes less constipation than morphine (61). Moreover, various studies have shown that methadone causes less constipation than morphine (29,62) and allows for a reduction in laxatives use (24). This may be due to different opioid affinities for gastrointestinal μ-receptors and maybe to the lipophilic nature of methadone.

Conclusions

Patients with advanced cancer are likely to have chronic constipation and will need continuous laxative treatment. Monitoring the results of this treatment is one of the more difficult and complex aspects of their management. It is important to keep records of the frequency, size, and consistency of bowel movements as well as to monitor symptoms associated with constipation. Occasionally, when the clinical assessment is equivocal or patients are not able to communicate, as may be the case in the presence of heavy sedation or cognitive failure, radiological monitoring may be required. Future randomized clinical trials are needed in order to compare different laxatives and/or prokinetic agents in the cancer patient population.

References

1. **Curtis EB; Krech R; Walsh TD.** Common symptoms in patients with advanced cancer. *Journal of Palliative Care* 1991;7:25–9.
2. **Twycross RG; Lack SA.** *Symptom Control in Far Advanced Cancer: Pain Relief.* London: Pittman, 1983.
3. **Bruera E; Suarez-Almazor M; Velasco A; Bertolino M; MacDonald SM; Hanson J.** The assessment of constipation in terminal cancer patients admitted to a palliative care unit: a retrospective review. *Journal of Pain and Symptom Management* 1994;9:515–19.
4. **Derby S; Portenoy RK.** Assessment and management of opioid-induced constipation. In: Portenoy RK; Bruera E, editors. *Topics in Palliative Care.* New York: Oxford University Press, 1997; 1: pp. 95–112.
5. **Read NW; Timms JM.** Defecation and the pathophysiology of constipation. *Clinical Gastroenterology* 1986;15:937–65.
6. **Kutchai HC.** Gastrointestinal system. In: Berne RM; Levy MN, editors. *Principles of Physiology.* St Louis: Mosby, 1990; 29: pp. 352–414.
7. **Sykes NP.** Constipation and diarrhoea. In: Doyle D; Hanks GWC; MacDonald N, editors. *Palliative Medicine.* Oxford: Oxford University Press, 1993: pp. 299–310.
8. **Connell AM.** The motility of the pelvic colon. *Gut* 1962;3:342–8.
9. **De Luca A; Coupar IM.** Insights into opioid action in the intestinal tract. *Pharmacological Therapies* 1996;69:103–15.
10. **Portenoy RK.** Constipation in the cancer patient: causes and management. *Medical Clinics of North America* 1987;71:303–11.
11. **Manara L; Bianchetti A.** The central and peripheral influences of opioids on gastrointestinal propulsion. *Annual Review of Pharmacology and Toxicology* 1985;25:249–73.
12. **Miller RJ; Hirning LD.** Opioid Peptides of the gut. In: Field M; Fritzell RA, editors. *Handbook of Physiology: The Gastrointenstinal System, Part II.* New York: Oxford University Press, 1989: pp. 631–60.
13. **Bianchi G; Ferretti P; Recchia M; Rocchetti M; Tavani A; Manara L.** Morphine tissue levels and reduction of gastrointestinal transit in rats. Correlation supports primary action site in the gut. *Gastroenterology* 1983;85:852–8.
14. **Margaritis J; Coupar IM; Bentley GA.** Studies to determine whether there is tolerance or cross-tolerance to the antisecretory effect of morphine and clonidine in the rat intestine. *Journal of Pharmacy and Pharmacology* 1991;43:655–8.
15. **Culpepper-Morgan JA; Inturrisi CE; Portenoy RK; Foley K; Houde RW; Marsh F; Kreek MJ.** Treatment of opioid-induced constipation with oral naloxone: a pilot study. *Clinical Pharmocology and Therapeutics* 1992;52:90–95.
16. **Sykes NP.** An investigation of the ability of oral naloxone to correct opioid-related constipation in patients with advanced cancer. *Palliative Medicine* 1996;10:135–44.
17. **Russel J ; Bass P; Goldberg LI.** Antagonism of gut, but not central effects of morphine with quarternary narcotic antagonists. *European Journal of Pharmocology* 1982;78:5–261.
18. **Daniel EE; Sutherland WH; Gogoch A.** Effects of morphine and other drugs on motility of the terminal ilium. *Gastroenterology* 1959;36:510–23.
19. **Parolaro D; Sala M; Gori E.** Effect of intracerebroventricular administration of morphine upon intestinal mortility in rat and its antagonism with naloxone. *European Journal of Pharmacology* 1957;46:329–38.
20. **Porreca E; Cowen A; Rafla RB; Tallarida RJ.** Ketazocines and morphine: effects on gastrointestinal transit after central and peripheral administration. *Life Sciences* 1983;32:1785–90.

21. **Galligan JJ; Burks TE.** Centrally mediated inhibition of small intestinal transit and motility by morphine in the rat. *Journal of Pharmacology and Experimental Therapeutics* 1983;226:356–61.
22. **Brown NJ; Coupar IM; Rumsey DE.** The effect of acute and chronic administration of morphine and morphine withdrawal on intestinal transit time in the rat. *Journal of Pharmacy and Pharmacology* 1988;40:844–8.
23. **Twycross RG; Harcourt JMV.** The use of laxative at a palliative care centre. *Palliative Medicine* 1991;5:27–33.
24. **Mancini I; Hanson J; Neumann C; Bruera E.** Opioid type and other clinical predictors of laxative dose in advanced cancer patients: a retrospective study. *Journal of Palliative Medicine* 2000;3:49–56.
25. **Fallon MT; Hanks GW.** Morphine, constipation and performance status in advanced cancer patients. *Palliative Medicine* 1999;13:159–60.
26. **Watanabe S; Bruera E.** Anorexia and cachexie, asthenia and lethargy. In: Cherny N; Foley K, editors. *Hematology/oncology Clinics of North America: Pain and Palliative Care.* Philadelphia: Saunders, 1996: pp. 189–206.
27. **Sykes NP.** The relationship between opioid use and laxative use in terminally ill cancer Patients. *Palliative Medicine* 1998;12:375–82.
28. **Maguire LC; Yon JL; Miller E.** Prevention of narcotic-induced constipation. *New England Journal of Medicine* 1981;305:1651.
29. **Daeninck PJ; Bruera E.** Reduction in constipation and laxative requirements following opioid rotation to methadone: a report of four cases. *Journal of Pain and Symptom Management* 1999;18:303–9.
30. **Radbruch L; Sabatowski R; Loick G; Kulbe C; Kasper M; Grond S; Lehmann KA.** Constipation and the use of laxatives: a comparison between transdermal fentanyl and oral morphine. *Palliative Medicine* 2000;14:11–19.
31. **Goldfinger SE.** Constipation and diarrhea. In: Wilson ID; Braunwald E; Isselbacher KJ, editors. *Harrison's Principles of Internal Medicine.* Toronto: McGraw-Hill, 1991: pp. 256–9.
32. **Pereira J; Bruera E.** Chronic nausea. In: Bruera E; Higginson I, editors. *Cachexia–Anorexia in Cancer Patients.* Oxford: Oxford University Press, 1996; 2: pp. 23–37.
33. **MacDonald A; Sheaver M; Patterson PJ; Finlay IG.** Relationship between outlet obstruction constipation and obstructed urinary flow. *British Journal of Surgery* 1991;78:693–5.
34. **Fadul CE; Lemann W; Thaler HJ; Posner JB.** Perforation of the gastrointestinal tract in patients receiving steroids for neurologic disease. *Neurology* 1988;38:348–52.
35. **Medalie JH; Rasen HR; Calkins E.** Confusion (delirium). In: Calkins E; Davis PJ; Ford AB, editors. *The Practice of Geriatrics.* Toronto: Saunders, 1986: pp. 210–13.
36. **Glare P; Lickiss JN.** Unrecognized constipation in patients with advanced cancer: a recipe for therapeutic disaster. *Journal of Pain and Symptom Management* 1992;7:369–71.
37. **Kim OD; Mobarhan S.** Constipation. In: Rakel RE, editor. *Conn's Current Therapy.* Toronto: Saunders, 1990: pp. 173–5.
38. **Starreveld JS; Pols MA; Vam Wijk HJ; Bogaard JW; Poen H; Smont AJPM.** The plain abdominal radiograph in the assessment of constipation. *Gastroenterology* 1990;28:335–8.
39. **Smith RG; Lewis S.** The relationship between digital examination and abdominal radiographs in elderly patients. *Age Ageing* 1990;9:142–3.
40. **McKay LF; Smith RG; Eastwood MA; Walsh SD; Cruikshank JG.** An investigation of colonic function in the elderly. *Age Ageing* 1983;12:105–10.
41. **Gaginella TS; Bris P.** Laxatives: an update on mechanism of pain. *Life Sciences* 1978;23:1001–10.
42. **Hardcastle JD; Wilkins JL.** The action of sennosides and related compounds on human colon and rectum. *Gut* 1970;11:1038–42.

43. **Leng-Peschlow E.** Effects of sennosides A+B and bisacodyl on rat large intestine. *Pharmacology* 1989;38:310–18.
44. **Binder HJ.** Pharmacology of laxatives. *Annual Review of Pharmacology and Toxicology* 1977;17:355–67.
45. **Tolman KG; Hammar S; Sannilla JJ.** Possible hepatotoxicity of doxidan. *Annals of Internal Medicine* 1976;84:290–2.
46. **Kreek MJ; Schaefer RA; Hahn EF; Fishman J.** Naloxone, a specific opioid antagonist, reverses chrome idiopathic constipation *The Lancet* 1983;I:261–2.
47. **Kreek MJ; Marsh F; Albeck H.,** ***et al.*** Effects of opioid antagonist naloxone on fecal evacuation in patients with idiopathic chronic constipation, irritable bowel syndrome, and narcotic induced constipation. Abstract. *Alcohol and Drug Research* 1986;6:168.
48. **Kromer W.** Endogenous and exagenous opioids in the control of gastrointestinal motility and secretion. *Pharmacological Reviews* 1988;40:123–50.
49. **Manara L; Bianchi G; Ferretti P; Tavani A.** Inhibition of gastrointestinal transit by morphine in rats results primarily from direct drag action on gut opioid sites. *Journal of Pharmacology and Experimental Therapeutics* 1986;237:945–9.
50. **Kreek MJ; Guggenheim FG; Ross JE; Tapley DF.** Glucuronide formation in the transport of testosterone and androstenedione by rat intestine. *Biochimica et Biophysica Acta* 1963;74:418–27.
51. **Yuan CS; Foss JF; O'Connor M.** Methylnaltrexone for reversal of constipation due to chronic methadone use. *Journal of the American Medical Association* 2000;283:367–72.
52. **Yuan CS; Foss JF.** Oral methylnatrexone for opioid-induced constipation. *Journal of the American Medical Association* 2000;284:1383–4.
53. **McCallum RW; Fink SM; Lerner E; Berkowitz DM.** Effects of metoclopramide and bethanechol on delayed gastric emptying present in gastroesophageal reflux patients. *Gastroenterology* 1983;84:1573–7.
54. **Lanfranchi GA; Marzio L; Cortini C; Osset EM.** Motor effect of dopamine on human sigmoid colon. Evidence for specific receptors. *American Journal of Digestive Diseases* 1978;23:257–63.
55. **Jacoby HI; Brodic DA.** Gastrointestinal actions in metoclopramide. An experimental study. *Gastroenterology* 1967;52:676–84.
56. **Harrington RA; Hamilton CW; Brodgen RN; Linkewich JA; Romankiewicz JA; Hell RC.** Metoclopramide. An updated review of its pharmacological properties and clinical use. *Drugs* 1983;25:451–4.
57. **Eisner M.** Gastrointestinal effects of metoclopramide in man. In vitro experiments with human smooth muscle preparation (preliminary communication). *British Medical Journal* 1968;4:679–80.
58. **Lechin F; Van Der Dijs B.** Effects of dopaminergic blocking agents on distal colon motility. *Journal of Clinical Pharmacology* 1979;19:617–25.
59. **Brogden RN; Carmine AA; Hecl RC.,** ***et al.*** Domperidone: a review of its pharmacological activity, pharmacokinetics and therapeutic efficacy in the symptomatic treatment of chronic dyspepsia and as an antiemetic. *Drugs* 1982;24:360–400.
60. **Schuurkes JAJ; Van Nueten JM.** Domperidone improves myogenically transmitted antroduodenal coordination by blocking dopaminergicreceptor sites. *Scandinavian Journal of Gastroenterology,* 1984;19:101–10.
61. **Hunt R; Fazekas B; Thorne D; Brooksbank M.** A comparison of subcutaneous morphine and fentanyl in hospice cancer patients. *Journal of Pain and Symptom Management* 1999;18:111–19.
62. **Mercadante S; Casuccio A; Groff L; Boffi R; Villari P; Gebbia V; Ripamonti C.** Switching from morphine to methadone to improve analgesia and tolerability in cancer patients. A prospective study. *Journal of Clinical Oncology* 2001;19:2898–904.

Chapter 10

Diarrhea, malabsorption

Sebastiano Mercadante

Diarrhea

Diarrhea is an abnormal looseness of the stools (increased liquidity or decreased consistency), and occurs when the intestine does not complete the absorption of electrolytes and water from the luminal content. Diarrhea is usually accompanied by an abnormal increase in daily stool weight. Patients often have associated symptoms of abdominal pain, urge to defecate, perianal discomfort, and fecal incontinence (1).

Diarrhea is a common complication in the oncologic population, and occurs in 5%–10% of patients with advanced cancer (2–4). The consequences of diarrhea can be troublesome, and include loss of water, electrolytes, albumin, failure to reach nutritional goals, declining immune function, risk of bedsores, or systemic infection. Diarrhea also causes additional work for the nursing staff or family who have to prevent maceration and bedsores. Moreover, loss of comfort and dignity have to be considered (5).

Several symptoms depend on dehydration, such as asthenia, anorexia, weight loss, and drowsiness, which limit the quality of life. Furthermore, it determines abnormal metabolic compartments influencing pharmacokinetic of drugs, blood renal flow, acid-base balance, as well as hypokaliemia and acidosis from massive potassium and bicarbonate loss (6).

Mechanisms

The presence in the lumen of unusual amounts of poorly absorbable, osmotically active solutes; intestinal ion secretion or inhibition of normal active ion absorption with or without exudation of mucus, blood, and protein from sites of inflammation; and deranged intestinal mobility constitute the principal mechanisms that produce diarrhea.

Osmotic diarrhea

The ingestion of a poorly absorbable solute causes osmotic diarrhea (Table 10.1), altering the osmolarity of the luminal content. The proximal small bowel is highly permeable to water and sodium, and water influx across the duodenum rapidly adjusts the osmolarity of the luminal fluid toward that of plasma, secreting water even though the osmolality values between luminal contents and plasma are similar. On the contrary, the mucosa of the ileum and colon has a low permeability to sodium and solutes. However, there is an efficient active ion transport mechanism that allows the reabsorption of electrolytes and water even against electrochemical gradients (5).

Table 10.1 Causes of osmotic diarrhea

◆ Carbohydrate malabsorption (generalized malabsorption, disaccharide deficiencies, specific sugar malabsorption)
◆ Excessive ingestion of poorly absorbed carbohydrate (lactulose, sorbitol in fruits, elixir, gum)
◆ Magnesium-induced diarrhea (food supplements, antacids, laxatives)
◆ Laxatives containing poorly absorbable anions (sodium sulphate, phosphate, citrate)

Carbohydrates and proteins are fermented by colonic bacteria and salvaged as short-chain fatty acids and gases. Anaerobic colonic flora are necessary for the fermentation of fiber into short-chain fatty acids and constitute the bulk of fecal mass. In the perioperative period cancer patients may receive massive antibiotic therapy, able to suppress normal colonic metabolism, thus resulting in diarrhea (7). When large amounts of lactulose, an unabsorbable sugar in the small intestine, are ingested, the protective role of colonic bacteria may be exhausted, resulting in severe diarrhea. Fecal volume in carbohydrate-induced diarrhea is proportional to the osmotic force of the malabsorbed saccharide (8). Osmotic diarrhea due to carbohydrate malabsorption is characterized by a low stool pH, due to the presence of short-chain fatty acids, a high carbohydrate content, high stool osmolality, and flatulence. In osmotic diarrhea caused by the ingestion of magnesium, sulfate and poorly absorbed salts there will be a normal pH. Osmotic diarrhea commonly subsides as the patient fasts or stops ingesting poorly absorbable solute laxatives, and is characterized by an osmotic gap in stool analysis, equivalent to the concentration of the osmotically active agents in fecal fluid that are causing the diarrhea (9).

Secretory diarrhea

An abnormal ion transport in intestinal epithelial cells, with a reduction in absorptive function or increase in the secretion of epithelial cells, is observed in secretory diarrhea. Secretory diarrhea is rarely present as the sole mechanism and is often associated with other mechanisms.

Differently from osmotic diarrhea, the anionic gap is small, eating does not markedly increase stool volume, and diarrhea usually persists during periods of fasting. Secretory diarrhea can result from bacterial toxins, or the presence of intraluminal secretagogues (such as bile acids or laxatives), circulating secretagogues (such as various hormones, drugs, and poisons), and other medical problems that compromise regulation of the intestinal function such as reduced absorptive surface area caused by disease or resection (10). Secretagogues are substances that stimulate the intestine to secrete fluid that acts mostly via the enteric nervous system (11). Endocrine tumors may cause diarrhea via the release of secretagogue transmitters (12,13). Diarrhea is a common manifestation of a carcinoid syndrome, occurring in about 70% of patients. Intestinal secretion seems to be mediated by serotonin and substance P. In the Zollinger–Ellison syndrome, secretory diarrhea is the consequence of gastric hypersecretion caused by a high concentration of circulating gastrin which overwhelms the intestinal absorptive capacity. Severe diarrhea with hypergastrinemia due to lansoprazole rather than gastrinoma has been reported (14). In a medullary carcinoma of the thyroid, circulating calcitonin is the major mediator of intestinal secretion.

Malabsorption is often associated with diarrhea. Malabsorption due to bile salts rendered insoluble by the low intraluminal pH is often associated with this. Ileal resection or a post-vagotomy state may result in watery diarrhea from the secretory effect of malabsorbed bile acids on colonic mucosa. Malabsorption due to lymphatic obstruction and fibrosis induced by the tumor may contribute to diarrhea (15) (see below).

Cancer treatment-related diarrhea caused by acute graft-versus-host disease (GVHD) and chemotherapeutic agents, particularly fluoropyrimidines, paclitaxel (16–21) and irinotecan, significantly affects morbidity and mortality. Diarrhea is a significant consequence of colorectal chemotherapy, with the majority of patients experiencing grades 3 or 4 diarrhea and 56% of all patients also modifying their chemotherapy treatment (22). These agents cause acute damage to the intestinal mucosa, necrosis, and extensive inflammation of the bowel wall. Mucosal and submucosal factors, produced directly or indirectly by the inflamed intestine, stimulate the secretion of intestinal fluid and electrolytes. Similar anatomical changes have been observed in patients with GVHD diarrhea, as well as chemotherapy and radiation enteritis (19).

Extensive necrosis of epithelial cells increases the risk of superinfection by oppurtunistic pathogens such as *Clostridium difficile, C. perfrigens, Bacillus cereus, Giardia lamblia, Cryptosporidium, Salmonella, Shigella, Campylobacter*, and rotavirus. This risk is highest in patients who may be neutropenic or immunosuppressed. Bacterial enterotoxins or other infective agents induce secretion probably by a local nervous reflex mediated by enteroendocrine cells or inflammation (5). The incidence of *C. difficile*-induced diarrhea is very high: 2.2% in patients receiving standard dose regimens and 20% in patients receiving high dose regimens (17,23,24).

Cancer patients who are immunocompromised or who have recently undergone surgery often are administered a long-term antibiotics therapy for resistant infections. These aggressive treatments, including ampicillin, clyndamicin, or cephalosporins, may result in a disruption of the normal flora and overgrowth of pathogens. *C. difficilis*, an anaerobic organism producing an enteric toxin, is the common cause of pseudo-membranous enterocolitis, which presents itself as a severe microbial diarrhea (5,25,26). Other infectious agents include *C. perfrigens, Staphylococcus aureus, Klebsiella oxytoca, Candida* species, and *Salmonella* species (24).

Some drugs, such as diuretics, caffeine, theophylline, antacids, antibiotics, and poorly absorbable laxative agents, e.g. osmotically active solutes, often chronically administered in a palliative care setting, may produce secretory diarrhea, mostly causing a reflex nervous secretion or directly activating the secretory cellular mechanism (1,6).

Deranged motility

When other measurable mechanisms are excluded, motility derangements should be suspected to be the cause of diarrhea. Even in the presence of a normal absorptive function of epithelial cells, defective motility may reduce the contact time between luminal content and epithelial cells. This commonly occurs in cancer patients with post-surgical disorders, such as post-gastrectomy dumping syndrome, post-vagotomy, ileocecal valve resection, or neoplastic and chronic diseases, such as malignant carcinoid syndrome, medullary carcinoma of the thyroid, and diabetes (27). The diabetic population can be affected by diarrhea as a result of severe neuropathy. The mechanism by which diabetic neuropathy causes dismobility is attributed to a sympathetic denervation of the bowel with a prevalence of cholinergic innervation. An iatrogenic autonomic neuropathy due to celiac plexus block, an antalgic procedure used in visceral abdominal cancer pain, has been described (28). The sympathetic denervation of the bowel may leave a cholinergic innervation unopposed leading to an increase in intestinal motility and diarrhea. This phenomenon is generally self-limiting (29,30). Abnormal reduced mobility may allow bacterial overgrowth which induces deconjugation of bile acids in the small bowel and thereby causes diarrhea and steatorrhea. Diarrhea secondary to dysmotility disorders commonly subsides after a 1 or 2 day fast, determining a small stool volume and an osmolality in the range of 250–300 mOsm.

Assessment

A document presenting the official recommendations of the American Gastroenterological Association for the evaluation and management of diarrhea has been approved recently (31). Dietary habits, alcohol consumption, or food intolerances or allergies should be investigated. The patient should be questioned in detail about the use of any prescription and any use of antibiotics in the preceding few months should be noted. The assessment of associated diseases or previous surgical intervention can provide important clues about the etiology.

Frequency, amounts, and consistency of the stools should be carefully obtained. When the stools are consistently large, light in color, watery or greasy, free of blood or containing undigested food particles, the underlying disorder is likely to be in the small bowel or the proximal colon, while small stool diarrhea in which frequent but small quantities of feces, dark in color, often containing mucus or blood, pass in spite of a sense of urgency is associated with a disorder of the left colon or rectum (5). These two patterns of diarrhea may occur simultaneously, because of widespread inflammation. A complete physical examination may reveal important clues as to the origin of the diarrhea, including abdominal mass, fever, postural hypotension, lymphadenopathy, ascites, abdominal distention, and deteriorated nutritional status. Fecal incontinence, change in stool caliber, rectal bleeding, and small, frequent but otherwise normal stools have to be distinguished. The passage of non-bloody diarrheal fluid, pus, or exudates indicates an inflammatory or infectious disease. Diarrhea associated with excessive flatus and mushy stools suggest carbohydrate malabsorption. Intermittent diarrhea and constipation are frequent in diabetic neuropathy, as well as in irritable bowel syndrome or subobstructive disorders. From a clinical point of view the suspicion of a partial obstruction should be raised in the case of sudden diarrhea after a period of constipation. Fecal impaction may cause apparent diarrhea because only liquids pass a partial obstruction. So, alternating diarrhea and constipation suggest fixed colonic obstruction. Abdominal X-ray will help the diagnosis. The presence of a mass suggests a possible malignancy, especially if associated with hepatosplenomegaly (6,32). Complaints of nocturnal diarrhea and fecal soiling are frequently reported by patients with autonomic neuropathy or anal sphincter dysfunction (Table 10.2).

Physical examination may reveal important clues to the cause of diarrhea, including abdominal mass, perianal fistula or abscess, signs of anemia, fever, postural hypotension, lymphadenopathy, neuropathy, hepatosplenomegaly, ascites, gaseous abdominal distension, reduced anal sphincter tone, and a rectal mass or impaction. Symptoms of dumping syndrome after gastric surgery, such as early nausea, abdominal distention, weakness, and diarrhea after a meal followed by hypoglycemia, sweating, dizziness, and tachycardia are typical. Secretory diarrhea combined with upper gastrointestinal symptoms caused by

Table 10.2 Signs and symptoms associated with diarrhea

Signs and symptoms	Diagnosis
Marked weight loss	Malabsorption
Lymphadenopathy—fever	Lymphoma—AIDS—enteric infections
Neuropathy—postural hypotension	Diabetes
Peptic ulcer disease	Zollinger–Ellison disease
Flushing—erythema	Carcinoid syndrome
Good response to antibiotics	Bacterial overgrowth (blind loop syndrome)
Good response to steroids	Chronic disease, Addison's disease

refractory peptic ulcer disease is suggestive of a gastrin-secreting tumor. High circulating serotonin levels in carcinoid syndrome cause other effects besides diarrhea, including hypotension, sweating, flushing, palpitations, and wheeziness (5). Peripheral or autonomic neuropathy confirms the possible concomitant visceral neuropathy secondary to these diseases.

The association of heat intolerance, palpitations, and weight loss suggest possible hyperthyroidism. Chronic bowel ischemia should be considered in the oldest patients with the clinical features of diffuse atherosclerotic disease. Of course the site of neoplasm and metastases is of paramount importance. The location of the tumor will be verified by CT, MRI scan, angiography, or laparoscopy. Intestinal dismotility or bacterial overgrowth due to diabetes, neoplastic conditions, or post-operative conditions may be associated with diarrhea (1).

Rectal examination and abdominal palpation should be performed to look for fecal masses and to exclude fecal impaction and intestinal obstruction. Rectal involvement is probable in the presence of little or no stool in spite of a sense of rectal urgency, commonly named tenusmus.

If feasible, collected diarrhea stool specimens should be submitted for qualitative study.

The initial assessment of treatment-related diarrhea should include evaluation of the duration of diarrhea and stool characteristics; stool cultures for bacterial, fungal, and viral pathogens; and formal evaluation of the gastrointestinal tract (19). Watery diarrhea is generally sustained by infective agents and efforts should be made for this purpose. Fever and abdominal tenderness may be present but are often absent in viral enteritis. Gram's stain of stool can diagnose the presence of *Staphylococcus*, *Campylobacter* or *Candida* infection. Multiple stool cultures should be obtained from patients with secretory diarrhea to rule out micro-organisms producing enterotoxins that stimulate intestinal secretion. The presence of a micro-organism in the stools is diagnostic (5). Chemotherapy-induced diarrhea typically occurs 2 to 14 days after therapy. Incidents of delayed diarrhea have been reported to be as high as 80% with irinotecan (20). The number of stools per day, the need for parenteral support or intensive care, nocturnal stools, and episodes of incontinence are common toxicity criteria to evaluate treatment-induced diarrhea. Stool volume, duration of diarrhea, stool consistency, and impact on quality of life should also be considered.

Radiation colitis is probable in patients receiving pelvic radiation for malignancies of the urogenital tract and of the prostate (5,9). The need for primary prevention is becoming urgent since evidence is emerging which suggests that the problem has an increasing frequency. The early acute syndrome, manifesting itself with diarrhea, is usually self-limiting and probably a consequence of inflammatory reactions.

The above data can also be helpful in differentiating the principal mechanisms involved in diarrhea. An anion gap of more than $50\,mmol\,l^{-1}$ (due to the reduction of stool content in sodium and potassium) is observed in osmotic diarrhea, while a value of less than $5\,mmol\,l^{-1}$ seems to indicate secretory diarrhea, characteristic of endocrine tumors showing an active secretion of salts and water (5). Osmotic diarrhea typically stops or reduces after fasting or stopping the drug previously used, while secretory diarrhea persists in spite of fasting. Positive findings in either the stool guaiac or leukocyte test would suggest an exudative mechanism, as happens in radiation colitis, colonic neoplasm, or infective diarrhea (1).

Treatment

Considering the different mechanisms involved in determining diarrhea in cancer patients, there is a consequent lack of a broadly accepted treatment protocol.

Current medication should be revised considering the use of laxatives, antacids, theophylline preparations, central nervous system drugs, antiarrhythmics, and antibiotics. In the majority of cases oral dietary therapy may provide effective symptom management.

Oral hydration solutions containing glucose, electrolytes, and water are the simplest and most common treatments. Adding glucose to electrolyte solutions takes advantage of the presence of the small intestinal sodium–glucose co-transporter to promote increased water and sodium absorption. Complex carbohydrate rather than monomeric forms improves water and electrolyte absorption (1).

A gluten-free diet can reduce abdominal cramping and bowel movement frequency in the presence of intestinal fermentation with bowel distention. Binders of osmotically active substances (kaolin–pectine) give a thicker consistency to loose stools producing a viscous colloidal absorbent solution, but their antidiarrheal effectiveness is disputable. Apples without the peel are particularly rich in pectine. Other dietary advice includes avoiding cold meals, milk, vegetables rich in fibers, fatty meat and fish, coffee, and alcohol.

Dietary sugar beet fiber may ameliorate the diarrhea induced by abdominal irradiation. The benefit depends on the effects on the luminal environment rather than on biochemical and histological changes in intestinal mucosa (33).

Sucralfate has been shown to mitigate diarrhea after pelvic radiation therapy. However, recent controlled studies were not able to demonstrate significant benefits. Moreover, some gastrointestinal symptoms, such as fecal incontinence, the need for protective clothing, and severity of nausea were worse among patients taking sucralfate (34).

Clinical signs of dehydration, such as orthostatic hypotension, decreased skin turgor, and a dry mouth, suggest the need of intensive hydration by intravenous route, especially in patients suffering from nausea and vomiting in which oral therapy is ineffective (6).

Colestyramine has been favorably used in radiation-induced diarrhea. However, real progress will come from the prevention of radiation enteritis rather than from changes in its management. In the same way, aspirin has been reported to be effective in post-radiotherapy diarrhea (35). It reduces prostaglandin synthesis thereby increasing water and electrolyte secretion which have a role in many kinds of diarrhea due to an inflammatory state. Silicate smectite has proved to be a promising drug in the prophylaxis of radiotherapy-induced diarrhea. Patients with a low irradiated small bowel volume show the greatest benefit, with a delay in the development of diarrhea after irradiation of the pelvis and abdomen (36).

Steroids may exert a positive effect on radiation enteritis. Corticosteroids can be useful in reducing edema in intestinal pseudo-obstruction. Furthermore, steroids can reduce hormone secretion in endocrine tumors, and the release and effect of the inflammation mediators, and promote salts and water absorption acting on sodium pump and sodium–hydrogen exchange (5). Steroids are also included in the pharmacological approach to GVHD-induced diarrhea (19). Budenoside, a topical active steroid, demonstrated a substantial activity in irinotecan and 5-fluorouracil induced diarrhea after the failure of loperamide treatment (37).

Antibiotics, such as norfloxacin and amoxicillin–clavulanic acid, are effective in the treatment of bacterial-overgrowth-related diarrhea (38). On the other hand, antibiotic-associated diarrhea (pseudo-membranous enterocolitis) requires the discontinuation of antibiotics and the commencement of either metronidazole or vancomycin (25). Diarrhea often subsides spontaneously after stopping the antibiotics. Bismuth subsalicylate in doses of 30–60 ml every 30 minutes for eight doses may bring mild symptomatic relief in patients with acute infectious diarrhea with an unknown effect (9). Probiotic bacteria, i.e. live bacteria that survive the passage through the gastrointestinal tract, may have beneficial effects on the host. In a recent review probiotic bacteria consistently shortened the diarrheal phase of rotavirus infection, although the evidence for other viral or bacterial infections was less strong (39,40).

Racecadotril, an enkephalinase inhibitor with antisecretory and antidiarrheal actions, has been found to be an effective and safe treatment for watery diarrhea, allowing for a reduction in oral rehydration, although no experience has been reported in cancer patients yet (41).

Clonidine, an alpha-2 agonist, has been reported useful in controlling diarrhea in diabetic patients or in patients with chronic idiopathic secretory diarrhea, who present a reduced intestinal sympathetic tone and denervation supersensitivity. The increase in salts and water absorption is probably due to an interaction with enterocyte receptors and the suppression of secretory transmitter release. However, hypotension and sedation may limit the usefulness of clonidine in advanced cancer patients (6).

The conventional management of diarrhea has centered on the use of empiric, non-specific therapy with opioids, such as loperamide, diphenoxylate, and codeine. Opioid receptors are represented at different sites, including smooth muscle, the myenteric plexus, the spinal cord and the brain; their activation influences intestinal motility and, as a consequence, secretion. However, the site of action appears to be neuronal rather than muscular. Loperamide shows the highest antidiarrheal–analgesic ratio among the opioid-like agents. It proved to be the drug of choice due to its few adverse side-effects. The standard dose of loperamide is 4 mg followed by 2 mg after every unformed stool. The dosage should be titrated against the effect and higher doses, 2 mg every 2 hours, have been recommended in conjunction with chemotherapic agents associated with a high incidence of diarrhea (42,43). A loperamide–simethicone combination was significantly more effective than the drugs taken alone in the treatment of acute diarrhea with gas-related abdominal discomfort (44).

However, the risk of producing paralytic ileus in the presence of continuous secretion should be considered as a life-threatening complication.

Refractory diarrhea that does not respond to specific therapy may present a challenging and serious clinical problem. Octreotide, an analogue of somatostatin with a more favorable pharmacokinetic profile, exerts a wide range of physiological effects on the gastrointestinal tract (6,45). Data from several clinical trials suggest that this antisecretory agent may be useful in the symptomatic treatment of diarrhea refractory to other medications. The mechanism by which octreotide produces these beneficial effects is probably multifactorial. It suppresses the secretion of many of the gut peptides implicated in the control of secretory and motor activity. Furthermore, it reduces splanchnic blood flow, inhibits exocrine secretions from the stomach, pancreas and small intestine thus impairing gastrointestinal motility and facilitating water and electrolyte absorptin (46.47).

Octreotide controls diarrhea due to carcinoid tumors, vipoma, gastrinoma, small-cell lung cancer, as well as AIDS-related diarrhea (47–50), although hormonal responses to the somatostatin analogue do not always parallel clinical responses, most probably because of the effects of co-secreted peptides. A dose–response effect of octreotide has been demonstrated (51). Octreotide seems to be an effective agent in the management of chemotherapy-related diarrhea and refractory GVHD-associated diarrhea (16,18,21,52–58). Finally, octreotide has been proved to be effective in the treatment of diarrhea induced by celiac plexus block, as well as diabetic diarrhea (29,30). Long-acting, biodegradable microsphere formulation of octreotide for monthly subcutaneous administration has been developed and could be evaluated for the prophylaxis of diarrhea in patients with a history of chemotherapy-induced diarrhea, in patients requiring high-dose chemotherapy, or those undergoing high-dose chemotherapy prior to autologous bone marrow cell transplantation.

Malabsorption

The term of malabsorption corresponds to an ineffective uptake of broken-down products in the small intestine. The digestive and absorptive processes are inextricably linked.

Mechanisms

Several cancer conditions may have multiple reasons for malabsorption. The digestion and absorption of nutrients may be affected by different mechanisms. Some conditions result in malabsorption due to a disturbed intraluminal environment of the proximal small intestine resembling that of the colon. In the intraluminal stage the hydrolosis of fat, protein, and carbohydrate by pancreatic enzymes, as well as the solubilization of fat by bile salts, may be alterated by several conditions (1). In pancreatic carcinoma or after pancreatic resection, decreased pancreatic enzyme and bicarbonate release may limit the digestion of fat and protein leading to a secondary pancreatic insufficiency. These diseases may be associated with the malabsorption of fat-soluble vitamins. The Zollinger–Ellison syndrome is characterized by an extreme acid hypersecretion causing a low luminal pH able to inactivate pancreatic enzymes with consequent fat malabsorption. Moreover, a decrease in intraluminal bile salts due to disruption of the enterohepatic circulation is often associated. A biliary tract obstruction (cholangiocarcinoma, pancreatic carcinoma), a terminal ileal resection, or cholestatic liver disease present a decreased bile salt formation or delivery to the duodenum. With limited resections (less than 100 cm) the malabsorbed bile acids dump into the colon thus determining the impairment of water and electrolyte absorption and resulting in choleretic diarrhea from increased intestinal bile salts loss. In massive resection, steatorrhea is caused by a diminished bile acid pool from an increased intestinal bile salts loss, loss of the absorptive intestinal surface, and bacterial overgrowth. A bile salt desconjugation has been reported in small bowel strictures, intestinal pseudo-obstruction, diabetes, and the elderly.

A large number of post-surgical disorders have been associated with a marked proliferation of intraluminal micro-organisms. An afferent loop of Billroth II partial gastrectomy, a surgical blind loop with end-to-side anastomosis or a recirculating loop with side-to-side anastomosis, loss or reservoir function with rapid emptying which dilutes pancreatic enzymes, obstruction or strictures, an autonomic neuropathy, and a resection of the ileocecal valve, are the most common disorders resulting in local stasis and recirculation of intestinal content with a consequent bacterial overgrowth. Bacterial overgrowth competes with the human host for some nutrients thus determining catabolism of carbohydrate by Gram-negative aerobes, deconjugation of bile salts by anaerobes, and the binding of cobalamin by anaerobes (58). Moreover, vitamin B_{12} malabsorption can result from intrinsic factor deficiency consequent to gastric resection.

Abnormalities of the small intestinal mucosa and an impaired epithelial cell transport may reduce the intestinal stage of absorption after radiotherapy due to radiation enteritis. After normal radiation doses, morphologic changes in the small intestine are evident but rarely cause symptoms. However, with a higher radiation dose, mucosal damage may be extensive with a loss of the epithelial barrier. Extensive fibrosis, strictures, and fistulae, with disruption of the mucosal surface, may develop, resulting in a chronically inflamed bowel with an impairment of mucosal function. Moreover, severe adhesions may develop between loops of intestine leading to the formation of fistulous tracts between adjacent bowel loops, and lymphatic obstruction (35).

Extensive surgical resection of the small intestine also reduces the epithelial surface area available for absorption. The extent and the specific level of resection are predictive of severe malabsorption and survival in short bowel syndrome (59). Resection of more than 50% of the small intestine usually results in significant malabsorption. The inclusion of the distal two-thirds of the ileum and ileocecal sphincter increases the risk also with minimal resection (less than 25%). In limited resections increased amounts of bile salts reach the colon and hepatic synthesis may compensate for the losses. Bile salts may enter the colon promoting water and electrolyte secretion and impairing their absorption. With massive resections hepatic synthesis is unable to compensate for the losses. Bile salts are insufficient for the solubilization of intraluminal fat. Fatty acids may enter the colon and have the same effect as bile acids. This difference has practical therapeutic implications regarding the use or not of salt-binding agents, such as cholestiramine. Enterostomy or intestinal fistulae may equally result in reduced absorption due to loss of the active surface or by flushing nutrients out. The preservation of the ileocecal sphincter is important because it may prevent contamination by the colonic flora and may increase the transit time of the intaluminal content. Bacterial metabolism of carbohydrates to produce short chain fatty acids which are rapidly absorbed is a well recognized process in the large intestine.

The loss of ileocolic absorptive capacity for NaCl may be the predominant cause of diarrhea in patients with these resections rather than the cathartic effect of unabsorbed bile acids from fat malabsorption (60). Large or carbohydrate-rich meals precipitate this motility disturbance reducing the exposure time and limiting an adequate absorption.

A vagotomy may increase the colonic content of bile acid due to an accelerated transit time and a low pH maintained by gastrinoma can reduce digestion and absorption. Moreover, blood levels of gastrin and cholecystokinin are increased after massive resection of the small intestine and colon. Transient gastric hypersecretion may follow massive intestinal resection. It is probably caused by the loss of an intestinal inhibitory factor. The consequent gastric hypersecretion may compromise intestinal absorption by inducing mucosal damage and impair lipid digestion and solubilization. The recovery from massive small bowel resection depends on the adaptive response of the remaining mucosa.

The lymphatic transport of chylomicrons and proteins is limited by a lymphatic obstruction. It causes dilatation of the intestinal lymphatic vessels. A rupture of the vessels may lead to an intestinal leakage of proteins, chylomicrons, and small lymphocytes. A localized ileal tumor, a diffuse intestinal lymphoma, a metastatic carcinoma, or metastatic carcinoid disease may produce a lymphatic obstruction leading to fat malabsorption and protein-losing enteropathy.

Malabsorption may be associated with diabetes. It results from intestinal dysmotility and bacterial overgrowth observed in this disease. Moreover, the elderly or those in an advanced stage of the illness show a decreased absorptive function although the mechanism is unclear. Poor intake and bacterial overgrowth are the major causes of malnutrition (15,58).

Assessment

History, physical examination, and laboratory and instrumental findings may help diagnosis and assessment. Patients with malabsorption syndrome usually suffer from diarrhea, weight loss, and malnutrition. The stools are bulky, greasy, and malodorous. Documentation of steatorrhea is the cornerstone of the diagnostic evaluation, although quantitative fecal fat is cumbersome to perform in cancer patients. D-xylose absorption tests may be used to assess the functional integrity of the intestinal mucosa. Xilose is largely excreted unchanged in the urine. Its absorption is decreased in small intestine involvement and not in pancreatic insufficiency. Analysis of 7a-hydroxy-4-cholesten-3-1 in serum may serve as a simple and sensitive method for the detection of bile acid malabsorption in patients with chronic diarrhea (61).

Small intestinal barium X-rays may define anatomic abnormalities after massive resection or causes associated with bacterial overgrowth (for example subobstruction or a blind loop). Biochemical examination of the material may provide information about the origin of a fistula (pancreatic or enteric). Prior radiotherapy or chemotherapy should be considered. Symptoms suggestive of some endocrine disorders, such as diabetes, and a careful drug history should be looked for. Colchicine, neomycin, and clyndamicin are the most common drugs capable of inducing malabsorption, although the pathophysiologic mechanisms are unknown. Among the chemotherapic drugs, methotrexate may impair absorption by damaging epithelial cells.

Diet phosphate absorption may be limited by aluminum-containing antacids resulting in hypophosphatemia and hypercalciuria. Resection of the proximal intestinal segment involves vitamins and divalent cations malabsorption. Certain signs are frequently associated with specific deficiency states secondary to malabsorption, such as glossitis in the case of folate or vitamin B_{12} deficiency, hypercheratosis, ecchimoses and hematuria due to fat vitamin deficiency (vitamins A and K). Anemia (chronic blood loss or malabsorption of iron, folate, or vitamin B_{12}), leukocytosis with eosinophilia, low blood levels of albumin, iron, cholestrol, and an extension of the prothrombin time are the most common laboratory findings in a state of malabsorption (1,58). Impaired absorption of Ca^{2+} and Mg^{+} may induce weakness, paresthesias, and tetany may develop. Osteopenia and bone pain, spontaneous fractures, and vertebral collapse due to vitamin D and calcium deficiency, may be probable features. Peripheral neuropathy may develop after gastric resection (vitamin B_{12} deficiency).

Weakness, severe weight loss, and fatigue result from caloric deprivation. In pancreatic carcinoma, floating, bulky, and malodorous stools due to high fat content and increased gas production are often associated with anorexia. Computerized tomography, endoscopic retrograde cholangiopancreatography, or eventually aspiration of the gland may confirm the pancreatic disease in the presence of fecal fat excretion.

Liver function tests and echographic imaging of the biliary tract may evidence a parenchimal liver dysfunction causing a decreased production of bile salts or a biliary tract obstruction with a decreased delivery.

Fluid loss is usually greatest during the first days after intestinal resection because of a shorter transit time. Diarrhea also results as a consequence of a disruption of the enterohepatic circulation of bile salts. High doses of cholestiramine bind bile salts thus limiting fat absorption.

Symptoms of dumping syndrome after gastrectomy include early nausea, abdominal distention, weakness, and diarrhea after a meal, followed by hypoglycemia, sweating, dizziness, and tachycardia.

Steatorrhea associated with peripheral lymphocytopenia, hypoalbuminemia, and peripheral edema are often observed in the abnormalities of lymphatic transport. Gastrointestinal symptoms and chylous ascites may complete the clinical picture.

While the early damage of intestinal mucosa may produce malabsorption and diarrhea, the late syndrome of chronic ischemic radiation enteritis may occur with intestinal stricture and fistula.

Treatment

After assessing the causes of malabsorption, therapy should be directed toward correcting the deficiencies, including enzyme replacement, bicarbonate supplements, vitamins, calcium, magnesium, and iron, according to the level and the mechanism of the recognized intestinal defect. Pancreatic enzyme replacement with a low-fat, high-protein diet is indicated in the case of malabsorption due to pancreatic insufficiency. The effectiveness of these substances is variable and depends on the gastric pH to prevent their degradation in the stomach before they act at the intestinal level (2,62). Large doses of pancreatic extract are required with each meal. Sodium and bicarbonate are mainly added to raise the duodenal pH.

Fat intake should be strictly limited, especially in short bowel syndrome. Medium chain triglycerides may be substituted for long-chain triglycerides. They improve fat absorption after a small intestinal resection and are useful in the presence of a lymphatic obstacle because they do not require intestinal lymphatic transport (35).

For patients with prominent dumping, dietary modification comprising frequent small, dry meals that are high in protein and low in carbohydrates and substances that prolong the absorption of carbohydrates such as pectin, may be useful (6). Pectin, a water-soluble fiber, stimulates epithelial growth in the colon and may reduce diarrhea in patients with a compromised colonic metabolism, observable during antibiotic therapy with enteral feeding devoid of dietary fibers (7).

In the presence of severe malnutrition and dehydration aggressive measures should be undertaken, especially after surgery. Parental nutrition is essential in the immediate post-operative period after massive intestinal resection. The weaning to oral nutrition depends on several variables, including the pre-operative nutritional conditions, the absorptive deficit, and the tolerance to oral intake, and should be initiated as soon as possible. The absorptive function improves with time and strictly depends on the early introduction of oral nutrients showing an important stimulatory effect on this response (32). Nutrients requiring minimal digestion for absorption should be chosen, using commercial preparations containing simple sugars, amino acids, or oligopeptides and medium-chain triglycerides. An excessive osmolar load should be avoided, initially diluting such hypertonic solutions. More complex food should be added gradually titrating it against the tolerance of the patient. Diet has to be individualized according to the different necessities dependent on the anatomic situation and adaptation after surgery. An increased caloric intake is necessary to maintain a reasonable weight in patients with massive resection. In such patients orally administered drugs may be poorly absorbed and frequently an alternative route is necessary.

Vitamin B_{12} should be replaced after terminal ileal resection. The dosage has to be adjusted to the severity of the malabsorption of the single substance considered.

There is also evidence that H2-blocking agents favorably influence the rate of adaptation of the remaining intestine after massive resection possibly by a mucosal trophic effect improving nutrient absorption. They are used to treat transient acid hypersecretion after extensive bowel resection. Large doses of H2-receptor antagonists revert the acid hypersecretion state in patients with gastrinoma (Zollinger–Ellison syndrome) (11). Omeprazole inhibits the hydrogen–potassium proton pump and produce a greater antisecretory effect than that achieved by H2-antagonist drugs. The use of cholestiramine should be carefully examined. While it is indicated in limited resections because it binds bile salts and prevents their irritant effects on the colon, in short bowel syndrome after massive resection it may strongly reduce the bile salt pool thus increasing fat malabsorption. Furthermore, cholestyramine have been favorably used in radiation-induced malabsorption (35). The dose suggested is 4 g three times before meals. Aluminum hydroxide exerts similar effects.

Antibiotic-associated malnutrition requires discontinuation of any implicated antimicrobial agents. However, if there is stasis with bacterial overgrowth caused by impaired motility or stricture, such as in radiation enteritis or blind loop syndrome, then broad-spectrum antibiotics should be administered. A 10-day course of a cephalosporin and metronidazole seems to be effective in suppressing the flora and correcting malabsorption. However, cyclic therapy may be needed (58).

Pharmacological treatment of patients affected by malabsorption with short bowel syndrome aims to reduce intestinal output or transit time, thereby increasing the chance of spontaneous closure and reducing the time of fistula closure or permitting an increase in the absorption time through a shorter intestinal surface.

Antidiarrheal agents may delay the transit time or reduce secretions. Codeine and loperamide are usually given, associated with H2-receptor antagonists with variable success depending on the possibility of absorption in specific situations (63). Somatostatin analogues, which have an antisecretory action, reduce gastric, pancreatic, and biliary secretions. They also reduce intestinal transit. These kinds of drugs create a situation analogous to the bowel rest state described for parenteral nutrition (30). Octreotide in doses of 0.2–0.6 mg daily have been advocated. It may reduce or shorten the use of parental administration in several post-operative conditions, such as enterocutaneous or pancreatic fistulae with severe short bowel syndrome and malabsorption either in short-term and long-term studies (63–66). Its use has been favorably reported also in terminally ill patients (30,67).

References

1. **Mercadante S.** Diarrhea, malabsorption, and constipation. In: Berger AM; Portenoy RK; Weissman DE., editors. *Principles and Practice of Supportive Oncology.* Philadelphia: Lippincott-Raven, 1998: pp. 191–206.
2. **Regnard CFB; Tempest S.** *A Guide to Symptom Relief in Advanced Cancer.* Manchester: Haigh & Hockland, 1992.
3. **Walsh TD; O'Shaughnessy C.** Diarrhoea. In: Walsh TD., editor. *Symptom Control.* Oxford: Blackwell, 1989: 99–116.
4. **Waller A; Caroline NL.** *Handbook of Palliative Care in Cancer.* Boston: Butterworth-Heinemann, 1996.
5. **Fine KD; Krejs GJ; Fordtran JS.** Diarrhea. In: Sleisenger MH; Fordtran JS., editors. *Gastrointestinal Disease.* Philadelphia: Saunders, 1993: pp. 1043–72.
6. **Mercadante S.** Diarrhea in terminally ill patients: pathophysiology and treatment. *Journal of Pain and Symptom Management* 1995;10:298–309.
7. **Schultz AA; Ashby-Highes B; Taylor R; Gillis DE; Wilkins M.** Effects of pectin on diarrhea in critically ill tube-fed patients receiving antibiotics. *American Journal of Critical Care* 2000;9:403–411.
8. **Clausen MR; Jorgensen J; Mortensen PB.** Comparison of diarrhea `induced by ingestion of fructooligosaccharide Idolax and disaccharide lactulose: role of osmolarity versus fermentation of malabsorbed carbohydrate. *Digest of Disease Science* 1998;43:2696–707.
9. **Krejs GJ. Diarrhea.** In: Wyngaarden JB; Smith LH; Bennett JC., editors. *Cecil Textbook of Medicine.* Philadelphia: Saunders 1992; pp. 680–7.
10. **Schiller LR.** Secretory diarrhea. *Current Gastroenterology Reports* 1999;1:389–97.
11. **Lundgren O; Pregrin AT; Persson K; Kordasti S; Uhnoo I; Svensson L.** Role of the enteric nervous system in the fluid and electrolyte secretion of rotavirus secretion. *Science* 2000;287:491–5.
12. **Lew EA; Lewin KJ; Zarchy T; Pisegna JR.** Adenocarcinoma of the colon with neuroendocrine features and secretory diarrhea. *American Journal of Gastroenterology* 1999;94:1692–4.
13. **Jensen RT.** Overview of chronic diarrhea caused by functional neuroendocrine neoplasms. *Seminars in Gastrointestinal Diseases* 1999;10:156–72.
14. **Goff JS.** Lansoprazole: a cause of secretory diarrhea. *American Journal of Gastroenterology* 1998;93:2298–9.
15. **Riley SA; Turnberg LA.** Maldigestion and malabsorption. In: Slesinger MH; Fordtran JE., editors. *Gastrointestinal Disease.* Philadelphia: Saunders, 1993: pp. 977–1008.
16. **Petrelli NJ; Rodriguez-Bigas M; Rustum Y; Herrera I; Creaven P.** Bowel rest, intravenous hydration, and continuous high-dose infusion of octreotide acetate for the treatment of chemotherapy-induced diarrhea in patients with colorectal carcinoma. *Cancer* 1993;72:1543–6.

17. **Husain A; Aptaker L; Springs DR; Barakat RR.** Gastrointestinal toxicity and Clostridium difficile diarrhea in patients treated with paclitaxel-containing chemotherapy regimens. *Gynecologic Oncology* 1998;71:104–7.
18. **Ippoliti C; Champlin R; Bugazia N.** Use of octreotide in the symptomatic management of diarrhea induced by graft-versus-host disease in patients with hematologic malignancies. *Journal of Clinical Oncology* 1997;15:3350–4.
19. **Kornblau S; Benson AB; Catalano R; Champlin RE; Engelking C; Field M; Ippoliti C; Lazarus HM; Mitchell E; Rubin J; Stiff PJ; Volkes E; Wadler S.** Management of cancer treatment-related diarrhea. Issues and therapeutic strategies. *Journal of Pain and Symptom Management* 2000;19:118–29.
20. **Marrouche Y; Extra JM; Abigerges D., *et al.*** High dose-intensity of irinotecan administered every 3 weeks in advanced cancer patients: a feasibility study. *Journal of Clinical Oncology* 1997;15:1080–6.
21. **Wasserman EI; Hidalgo M; Hornedo J; Cortes-Funes H.** Octreotide (SMS 201-995) for hematopoietic support-dependent high-dose chemotherapy (HSD-HDC)-related diarrhea: dose finding study and evaluation of efficacy. *Bone Marrow Transplant* 1997;20:711–14.
22. **Arbuckle RB; Huber SL; Zacker C.** The consequences of diarrhea occurring during chemotherapy for colorectal cancer: a retrospective study. *Oncologist* 2000;5:250–9.
23. **Goodman L; Segreti J.** Infectious diarrhea. *Disease-a-Month* 1999;45:268–99.
24. **Hogenauer C; Hammer HF; Krejs GJ; Reinsinger EC.** Mechanisms and management of antibiotic-associated diarrhea. *Clinical Infectious Diseases* 1998;27:702–10.
25. **Gorenek L; Dizer U; Besirbellioglu B; Eyigun CP; Hacibektasoglu A; Van Thiel DH.** The diagnosis and treatment of Clostridium difficile in antibiotic-associated diarrhea. *Hepatogastroenterology* 1999;46:343–8.
26. **Schiller LR.** Diarrhea. *Medical Clinics of North America* 2000;84:1259–74.
27. **Mercadante S.** Assessment and management of dysmotility disorders. In: Dunlop R., editor. *Concise Oxford Textbook of Palliative Care.* Oxford: Oxford University Press, in press.
28. **Lysy J; Israeli E; Goldin E.** The prevalence of chronic diarrhea among diabetic patients. *American Journal of Gastroenterology* 1999;94:2165–70.
29. **Dean AP; Reed WD.** Diarrhea—an unrecognized hazard of coeliac plexus block. *Australian and New Zealand Journal of Medicine* 1991;21:47–8.
30. **Mercadante S.** The role of octreotide in pallative care. *Journal of Pain and Symptom Management* 1994;9:406–11.
31. American Gastrointestinal Association medical position statement: guidelines for the evaluation and management of chronic diarrhea. *Gastroenterology* 1999;116:1461–3.
32. **Sykes NP.** Constipation and diarrhea. In: Doyle D; Hanks GW; MacDonald N., editors. *Oxford Textbook of Palliative Medicine.* Oxford: Oxford University Press, 1993: pp. 299–310.
33. **Ishizuka S; Ito S; Kasai T; Hara H.** Dietary sugar beet fiber ameliorates diarrhea as an acute gamma-radiation injury in rats. *Radiation Research* 2000;154:261–7.
34. **Martenson JA; Bollinger JW; Sloan JA; Novotny PJ; Uria RE; Michalak JC; Shanahan TG; Maillard JA; Levitt R.** Sucralfate in the prevention of treatment-induced diarrhea in patients receiving pelvic radiation therapy: a North Central Cancer Treatment Group phase III double-blind placebo-controlled trial. *Journal of Clinical Oncolology* 2000;18:1239–45.
35. **Earnest DL; Trier JS.** Radiation enteritis and colitis. In: Sleisinger MH; Fordtran JS., editors. *Gastrointestinal Disease.* Philadelphia: Saunders, 1993: pp. 1257–69.
36. **Hombrick J; Frohlich D; Glazel M; Krauss A; Thiel HJ; Meier J; Hamann D; Mucke R; Glaser FH; Kost S.** Prevention of radiation-induced diarrhea by smectite. Results of a double-blind randomized, placebo-controlled multicenter study. *Strahlentherapie Onkologie* 2000;17:173–9.

37. **Lenfers BH; Loeffler TM; Droege CM; Hausamen TU.** Substantial activity of budesonide in patients with irinotecan (CPT-11) and 5-fluorouracil induced diarrhea and failure of loperamide treatment. *Annals of Oncology* 1999;10:1251–3.

38. **Attar A; Flourie B; Ranbaud JC; Franchisseur C; Ruszniewski P; Bouhnik Y.** Antibiotic efficacy in small intestinal bacterial overgrowth-related chronic diarrhea: a crossover, randomized trial. *Gastroenterology* 1999;117:794–7.

39. **de Roos NM; Katan MB.** Effects of probiotic bacteria on diarrhea, lipid metabolism, and carcinogenesis: a review of papers published between 1988 and 1998. *American Journal of Clinical Nutrition* 2000;71:405–11.

40. **Saavedra J.** Probiotics and infectious diarrhea. *American Journal of Gastroenterology* 2000;95:S16–S18.

41. **Salazar-Lindo E; Santisteban-Ponce J; Chea-Woo E; Gutierrez M.** Racecadotril in the treatment of acute watery diarrhea in children. *New England Journal of Medicine* 2000;17:463–7.

42. **Taplin SC; Blanke CD; Baughman C.** Nursing strategies for the management of side effects in pateints treated for colorectal cancer. *Seminars in Oncology* 1997;24:S18–S70.

43. **Cascinu S; Bichisao E; Amadori D; Slingardi V; Giordani P; Sansoni E; Luppi G; Catalano V; Agostinelli R; Catalano G.** High-dose loperamide in the trreatment of 5-fluorouracil-induced diarrhea in colorectal cancer patients. *Supportive Care in Cancer* 2000;8:65–7.

44. **Kaplan MA; Prior MJ; Ash RR; McKonly KI; Helzner EC.** Loperamide–simethicone vs loperamide alone, simethicone alone, and placebo in the treatment of acute diarrhea with gas-related abdominal discomfort. A randomized controlled trial. *Archives of Family medicine.* 1999;8:243–8.

45. **Fried M.** Octreotide in the treatment of refractory diarrhea. *Digestion* 1999;60(Suppl. 2):42–6.

46. **Harris AG.** Octreotide in the treatment of disorders of the gastrointestinal tract. *Drugs* 1992;4(Suppl. 3):1–54.

47. **Cello JP; Grendell JH; Basuk P., *et al.*** Effect of octreotide on refractory AIDS-associated diarrhea: a prospective, multicenter clinical trial. *Annals of Internal Medicine* 1991;115:705–10.

48. **Fuessl HS; Carolen G; Williams G., *et al.*** Effect of long-acting somatostatin analogue (SMS 201-995) on postprandial gastric empying of 99mTC-tin colloid and mouth-to-caecum transit time in man. *Digestion* 1987;36:101–7.

49. **Kvols LK.** Therapy of malignant carcinoid syndrome and metastatic islet cell carcinoma. In: D'Orisio TM., editor. *Sabdostatin in the Treatment of Gastroenteropancreatic Endocrine Tumors: a Consensus Roundtable.* Berlin: Springer-Verlag, 1987: pp. 65–82.

50. **Goumas P; Naxakis S; Christopoulou A; Chrysanthopoulos C; Nikolopoulou V; Kalonos HP.** Octreotide acetate in the treatment of fluorouracil-induced diarrhea. *Oncologist* 1998;3:50–3.

51. **Cascinu S; Fedeli A; Fedeli SL; Catalano G.** Control of chemotherapy-induced diarrhea with octreotide in pateints receiving 5-fluorouracil. *European Journal of Cancer* 1992;28:482–3.

52. **Cascinu S; Fedeli A; Fedeli SL; Catalano G.** Octreotide versus loperamide in the treatment of fluorouracil-induced diarrhea: a randomized trial. *Journal of Clinical Oncology* 1993;11:148–51.

53. **Cascinu S; Fedeli A; Fedeli SL; Catalano G.** Control of chemotherapy-induced diarrhea with octreotide. *Oncology.* 1994;51:70–3.

54. **Wadler S; Haynes H; Wiernik PH.** Phase I trial of the somatostatin analog octreotide acetate in the treatment of fluoropyrimidine-induced diarrhea. *Journal of Clinical Oncology* 1995;13:222–6.

55. **Gebbia V; Carreca I; Testa A.** Subcutaneous octreotide versus oral loperamide in the treatment of diarrhea following chemotherapy. *Anticancer Drugs* 1993;4:443–5.

56. **Crouch MA; Restino MS; Cruz JM.** Octreotide acetate in refractory bone marrow transplant-associated diarrhea. *Annals of Pharmatherapy* 1996;30:331–6.

57. **Beckman RA; Siden R; Yanik GA; Levine JE.** Continuous octreotide infusion for the treatment of secretory diarrhea caused by acute intestinal graft-versus-host disease in a child. *Journal of Pediatric Hematology, and Oncology* 2000;22:344–50.

58. **Toskes PP.** Malabsorption. In: Wyngaarden JB; Smith LH; Bennett JC, editors. *Cecil Textbook of Medicine.* Philadelphia: Saunders, 1992: pp. 667–99.
59. **Westergaard H; Spady DK.** The short bowel syndrome. In: Sleisenger MH; Fordtran JS, editors. *Gastrointestinal Disease.* Philadelphia: Saunders, 1993: pp. 1249–56.
60. **Arrambide KA; Santa Ana CA; Achiller LR., *et al.*** Loss of absorptive capacity for sodium chloride as a cause of diarrhea following partial ileal and right colon resection. *Digestive Diseases and Science* 1989;34:193–201.
61. **Sauter GH; Munzing W; von Ritter C; Paumgartner G.** Bile acids malabsorption as a cause of chronic diarrhea: diagnostic value of 7a-hydroxy-4-cholesten-3-one in serum. *Digestive Diseases and Science* 1999;44:14–19.
62. **Nightingale JMD; Walker ER; Farthing MJG; Lennard-Jones JE.** Effect of omeprazole on intestinal output in the short bowel syndrome. *Alimentary Pharmacological Therapeutics* 1991;5:405–12.
63. **Nightingale JMD; Walker ER; Burnham WR., *et al.*** Short bowel syndrome. *Digestion* 1990;45(Suppl. 1):77–83.
64. **Cooper JC; Williams NS; King RFGJ; Barker MCJ.** Effects of a long acting somatostatin analogue in patients with severe ileostomy diarrhoea. *British Journal of Surgery* 1986;73:128–31.
65. **Ladefoged K; Christensen KC; Hegnhoj J; Jarnum S.** Effect of a long acting somatostatin analogue SMS 201-995 on jejunostomy effluents in patients with severe short bowel syndrome. *Gut* 1989;30:943–9.
66. **Nightingale JMD; Lennard-Jones JE; Walker ER; Fathing MJG.** Jejunal efflux in short bowel syndrome. *Lancet* 1990;336:765–8.
67. **Mercadante S.** Treatment of diarrhoea due to enterocolic fistula with octreotide in a terminal cancer patient. *Palliative Medicine* 1992;6:257–9.

Chapter 11

Abdominal pain

Sebastiano Mercadante

Introduction

Excluding pain directly originating from the abdominal wall, which has somatic characteristics, abdominal pain in cancer is due predominantly to a visceral involvement. Visceral cancer pain originates from a primary or metastatic lesion involving the abdominal or pelvic viscera. In a survey on prevalence, causes, and mechanisms of pain in advanced cancer patients followed at home, abdominal pain was found to have an incidence of 45%. Two-thirds of patients presented a visceral pain, although mixed pain syndromes were observed in more than half of these patients (1).

The viscera have a complex peripheral nervous system and different neurophysiological understandings of visceral pain have been reported. Unlike their cutaneous counterparts, visceral nociceptors appear not to be a simple acute warning system. Many viscera are innervated by receptors that do not evoke conscious perception. Visceral nociceptors, however, have a wide range of response, and may be activated in the presence of inflammation or tissue injury. Therefore, visceral afferents are considered polymodal, giving excitatory responses to different stimuli, including inflammation, stretching, and distension (2).

Neurons that transmit visceral sensory information to the spinal cord cell bodies reside in the dorsal root ganglia. These primary afferents travel through the paravertebral ganglia, through the paravertebral ganglia, and have sensory endings in the viscera themselves. These afferents are in conjunction with motor fibers of the parasympathetic and sympathetic nervous system. Most visceral afferents have relatively slow conduction velocities.

Recent studies suggest possible autonomic visceral pain pathways in the dorsal column of the spinal cord. In animals, the responses of neurons in the ventral posterolateral thalamic nucleus to noxious colorectal distension are dramatically reduced after a lesion at T10, but not by interruption of the spinothalamic tract. This observation is explainable in light of strong evidence in support of the existence of a visceral pain pathway that ascends in the dorsal column of the spinal cord (3).

Pathophysiology of visceral pain

Experiments using distension most likely measure the effects of a mixture of visceral stimuli, including the stimulation of stretch receptors in the intestinal wall and a concomitant excitation of mesenteric mechanoreceptors. A good correlation between the size of the response and the stimulus intensity has been observed (4). Traction on mesentery is another suitable method to investigate acute visceral nociception (5).

Nociceptors

Two distinct classes of nociceptive sensory receptors that innervate internal organs have been proposed: high-threshold receptors, mostly mechanical, activated by stimuli within the noxious range, and low-threshold receptors activated in the range of stimulation intensity from innocuous to noxious. According to this theory, high-threshold receptors would contribute to the peripheral encoding of noxious events in the viscera. Other prolonged and intense stimuli, such as hypoxia or tissue inflammation, would result in the sensitization of these receptors and bring into play previously silent receptors, normally unresponsive to innocuous stimuli (6). The activity of afferents and the excitability of dorsal horn neurons are increased with repeated or persistent stimuli due to a process of sensibilization of afferents which occurs secondary to the local release of chemical substances in tissues damaged or ischemic. A critical level of preceding activity in the afferents is required to induce facilitation of dorsal horn neuronal responses via the central mechanism (7). Moreover, the normal pattern of motility and secretion is altered by the local damage produced by inflammation, producing changes in the environment surrounding the nociceptor endings. This is consistent with the continuous and increasing input in the presence of an abdominal cancer disease.

Pathophysiologic characteristics of visceral pain

Visceral pain tends to be diffuse because of the absence of a separate visceral sensory pathway and the low proportion of visceral afferent nerve fibers compared with those of somatic origin. Thus, the neurological mechanisms of visceral pain differ from those involved in somatic pain. The characteristics of visceral pain are listed in Table 11.1

The nature of referred pain is not clearly defined. Different groups of spinal neurons may play a role. Some spinal neurons are involved in the localization of pain and project to the brain, while another group of neurons has short ascending projections with collaterals into multiple spinal segments. The activation of visceral efferents should lead to changes in the excitability of multiple spinal units, including those responsible for somatic nociceptive sensory pathways, or a direct activation of neurons receiving both visceral and somatic inputs. Alternatively, the brain may misinterpret activity in the viscerosomatic neurons. Convergent receptive fields are generally described as multidermatomal, centered in the dermatome corresponding to the spinal segment stimulated, and are significantly larger than the receptive fields of spinal neurons receiving only somatic input (7). These

Table 11.1 Characteristics of visceral pain

- Not evoked from all viscera: most solid viscera and paranchyma are not sensitive to pain
- Independent of typical injury, such as cutting
- Diffuse, poorly localized, and referred to other locations
- Associated with motor and autonomic reflexes

observations explain why visceral pain is difficult to localize and often referred to other areas of the body. Pain originating from any viscera cannot easily be differentiated from pain originating in another viscus, although descriptions of some visceral pains have been associated with specific etiologies, such as in cases of pancreatic pain or peptic ulcer.

Nociceptive stimuli in clinical conditions

Mechanic stimuli, such as torsion or traction of mesentery, distension of hollow organs, stretch of serosal and mucosal surfaces, and compression of some organs produce pain in humans. These conditions are frequently observed in cancer patients with abdominal diseases and intraperitoneal masses.

Human studies have revealed that pain is produced when the intraluminal pressure of hollow organs is maintained above certain pressure thresholds. Obstruction or inflammation within the biliary tract or pancreatic duct induces pain directly related to an increased intraluminal pressure with consequent inflammation, and release of pain-producing substances. Capsular stretch of the liver due to cancer growth produces pain. Distension or traction on the gall bladder leads to deep, epigastric pain, inspiratory distress, and vomiting. Spontaneous spasm of the sphincter of Oddi or that induced by morphine leads to increases in pain sensation, resulting in a paradoxical opioid-induced pain. On the other hand, morphine and other opioids increase the pressure threshold necessary to produce the sensation of pain due to distension of the biliary system. Renal colic is commonly secondary to ureteral obstruction and subsequent distension of the ureter and renal pelvis. This may be evident in circumstances in which an abdominal–pelvic mass compresses or invades the ureter, as often occurs in gynecological cancers. Reports of pain appear to be directly related to the pressure of urinary bladder. Bladder distension may also activate mechanisms related to the phenomena of counter-irritation.

The etiology of pain from visceral tissues may also be related to ischemia, particularly in metastatic or recently damaged tissues (post-surgical). Ischemia may act as a modulator of mechanoreceptive visceral inputs. The variability in responses to ischemia may be due to the pre-existing pathology or cancer-related mechanical distortion of the viscera secondary to local changes.

Chemical stimuli and algogenic tumor-mediated substances may give serosal or mucosal irritation. However, these seem to act as a modulator or co-stimulant of visceral sensory systems rather than as a primary stimulus, as frank tissue damage (e.g. cutting and burning) does not reliably produce reports of the visceral pain, despite resulting in the production of bradykinin. However, if a viscous is inflamed, stimuli that are normally non-painful, such as pressure, or stimuli applied for a period of time, will cause pain, assuming the pathophysiologic condition of summation. A better localization of stimulus occurs when the disease extends to a somatically innervated structure such as the parietal peritoneum. Thus, initially, visceral pain is poorly localized and dull because of the wide divergence of visceral afferents in the spinal cord. Poorly localized visceral pain becomes localized as visceral afferent input increases due to spinal facilitation or the activation of visceral nociceptors. The greatest localization occurs when somatic structures, such as the peritoneum, become involved, Somatic structures may also be involved with an indirect mechanism. For example, diaphragmatic irritation due to abdominal distension produced by large subdiaphragmatic masses may induce shoulder pain often associated to hiccup (8).

Clinical implications in cancer pain

Because of these qualities, visceral pain is generally separated as a special case of deep pain. Visceral pain is often referred to somatic structures. Moreover, it is not amenable to the localization of a precise point tenderness until the cancer process spreads and involves the abdominal wall peritoneum. Cutaneous and deep tissue hyperalgesia also occurs in association with visceral pain. Common examples of referred pain in cancer patients include back pain, which occurs with pancreatic cancer, and right shoulder pain, which occurs with liver cancer or metastases.

The models of visceral pain are useful in explaining the outcome of some neurolytic blocks for abdominal cancer pain and the response to analgesic drugs (9). The failure or partial success of celiac or hypogastric plexus block may be attributed to the fact that the tumor has metastatized beyond the nerves that conduct pain via the celiac plexus and the component nerves that form it. Somatic pain may arise from parietal peritoneum and abdominal wall involvement as well as retroperitoneal nodal involvement or bone metastases. Finally, a neuropathic pain from radiculopathy related to retroperitoneal spread, post-chemotherapy pain from mucositis, liver chemoembolization as well as post-operative pain and post-radiation pain may be associated (10). These phenomena occur generally in the late stage of pancreatic disease while it may occur earlier with other abdominal malignancies (11,12). Concomitant pain of somatic origin, due to significant peritoneal involvement, requires other therapeutic measures.

Treatment

Most pain in cancer responds to pharmacological management using orally administered analgesics. Current treatment is based on the analgesic ladder, which involves a stepwise approach to the use of analgesic drugs and is essentially a framework of principles rather than a rigid protocol (13). When cancer patients experience severe pain, opioids are the mainstay of therapy. There is a large variety of options for the delivery of opioids in the management of cancer pain. In some instances there are clear indications for using one preparation or delivery system over another, according to the ability of the patient to use a specific type of delivery system, the efficacy of that system to deliver acceptable analgesia, the ease of use by the patient and his or her family, and the potential or actual complications associated with that system. Cost is another important consideration for patients who must purchase their own medications.

Oral route

The oral route is the most common, least invasive, and easiest route for opioid administration for most patients with cancer pain. In all patents who can take oral medications, this route should be considered first. The main problem with the oral route is the first-pass biotransformation of opioids in the liver. All opioids given orally are absorbed via the gastric and duodenal mucosa and then transported to the liver via the portal venous system. In the liver, these medications undergo 'first-pass metabolism' before entering the systemic circulation. This has a major impact on the systemic plasma concentrations of drugs. Bioavailability is defined as the percentage of administered medication that reaches the systemic circulation. For example, the dose of an opioid given orally to a patient with cancer pain must be three times the intravenous or intramuscular dose of morphine and twice the parenteral dose of methadone. Oxycodone, while roughly equipotent to morphine if given parenterally, appears to be approximately twice as potent as morphine when given orally because of less first-pass metabolism. Morphine, the most commonly used medication in the world to treat cancer pain, has a terminal elimination plasma half-life of about 3 hours. To provide longer-lasting analgesia, several preparations have become available. The bioavailability of these slow-release preparations is the same as that of immediate-release preparations, but time to peak plasma drug concentrations is longer, and peak plasma concentrations is decreased. These preparations are recommended by the manufacturer to be administered every 12 hours. Clinicians occasionally use an 8-hour schedule if necessary to provide adequate analgesia. Other preparations, such as a morphine pellet coated with a polymer, is manufactured to be administered once every 24 hours. If additional analgesia is needed for 'breakthrough' pain, then doses of a fast-onset, short-acting opioid preparation should be available to the patient. However, immediate–release oral opioid preparations usually require approximately 30 minutes to onset of analgesic action when taken on an empty stomach, and faster routes may be required. Oxycodone, methadone, and hydromorphone are possible alternatives to oral morphine (13).

Parenteral routes

Many patients, even with abdominal masses, will develop tolerance to most of the undesirable side-effects of opioids (such as nausea/vomiting or sedation) over a period of several days; therefore, a medication should not be labelled 'intolerable' until a reasonable trial has been undertaken. However, certain patients may not be able to tolerate oral medications because of esophageal motility problems or gastrointestinal obstruction (e.g. head and neck or esophageal cancer) or may present nausea and vomiting, limiting the utility of the oral route. Females seem to be more predisposed to these opioid-induced symptoms. Finally, some patients are unable to swallow due to the site of their cancer or because they are receiving end-of-life care, when an inability to take oral medications may arise. In these cases an alternative form of analgesia must be used. Alternative routes, including intravenous and subcutaneous, as well as the transdermal ones, have been advocated in such circumstances.

The intravenous route of administration is indicated for those patients whose pain cannot be controlled by a less invasive route or having a central venous access. The major disadvantage of this route is that it is more complex to manage, especially at home, and requires some expertise. On the other hand, this route is the fastest one, allowing for an immediate effect in emergency conditions. Different opioids are available in intravenous solution in the majority of countries, including morphine, hydromorphone, fentanyl, alfentanil, sufentanil, and methadone. Fentanyl is approximately 80–100 times more potent than morphine, and sufentanil is approximately 1000 times more potent. The main drawback to their use in the practise of oncology is their high cost compared with the cost of morphine. Intravenous opioid infusions can be given as continuous infusions or by a patient-controlled analgesia (PCA) device, which provides continuous infusion plus on-demand boluses. Confused or not collaborating patients may not be the best candidates for PCA use (14).

For patients requiring parenteral opioids who do not have in-dwelling intravenous access, the subcutaneous route can be used. This simple method of parenteral administration involves inserting a small plastic cannula on an area of the chest, abdomen, upper arms, or thighs and attaching the tubing to an infusion pump. The limiting factor is the volume of fluid that can be injected per hour, often requiring more concentrated solutions. The subcutaneous route can be used in conjunction with a PCA device. Most drugs used by the intravenous route can also be used by subcutaneous infusion except methadone which could induce local toxicity. The main advantages of subcutaneous over intravenous route is that there is no need for vascular access, changing sites can be easily accomplished, and problems associated with in-dwelling intravenous catheters are avoided. The oral–parenteral ratio for morphine is 2:1 or 3:1 (13,14).

Transdermal route

For patients with abdominal cancers unable to take oral medications , the transdermal route is a non-invasive option for maintaining continuous plasma concentrations of opioids. This delivery system consists of a reservoir of fentanyl and alcohol that contains a three-day supply of fentanyl. The patch releases fentanyl at a constant rate until the reservoir is depleted. Upon initial application of the patch, a subcutaneous 'depot' is formed as fentanyl saturates the subcutaneous fat beneath the patch. After approximately 12 hours, steady-state plasma fentanyl concentrations are reached, which are maintained for about 72 hours. Fentanyl patches are currently available in 25, 50, 75, and 100 $\mu g\,h^{-1}$ dosages. The bioavailability of transdermal fentanyl is very high, approximately 90%. Several pharmacokinetic properties concerning transdermal fentanyl are of interest to the clinician. Because of the slow depot formation and slow rise in plasma concentrations, this system is not suitable for rapid titration of pain. Because of the prolonged elimination after removal of a system, the opioid side-effects will take many hours to resolve. Thus, the transdermal fentanyl system is best suited for patients with stable pain in whom the 24-hour opioid requirement has already been determined. Vigorous exercise and elevation of body temperature secondary to fever or bathing will increase blood flow to the skin and increase drug diffusion into the systemic circulation. Adverse effects of the fentanyl patch include skin reactions and the typical opioid side-effects, e.g. nausea/vomiting, constipation, somnolence, and confusion. In general, this delivery system is well tolerated by cancer patients with relatively constant pain who are on stable doses of opioids. In patients unable to use the oral route, the transmucosal or rectal route is available for 'breakthrough' administration of fast-acting opioids (14).

The transmucosal/sublingual routes

The sublingual administration of opioids is particularly beneficial in the patient with cancer who is unable to tolerate oral administration because of nausea/vomiting or dysphagia. It may also be attractive in patients who cannot receive parenteral opioids because of lack of venous access or who present with typical contraindications for subcutaneous drug administration. Because sublingual venous drainage is systemic rather than portal, hepatic first-pass elimination can be avoided. On the other hand, the transmucosal or sublingual also offers the potential for more rapid absorption and onset of action relative to the oral route. This is particularly useful for treating breakthrough pain. Lipophilic drugs are better absorbed than hydrophilic drugs. For these reasons fentanyl and buprenorphine are mainly used by this route. This route is simple and requires little expertise. Both the plasma fentanyl concentration and bioavailability of fentanyl will vary depending on the fraction of the dose absorbed through the oral mucosa and the fraction swallowed. Approximately 25% of the total dose is rapidly absorbed from the buccal mucosa and becomes systemically available. The remaining 75% is swallowed, is slowly absorbed from the stomach, and then undergoes first-pass metabolism in the liver, with a bioavailability of 33%. Thus, the overall observed bioavailability of transmucosal fentanyl is approximately 50% of the total dose. The onset of action is within about 15 minutes. Transmucosal fentanyl is the only medication that has been found to be a very useful tool in the management of breakthrough pain in cancer patients in different controlled studies (14).

Rectal route

This route may be a simple alternative when the oral route is not possible because of vomiting, obstruction, or altered consciousness. Its principal advantage is that it is independent of gastrointestinal tract motility and rate of gastric emptying. However, the rectal route also has several disadvantages. There may be a great deal of variation among individuals regarding the necessary dose, as the amount of drug drained from the rectum is highly variable. Absorption may be delayed or limited by the small surface area of the rectum and may be interrupted by defecation. Constipation may prevent contact of drug with rectal mucosa and cause subsequent absorption into feces. All these factors may affect bioavailability. The rectal route is uncomfortable for prolonged use and contraindicated if the patient has painful anal conditions such as fissures or inflamed hemorrhoids. The usual recommendation for intial doses of morphine and most other opioids given rectally is the same does as that given orally (14).

Spinal route

A small number of patients may still fail to obtain adequate analgesia with large systemic opioid doses, or they may suffer from uncontrollable side-effects such as nausea, vomiting, or oversedation. These patients may be candidates for the administration of a combination of opioids, local anesthetics, and clonidine via the spinal (epidural or intrathecal) route. The goal of spinal opioid therapy is to place a small dose of an opioid and/or local anesthetic close to the spinal opioid receptors located in the dorsal horn of the spinal cord to enhance analgesia and reduce systemic side-effects by decreasing the total daily opioid dose. Use of this route to deliver opioids requires placing a catheter into the epidural or intrathecal space and using an external of implantable infusion pump to deliver the medications. Deciding between epidural versus intrathecal placement or external versus implantable pumps to deliver the opioid is based on multiple factors including duration of therapy, type and location of the pain, disease extent and central nervous system involvement, opioid requirement, and individual experience. The daily epidural opioid requirement is approximately 10 times that of intrathecal administration. Intrathecal opioid administration has the advantage of allowing a higher concentration of drug to be localized at the receptor site while minimizing systemic absorption, thus possibly decreasing drug-related side-effects. Morphine remains the drug of choice for the spinal route, because of its relatively low lipid solubility. It has a slow onset of action, but a long duration of analgesia when given via intermittent bolus. The starting dose is quite difficult to calculate and should take into consideration various factors, including the previous opioid dose, age, and the pain mechanism. Adding a local anesthetic (bupivacaine or ropivacaine) to morphine via the spinal route has been successful in providing good analgesia in patients whose pain was resistant to epidural morphine alone, despite high doses. Further clinical studies and trials will still be required to judge the safety, efficacy, and extended role of the spinal route in chronic cancer pain and, more importantly, to define in which patients this technique is best indicated. Clonidine, an alpha-adrenergic agonist that acts at the dorsal horn of the spinal cord to produce analgesia, has been used in cancer patients in combination with epidural (or intrathecal) morphine infusions. There is some evidence to suggest that neuropathic pain may be somewhat more responsive to the combination of clonidine/morphine than to morphine alone, although orthostatic hypotension is of concern. Procedural and surgical complications, system malfunction, and pharmacological adverse effects are the main categories of complications associated with spinal drug delivery (15).

In conclusion, for the patient with cancer pain, the oral route of opioid delivery should be the first choice. If the oral route cannot be used because of gastrointestinal obstruction and/or severe nausea/vomiting, the rectal route is equivalent, although unsuitable for prolonged use. Another non-invasive alternative to the oral route is the transdermal route, which at present is available only for continuous administration of fentanyl. For the treatment of breakthrough pain in a patient unable to take oral or rectal medications, a transmucosal preparation of fentanyl is available. For those patients in whom oral or transdermal opioids are not appropriate, intravenous or subcutaneous administration is effective, the latter route being relatively easier to administer. The spinal route can be attempted when the oral and other parenteral routes have been unsuccessful. This route may be most successful when opioids and local anesthetics and/or clonidine are used in combination. Whatever route is used, the administration of opioids to manage cancer pain requires knowledge of potency relative to morphine and bioavailability of the route chosen. Dose-equivalent tables are only close approximations and substantial interpatient variability is often observed. Therefore, patients should be closely followed and doses titrated to minimize side effects whenever the opioids, route, or dose is changed.

Response to analgesics

Pharmcological studies of visceral pain have demonstrated that most analgesics are effective in this type of pain. Non-steroidal anti-inflammatory drugs (NSAIDs), opioids, and clonidine produce a dose-dependent inhibition of viscero responses to distension of the gut (16). NSAIDs have been claimed to have a major role in the management of some specific cancer pain syndromes, including pain from bone metastasis, soft-tissue infiltration, arthritis, and recent surgery. However, it has been shown that the analgesic effect of NSAIDs is similar to that produced by opioids in experimental visceral pain. In patients with cancer pain, NSAIDs were useful both for somatic and visceral pain as the first step on the analgesic ladder, and were also useful in combination with opioids, regardless of the pain mechanism involved (17). Administration of analgesics resulted in an equal pain relief until death, although with more unpleasant adverse effects and deterioration of quality of life than when using celiac plexus block (9,18).

Of concern is that morphine and other opioids, as opposed to meperidine, which has spasmolytic properties, may induce spasm at the level of the intestinal valves and sphincters, and may paradoxically worsen the clinical picture in the presence of distended intestinal loops.

Sympathetic blocks

A neurolytic celiac plexus block (NCBP) is indicated for abdominal pain from pancreatic cancer, sovramesocolic viscera, painful retroperitoneal tumors or metastases, and chronic abdominal pain unresponsive to treatment. The use of neurolytic agents provides long-term relief that may match the life expectancy of cancer patients. The point at which the procedure should be considered has not been well established in cancer patients. Several techniques have been devised that differ significantly in the site of approach, solution injected, instruments used, and radiologic guidance methods. The choice of technique should be individualized to the available facilities and clinician's experience, the patient's physical condition, as well as the extent of malignancy, since the analgesic results seem to be independent of the principal techniques used. The retrocrural or deep splanchnic technique is the most known one. The needles are bilaterally inserted at the lower border of the twelth rib, about 7 cm from the spinous process of the L1 vetebra to the spine, advanced at an angle of about 45° from horizontal, and cephalad of about 15°, to contact the lateral part of the L1 vertrebral body. The needle is withdrawn and then laterally redirected to walk-off the vertebral body 1–2 cm anteriorily. The position of the needle is checked using imaging in the posteroanterior and lateral positions during the procedure. When the position of the needle is deemed satisfactory, 3–5 ml of contrast medium is injected through each needle and its spread observed radiographically, after negative aspiration. This classic method allows for the bathing of the neurolytic agent at the celiac neural axis in addition to producing splanchnic neurolysis. The diaphragmatic crura may prevent the solution from extending around the celiac plexus, facilitating the involvement of the splachnic nerves, although it may diffuse via the aortic hiatus of the diaphram or flow through the gaps present in the diaphragmatic crura and spread anteriorly to the aorta to also bath the plexus, when high volumes of neurolytic solution are injected. This passage may be impeded by the distortion of anterocrural structures. However, this classic method is more likely to produce splanchnic nerve block, as the injectate appears to preferentially spread to the retroaortic celiac fibers and rostrally to the splanchnic nerves.

The specific technique for a splanchnic nerve block differs markedly from the classic retrocrural approach. The needles are more cephalad to the anterolateral margin of the T12 vertebral body. This site can be reached using a paramedian approach, placing the needle tips at the anterolateral margin of the T12 body. Splanchnic neurolysis is better preserved in patients with an upper abdominal malignancy. Moreover, visceral sympathetic pathways can be blocked with a smaller volume of neurolytic solution, when considering that the anterocrural space contains the celiac plexus surrounded by a large amount of adipose tissue.

In the transcrural approach the needles are advanced another 1–2 cm with respect to the retrocrural technique, so that their points lie laterally to and approximately at the anterior wall of the aorta on the left, and at the same depth on the right. The transaortic approach is a single needle technique in which a needle is introduced on the left side intentionally to pierce the aorta until no blood can be aspirated to locate the centre of the celiac plexus.

The anterior abdominal approach involves placing the needle just anterior to the diaphragmatic crus at or between the levels of the celiac and superior mesenteric arteries. Although this technique involves the passage of fine needles through the liver, stomach, small and large bowels, and pancreas to reach the celiac ganglia, it is associated with very low rates of complications. The theoretical advantages of this approach include reduced discomfort during the procedure thus avoiding a prolonged prone position and a lower risk of neurologic injury related to the spread of neurolytic solution to the somatic nerve roots. Ultrasound or CT guidance are commonly used. The use of a radiological contrast medium is essential to enhance imaging capabilities, to better determine the correct needle localization, and to ensure that the material to be injected spreads as expected, excluding an aberrant spread of injectate into areas not to be included in the block, such as vessels, somatic nerves, and organs.

A fluoroscopy compared with CT is of little or no value in establishing whether the needle has punctured an organ, provides the exact distance point is located anterior to the first vertebra, and the exact spread of the injected solution. A CT guide technique allows accurate placement of the needles and theoretically further reduces the risk of organ injury and is especially preferred when the normal anatomy might be distorted. It is particularly useful when the anterior and transcrural approaches are planned. A better overall resolution is possible.

The most common adverse effects, including local pain reported in 96% of patients, diarrhea in 44%, and hypotension in 38%, are transient. However, the frequency of these effects is difficult to evaluate due to the inconsistency in reporting them in several studies. Paraplegia following an NCPB has been reported, due to vascular ischemia of the spinal cord or an unintentional subarachnoid or epidural.

An NCPB offers other non-analgesic advantages. Depression of the sympathetic tone induces increased bowel motility with decreased constipation and less nausea with increased appetite, mainly secondary to an irritation of the vagus nerve by malignant processes. Increased weight gain has also been reported. This also results from a decrease in opioid dosage due to better pain relief. The decrease in opioid doses or the suspension of opioid therapy make the patient less sedated, more alert and satisfied.

An NCPB is claimed to be an effective treatment for pancreatic cancer pain, but assessment of the course and effectiveness of this block have been questioned by some. Critical analysis revealed major deficiencies in all the reports reviewed. A meta-analysis of the literature has revealed inconsistencies in the nature and completeness of the data reported. In studies reporting a long-term outcome (more than three months) approximately 90% of patients maintained acceptable pain relief. The majority of patients experience relatively pain-free deaths, occurring in most cases within one month after the block. Many patients could be weaned from opioids or, at least, have their dose reduced. The effectiveness and duration of an NCPB has been compared with traditional treatment with analgesics taking into consideration the previous and subsequent consumption of opioids until the patient's death, in a randomized, controlled study. The NCPB made it possible to maintain a reduced opioid consumption and fewer problems ascribed to treatment when compared with the use of analgesics only. It has been reported that the NCBP may prevent a deterioration in the quality of the life by the long-lasting analgesic effect, limitation of side-effects, and the reduction of morphine consumption when compared with treatment with analgesics (9).

The probability of patients remaining completely pain-free diminished with increased survival time. Failure of the block may be attributed to the fact that the tumor has metastatized beyond the nerves that conduct pain via the celiac plexus and the component nerves that from it. This phenomenon occurs generally in the late stage of pancreatic disease, while it may occur earlier with other abdominal malignancies. Abdominal pain is only one component of pancreatic cancer pain and other pain sites cannot be relieved by the NCPB. Concomitant pain of somatic origin, frequently observed in upper gastrointestinal cancer, due to large peritoneal involvement, requires other therapeutic measures, although it is difficult to differentiate between a somatic and a visceral component in such circumstances. Other causes of the failure of an NCPB include technical problems, the presence of a tumor in the area of the celiac plexus preventing the spread of the neurolytic substance, or the presence of metastases. However, it may still decrease pain, analgesic requirements and their side-effects by reducing the visceral component of pain. The NCPB was effective in controlling pancreatic cancer pain in a higher percentage of cases if performed early after the pain onset, when the pain was still only or mainly of a visceral type and responded to antinflammatory drugs (19,20). However, despite the impression that the celiac plexus block is less likely to be successful when the tumor has extended beyond the innervation of the celiac plexus, and more effective when performed earlier, it is not yet possible to correlate outcome with pain characteristics.

Clinical problems concerning neurolytic superior hypogastric block are nearly the same as for celiac plexus block. Both control visceral pain. However, the less favorable results obtained with the hypogastric plexus block may be due to the greater tendency of pelvic tumors to infiltrate somatic structures and nerves compared with pancreatic tumors where the celiac plexus block is usually used. Other than with visceral pain, pelvic cancers are more often associated with myofascial involvement, and as a consequence, with a somatic pain mechanism, although pain seems prevalently caused by pressure on the sciatic nerve. Thus, pelvic cancer pain can arise, among other reasons, from visceral and peritoneal involvement as well as from the involvement of muscles in the peritoneal floor with nerve entrapment and muscle necrosis. Due to the location of the piriformis muscle deep in the pelvic floor, pain may be a complication of a primary tumor or relapse, surgery, or radiotherapy. Buttock or rectal pain with or without posterior thigh pain, aggravated by sitting or activity, may be due to the compression of the piriformis muscle. As a consequence, it may be associated with referred/localized pain of somatic origin. Motor reflexes may lead to muscle spasm and the additional component of somatic pain. The clinical picture is often mixed. In pelvic cancer lumbar pain may also be due to ileopsoas muscle involvement. Nerve trunk pain, often radiating to the lower limbs, may be observed due to the involvement of lumbosacral plexus in the presacral area, or radiculopathy related to retroperitoneal spread. As a consequence, patients who might be candidates for hypogastric plexus block, a sympathetic block performed for visceral pelvic pain, have to be strictly selected. On the other hand, retroperitoneal invasion may result in a limited spread of neurolytic solution and may be another reason for a lack of success (11).

The choice of performing such blocks should be on the preference of patients after being given a full explanation of the possible advantages and complications. These blocks should be considered as an adjuvant treatment and not as a last resort, when the advantages of the block seem to be minimal.

References

1. **Mercadante S.** Prevalence, causes, and mechanisms of pain in home-care patients with advanced cancer. *Pain Clinic* 1994;7:131–136
2. **Cervero F; Laird JMA.** Visceral pain. *Lancet* 1999;353:2145–8.
3. **Willis WD; AI Chaer ED; Quast MJ; Westlund KN.** A visceral pain pathway in the dorsal column of the spinal cord. *Proceedings of the National Academy of Sciences of the United States of America* 1999;96:7675–9.
4. **Ness TJ; Gebhart GF.** Colorectal distension as a noxious visceral stimulus: physiologic and pharmacologic characterization of pseudoaffective reflexes in the rat. *Brain Research.* 1988;450:153–69.
5. **Holzer-Petsche U; Brodacz B.** Traction on the mesentery as a model of visceral nociception. *Pain* 1999;80:319–28.
6. **Ness TJ; Gebhart GF.** Visceral pain: a review of experimental studies. *Pain* 1990;41:167–234.
7. **Cervero F.** Visceral pain: mechanisms and update. In Max M., ed. *Pain* 1999—*An Update Review.* Seattle: IASP Press, 1999: pp. 39–46.
8. **Payne R; Gonzales G.** Pathophysiology of pain in cancer and other terminal diseases. In: Doyle D; Hanks GW; MacDonald N., editors. *Oxford Textbook of Palliative Medicine.* Oxford: Oxford Medical Publications Oxford University Press, 1993: pp. 140–8.
9. **Mercadante S.** Celiac plexus block: a reapprisal. *Regional Anesthesia and Pain Medicine* 1998;23:37–48.
10. **Caraceni A; Portenoy RK.** Pain management in patients with pancreatic carcinoma. *Cancer* 1996;78:639–53.
11. **Mercadante S.** Celiac plexus block versus analgesics in pancreatic cancer pain. *Pain.* 1993;52:187–92.
12. **Orlandini G.** Selection of patients undergoing neurolytic superior hypogastric plexus block. *Pain* 1994;56:121.
13. Hanks GW and the Expert Working Group of the Research Network of the European Association for Palliative Care (EAPC). Morphine and alternative opioids in cancer pain: the EAPC recommendations. *British Journal of Cancer* 2001;84:587–93.
14. **Mercadante S.** Alternative to oral morphine in cancer pain. *Oncology* 1999;13:215–25.
15. **Mercadante S.** Problems of long-term spinal opioid treatment in advanced cancer patients. *Pain* 1999;79:1–13.
16. **Mercadante S; Casuccio A; Agnello A; Pumo S; Kargar J; Garofalo S.** Analgesic effects of nonsteroidal anti-inflammatory drugs in cancer pain due to somatic or visceral mechanisms. *Journal of Pain and Symptom Management* 1999;17:351–6.
17. **Colburn RW; Coombs DW; Degnen CC; Rogers LL.** Mechanical visceral pain model: chronic intermittent intestinal distension in the rat. *Physiological Behavior.* 1989;45:191–7.
18. **Kawamata M; Ishitani K; Ishikawa K; Sasaki H; Ota K; Omote K; Namiki A.** Comparison between celiac plexus block and morphine treatment on quality of life in patients with pancreatic cancer pain. *Pain* 1996;64:597–602.
19. **Lillemoe KD; Cameron JL; Kaufman HS; Yeo CJ; Pitt HA; Sauter PK.** Chemical splanchnicectomy in patients with unreasonable pancreatic cancer. A prospective randomized trial. *Annals of Surgery* 1993;217:447–57.
20. **Polati E; Finco G; Gottin L; Bassi C; Pederzoli P; Ischia S.** Prospective randomized double blind trial of neurolytic coeliac plexus block in patients with pancreatic cancer. *British Journal of Surgery* 1998;85:199–201.

Chapter 12

Malignant bowel obstruction

Carla Ripamonti

Introduction

Malignant bowel obstruction (MBO) is a distressing outcome in patients with abdominal and pelvic primary and/or metastatic cancer. MBO may be the first manifestation of the abdominal disease or the consequence of advanced disease due to the failure of anticancer treatments. The exact frequency of MBO in cancer patients is not known. In highly selected groups of patients, retrospective and autoptic studies have estimated that MBO occurs in 4%–28.4% of patients with gastrointestinal cancer and in 5%–51% of patients with gynecological disease, in particular with ovarian cancer, where it is a major cause of death (1,2).

The obstruction may be partial or complete and reduces or blocks the movement of bowel contents through the intestinal passage. Bowel obstruction can be single or multiple, due to benign or malignant causes. The frequency of benign causes (e.g. adhesions, post-irradiation bowel damage, inflammatory bowel disease, hernia) ranges from 6.1% in ovarian and other gynecological cancers to 48% in colorectal cancer. The small bowel is more commonly involved than the large bowel (61% versus 33%) and both are involved in over 20% of patients (2–7).

Pathophysiology, signs, and symptoms

Several mechanisms may be involved in the onset of bowel obstruction (Table 12.1) (2) and there is variability in both presentation and etiology. As a consequence of the partial or complete occlusion of the lumen, there is an accumulation of unabsorbed secretions causing the sequence of distension–secretion–motor activity. The gastrointestinal (GI) symptoms caused by this sequence in the obstructed bowel are nausea, vomiting, pain, and colicky activity (not present in functional obstruction) to surmount the obstacle that causes intermittent colicky pain (Figure 12.1). Those symptoms occur in different combinations and intensity depending on the site of the obstruction and tend to worsen (Table 12.2).

Abdominal distension may be absent in high obstruction, i.e. of the duodenum or proximal jejunum, and when the bowel is 'plastered' down by extensive mesenteric spread. The symptoms noted by the patient should be monitored daily. Vomiting can be evaluated in terms of quantity, quality, and number of daily episodes. Others symptoms, such as nausea, pain, dry mouth, drowsiness, dyspnea, hunger, and thirst, can be assessed by numerical or verbal scales.

Table 12.1 Pathophysiological mechanisms of MBO

Mechanical obstruction is caused by:

1 extrinsic occlusion of the lumen due to an enlargement of the primary tumor or recurrence, mesenteric and omental masses, abdominal or pelvic adhesions (caused either by the tumor or secondary to surgery), post-irradiation fibrosis

2 intraluminal occlusion of the lumen due to neoplastic mass or annular tumoral dissemination

3 intramural occlusion of the lumen due to intestinal linitis plastica

Functional obstruction (or adynamic ileus) is caused by intestinal motility disorders as a result of:

1 tumor infiltration of the mesentery or bowel muscle and nerves (carcinomatosis), malignant involvement of the coeliac plexus

2 paraneoplastic neuropathy in patients with lung cancer

3 chronic intestinal pseudo-obstruction (CIP) mainly due to diabetes mellitus, previous gastric surgery, and other neurological disorders

4 paraneoplastic pseudo-obstruction

Other causes such as inflammatory edema, fecal impaction, constipating drugs (such as opioids, anticholinergics, etc.), and dehydration, are likely to contribute to the development of bowel obstruction or to worsen the clinical picture

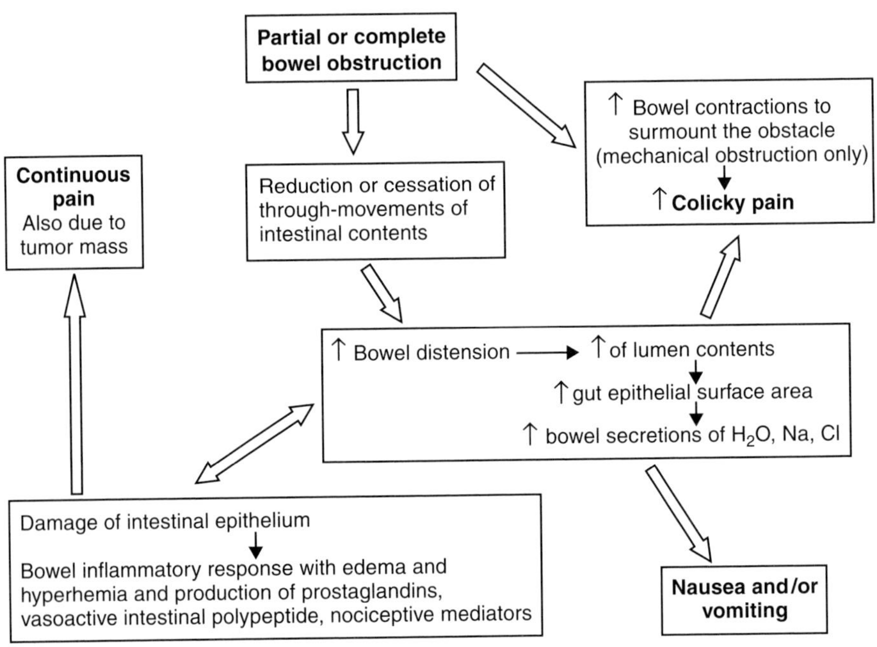

Figure 12.1

Table 12.2 Common symptoms in cancer patients with MBO

Vomiting	Intermittent or continuous	It develops early and in great amounts in gastric, duodenum and small bowel obstruction and develops later in large bowel obstruction	Biliary vomiting is almost odorless and indicates an obstruction in the upper part of the abdomen. The presence of bad smelling and fecaloid vomiting can be the first sign of a ileal or colic obstruction
Nausea	Intermittent or continuous		
Colicky pain	Variable intensity and localization due to distension proximal to the obstruction; secondary to gas and fluid accumulation most of which are produced by the gut	If it is intense, periumbelical and occurring at brief intervals, may be an indication of an obstruction at the jejunum–ileal level. In large bowel obstruction the pain is less intense, deeper, occurring at longer intervals and spreads toward the colon wall	An overall acute pain that begins intensely and becomes stronger, or a pain that is specifically localized, may be a symptom of a perforation or an ileal or colic strangulation. A pain that increases with palpation may be due to peritoneal irritation or the beginning of a perforation
Continuous pain	Variable intensity and localization	It is due to abdominal distension, tumor mass and/or hepatomegaly	
Dry mouth		It is due to severe dehydration, metabolic alterations, but above all to the use of drugs with anticholinergic properties and poor mouth care	
Constipation	Intermittent or complete	In the case of complete obstruction there is no evacuation of feces and no flatus	In the case of partial obstruction the symptom is intermittent
Overflow diarrhea		It is the result of bacterial liquefaction of fecal material	

Differential diagnosis

When a cancer patient presents suspected bowel obstruction, all the possible causes of constipation (see Chapter 9 by Mancini and Bruera) nausea and vomiting (8,9; see also Chapter 8 by Ripamonti and Bruera) and abdominal pain (see Chapter 11 by Mercadante) have to be ruled out. Possible metabolic alterations, the type and dosages of drugs taken as well as the state of hydration and nutrition must be assessed. The patient must be investigated regarding a relapse or a disease progression, bowel movements, and the presence of overflow diarrhea which could lead to underestimating the problem.

The type, frequency as well as the amount of vomiting have to be monitored because these indicate the presence and the level of the gastrointestinal occlusion.

Abdominal examination can show the presence of abdominal cancer or fecal masses, distension to all the abdomen or above the obstacle, the eventual presence of ascite as well as painful sites. Rectal exploration can show the absence or presence of feces in the rectal ampulla.

An abdominal X-ray taken in a supine or a standing position is the first investigation in patients with suspected small bowel obstruction to document the dilated loops of the bowel, air–fluid interfaces, or both. Contrast radiography helps to evaluate dysmotility, partial obstruction, and to define the site and extent of the obstruction. Retrograde transrectal radiographic contrast studies should be used to rule out or to diagnose isolated or concomitant obstruction of the large bowel.

An abdominal CT is useful for evaluating the global extent of disease, to perform staging, and to assist in the choice of surgical, endoscopic, or simple pharmacological palliative intervention for the management of the obstruction.

Management

The management of patients with MBO is one of the greatest challenges for physicians who care for cancer patients. A number of treatment options are available for the management of cancer patients who develop bowel obstruction. However, a number of questions arise when the obstruction occurs in advanced and terminal cancer patients:

- Is the patient fit for surgery?
- Is there a place for stenting?
- Is it necessary to use a venting nasogastric tube in inoperable patients?
- Which drugs are indicated for symptom control, what is the proper route of their administration, and what drugs can be administered in association?
- When should a venting gastrostomy be considered?
- What is the role of total parenteral nutrition (TPN) and parenteral hydration (PH)?

A multidisciplinary working group was established by the European Association for Palliative Care with the aim to review issues relating to bowel obstruction in end-stage cancer and to produce clinical-practice recommendations for management (2).

The first recommendation is the need for a collaborative approach by surgeons and physicians of other specialities in the care of each patient with end-stage cancer and MBO. The second one is the need to implement an individualized symptom management plan with the goals of therapy agreed upon by all concerned: doctors, nurses, patient and family.

Moreover, because the obstruction of the lumen develops slowly and often remains partial, MBO in advanced cancer patients is rarely an emergency event and intestinal strangulation is uncommon. Thus there is time to evaluate the most suitable therapeutic intervention for each patient. The following clinical-practice recommendations have been developed and published (2).

Palliative surgical intervention

This should be considered but not routinely undertaken in all patients with bowel obstruction. However, it is important to consider whether palliative surgery is technically feasible and whether the patient is likely to benefit from surgery (2,10).

Published data show that in advanced cancer, the operative mortality (defined as death from any cause within 30 days of the operation) is 30%–40% and complication rates vary from 27% to 90% (2). Since these recently published results are no better than those published in the past, improvements in surgical techniques and perioperative care appear not to influence the outcome.

Surgical palliation in advanced cancer patients is a complex issue, and the decision to proceed with surgery must be evaluated carefully for each individual patient. Surgery must be justified on the basis of more benefit than burden to the patient. Consent for surgery should include discussion of the surgical risks, possible complications, and symptomatic therapeutic strategies.

Based on retrospective data, several authors have derived clinical parameters that indicate low likelihood of clinical benefit from the surgical management of bowel obstruction:

1. obstruction secondary to cancer (11),
2. intestinal motility problems due to diffuse intraperitoneal carcinomatosis (12–16),
3. widespread tumor (17),
4. patients over 65 (17) in association with cachexia (12,18),
5. ascites requiring frequent paracentesis (14–20),
6. low serum albumin level (18) and low serum pre-albumin level (21),
7. previous radiotherapy of the abdomen or pelvis (17,22),
8. patients with nutritional deficits (23),
9. palpable intra-abdominal masses (14,18) and liver involvement,
10. distant metastases, pleural effusion, or pulmonary metastases (17,19,24),
11. multiple partial bowel obstruction with prolonged passage time on radiograph examination (18,19),
12. elevated blood urea nitrogen levels, elevated alkaline phosphatase levels, advanced tumor stage, and short diagnosis to obstruction interval (18,19),
13. poor performance status (25).

According to Krebs and Gloperud (17), the operative mortality was 44% in the group of patients with ovarian carcinoma and two or more of factors 3, 4, 5, and 7; and it was significantly higher than the 13% operative mortality among 32 patients who had no more than one risk factor. In the study of Jong *et al.* (26) successful palliation (defined as patient survival >60 days after surgery, the ability to return home, and relief of obstruction postoperatively >60 days) was significantly associated with four prognostic factors: absence of palpable abdominal or pelvic masses, volume of ascites less than 3 l, unifocal obstruction, and pre-operative weight loss less than 9 kg.

According to the multidisciplinary working group the absolute contraindication factors to surgery include:

1 a previous laparotomy/surgery that showed diffuse metastatic cancer making the patient unfit for surgery,
2 multiple partial bowel obstructions,
3 severe motility problems due to intraperitoneal carcinomatosis,
4 massive ascites which rapidly recur after drainage,
5 extra-abdominal metastases producing symptoms difficult to control, such as severe dyspnea.

Each of these is considered as a 'stand-alone' contraindication (2).

Realizing that not all advanced cancer patients are suitable for surgery, the physician has to deal with patients suffering from nausea, vomiting, and pain, with a short life-expectancy, who can only be treated with self-expanding metallic stents or with venting procedures and/or pharmacological palliative therapies.

Self-expanding metallic stents

Stents are an option in malignant obstruction of the gastric outlet, proximal small bowel, and colon. The stents may be useful in the management of patients who are at surgical risk or in those presenting large bowel obstruction in which decompression by a stent allows treatment of coexisting medical complications to enable surgery to be carried out at a later date, after staging of the disease and an optimal colonic preparation (27). Flexible, self-expanding metallic stents may be inserted using radiological or endoscopic techniques. The major limiting factor in the use of the endoscopic technique is the inability to pass the endoscope through the stricture.

Several authors report relief from malignant gastric and/or duodenal obstruction in the majority of patients treated by peroral (28–30) or percutaneous insertion of a metal stent (31–35). Most of patients had an immediate benefit and were able to eat small amounts of food without vomiting. No recurrence of gastric outlet obstruction was noted in the follow-up period of 1–5 months (30,32,33).

As with any procedure, complications are possible. The major complications reported were gastric ulceration, bowel perforation after balloon dilatation of the stent, and stent migration. According to some less recent reports, however, complications such as chest pain, blockage, gastroesophageal reflux, migration, perforation, and delayed massive bleeding occur in about 40%–53% of patients (36–38).

Seventy per cent of colon and rectal cancers are left-sided and are considered accessible to stent placement (39). Positive results have been reported by various authors after the insertion of colonic stents in colorectal obstruction (27,39–46).

Complications, which potentially include perforation, bleeding, and stent migration, have been reported in fewer than 3% of cases (39–42) and only in a few patients treated with self-expanding mesh stents was there a recurrent obstruction due to tumor ingrowth (46). Temporary incontinence may be observed (46). Canon *et al.* (47) report that stent placement was successful in 2 out of 4 patients who needed standard bowel cleansing before surgical resection with primary anastomosis, and in 5 out of 9 patients who had a stent as palliation of non-resectable tumors. Although colonic obstruction was relieved in 12 of 13 patients, 7 (54%) had some type of complication.

Mainar *et al.* (39) recommend self-expandable stents instead of balloon-expandable stents due to the risk of bowel perforation secondary to the excessive manipulation of balloon dilation on the friable tumoral areas. According to Feretis *et al.* (43) one of the possible disadvantages of the method may be the difficulty of treating tumor bleeding, since laser and thermal methods of hemostasis cannot be safely applied to a tumor that is covered by an endoprosthesis.

Normal bowel contractions could cause stent migration, especially if the stent diameter is too small, if the stent length is too short, or if the stent is placed too distal in the lesion. Migration into the rectal ampulla can result in obstruction and in painful spasm. According to Wholey *et al.* (48) it is possible to retrieve stents from the rectum using fluoroscopic guidance.

According to Canon *et al.* (47), before a patient is selected as a candidate for having an expandable metal stent placed in the colon, three factors should be determined: the location of the lesion within the colon; the length of the tumor; and the presence or absence of a synchronous carcinoma. Thus, meticulous evaluation of the digestive tract downstream is mandatory to avoid pointless stent placement.

Contraindications for the position of self-expanding stent are the presence of multiple stenoses, peritoneal carcinomatosis located distally in the small bowel that may be undiagnosed at the preprocedural opacification because of the severity of the duodenal stenosis. Failure to relieve the obstruction may be secondary to an inability to cross the stricture, incomplete opening of the stent, or stent malposition that fails to traverse the entire stricture. In this case it is necessary to apply additional stents across the remaining obstruction.

The usefulness of stents in patients with end-stage cancer has not yet been formally evaluated. Further studies are necessary to identify those patients with advanced and terminal cancer and MBO who may benefit in terms of symptom control and quality of life after these procedures.

Venting procedures

Nasogastric suction is the usual hospital treatment to reduce secretions, vomiting, pain, and abdominal distension. However, long-term use of nasogastric tube (NGT) is very uncomfortable, often creates complications and thus it should only be considered to reduce large amount of secretions before starting pharmacological treatment, or when drugs for symptom control are ineffective, or when a venting gastrostomy cannot be performed.

Gastrostomy is a much more acceptable and well-tolerated method for the middling to long-term decompression of the obstructed GI tract (49). Operative or percutaneous endoscopic gastrostomy (PEG) are much more acceptable methods for longer term decompression of an obstructed GI tract rather than a NGT (2,50).

Percutaneous gastrostomy (PG) is the insertion of a tube into the stomach through the abdominal wall under fluoroscopic, ultrasound, or endoscopic guidance (51,52). The addition of transcutaneous ultrasonography at the time of endoscopy permits accurate localization of the optimal site for PEG placement in patients with diffuse intra-abdominal disease and multiple prior surgeries (53,54). The procedure may be performed under intravenous sedation and local anesthesia (55). Overall, this approach has been reported to control nausea and vomiting due to bowel obstruction in 83%–93% of cases (56–58). Intermittent venting of the gastrostomy allows the patient to continue oral intake and maintain an active lifestyle without the inconvenience of a nasal tube, thus giving significant psychological benefit. PG should be avoided in patients with portal hypertension, large volume ascites, in those predisposed to bleed or those taking anticoagulants, and those with active gastric ulceration (49). Other relative contraindications are multiple previous abdominal surgeries, carcinomatosis, a colostomy, or open/infected abdominal wounds.

In some patients with gastric outlet or proximal small bowel obstruction, some authors have described experience with the insertion of a draining gastrostomy with a concurrent feeding jejunostomy (59).

Pharmacological palliative treatment

The pharmacological management of bowel obstruction due to advanced cancer focuses on the treatment of nausea, vomiting, pain, and other symptoms without the use of a NGT. Drug therapy comprising analgesics, antisecretory drugs, and antiemetics was first described by Baines *et al.* (60). Several authors have confirmed the efficacy of this approach (2). Medications should be tailored to each patient regarding both the drugs to be administered, the dosages, the drug associations and the route of their administration (Figure 12.2) (2). In most bowel-obstructed patients, oral administration is not suitable and alternative routes have to be considered. If a central venous catheter has been previously inserted, this can be used to administer drugs for symptom control. Continuous subcutaneous infusion of drugs using a portable syringe driver allows the parenteral administration of different drug combinations, produces minimal discomfort for the patient, and is easy to use in a home setting. Most of the recommended drugs can be administered in association via parenteral continuous infusion (2). Rectal, sublingual, and transdermal medications are useful alternatives to intravenous and subcutaneous ones.

Pain

To relieve continuous abdominal pain, opioid analgesics via continuous parenteral infusion are necessary in most patients. The dosage has to be titrated for each patient until pain relief is achieved. Anticholinergics such as scopolamine, scopolamine butylbromide, scopolamine hydrobromide, glycopyrrolate, and loperamide hydrochloride may be administered in association with opioids to control colicky pain (see Chapter 11 by Mercadante) if opioids alone fail.

Nausea and vomiting

Vomiting should be reduced to an acceptable level for the patient (e.g. once or twice a day). It can be managed using two different pharmacological approaches:

- drugs such as anticholinergics or/and octreotide that reduce GI secretions;
- antiemetics acting on the central nervous system, alone or in association with drugs to reduce GI secretions.

Drugs used to reduce GI secretions Among the anticolinergics, scopolamine butylbromide (SB) is frequently used by some palliative care centers to relieve both vomiting and colicky pain (2,61). This drug differs from both atropine and scopolamine hydrobromide in having a low lipid solubility. It does not penetrate the blood–brain barrier as well as these

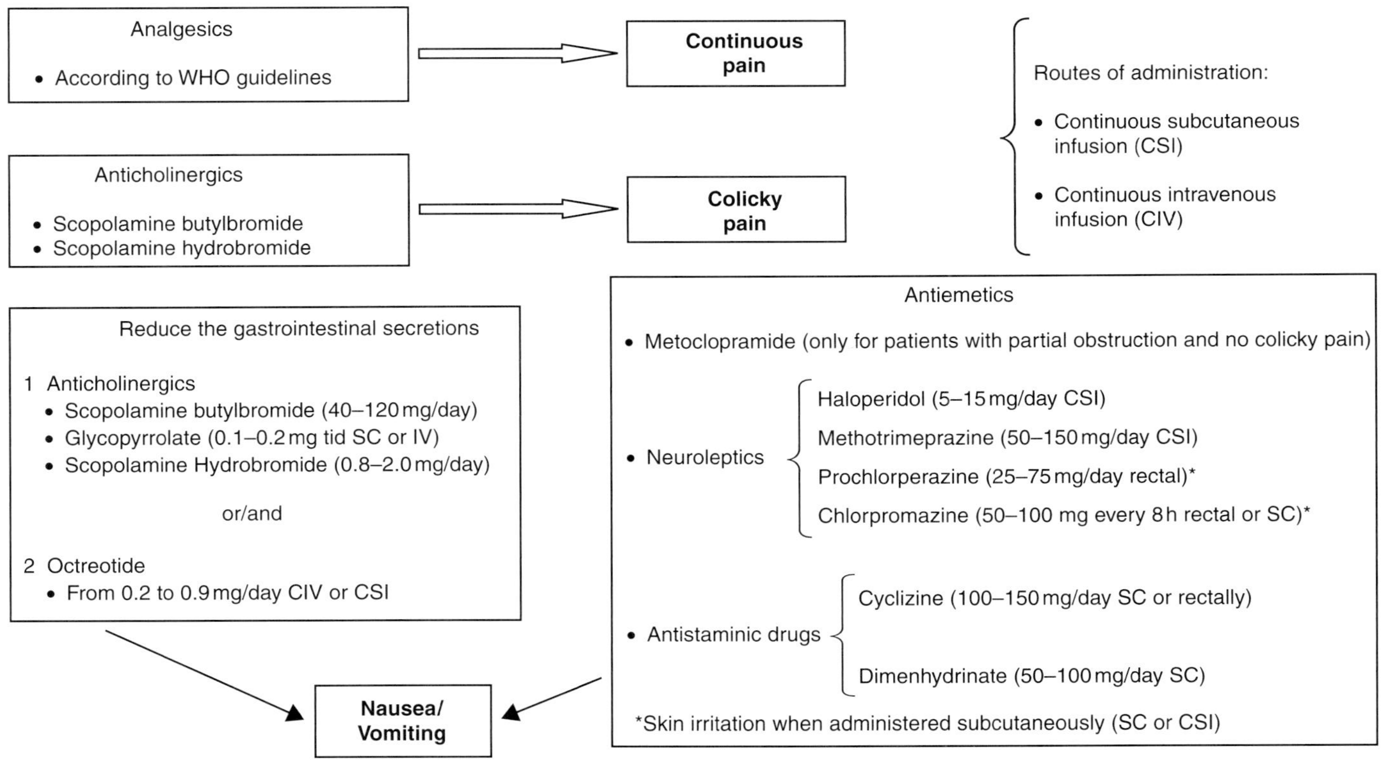

CSI: continuous subcutaneous infusion; CIV: continuous intravenous infusion; SC: subcute; IV: intravenous.

Figure 12.2 Symptomatic pharmacological approach. Reference (2).

other drugs and, consequently, may produce fewer side-effects, such as somnolence and hallucinations, when administered in combination with opioids. The anticholinergic activity of SB decreases the tonus and peristalsis in smooth muscle both by competitive inhibition of muscarinic receptors at the smooth muscle level and by impairment of ganglionic neural transmission in the bowel wall. Muscarinic cholinergic receptors have also been observed on mucosal cells of the intestinal lumen and in human salivary glands, which explains its analgesic effect on the colicky pain while reducing intestinal secretions. The antiemetic, antisecretory as well the analgesic role of SB administered subcutaneously by a syringe driver has been well documented by different authors (2). A dry mouth is reported to be the most significant side-effect, but patients tolerated it by sucking ice cubes and drinking small sips of water. In some countries where SB is not available, glycopyrrolate can be used instead (62). It is a quaternary ammonium anticholinergic with a limited lipid solubility that reduces both central nervous system and ocular effects. The onset of its action when given subcutaneously is 35–45 minutes and 1 minute via intravenous route. Glycopyrrolate is not compatible with diazepam, methylprednisolone, dexamethasone, dimenhydrinate, and phenobarbital (63).

Among the somatostatine analogues; octreotide, a synthetic analogue that has a more potent biological activity and a longer half-life, has also been used to manage the symptoms of bowel obstruction. Somatostatin and its analogues have been shown to inhibit the release and activity of GI hormones, modulate GI function by reducing gastric acid secretion, slow intestinal motility, decrease bile flow, increase mucous production, and reduce splanchnic blood flow. It reduces GI secretions and increases the absorption of water and electrolytes at the intracellular level, via cAMP and calcium regulation (64).

Submucosal somatostatin-containing neurons, activated by octreotide, inhibit excitatory nerves, mainly by inhibiting acetylcholine output. As a result, muscle relaxation can occurs, ameliorating the spastic activity responsible for colicky pain. The inhibitory effect of octreotide on both peristalsis and GI secretions reduces bowel distension and the secretion of water and sodium by the intestinal epithelium, thereby reducing vomiting and pain. The drug may therefore break the vicious circle represented by secretion, distension, and contractile hyperactivity.

Pre-clinical studies show that the pro-absorptive effects of somatostatin and octreotide reduce intestinal distension, electrolyte losses, and ischemia in animal models of bowel obstruction (65). Octreotide may be administered by subcutaneous bolus or continuous subcutaneous infusion. Its half-life is about 1.5 hours after intravenous or subcutaneous administration, and its kinetics are linear. The recommended starting dose is 0.3 mg/day subcutaneously. The dose can be titrated upward until symptom control is achieved, generally at 0.6–0.9 mg/day.

In retrospective studies and in case reports octreotide was shown to be effective where other drugs failed (Tables 12.3 and 12.4) (66–71).

Two randomized controlled studies have been carried out comparing the antisecretory effects of octreotide and SB in patients with inoperable MBO (72,73). Octreotide was significantly more effective and faster than SB in reducing the amount of GI secretions, the intensity of nausea, and the number of vomiting episodes. Octreotide was also effective in patients with upper abdominal obstruction where SB had failed. Moreover, octreotide may prevent the development of irreversible bowel obstruction in patients with recurrent episodes of obstruction (74).

Table 12.3 Role of octreotide in malignant bowel obstruction: prospective studies

Author(s)	Number of patients	Site of cancer(s) Site of obstruction	Symptom(s)	OCT dose/route ± other drugs	Results
Mercadante *et al.* (66)	14	Various intra-abdominal Small and/or large bowel	Nausea, vomiting unresponsive to haloperidol or chlorpromazine	0.3–0.6 mg/day SCB or CSI +haloperidol +analgesics	Vomiting was controlled in 12 patients and reduced in 2 In 2 out of 3 patients NGT was removed and the symptoms controlled No important toxicity was reported
Riley *et al.* (67)	24	Various intra-abdominal Small and/or large bowel	Intractable vomiting not responsive to a combination of antiemetics, steroids and/or NGT drainage for 24 h	0.1–1.2 mg/day SCB or CSI	14 patients had no further vomiting and 4 patients showed some improvements with a dose from 0.1–0.6 mg/day There was a reduction of aspirate in all 5 patients with NGT 6 patients did not respond despite dosages of 0.6–1.2 mg/day No adverse effects were reported also at higher dosages
Mangili *et al.* (68)	13	Ovary Small and/or large bowel	Vomiting not responsive to metoclopramide and haloperidol	0.3–0.6 mg/day SCB or CSI ± analgesics	Vomiting was controlled in all cases within 3 days (range 1–6) In 8 patients with a NGT there was a significant reduction of secretions and NGT was removed No adverse effects were reported

OCT: octreotide; SCB: subcutaneous bolus; CSI: continuous subcutaneous infusion; IV: intravenous; NGT: Nasogastric tube

Table 12.4 Role of octreotide in malignant bowel obstruction: case reports

Author(s)	Number of patients	Site of cancer(s) Site of obstruction	Symptom(s)	OCT dose/route ± other drugs	Results
Khoo *et al.* (69)	5	Various intra-abdominal Small bowel	Intractable vomiting unresponsive to conventional therapy	0.1–0.5 mg/day SCB at start then CSI	Vomiting stopped within 1 h of start of treatment The only patient with a NGT presented a reduction in aspirate from 2000 ml/day to under 300 ml/day No important toxicity was reported
Mercadante *et al.* (70)	1	Intra-abdominal Small and/or large bowel ±Carcinomatosis	Abdominal pain and vomiting	0.3–0.2 mg/day + 0.9 mg buprenorphine CSI	Pain and vomiting disappeared within 24 h after NGT was removed No adverse effects were reported
	1		Colic pain and vomiting despite the use of NGT and Haloperidol	0.9 mg/day + 3 mg haloperidol	Within 24 h NGT secretions decreased from 2600 to 350 ml/day and vomiting disappeared. NGT was removed. No adverse effects were reported No further need for analgesics or IV
Steadman *et al.* (71)	1	Pancreas Small bowel	Vomiting and drowsiness with Diamorphine, cyclizine, hyoscine	0.2 mg/day + diamorphine	Switching to octreotide produced good symptom relief without causing unwanted uncomfortable drowsiness NGT was removed

OCT: octreotide; SCB: subcutaneous bolus; CSI: continuous subcutaneous infusion; IV: intravenous; NGT: Nasogastric tube

In a randomized, double-blind clinical trial carried out on 54 consecutive patients with mechanical bowel obstruction, 27 patients received somatostatin pre-operatively and 27 did not (75). In the latter group 44% of patients were operated on, while only 22% of those who received somatostatin required surgery. Moreover, 16% of patients treated with somatostatin presented severe dilatation and necrosis of the bowel proximal to the area of obstruction as compared with 83% of those patients who did not receive somatostatin pre-operatively.

Mercadante *et al.* (76) studied the effect of octreotide administered at the dose of 0.3 mg/day for 2–5 days pre-operatively in three cancer patients undergoing surgery for bowel obstruction caused by extrinsic occlusion of the lumen. During surgery, the diameter of the bowel above the obstruction was observed to be normal, and there was no local significant pathological findings such as edema, vessel congestion, or necrosis of the bowel above the obstruction due to the accumulation of fluids in the lumen. The study of some samples of the intestine above and below the obstruction showed a normal anatomical and biochemical pattern.

The association of octreotide and scopolamine butylbromide may reduce GI secretions and vomiting whenever one drug alone is ineffective (72,77).

Octreotide is an expensive drug and its cost–benefit ratio should be carefully considered, especially for prolonged treatment. However, the cost of the drug should be interpreted in the widest possible sense; that is, whether the use of the drug results in a more rapid improvement of GI symptoms which potentially limits the bed stay or the admission to an in-patient unit in addition to a better quality of life of the patient.

Vapreotide is a long-acting preparation of somatostatin analogue with similar clinical properties to somatostatin but a longer duration of action. In a patient with MBO due to pancreatic cancer, Stiefel and Morant (78) injected 4 mg of vapreotide 5 times at weekly interval. The patient vomited only 6 times in 29 days and reported good symptom control until death. The drug is not available in most countries.

Antiemetics Among the antiemetics, parenteral metoclopramide is the drug of choice in patients with functional bowel obstruction and no colic. It is not indicated in patients with complete bowel obstruction due to its prokinetic activity, tending to increase nausea, vomiting, and colicky pain (2).

Other antiemetics are the butyrophenones, antihistaminic–antiemetics, and phenothiazines. There are no studies comparing the different antiemetics in patients with inoperable bowel obstruction. Haloperidol is considered the antiemetic of first choice and can be combined with SB and opioid analgesic in the same syringe. It causes less sedation and fewer anticholinergic effects compared with phenothiazines.

In some countries, antihistaminic–antiemetics (e.g. cyclizine, dimenhydrinate, diphenhydramine, meclozine) are used as the first-line drug. Cyclizine can be added to prochlorperazine suppositories and to haloperidol subcutaneously. Crystallization may occur at higher doses or in association with other drugs (2,3).

Among the phenothiazines, methotrimeprazine, chlorpromazine, and prochlorperazine are all used and have been found to be effective. Chlorpromazine and prochlorperazine are not recommended for continuous subcutaneous infusions because they cause skin irritation (60,79). A combination of antiemetics with different sites of action may be more effective than a single agent (7).

The role of corticosteroids in treating bowel obstruction is still controversial (1). Several authors recommend the use of corticosteroids for symptoms due to bowel obstruction because it can reduce peritumoral inflammatory edema, thus improving intestinal motility. No controlled clinical trials have been carried out and administration routes and dosing of these drugs have not been standardized as yet. According to Fainsinger *et al.* (80), dexamethasone (from 8 mg to 60 mg/day) is a very useful agent in managing nausea and vomiting; however, its role in preventing progression to complete bowel obstruction was impossible to determine in their study.

Parenteral nutrition and hydration

The role of total parenteral nutrition (TPN) in patients with MBO should not be considered a routine part of a terminal care regimen but should be used in selected patients who may die of starvation rather than from tumor spread (81,82). A favorable criteria for selecting these patients is a Karnofsky Performance Status > 50 (81).

The need to treat dehydration in terminally ill patients remains a controversial issue (see Chapter 23 by MacDonald and Chapter 22 by Fainsinger). The intensity of dry mouth and thirst are independent of the quantity of parenteral hydration, whereas the intensity of nausea and drowsiness is significantly lower in inoperable obstructed patients treated with more than 1 litre per day of parenteral fluids (72,73). Because a high level of hydration may increase GI secretions, it is necessary to keep a balance between the efficacy of the treatment and the adverse effects.

Intravenous (IV) hydration can be difficult and uncomfortable for terminal cancer patients who do not have a central venous catheter previously inserted. Hypodermoclysis (83) is a valid alternative with few problems and several potential advantages over the IV route: it is a simple and inexpensive way of managing patients both at hospital and at home and can be started by any staff member able to give a subcutaneous injection.

Conclusion

The optimal treatment of bowel obstruction in patients with advanced cancer is still an open and widely debated issue. Patients are usually considered suitable candidates for surgery when survival is expected be more than two months. Studies of prognostic indicators of survival in advanced cancer patients are necessary to assist doctors in making appropriate therapeutic decisions, together with the patient and family members. Medical treatment by the continuous subcutaneous or intravenous administration of opioids, anticholinergic drugs, octreotide, and antiemetic drugs can be an effective approach for controlling pain, nausea, and vomiting in most patients with inoperable GI obstruction. Nasogastric suction or percutaneous gastrostomy may be considered for patients with refractory symptoms and/or upper bowel obstruction who do not respond satisfactorily to pharmacological measures alone. The efforts of the doctor/nurse team must be aimed at both symptom control and other aspects of the patient's suffering, including psychological distress and spiritual concerns.

References

1. **Feuer DJ; Broadley KE.** With members of the Systematic Review Steering Committee. Systematic review and meta-analysis of corticosteroids for the resolution of malignant bowel obstruction in advanced gynaecological and gastrointestinal cancers. *Annals of Oncology* 1999;10:1035–41.

2. **Ripamonti C; Twycross R; Baines M., *et al.*** Clinical-practice recommendations for the management of bowel obstruction in patients with end-stage cancer. Working Group of the European Association for Palliative Care. *Supportive Care in Cancer* 2001;9:223–33.
3. **Baines M.** The pathophysiology and management of malignant intestinal obstruction. In: Doyle D; Hanks GWC; MacDonald N., editors. *The Oxford Text Book of Palliative Medicine.* 2nd edn. Oxford: Oxford Medical Publications, Oxford University Press, 1998: pp. 526–34.
4. **Ripamonti C.** Management of bowel obstruction in advanced cancer. *Current Opinion in Oncology* 1994;6:351–7.
5. **Ripamonti C.** Bowel obstruction. In: Berger A; Portenoy RK; Weissman DE., editors. *Principles and Practice of Supportive Oncology.* Philadelphia: Lippincott-Raven, 1998; 14: pp. 207–16.
6. **Krebs HB; Goplerud DR.** Mechanical intestinal obstruction in patients with gynecologic disease: A review of 368 patients. *American Journal of Obstetrics and Gynecology* 1987;157:577–83.
7. **Twycross RG; Lack SA.** Gastrointestinal obstruction. In: Twycross RG; Lack SA., editors. *Symptom Control in Advanced Cancer: Alimentary Symptoms.* London: Pitman, 1986; 11: p. 239.
8. **Pisters KMS; Kris MG.** Treatment-related nausea and vomiting. In: Berger A., *et al.*, editors. *Principles and Practice of Supportive Oncology.* Philadelphia: Lippincott-Raven, 1998; 11: pp. 165–77.
9. **Twycross R; Back I., *et al.*** Nausea and vomiting in advanced cancer. *European Journal of Palliative* Care 1998;5(2):39–45.
10. **Feuer DJ; Broadley KE; Shepherd JH; Barton DPJ.** Systematic review of surgery in malignant bowel obstruction in advanced gynecological and gastrointestinal cancer. *Gynecologic Oncology* 1999;75:313–22.
11. **Buther JA; Cameron BL; Morrow M; Kahng K; Tom J.** Small bowel obstruction in patients with a prior history of cancer. *American Journal of Surgery* 1991;162:624–8.
12. **Aabo K; Pedersen H; Bach F., *et al.*** Surgical management of intestinal obstruction in the late course of malignant disease. *Acta Chirurgica Scandinavica* 1984;150:173–6.
13. **Turnbull ADM; Guerra J; Starners HF.** Results of surgery for obstructing carcinomatosis of gastrointestinal, pancreatic, or biliary origin. Journal of Clinical Oncology 1989;7:381–6.
14. **van Oojen B; van der Burg MEL; Planting AST., *et al.*** Surgical treatment or gastric drainage only for intestinal obstruction in patients with carcinoma of the ovary or peritoneal carcinomatosis of other origin. *Surgery Gynecology and Obstetrics* 1993;176:469–73.
15. **Larson JE; Podczaski ES; Manetta A; Whitney CW; Mortel R.** Bowel obstruction in patients with ovarian carcinoma: analysis of prognostic factors. *Gynecologic Oncology* 1989;35:61–5.
16. **Gallick HL; Weaver DW; Sachs RJ., *et al.*** Intestinal obstruction in cancer patients. An assessment of risk factors and outcome. *American S*urgeon 1986;52:434–7.
17. **Krebs HB; Goplerud DR.** Surgical management of bowel obstruction in advanced ovarian carcinoma. *Obstetrics and Gyn*ecology 1983;61:327–30.
18. **Fernandes JR; Seymour RJ; Suissa S.** Bowel obstruction in patients with ovarian cancer: a search for prognostic factors. *American Journal of Obstetrics and Gynecology* 1988;158:244–9.
19. **Glass RL; LeDuc RJ.** Small intestinal obstruction from peritoneal carcinomatosis. *American Journal of Surgery* 1973;125:316–7.
20. **Yazdi GP; Miedema BW; Humphrey LJ.** High mortality after abdominal operation in patients with large-volume malignant ascites. *Journal of Surgical Oncology* 1996;62:93–6.
21. **Rapin ChH; Chatelain C; Weil R; Guggisberg E; Feuz A.** Pour une meilleure qualité de vie en fin de vie: nutrition et hydratation. *Age et Nutrit*ion 1990;1:22–8.
22. **Castaldo TW; Petrilli ES; Ballon SC., *et al.*** Intestinal operations in patients with ovarian carcinoma. *American Journal of Obstetrics and Gynecology* 1981;139:80–4.

23. **Clarke-Pearson DL; DeLong ER; Chin EN., *et al.*** Surgical management of intestinal obstruction in ovarian cancer II. Analysis of factors associated with complications and survival. *Archives of Surgery* 1988;123:42–5.
24. **Tunca JC; Buchler DA; Mack EA; Ruzicka FF; Crowley JJ; Carr WF.** The management of ovarian-cancer-caused bowel obstruction. *Gynecologic Oncology* 1981;12:186–92.
25. **Weiss SM; Skibber JM; Rosato FE.** Bowel obstruction in cancer patients: performance status as a predictor of survival. *Journal of Surgical Oncology* 1984;25:15–17.
26. **Jong P; Sturgeon J; Jamieson CG.** Benefit of palliative surgery for bowel obstruction in advanced ovarian cancer. *Canadian Journal of Surgery* 1995;38(5):454–7.
27. **Wallis F; Campbell KL; Eremin O; Hussey JK.** Self-expanding metal stents in the management of colorectal carcinoma—a preliminary report. Comments. *Clinical Radiology* 1998;53:251–4.
28. **Scott-Mackie P; Morgan R; Farrugia M; Glynos M; Adam A.** The role of metallic stents in malignant duodenal obstruction. *British Journal of Radiology* 1997;70:252–5.
29. **Pinto IT.** Malignant gastric and duodenal stenosis: palliation by peroral implantation of a self-expanding metallic stent. *Cardiovascular Intervention Radiology* 1997;20:431–4.
30. **Park HS; Do YS; Suh SW., *et al.*** Upper gastrointestinal tract malignant obstruction: initial results of palliation with a flexible covered stent. *Radiology* 1999;210:865–70.
31. **Keymling M; Wagner H-J; Vakil N; Knyrim K.** Relief of malignant duodenal obstruction by percutaneous insertion of a metal stent. *Gastrointestinal Endoscopy* 1993;39(3):439–41.
32. **Feretis C; Benakis P; Dimopoulos C; Manouras A; Tsimbloulis B; Apostolidis N.** Duodenal obstruction caused by pancreatic head carcinoma: palliation with self-expandable endoprostheses. *Gastrointestinal Endoscopy* 1997;46:161–5.
33. **de Baere T; Harry G; Ducreux M., *et al.*** Self-expanding metallic stents as palliative treatment of malignant gastroduodenal stenosis. *American Journal of Roentgenology* 1997;169:1079–83.
34. **Sebastian JJ; Zaragozano R; Vicente J; Gallego O; Trufero JM.** Duodenal obstruction secondary to a metastasis from an adenocarcinoma of the cecum: a case report. *American Journal of Gastroenterology* 1997;92:1051–2.
35. **Howden CW; Woods BL.** Self-expanding metal stents for palliative treatment of malignant biliary and duodenal stenoses. *Gastrointestinal Endoscopy* 1995;42:104–5.
36. **Song HY; Do YS; Han YM., *et al.*** Covered, expandable esophageal metallic stent tubes: experiences in 119 patients. *Radiology* 1994;193:689–95.
37. **Saxon RR; Barton RE; Katon RM., *et al.*** Treatment of malignant esophageal obstructions with covered metallic Z stents: long-term results in 52 patients. *Journal of Vascular and Interventional Radiology* 1995;6:747–54.
38. **Feins RH; Johnstone DW; Baronos ES; O'Neil SM.** Palliation of inoperable esophageal carcinoma with the Wallstent endoprosthesis. *Annals of Thoracic Surgery* 1996;62:1603–7.
39. **Mainar A; Tejero E; Maynar M; Ferral H; Castaneda-Zuniga W.** Colorectal obstruction: treatment with metallic stents. *Radiology* 1996;198:761–4.
40. **Arnell T; Stamos MJ; Takahashi P; Ojha S; Sze G; Eysselein V.** Colonic stents in colorectal obstruction. *American Surgeon* 1998;64:986–8.
41. **Tejero E; Fernandez-Lobato R; Mainar A., *et al.*** Initial results of a new procedure for treatment of malignant obstruction of the left colon. *Diseases of the Colon and Rectum* 1997;40:432–6.
42. **Saida Y; Sumiyama Y; Nagao J; Takase M.** Stent endoprosthesis for obstructing colorectal cancers. *Diseases of the Colon and Rectum* 1996;39:552–5.
43. **Feretis C; Benakis P; Dimopoulos C; Georgopoulos K; Manouras A; Apostolidis N.** Palliation of large-bowel obstruction due to recurrent rectosigmoid tumor using self-expandable endoprostheses. *Endoscopy* 1996;28:319–22.

44. **Vandervoort J; Weiss EJ; Somnay K; Tham TC; Wong RC; Carr-Locke DL.** Self-expanding metal stent for obstructing adenocarcinoma of the sigmoid. *Gastrointestinal Endoscopy* 1996;44:739–41.
45. **Rey JF; Romanczyk T; Greff M.** Metal stents for palliation of rectal carcinoma: a preliminary report on 12 patients. *Endoscopy* 1995;27:501–4.
46. **Dohmoto M; Hunerbein M; Schlag PM.** Application of rectal stents for palliation of obstructing rectosigmoid cancer. *Surgery and Endoscopy* 1997;11:758–61.
47. **Canon CL; Baron TH; Morgan DE; Dean PA; Koehler RE.** Treatment of colonic obstruction with expandable metal stents: radiologic features. *American Journal of Roentgenology* 1997;168:199–205.
48. **Wholey MH; Ferral H; Reyes R; Lopera J; Castaneda-Zuniga W; Maynar M.** Retrieval of migrated colonic stents from the rectum. *Cardiovascular Intervention Radiology* 1997;20:477–80.
49. **Forgas I; Macpherson A; Tibbs C.** Percutaneous endoscopic gastrostomy. The end of the line for nasogastric feeding? *British Medical Journal* 1992;304:1395–6.
50. **Gemlo B; Rayner AA; Lewis B.** Home support of patients with end-stage malignant bowel obstruction using hydration and venting gastrostomy. *American Journal of Surgery* 1986;152:100–4.
51. **Malone JM; Koonce T; Larson DM; Freedman RS; Carrasco CHO; Saul PB.** Palliation of small bowel obstruction by percutaneous gastrostomy in patients with progressive ovarian carcinoma. *Obstetrics and Gynecology* 1986;68:431–3.
52. **George J; Crawford D; Lewis T., *et al.*** Percutaneous endoscopic gastrostomy: a two year experience. *Medical Journal of Australia* 1990;152:17–20.
53. **Vargo JJ; Germain MM; Swenson JA; Harrison CR.** Ultrasound-assisted percutaneous endoscopic gastrostomy in a patient with advanced ovarian carcinoma and recurrent intestinal obstruction. *American Journal of Gastroenterology* 1993;88(11):1946–8.
54. **Cannizzaro R; Bortoluzzi F; Valentini M; Scarabelli C; Campagnutta E; Sozzi M; Fornasarig M; Poletti M.** Percutaneous endoscopic gastrostomy as a decompressive technique in bowel obstruction due to abdominal carcinomatosis. *Endoscopy* 1995;27:317–20.
55. **Adelson MD; Kazowits MH.** Percutaneous endoscopic drainage gastrostomy in treatment of gastrointestinal obstruction from intraperitoneal malignancy. *Obstetrics and Gynecology* 1993;81:467–9.
56. **Herman LL; Hoskins WJ; Shike M.** Percutaneous endoscopic gastrostomy for decompression of the stomach and small bowel. *Gastrointestinal Endoscopy* 1992;38:314–18.
57. **Cunningham MJ; Bromberg C; Kredentser DC; Collins MB; Malfetano JH.** Percutaneous gastrostomy for decompression in patients with advanced gynecologic malignancies. *Gynecologic Oncology* 1995;59:273–6.
58. **Campagnutta E; Cannizzaro R; Gallo A; Zarrelli A; Valentini M; De Cicco M; Scarabelli C.** Palliative treatment of upper intestinal obstruction by gynecological malignancy: the usefulness of percutaneous endoscopic gastrostomy. *Gynecologic Oncology* 1996;62:103–5.
59. **Sriram K; Sridhar K; Sridhar R.** Gastroduodenal decompression and simultaneous nasoenteral nutrition: 'extracorporeal gastrojejunostomy'. Clinical conference. (Published erratum appears in *Nutrition* 1996 Oct;12(10):747.) *Nutrition* 1996;12:440–1.
60. **Baines M; Oliver DJ; Carter RL.** Medical management of intestinal obstruction in patients with advanced malignant disease: a clinical and pathological study. *The Lancet* 1985;2:990–3.
61. **De Conno F; Caraceni A; Zecca E; Spoldi E; Ventafridda V.** Continuous subcutaneous infusion of hyoscine butylbromide reduces secretions in patients with gastrointestinal obstruction. *Journal of Pain and Symptom Management* 1991;6(8):484–6.
62. **Davis MP; Furste A.** Glycopyrrolate: a useful drug in the palliation of mechanical bowel obstruction. *Journal of Pain and Symptom Management* 1999;18(3):153–4.

63. **Twycross R; Wilcock A; Thorp S.** *Palliative Care Formulary.* Oxford: Radcliffe Medical Press, 1998; pp. 175–88.
64. **Fallon MT.** The physiology of somatostatin and its synthetic analogue, octreotide. *European Journal of Palliative Care* 1994;1(1):20–2.
65. **Ripamonti C; Panzeri C; Groff L; Galeazzi G; Boffi R.** The role of somatostatin and octreotide in bowel obstruction: pre-clinical and clinical results. *Tumori* 2001;87:1–9.
66. **Mercadante S; Spoldi E; Caraceni A; Maddaloni S; Simonetti MT.** Octreotide in relieving gastrointestinal symptoms due to bowel obstruction. *Palliative Medicine* 1993;7:295–9.
67. **Riley J; Fallon MT.** Octreotide in terminal malignant obstruction of the gastrointestinal tract. *European Journal of Palliative Care* 1994;1:23–8.
68. **Mangili G; Franchi M; Mariani A; Zanaboni F; Rabaiotti E; Frigerio L., *et al.*** Octreotide in the management of bowel obstruction in terminal ovarian cancer. *Gynecologic Oncology* 1996;61:345–8.
69. **Khoo D; Riley J; Waxman J.** Control of emesis in bowel obstruction in terminally ill patients. *The Lancet* 1992;339:375–6.
70. **Mercadante S; Maddaloni S.** Octreotide in the management of inoperable gastrointestinal obstruction in terminal cancer patients. *Journal of Pain and Symptom Management* 1992;7(8):496–8.
71. **Steadman K; Franks A.** A woman with malignant bowel obstruction who did not want to die with tubes. *The Lancet* 1996;347:944.
72. **Ripamonti C; Mercadante S; Groff L; Zecca E; De Conno F; Casuccio A.** Role of octreotide and scopolamine butylbromide, and hydration in symptom control of patients with inoperable bowel obstruction and nasogastric tubes: a prospective randomized trial. *Journal of Pain and Symptom Management* 2000;19:23–34.
73. **Mercadante S; Ripamonti C; Casuccio A; Zecca E; Groff L.** Comparison of octreotide and hyoscine butylbromide in controlling gastrointestinal symptoms due to malignant inoperable bowel obstruction. *Supportive Care in Cancer* 2000;8:188–91.
74. **Mercadante S; Kargar J; Nicolosi G.** Octreotide may prevent definitive intestinal obstruction. *Journal of Pain and Symptom Management* 1997;13:352–5.
75. **Bastounis E; Hadjinikolau L; Ioannou N., *et al.*** Somatostatin as adjuvant therapy in the management of obstructive ileus. *Hepato-Gastroenterology* 1989;36(6):538–9.
76. **Mercadante S; Avola G; Maddaloni S; Salamone G; Aragona F; Rodolico V.** Octreotide prevents the pathological alterations of bowel obstruction in cancer patients. *Supportive Care in Cancer* 1996;4:393–4.
77. **Mercadante S.** Scopolamine butylbromide plus octreotide in unresponsive bowel obstruction. *Journal of Pain and Symptom Management* 1998;16(5):278–9.
78. **Stiefel F; Morant R.** Vapreotide, a new somatostatin analogue in the palliative management of obstructive ileus in advanced cancer. *Supportive Care in Cancer* 1993;1:57–8.
79. **Dover SB.** Syringe driver in terminal care. *British Medical Journal* 1987;294:553–5.
80. **Fainsinger RL; Spachynski K; Hanson J; Bruera E.** Symptom control in terminally ill patients with malignant bowel obstruction (MBO). *Journal of Pain and Symptom Management* 1994;9(1):12–18.
81. **Cozzaglio L; Balzola F; Cosentino F., *et al.*** Outcome of cancer patients receiving home parenteral nutrition. *Journal of Parenteral and Enteral Nutrition* 1997;21:339–42.
82. **Bozzetti F; Amadori D; Bruera E; Cozzaglio L; Corli O; Filiberti F., *et al.*** Guidelines on artificial nutrition versus hydration in terminal cancer patients. *Nutrition* 1996;12/3:163–7.
83. **Fainsinger RL; MacEachern T; Miller MJ; Bruera E; Spachynski K; Kuehn N; Hanson J.** The use of hypodermoclisis for rehydration in terminally ill cancer patients. *Journal of Pain and Symptom Management* 1994;9:298–302.

Chapter 13

Enteric fistulae

Brett Gemlo

Introduction

Enteric fistulae represent an especially difficult clinical challenge for clinicians caring for patients with malignant as well as benign disease, and result in significant morbidity and mortality (1). Patients with inflammatory bowel disease commonly present with entero-entero and enterocutaneous fistulae, and other patients who have suffered post-operative complications such as anastomotic leak or unrecognized enterotomies can fistulize and be challenging to manage, but are beyond the scope of this chapter. We will concentrate on the evaluation, diagnosis, and treatment of fistulae in patients with underlying malignancies that have resulted in the development and perpetuation of those fistulae.

Background

Fistulae from the gastrointestinal (GI) tract to other body cavities or the skin are the result of a disruption of the integrity of the GI tracts wall anywhere from the oral cavity to the anus. Oropharyngeal-cutaneous fistulae can be seen after the surgical treatment of oral malignancies. Esophago-bronchial and esophago-pleural fistulae are seen with locally aggressive esophageal cancers. Gastrocoloic fistulae can result from invasion of the transverse colon by perforating gastric cancer, or conversely by colon cancer invading the stomach. Curative resection of colon cancer in nutritionally depleted or otherwise immunocompromised patients runs the risk of leak at the anastomosis and subsequent intra-abdominal abscess, the percutaneous drainage of which can result in a colocutaneous fistula. Recto-perineal fistulae can develop when a locally aggressive rectal cancer 'necessitates', or erodes, through the perineal skin.

The critical elements of a fistula are a source organ, a track, and a target organ. The source organ loses integrity of its wall due to trauma, usually surgical, or local progression of a neoplasm. In the absence of free perforation and peritonitis requiring emergent surgical intervention, the body tries to contain and wall off the perforation. It is this close adherence of other structures that lead to fistula formation. The anatomy of the subsequent fistula track is determined by the path of least resistance, and generally flows from a higher-pressure source to a lower-pressure reservoir. Often this is through a previous surgical wound. The target organ is usually a hollow viscus like another loop of bowel or the skin.

Once established, the natural history of simple fistulae is that they will heal spontaneously with time. Several factors, however, can contribute to persistence of a fistula (2,3).

The presence of malignancy or foreign body at the origin of the fistula generally prevents the source organ from re-establishing the integrity of its wall. Another significant factor is the presence of obstruction in the GI track distal to the source of the fistula. Any degree of distal obstruction can lead to non-healing of even simple fistulae by diverting intestinal contents through the fistula rather than through the lumen of the GI track. The presence of complete obstruction distal to the fistula converts what can be thought of as 'side' fistula to an 'end' fistula, receiving the entire flow of intestinal contents, and perpetuating the fistula. Finally, the nutritional and immune status of the patient has a profound effect on the body's ability to wall off, control, and heal enteric fistulae.

Assessment

The assessment of a patient suspected of having an enteric fistula must be thorough and multidisciplinary. In the case of a patient with known or suspected malignancy, the stage and extent of the tumor must be determined, as well as the patient's prognosis, since this may influence the vigor by which the situation is pursued. If the patient has been operated on, a careful review of the surgical notes is required to understand the patient's previous surgery and current anatomy, extent of residual tumor if present and potential for subsequent obstruction, and whether any events during surgery, like enterotomies or other organ injuries, may serve as sources of a fistula.

The patient's GI functional status must be carefully evaluated, including the nature and amount of current oral intake or any symptoms of obstruction like nausea, vomiting, bloating, or cramping. If vomiting is present, then a feculent nature may suggest the presence of high-grade obstruction of a communication between the stomach and the colon. The patient's bowel function, along with any recent changes, should be carefully noted as some internal fistulae may present as no more than the new onset diarrhea as the intestinal contents bypass much of the GI tract. See Figure 13.1.

Nutritional status and immune competence should be determined as they can influence the body's ability to heal fistulae and withstand future therapeutic interventions. The nature and proximity of chemotherapy or radiation therapy can influence the formation and persistence of fistulae as well.

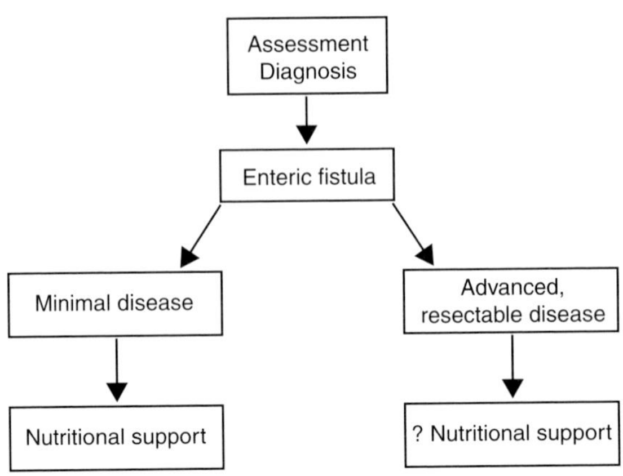

Figure 13.1

Physical examination should be thorough, systematic, and include the entire body. Enterocutaneous fistulae have communicated with the skin as far from the abdominal cavity as the thigh and popliteal fossa. After a careful head, neck, and chest examination, special attention should be focused on the abdomen. The size and location of surgical scars is very helpful, especially in cases where previous medical records are unavailable. If a draining fistula site is present, its location and the nature and daily volume of the drainage should be carefully noted, as well as the condition of the skin surrounding the fistula.

Biochemical assessment should include serum electrolyte and nutritional panels to determine if fluid and electrolyte losses through the fistulae are affecting homeostasis. Hematologic evaluation may help detect the presence of ongoing sepsis and evaluate immunocompetence.

Finally, a careful psychosocial evaluation needs to be made. The patient's prognosis, code status, support structures and quality of life provide a frame of reference from which to assess the impact of an enteric fistula. Many fistulae are minimally symptomatic and deserve little attention. Others can actually be beneficial in relieving obstructive symptoms. Generally, however, fistulae exert a significant negative effect on quality of life, but they have to be viewed in the context of the entire clinical situation to determine which therapeutic approach is most suitable.

Diagnosis

After careful assessment of the patient, the goal of any diagnostic maneuvers should be to confirm the presence of an enteric fistula and delineate its anatomy. The gold standard is radiographic visualization of extravasation of contrast from the GI tract and flow into the target organ. Typically this is done under fluoroscopy after the ingestion of oral water-soluble contrast or the instillation of rectal contrast. Important factors to determine are the site of the fistula in the GI tract, the condition of the source organ, and the length and course of the fistula itself. Occasionally retrograde studies through an enterocutaneous fistula tract are useful, especially if the patient is clinically obstructed or has an ileus. It is important during these studies to also ascertain the status of the GI tract distal to the site of the fistula as the degree of obstruction, if present, can have an impact on how the fistula can be treated.

In those patients in whom contrast studies fail to demonstrate the presence of an enterocutaneous fistula, ingestion of powdered charcoal or methylene blue can be useful in confirming that a communication between the bowel and skin does in fact exist.

Computerized tomography (CT) and magnetic resonance imaging (MRI) are usually not useful in establishing the presence or anatomy of enteric fistulae. They are useful in documenting the extent of residual tumor if present, and in the percutaneous drainage of associated intra-abdominal abscesses.

Endoscopic evaluation of patients with suspected enteric fistulae is generally unrewarding. Fistulae can be quite small and hard to visualize, and the associated insufflation of air has the potential to disrupt the fistula track and cause free perforation. The one setting in which endoscopy is useful is in determining if the source of a fistula is associated with malignancy or not. For instance, colonoscopy and biopsy can be very useful in differentiating between a colo-vesical fistula secondary to diverticular disease and one secondary to a perforated cancer.

In cases where the presence of malignancy in the source organ is uncertain, curettage of the fistula track and cytologic evaluation of the scrapings can help make a diagnosis.

Treatment

Prior to embarking on a discussion of the options available for treating enteric fistulae in cancer patients, several observations should be made. Most reports in the literature concerning the treatment of enteric fistulae are based on experience with patients who, if they have cancer, have been resected and now are experiencing a fistula as a post-operative complication. The concern in these patients is to treat them as expeditiously as possible to enable the use of post-operative adjuvant chemotherapy, the administration of which while the fistula exists may antagonize efforts to heal the fistula. The reported experience with true malignant fistulae, with tumor in the target organ as the source of the fistula, is much smaller, and difficult to separate from benign fistula, even those with a malignant distal bowel contributing to the fistula. Patients with no or minimal disease and benign fistulae should be treated aggressively.

In those patients with widely metastatic disease and enteric fistulae, surgical intervention is often not feasible or appropriate, nor are long-term efforts at nutritional support or other non-interventional methods. In these patients minimizing the impact of the fistula and maximizing quality of life should be the goals.

Surgical correction of enteric fistulae with takedown of the fistula, resection of diseased bowel, relief of distal obstruction, and restoration of intestinal continuity with acceptable morbidity and mortality remains the gold standard. After a period of homeostatic and nutritional resuscitation, surgical intervention can be associated with success rates as high as 94%, and is superior to non-operative approaches in terms of healing (4,5). Very often, surgery is not an option because of the condition of the patient or conditions in their abdomen, and a variety of alternative surgical approaches have been described, including internal bypass (6), alternative methods for entering a frozen abdomen (7), and various external flap procedures that do not require entering the peritoneal cavity (8,9). However, the impact of subsequent oncologic treatment like chemotherapy remains unclear.

With the advent of hyperalimentation in the late 1970s, it became clear that not all enteric fistulae required surgery, and that a significant number would heal with prolonged bowel rest and parental feeding. These beneficial effects were thought to be attributable to the correction of underlying nutritional deficits, as well as allowing the cessation of oral intake and thus minimizing the volume of enteric contents exposed to the fistula. The majority of reports concern post-operative fistulae, with healing rates ranging from 50% to 64% (10–13). Enteral nutritional support has a number of theoretical advantages over parenteral nutrition, and Levy *et al.* were able to achieve a 38% healing rate, even in high output enteric fistulae (14). While the advisability of prolonged nutritional support is controversial in patients with malignant fistulae or extensive metastatic disease, its preliminary use while the patient is being evaluated for other interventions is appropriate, and may even lead to healing or a reduction in symptoms related to the fistula.

Prospects for the non-operative management of enteric fistulae brightened in the late 1980s with the release of octreotide, an analogue of somatostatin. Its properties included reductions in GI secretion and relaxation of the small bowel musculature, reducing motility and promoting the healing of fistulae. Early reports were enthusiastic about reductions in fistula outputs and improvement in healing rates (15–17), but the uncontrolled nature of these studies called their impact into question. Scott reported the first prospective, randomized double-blind study comparing octreotide with placebo in 19 patients over 12 days of infusion (18). Patients with malignancy or a history of radiation were excluded. No difference in fistula output was found, and spontaneous healing was seen in only one octreotide patient and three placebo patients. This study has been questioned because of strict exclusion criteria and a single institution, leading to less accrual and small numbers. A multicenter randomized prospective double-blind trial was reported by Sancho in 1995. The trial comprised 26 enterocutaneous fistulae and 5 pancreatic fistulae started on total parenteral nutrition (TPN) and either octreotide or placebo at the onset of the study. Reductions in fistula output were approximately 60% in each group, and not significantly different. Healing rates were also similar, 57% for octreotide and 35% for placebo, $p=0.4$ (19). Finally, Alvarez found that 13 patients treated with octreotide experienced a significant reduction in fistula output when compared with case matched controls, but there was no increase in fistula healing (20).

While the benefit of octreotide has not been substantiated by prospective studies, anecdotal evidence of success, even in malignant fistulae, exist, as found by Ayache after treatment of a retroperitoneal angiosarcoma. A lack of demonstrable clinical effect may also be due to downregulation of somatostatin receptors by octreotide after 7 days, as has been pointed out by Jenkins (21). Further large studies may yet demonstrate a role for octreotide in the management of enteric fistulae.

Interventional radiologic control of enteric fistulae has been described since the early 1980s (22), and generally involves minimally invasive intubation and control of the fistula tracks with catheters, allowing local sepsis to abate and a mature fistula track to develop, and subsequently close. Sammarco described using absolute alcohol and hyperosmolar contrast media to sclerose a fistula track and achieve healing (23). LaBerge and his colleagues achieved a 57% fistula closure rate in 53 patients with a variety of enterocutaneous fistulae, 85% with 2 months of treatment. D'Harcour used percutaneous catheters to aggressively control local sepsis and drain high-output fistulas in 147 patients, and was able to successfully heal an amazing 81% of them. Interventional radiology may be an underutilized modality in the management of these fistulas. Even when healing is not achieved, cannulation and control of drainage made lead to significant palliation.

Endoscopic efforts to treat enteric fistulae can be divided into two areas. Endoscopic balloon dilation or endoluminal stent placement can be used to relieve distal obstructions and promote the healing of more proximal fistulae, usually in conjunction with other non-invasive measures. An alternative use for the endoscope is the instillation of tissue adhesives like fibrin glue into the fistula track, either percutaneously (24) or intraluminaly (25). Both small early series achieved excellent healing rates with minimal morbidity. Hwang conducted a prospective randomized trial of TPN plus fibrin glue injection versus TPN alone (26). While all fistulae in each group healed, it was achieved in a significantly shorter period of time in the fibrin glue group. More recently, injection with biological glue, *N*-butyl-2-cyanoacrylate (Histoacryl), was been reported with two groups with similar results (27,28).

A large proportion of patients do not suffer significant fluid or electrolyte abnormalities as a result of their fistula, and can be successfully palliated by thoughtful, persistent, and innovative nursing care. Numerous reports can be found detailing the use of custom-made or commercial products to locally control fistula effluents and avoid skin irritation and breakdown (29–31). Dearlove has written an excellent review article about the nursing challenges associated with enteric fistulae (32). These patients are extremely challenging problems for nurses, and the opportunity for huge improvements in quality of life rely on their efforts.

The key to the optimal care of patients with enteric fistulae, especially those for whom definitive surgical repair is not an option, is an experienced multidisciplinary team. Such a team needs to meet not only the medical, surgical, and pharmacologic needs of the patient, but their nursing, homecare, psychosocial, and spiritual needs as well.

Future improvements in the treatment of patients with enteric fistulae will come in two different areas. Advances in the pharmacologic management of these patients should al low better control of GI secretion and promotion of fistula healing. Immune modulators-like anti-TNF alpha have proven useful in the treatment of fistulas associated with Crohn's disease, and parallel advances may be possible in other enteric fistulae. Secondly, improvements in interventional radiology may obviate the need for surgical intervention, especially in cases of unresectability and limited life expectancy.

References

1. **Chamberlain RS; Kaufman HL; Danforth DN.** Enterocutaneous fistula in cancer patients: etiology, management, outcome, and impact on further treatment. *American Surgeon* 1998;64(12):1204–11.
2. **Berry SM; Fischer JE.** Classification and pathophysiology of enterocutaneous fistulas. *Surgical Clinics of North America* 1996;76(5):1009–18.
3. **Hugh TB; Coleman MJ; Cohen A.** Persistent postoperative enterocutaneous fistula: pathophysiology and treatment. *Australia and New Zealand Journal of Surgery* 1986;56(12):901–6.
4. **Conter RL; Roof L; Roslyn JJ.** Delayed reconstructive surgery for complex enterocutaneous fistulae. *American Surgeon* 1988;54(10):589–93.
5. **Borison DI; Bloom AD; Pritchard TJ.** Treatment of enterocutaneous and colocutaneous fistulas with early surgery or somatostatin analog. *Diseases of the Colon and Rectum* 1992;35(7):635–9.
6. **Schirmer CC; Gurski RR; Gugel FL; Lazzaron AR; Brentano L; Kruel CD.** Alternative surgical treatment for complex enterocutaneous fistula. *International Surgery* 1999;84(1):29–34.
7. **Bosscha K; van Vroonhoven TJ.** Novel approach to the treatment of intestinal fistula in the inaccessible abdomen: transbursal end-to-side duodenogastrostomy. *British Journal of Surgery* 1998;85(2):276–8.
8. **Chang P; Chun JT; Bell JL.** Complex enterocutaneous fistula: closure with rectus abdominis muscle flap. *Southern Medical Journal* 2000;93(6):599–602.
9. **Kearney R; Payne W; Rosemurgy A.** Extra-abdominal closure of enterocutaneous fistula. *American Surgeon* 1997;63(5):406–9.
10. **Alhan E; Calik A; Kucuktulu U.** The management of enterocutaneous fistulas with parenteral hyperalimentation. *Zeitschrift feur Gastroenterologic* 1993;31(11):657–60.
11. **Dardai E; Pirityi S; Nagy L.** Parenteral and enteral nutrition and the enterocutaneous fistula treatment. II. Factors influencing the outcome of treatment. *Acta Chiruorgica Hungaricae* 1991;32(4):305–18.
12. **Dardai E; Bite A.** Treatment of enterocutaneous small intestine fistula using parenteral nutrition therapy. *Deutsche Zeitschrift fuer Verdauungs—und Stoffwechselkr-ankheiten* 1984;44(4):149–52.
13. **Zera RT; Bubrick MP; Sternquist JC; Hitchcock CR.** Enterocutaneous fistulas. Effects of total parenteral nutrition and surgery. *Diseases of the Colon and Rectum* 1983;26(2):109–12.
14. **Levy E; Frileux P; Cugnenc PH; Honiger J; Ollivier JM; Parc R.** High-output external fistulae of the small bowel: management with continuous enteral nutrition. *British Journal of Surgery* 1989;76(7):676–9.

15. **Nubiola P; Badia JM; Martinez-Rodenas F; Gil MJ; Segura M; Sancho J., *et al.*** Treatment of 27 postoperative enterocutaneous fistulas with the long half-life somatostatin analogue SMS 201–995. Published erratum appears in *Annals of Surgery* 1990 Feb;211(2):246. *Annals of Surgery* 1989;210(1):56–8.
16. **Planas M; Porta I; Angles R; Baena JA; Serra J; Padro JB.** Somatostatin and/or total parenteral nutrition for the treatment of intestinal fistulas. *Revista Espanola de las Enfermedalles del Aparato Digestivo* 1990;78(6):345–7.
17. **Spiliotis J; Briand D; Gouttebel MC; Astre C; Louer B; Saint-Aubert B., *et al.*** Treatment of fistulas of the gastrointestinal tract with total parenteral nutrition and octreotide in patients with carcinoma. *Surgery Gynecology and Obstetrics* 1993;176(6):575–80.
18. **Scott NA; Finnegan S; Irving MH.** Octreotide and postoperative enterocutaneous fistulae: a controlled prospective study. *Acta Gastro-Enterologica Belgica* 1993;56(3–4):266–70.
19. **Sancho JJ; di Costanzo J; Nubiola P; Larrad A; Beguiristain A; Roqueta F., *et al.*** Randomized double-blind placebo-controlled trial of early octreotide in patients with postoperative enterocutaneous fistula. Comments. *British Journal of Surgery* 1995;82(5):638–41.
20. **Alvarez C; McFadden DW; Reber HA.** Complicated enterocutaneous fistulas: failure of octreotide to improve healing. *World Journal of Surgery* 2000;24(5):533–7; discussion 538.
21. **Jenkins SA; Javle P; Parsons KF; Balan KK; Berein A.** Randomized double-blind placebo-controlled trial of early octreotide in patients with postoperative enterocutaneous fistula. Letter; comment. *British Journal of Surgery* 1995;82(11):1576.
22. **McLean GK; Mackie JA; Freiman DB; Ring EJ.** Enterocutaneous fistulae: interventional radiologic management. *American Journal of Roentgenology* 1982;138(4):615–19.
23. **Sammarco G; Iaccarino V; Liguori G; Aloi V; Cavalcanti BS; Cristofaro MG., *et al.*** Fistula following emergency total colectomy: an efficient method of treatment. *Minerva Chirurgica* 1990;45(8):599–602.
24. **Lange V; Meyer G; Wenk H; Schildberg FW.** Fistuloscopy—an adjuvant technique for sealing gastrointestinal fistulae. *Surgical Endoscopy* 1990;4(4):212–16.
25. **Eleftheriadis E; Tzartinoglou E; Kotzampassi K; Aletras H.** Early endoscopic fibrin sealing of high-output postoperative enterocutaneous fistulas. *Acta Chirurgica Scandinavica* 1990;156(9):625–8.
26. **Hwang TL; Chen MF.** Randomized trial of fibrin tissue glue for low output enterocutaneous fistula. *British Journal of Surgery* 1996;83(1):112.
27. **Santos F; Campos J; Freire J; Andrade A; Tavora I; Castelo HB.** Enterocutaneous fistulas: an unusual solution. *Hepatogastroenterology* 1997;44(16):1085–9.
28. **Dalton D; Woods S.** Successful endoscopic treatment of enterocutaneous fistulas by histoacryl glue. *Australia and New Zealand Journal of Surgery* 2000;70(10):749–50.
29. **Medeiros ADC; Soares CE.** Treatment of enterocutaneous fistulas by high-pressure suction with a normal diet. *American Journal of Surgery* 1990;159(4):411–13.
30. **Slauf P; Antos F; Vedral J.** Use of the Convatec Wound Manager and Stomahesive flanges in local treatment of external gastrointestinal fistulas. *Rozhledy Chirurgia* 1993;72(7):324–7.
31. **Hyon SH; Martinez-Garbino JA; Benati ML; Lopez-Avellaneda ME; Brozzi NA; Argibay PF.** Management of a high-output postoperative enterocutaneous fistula with a vacuum sealing method and continuous enteral nutrition. In Process Citation. *Asaio Journal* 2000;46(4):511–14.
32. **Dearlove JL.** Skin care management of gastrointestinal fistulas. *Surgical Clinics of North America* 1996;76(5):1095–109.

Chapter 14

Gastrointestinal bleeding in advanced cancer patients

Isabelle Mancini, Alain Hendlisz, and
Jean-Jacques Body

Incidence

There are few data concerning the frequency of symptomatic gastrointestinal (GI) bleeding in patients with advanced cancer. In a survey of 800 advanced cancer patients admitted in a palliative care program, the incidence of GI bleeding was 2.25% (1). In the general population, hospitalization for acute GI bleeding is 1 per 1000 (2). The incidence among men is approximately double that among women, and the rate increases markedly with age and with the use of non-steroidal anti-inflammatory drugs (NSAIDs) (3).

Although infrequent, it is feared by clinicians, causing real clinical challenges in many cases.

Causes of GI bleeding in advanced cancer patients

GI bleeding is due to upper or lower GI tract lesions. Hemostatic abnormalities, due to cancer itself or its treatment, can exacerbate this complication. The different causes of GI bleeding in advanced cancer patients are listed in Table 14.1.

Upper GI bleeding

Peptic disease

As in the general population, and despite the widespread use of H_2-receptor antagonists and proton-pump inhibitors, bleeding from hemorrhagic gastritis and peptic ulcer remains the most common cause of upper GI bleeding, accounting for approximately 50% of the cases with severe upper GI hemorrhage (4).

Portal hypertension

Portal hypertension and esophageal varices can develop in cancer patients who have chronic liver disease, i.e. chronic viral hepatitis or alcohol cirrhosis, as well as a tumor-related complication. Esophageal or gastric variceal bleeding in the absence of previous liver disease strongly suggests portal vein thrombosis, or massive metastatic (or tumoral) involvement of the liver (5).

Table 14.1 Causes of GI bleeding in advanced cancer patients

Upper GI bleeding	Lower GI bleeding
Gastric and duodenal ulcer	Colonic diverticulosis
Esophagitis, gastritis and duodenitis	Angiodysplasia
Esophageal varices	Arteriovenous malformation
Neoplasm	Neoplasms and polyps
Mallory–Weiss tear	Radiation proctitis
Stress ulcerations	Hemorrhoids
Angiodysplasia	Infectious diarrhea
Arteriovenous malformation	Small and large bowel ulcerations
Dieulafoy's lesions	Chronic inflammatory bowel disease
Aortoenteric fistula	Meckel's diverticulum
	Ischemic colitis
	Massive upper GI bleeding
	Aortoenteric fistula
Risk factors for developing GI bleeding	
Systemic changes	
Thrombocytopenia	
Liver failure	
Medications	
NSAIDs	
Anticoagulants	
(Corticosteroids)	

Gastroduodenal tumors

The proportion of patients presenting with upper GI bleeding who were found to bleed from gastric malignancies varies from 1% to 5% (6–8). Seventy per cent of patients presenting with bleeding gastric tumors have stage IV disease at presentation, i.e. disseminated malignancy or local malignant infiltration to adjacent structures (8). The reason is probably that these gastric cancers that bleed acutely may develop in the body of the stomach and then develop insidiously with relatively minor symptoms, as opposed to cardial or antral lesions. By the time of symptomatic presentation, the underlying lesions are often too advanced for radical surgical ablation (9). The majority of gastric bleeding tumors consist of adenocarcinomas (8).

Other causes

Esophagitis and Mallory–Weiss tears are other relatively frequent causes of upper GI bleeding in cancer patients. Gastric angiodysplasias, arteriovenous malformation, Dieulafoy's lesions, aortoduodenal fistulas following infection, and breakdown of a retroduodenal aortic graft anastomosis are rare but ominous sources of bleeding (6,7).

Causes of lower GI bleeding

Diverticulosis

The commonest cause of lower GI bleeding in the general population and in cancer patients is diverticulosis (10) (accounting for approximatively 70% of all causes). Bleeding is usually painless and acute, producing marron stools or bright red hematochezia. Blood loss is usually significant and badly tolerated if patient condition is poor (11).

Vascular malformations

The next most frequent sources are colonic angiodysplasia and arteriovenous malformations. The clinical presentation of lower GI bleeding from angiodysplasia is usually less dramatic, more chronic and occult than in diverticular disease. Bleeding can, however, be massive in both conditions (12).

Cancer-related causes

Neoplasms and polyps, both benign and malignant, are fairly common and occur more often in elderly patients. Between 10% and 20% of patients with neoplasms or polyps will bleed, but bleeding is usually slow and chronic (12). Bleeding can be acute but is usually self-limiting. Advanced lesions will often have other symptoms such as obstruction. Bleeding from metastases by highly vascularized tumors such as renal cell carcinoma and breast carcinomas are rare (13).

Cancer treatment can also lead to GI bleeding. Rectal bleeding is common in radiation proctitis. This condition can occur after radiotherapy for gynecologic, prostatic, rectal, or anal margin malignancies. Bleeding is due to the neoformation of fragile mucosal vessels (angiodysplasia) in the mucosal areas exposed to radiation. The median time to occurrence of rectal bleeding ranges from 9 to 15 months after radiotherapy but can be delayed by 3 years or more (13).

Other causes

External hemorrhoids are extremely common and usually cause only minor ano-rectal bleeding, except in rare instances of liver disease and portal hypertension where massive bleeding can occur due to a ruptured rectal varice (13). Following passage of a hard stool or excessive straining, internal hemorrhoids can bleed painlessly, leaving blood around the stool but not mixed in the stool. Anal fissure can have a similar bleeding pattern, but is painful (12–14).

Infectious diarrhea can also cause bleeding. The offending agents are most often *Campylobacter Jejuni*, *Salmonellea*, *Shigella*, *Escherischia coli* or *Clostridium difficile.* Immunocompromised patients may present with bloody diarrhea caused by a large number of organisms, but cytomegalovirus is a common offender (14).

Small and large bowel ulcers of variable etiology, including uremic stress ulcers, are unusual bleedings sources, as are chronic inflammatory bowel diseases and Meckel's diverticulum. Other rare causes of lower GI bleeding are post-radiation telangiectasias, ischemic colitis, massive upper GI bleeding, and various small bowel lesions (15). Aortoenteric fistulas essentially occur in elderly patients with abdominal aortic aneurism or aortic grafts. Fistulas develop as a result of inflammation between the bowel and the aneurysm or graft. Bleeding is most often devastating in these cases (13,14).

Risk factors

Risk factors for developing GI bleeding in advanced cancer patients essentially consist of systemic changes in blood coagulation ability induced directly or indirectly by the malignancy (16) and the use of concomittant medications such as NSAIDS (17) and anticoagulants (18) (Table14.1).

Systemic changes

Possible systemic disorders are numerous and their influence is variable. They include disorders of hemostasis resulting from bone marrow failure, diffuse intravascular coagulopathy, liver or renal failure with clotting dysfunction, and thrombocytopenia secondary to the malignancy itself or its treatment (16). We will briefly review the last two conditions.

Thrombocytopenia

Thrombocytopenia may be seen in the palliative care setting in patients with extensive bone marrow involvement, disseminated coagulopathy, splenomegaly, advanced hematological malignancy, or following myelotoxic therapy (16). Platelet dysfunction may be caused or aggravated by several medications including aspirin, NSAIDs and semisynthetic penicillins, by metabolic disorders such as uremia, increased fibrinolysis secondary to disseminated intravascular coagulation, or an underlying hematological malignancy (16).

There is only one study that has specifically reviewed bleeding associated with thrombocytopenia (19). Of 458 consecutive patients referred for esophagogastroduodenoscopy, only 7 (1.5%) had GI bleeding associated with profound thrombocytopenia ($<20\,000$ platelets mm^{-3}). The endoscopy, performed within one day after correction of the profound thrombocytopenia, revealed numerous superficial upper GI lesions consisting of petechiae, ecchymoses, and erosions without any other upper GI pathology. Bleeding of these lesions was attributed by the authors to the profound thrombocytopenia.

Liver failure

Patients with liver cancer or hepatic metastases constitute a group at higher risk of developing GI bleeding during the course of illness. In a recent survey, Mercadante (1) showed that their risk was more than 20-fold in comparison with other cancer patients (15% versus 0.7%). This increased risk is due to several factors. Patients with liver disease commonly develop excessive fibrinolysis, disseminated intravascular coagulation, and thrombocytopenia notably due to congestive splenomegaly, platelet pooling, and antiplatelet autoantibodies (20). In addition, patients with liver disease have a decreased ability to synthesize all coagulation proteins except factor VIII (18). The vitamin K dependent factors II, VII, and X have been shown to decrease first in progressive liver disease, whereas factor IX may initially remain in the normal range (18). Factor V also decreases early in liver disease, and this decrease has been shown to correlate with the extent of liver damage (18). These factors are essential for the extrinsic and common coagulation pathways. This explains why prothrombin time (PT) is often prolonged in patients with liver disease. The partial thromboplastin time (PTT) will be prolonged when coagulation factors decline further with progressive liver disease. Intravascular or subcutaneous administration of 5–10 mg of vitamin K once or twice a week could potentially prevent some hemorrhagic complications in these patients (18).

Medications with potential GI toxicity

NSAIDs

NSAIDs are often used as a first-line treatment in cancer pain and as adjuvants to opioids in patients with severe pain (21). These agents have both a peripheral effect on inflammation and a role in attenuating central pain pathways. Unfortunately, NSAIDs are well-known agents to cause upper GI complications, ranging from dyspeptic symptoms in up to 40% of patients to life-threatening complicated ulcers (hemorrhage, perforation, or pyloric obstruction) (17). The prevalence of peptic ulceration in chronic NSAID users is 20%–30%, with gastric ulcers approximately six times more common than duodenal ulcers (22).

Factors increasing the risk of NSAID-induced gastroduodenal (GD) damage are listed in Table 14.2. The elderly are clearly at greater risk of NSAID-induced GD toxicity. This may be related to impaired mucosal defenses, but may also be associated with a reduced renal clearance of the drug leading to increased plasma levels. Gender, smoking, alcohol intake, and cardiovascular disease have also been reported to be risk factors in some studies. *Helicobacter pylori* gastric infection does not by itself increase the risk of ulceration in NSAID users, but it is associated with 60%–80% of gastric ulcers and 70%–100% of duodenal ulcers (23). Moreover, eradication of H. pylori with antibiotics lowers the incidence of ulcer recurrence and rebleeding (24). The effect of severe illness on the risk of NSAID-induced GD toxicity is unclear. A recent audit of the use of NSAIDs in the palliative care setting showed this population to be at very high risk of GD toxicity. NSAID use was common (36% of the patients reviewed in the audit) and additional risk factors were frequently present (25). In particular, the co-administration of corticosteroids was noted in 62.5% of patients taking NSAIDs (25). NSAIDs vary considerably in their intrinsic potential to damage the GD mucosa. Among classical NSAIDs, ibuprofen appears to be associated with the lowest incidence of GD toxicity, whereas the use of azapropazone and piroxicam carries

Table 14.2 Risk factors for NSAID-associated gastrotoxicity

Patient factors
Advanced age
Alcoholism
Coffee consumption
Family history
Female gender
General poor health
History of ulcer
Occupation
Prostaglandin deficiency
Smoking
Medication factors
Corticosteroids
Antineoplastic agents
Anticoagulants
Oral bisphosphonates such as alendronate

much greater risk (17). Prophylaxis is warranted if any of these risk factors is identified, with the possible exception of age alone (17). According to the current evidence (26–30), the prophylactic agent should either be a proton-pump inhibitor or misoprostol but not the standard dose of H_2 antagonists (26) or sucralfate (31). New generation NSAIDs, including highly selective CoX-2 inhibitors, will have a major impact on NSAID safety since the incidence of GD ulcers is two or three times less (32). However, there are no data yet on their use in the palliative care setting.

Anticoagulants

Thromboembolic complications requiring anticoagulants are quite common in patients with advanced cancer (16). Bleeding is a major risk associated with anticoagulation therapy and the GI tract is the most common site of bleeding. Acute GI hemorrhage in anticoagulated patients is a real therapeutic challenge (18). When managing a patient who bleeds and receives warfarin, one must first reconsider the need for anticoagulation therapy in order to take further therapeutic decisions. Short-term replacement of coagulation factors may be accomplished with fresh frozen plasma transfusions (18). If they are ineffective and the bleeding is life-threatening, prothrombin complex concentrates may be helpful. For longer-term control of the coagulopathy, a dose of 0.5–1 mg of vitamin K, given intravenously or subcutaneously, can lower the international normalized ratio value and allow for safe reanticoagulation after the acute event is over. However, if larger (10 mg) doses of vitamin K are given, reanticoagulation with warfarin becomes extremely difficult (18).

Corticosteroids and peptic ulcerations

The relationship between corticosteroids and peptic ulcerations is less important than commonly thought (33). It remains that corticosteroids clearly increase the risk of severe complications (i.e. bleeding or intestinal perforations). Risk factors include the total dose of corticosteroids, a previous history of peptic ulceration, the presence of an advanced malignant disease, and the concurrent administration of NSAIDs (33). Corticosteroids are widely prescribed in palliative care for different indications. The same prophylaxis as for NSAIDs should be considered for patients with two or more risk factors (33).

Clinical presentation

Clinical presentation patterns are classically divided into five categories (3).

1 Hematemesis is bloody vomitus, and can be fresh and bright red or older and 'coffee-ground' in character.

2 Melena is black, tarry, foul-smelling stool. It results from the degradation of blood and must not be confused with the effects of exogenous stool darkeners such as iron and bismuth.

3 Hematochezia is the passage of right red or maroon blood from the rectum in the form of pure blood, blood intermixed with formed stool, blood clots, or bloody diarrhea.

4 GI blood loss is frequently occult: blood is only identified by special examination of the stools.

5 Finally, patients may present without any objective sign of GI bleeding but rather with symptoms of major blood loss, such as palor, syncope, dyspnea, angina, or even shock.

Hematemesis and melena are the most common manifestations of an acute episode of upper GI bleeding. Wara and Stodkilde correlated various patterns of these findings with clinical outcome and found that dark hematemesis or melena alone is predictive of massive bleeding in 5%–10% of cases in a general patient population (34). On the other hand, fresh hematemesis alone, dark hematemesis with melena, and fresh hematemesis with melena were predictive of massive bleeding in 21%, 24%, and 27% of cases, respectively (2).

In the survey of Mercadante (1), all bleeding patients presented with hematemesis, melena, or both, suggesting that the upper GI tract is the main source of bleeding in patients with advanced cancer.

Clinical approach of GI bleeding in advanced cancer patient

In patients with advanced cancer, the decision regarding the management of GI bleeding needs to be individualized and the decision-making process needs to consider factors such as the extent of disease, the expected survival, the disease burden, the invasiveness of planned treatment strategies, and the patient's own wishes. A balance needs to be achieved between aggressive management with increased iatrogenicity and the failure to use treatments that have potential symptomatic benefits (35).

The management of GI bleeding in advanced cancer patients starts with a precise assessment of the patient followed by diagnostic evaluation maneuvers and treatment.

Assessment

The initial assessment of the patient with upper GI bleeding should evaluate the severity of the bleeding and the patient's hemodynamic status (36). The first assessment includes a rapid measurement of resting blood pressure and pulse, and a check for orthostatic hypotension (blood pressure is maintained on recumbency but falls by more than 15–20 mm Hg when the patient sits up), which is an early sign of severe blood loss. Blood pressure and heart rate reflect the importance and rapidity of blood loss, as well as the cardiac and vascular compensation. Tachycardia and vasoconstriction first ensue to compensate, but, finally, recumbent hypotension results. Vascular collapse and shock will follow. As in any emergency setting, a direct history and physical examination are performed to try to identify a specific diagnosis and the site of bleeding. The assessment includes a search for systemic bleeding whose manifestations can be purpura, petechiae, epistaxis, melena, hematuria, vaginal bleeding, and excessive bleeding after procedures such as venipuncture or the insertion of a subcutaneous needle. Accurate information on the stage of the cancer, its location, its possible role in the bleeding, on therapy for the cancer itself or its palliation, and on the patient's wishes are all important for planning the treatment of bleeding. Bad prognostic factors (see below) must be identified in order to avoid unhelpful and uncomfortable rescussitation maneuvers.

Diagnostic investigations

Upper GI bleeding

Urgent upper endoscopy identifies the bleeding source in 90%–95% of patients with acute upper GI bleeding (37,38). Barium upper GI studies should be avoided as they are helpful in less than 50% of cases (39). This is explained by various factors:

1 endoscopy is more sensitive than upper GI barium radiograph and permits mucosal biopsy as well as hemostatic therapy (40);

2 endoscopy visualizes the source of active bleeding or stigmata of recent hemorrhage, providing important prognostic information, whereas barium studies only identify potential bleeding sites;

3 barium studies interfere with subsequent diagnostic tests such as endoscopy or angiography; and

4 now that most ulcer diseases can be cured by treating *H. pylori* infection, it is important to make this diagnosis rather than to treat blindly with antisecretory therapy.

The accuracy of endoscopy has much lowered the need for angiography. Sometimes, however, bleeding may be so massive that endoscopy cannot be safely or satisfactorily performed and surgery is contraindicated. Selective mesenteric angiography localizes the site of bleeding in about 75% of such patients, and provides a therapeutic option. According to animal studies, a rate of about 0.5 ml min^{-1} of blood loss is necessary to be seen on radiography (41).

Radionuclide imaging studies are rarely used in upper GI bleeding. These are less sensitive than angiography or endoscopy for small bleedings and poorly helpful in massive hemorrhage (42–43).

Lower GI bleeding

For the 90% of patients whose bleeding has ceased spontaneously, an elective colonoscopy after standard preparation is the procedure of choice (44). Urgent colonoscopy following a rapid oral purge can define the source of bleeding in 74% of cases (45). A colonoscopy during acute lower GI severe hemorrhage is technically difficult and almost always non-contributive. It is more reasonable to perform colonoscopy within 24 hours after hemodynamic stability is achieved. With more severe or ongoing hematochezia, fluid resuscitation and more urgent evaluation is indicated if appropriate. Hemodynamically unstable patients have lost more than 15% of their blood volume; after fluid administration and transfusions if needed, a nasogastric tube (NGT) should be inserted and the gastric aspirate observed for visible blood. Although a non-bloody aspirate does not rule out an upper GI source of bleeding, a bilious aspirate makes it less likely. Upper endoscopy should be performed if the nasogastric aspirate is positive. In patients having upper endoscopy, 11% have lesions in the stomach or duodenum responsible for the severe hematochezia (46).

Barium enema should not be performed in the evaluation of a lower GI bleeding because, as for upper GI bleedings, it is unable to detect sites of active bleeding and obscures subsequent colonoscopy or angiography.

Angiography may detect the site of bleeding and, in some cases, determine if the lesion is a diverticulum, a vascular anomaly, or a tumor. In the case of massive bleeding, it must be considered as the gold standard.

The Tc-labeled red blood cell scan (46) is another test potentially helpful for the diagnosis of lower GI bleeding. If an active site of bleeding is seen, it directs the angiographer to the most likely source of bleeding. If subsequent angiography is negative, the radionuclide scan provides a clue for subsequent colonoscopy or surgery. However, radionuclide scans may be normal in up to 70% of patients later documented to have a lower GI source of bleeding (42). Moreover, a positive scan may identify the wrong bleeding source in as many as 30%–50% of bleeding colonic lesions (42). It is thus more reasonable to obtain an arteriography without delay in patients with major lower GI bleeding in whom colonoscopy is unrevealing or cannot be performed.

Treatment of GI bleeding in advanced cancer patients

Massive bleeding

In the patient with advanced cancer who has a life-threatening bleed and presents with bad prognostic factors, resuscitation and investigations are generally not appropriate. A massive hemorrhage is extremely distressing for the patient and his family. If death is not immediate, sedation may be required in order to spare great distress. The benzodiazepine Midazolam can be used in that setting. It can be given subcutaneously, intramuscularly, or intravenously and is effective within second to a few minutes (47). The anxiogenic effect of seeing large amounts of blood can be reduced for patients, family members, and care-givers by the use of dark green (surgical) towels or sheets. When possible, issues regarding resuscitation orders need to be discussed with the patient and family.

Pharmacologic approaches

Antiacid therapy

Pharmacologic approaches to upper GI tract bleeding have been aimed at reducting or neutralizing gastric acid secretion. No single trial has convincingly demonstrated an overall benefit of H_2-receptor antagonists, such as ranitidine, in stopping active bleeding or the prevention of rebleeding. In a meta-analysis of 27 randomized controlled trials that evaluated the use of histamine H_2-antagonists in the management of upper GI hemorrhage in more than 2500 patients, there was no statistically significant decrease in bleeding and only marginally significant decreases in the need for surgery and in the number of deaths (48). There are, however, no specific trials in cancer patients.

The use of proton-pump inhibitors in patients with bleeding peptic ulcers has been evaluated in several trials. In a large, multicenter, placebo-controlled study, Daneshmend and colleagues (49) found that the use of intravenous bolus injections of omeprazole (80 mg intravenously followed by three doses of 40 mg intravenously at 8-hourly intervals, and then 40 mg orally at 12-hourly intervals) had no effect on the outcome of upper GI bleeding. However, after endoscopic treatment of bleeding peptic ulcers, a high-dose infusion of omeprazole (bolus intravenous injection of 80 mg followed by an infusion of 8 mg per hour for 72 hours) reduced the rate of recurrent bleeding, decreased the need for endoscopic retreatment and of blood transfusions, and shortened the length of hospitalization (50).

Somatostatin and octreotide

Somatostatin (ST) and octreotide (OT), its synthetic analogue, are relatively specific splanchnic arterial vasoconstrictors that avoid many of the side-effects of vasopressin (51). Somatostatin analogues have been found to be effective in 80%–100% of patients with bleeding ulcers in randomized controlled studies. However, some studies were negative. The effectiveness of these agents is more evident in the management of variceal bleeding. ST or OT is as affective as sclerotherapy for initial variceal bleeding control (52,53). Therefore, if endoscopic treatment is not feasible or not available, ST/OT should be prescribed to control active variceal bleeding. Generally, a starting dose of 50–100 μg of octreotide given subcutaneously twice daily seems appropriate. The dose should be increased according to the clinical response and seldom needs to exceed 600 μg day^{-1}. Non-selective beta-blockers have no role in acute variceal hemorrhage, but propanolol and similar drugs are useful for the prevention of recurrence (54).

Tranexamic acid

Tranexamic acid (TA) is a synthetic antifibrinolytic agent that acts by blocking the lysine binding sites of plasminogen. This interaction inhibits the conversion of plasminogen into plasmin by tissue plasminogen activator, thereby inihibiting the lysis of fibrin clots (55). Tranexamic acid has been successfully used for the management of GI bleeding from different origins and has also been used as rectal instillation for colonic bleeding (56). The recommended oral dose of TA is 1–1.5 g two to four times daily orally or 10 mg kg^{-1} IV daily (57). The optimal duration of therapy is unknown and no study concerning the prolonged use of these agents has been reported. In the interim, it is suggested that these agents should be continued until clinical symptoms resolve. The most common side-effects of these medications, occurring in about 25% of the cases, include nausea, vomiting, diarrhea and, more rarely, thromboembolic complications (57).

Platelet transfusions

The bleeding time increases linearly as the platelet count falls from 100 000 to 10 000 per μl (58). The frequency and severity of hemorrhage also increase as the platelet count declines below 20 000 per μl (58). A recommended threshold of 20 000 per μl has been proposed for the administration of prophylactic platelet transfusions. However, prophylactic platelets transfusions based on strict cut-off criteria have been criticized (58). In advanced cancer patients, the aim is to control symptoms, and transfusions of platelets should only be considered when symptoms are distressing. Lassauniere proposed some criteria for platelet transfusions in patients with advanced hematologic malignancies (59). These criteria include continous bleeding of the mouth or gums, epistaxis, extensive and painful hematomas, severe headaches or disturbed vision of recent onset, as well as continuous bleeding through the GI, gynecological, or urinary systems. Although specifically reported for patients with hematological malignancies, these criteria may serve as guidelines for thrombocytopenic patients with other malignancies. A single platelet concentrate should increase the peripheral platelet count in a 75 kg recipient by approximately 6000 per μl. The transfusion of 4 to 6 units of platelet concentrates should be adequate to control bleeding in most patients (58). These estimates assume normal splenic pooling. Clinicians with limited palliative care experience tend to prolong the infusions indefinitely. In these cases, the limited role of platelet transfusions should be discussed with the patient and the family. The discontinuation of further transfusions needs to be accompanied by psychological support and the possible occurrence of massive bleeding has to be considered (see above).

Local interventions

Endoscopy

The endoscopic modalities include active methods (laser, electrocoagulation, heater probe), topical or injectable methods (sclerotherapy, tissue glue), or mechanical methods (endoscopic stapling, band ligation).

Modern endoscopic interventional techniques have greatly reduced the number of patients requiring surgery for peptic ulcer disease. The aspect of the ulcer at the time of initial endoscopy provides the most reliable prognostic information on the risk of recurrent bleeding. Ulcers may have a clean base, a flat pigmented spot, an adherent clot, oozing, a visible vessel, or an actively bleeding vessel. A clean base is a factor of good prognosis, whereas rebleeding occurs in approximately 85–100% of untreated patients with visible vessels (60–65).

The data concerning the effectiveness of endoscopic hemotasis of bleeding upper GI tumors are controversial. In the survey of Loftus *et al.* (66) at the Mayo Clinic, endoscopy therapy for patients with major bleeding from advanced gastroduodenal malignant lesions seemed to provide limited benefit: the endoscopic hemostasis rate was 67%, with rebleeding rate of 80% in patients with initially successful endoscopic hemostasis. Moreover, the endoscopy-related mortality was 6%. In opposition, in the survey of Savides (8), the endoscopic hemostasis rate of 100% and the rebleeding rate of 33% are much more encouraging.

The management of bleeding from esophageal or gastric varices consists of sclerotherapy, glue injections, variceal ligation and the use of somatostatin and its synthetic analogue, octreotide. Post-systemic gradient is the most reliable predictor of future variceal hemorrhage, but an indirect sign is variceal size. Endoscopic sclerotherapy (ES) or glue injection is performed by injecting a sclerosing agent via a needle passed through the endoscope into a bleeding varix and is a widely accepted treatment for acutely bleeding esophageal varices. ES will control acute hemorrhage in 75%–95% of cases (67). Endoscopic variceal ligation (EVL) or banding consists of the endoscopic ensnaring of esophageal varices with elastic bands. A meta-analysis (36) combined the results obtained in 547 patients from seven studies comparing ES with EVL and demonstrated that EVL better reduced the bleeding rate, the mortality rate, and mortality secondary to bleeding as compared with sclerotherapy. The combination of sclerotherapy and banding did not decrease the rate of rebleeding, number of transfusions or treatments required, or mortality rate (68).

For lower hemorrhage, colonoscopy may occasionally permit the definitive treatment of some identified lesions by heater probe, injection therapy, laser photocoagulation, electrocautery, or snare cautery. If vision if obscured by blood, angiography may be needed (69).

Embolization

When endoscopy is not feasible or is a technical failure, diagnostic angiography is the next logical procedure to demonstrate the bleeding site. Angiography should be undertaken as soon as possible as active bleeding provides the best chance for arteriography to demonstrate the site of extravasation. Transfemoral catheterization is most often used and then examination should include selective studies of the coeliac axis, the left gastric artery, and the gastroduodenal artery (70). The preferred emboli material for most GI bleeding sources consists of gelfoam particules. Gelfoam embolization is carried out until the area is occluded and extravasation is no longer detectable. The procedure is generally well tolerated and requires only mild sedation. Limiting factors include the availability of radiologists with appropriate expertise and skills and the presence of bleeding disorders. Embolization is obviously restricted to areas where the catheter can be easily guided into a blood vessel and where embolization of such a blood vessel does not result in devastating adverse consequences.

Radiotherapy

There are few data on the success of radiotherapy to control tumor-induced bleeding from the upper GI tract. In the case of rectal carcinoma, an overall response rate of 85% with a complete control rate of 63% has been reported after palliative irradiation (71).

Surgical methods

Surgical intervention in the context of GI bleeding in an advanced cancer patient is rarely appropriate and must be considered only if other measures have failed and if the patient continues to bleed. If transfusion requirement exceeds four units in the first 24 hours, there is a 50% chance that operation will have to be considered (44,69).

The decision to perform a surgical intervention needs, however, to be individualized. The specific needs and hopes of the patient and family, including the level of distress, and life expectancy have to be taken into account.

Prognosis

The prognosis of GI bleeding depends on many factors including host factors, patient course, and endoscopic findings (72).

Factors that increase morbidity and mortality include: age greater than 60 years; bad performance status; underlying co-morbidity such as pulmonary disease, liver disease, renal disease, encephalopathy or cancer; physiologic stress from major surgery, trauma or sepsis; coexisting disease in three organ systems; low hematocrit, melena or hematochezia; and prolonged prothrombin time. Patients with advanced cancer most often present several of these poor prognosis factors. This explains why the mortality rate after GI bleeding in this setting is so high [10/18 patients in the survey of Mercadante (1)].

Whereas patients with brown stool and a clear nasogastric aspirate have 5%–8% mortality rate, patients presenting with bright red blood per rectum and a bloody or 'coffee ground' nasogastric aspirate have about a 30% mortality rate (73).

Hematochezia usually is a manifestation of a lower GI source of bleeding and may reflect either a major or minor bleeding episode. If hematochezia is from an upper GI source, it reflects major bleeding, with attendent hemodynamic intability and often poor prognosis. Most lower GI bleeding episodes are, however, self-limited and not severe. Shock is less likely than for upper GI bleeding (19% versus 35%, respectively 69).

Conclusion

GI bleeding, although relatively uncommon in patients with advanced cancer, presents a significant stress for the patient, the family, and the care-givers. The causes of GI bleeding are quite similar to those encountered in the general population, but the multiple poor risk factors often presented in the advanced cancer patient lower the chances of therapeutic success. The management of GI hemorrhage starts with a precise assessment of the severity of the bleeding, followed by the identification of its source and review of the different prognostic factors.

We propose an algorithm for the management of GI bleeding (Figure 14.1) but the treatment always requires an individualized approach which recognizes the specific needs of the patient and family, including the level of distress, stage of disease, as well as the available expertise.

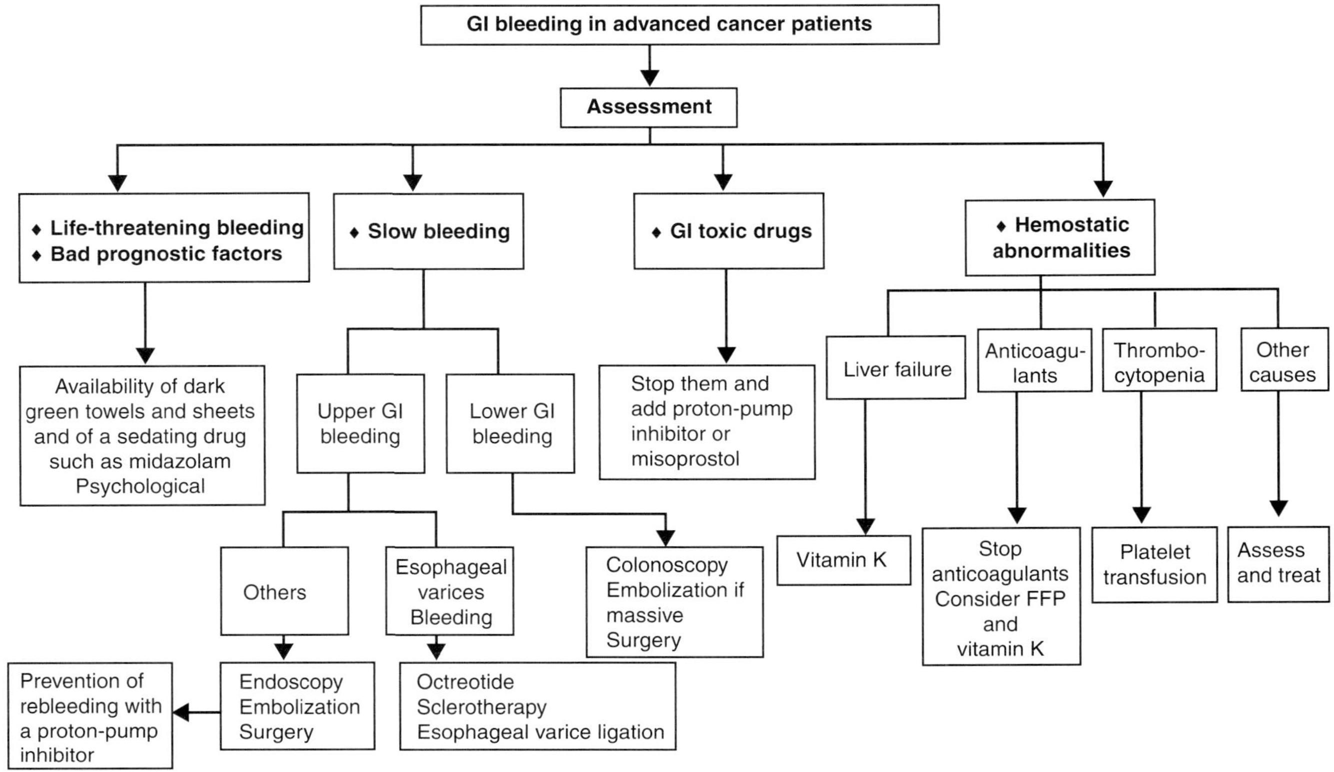

Figure 14.1 Algorithm for the management of GI bleeding in advanced cancer patients.

References

1. **Mercadante S; Barresi L; Casuccio A; Fulfaro F.** Gastrointestinal bleeding in advanced cancer patients. *Journal of Pain and Symptom Management* 2000;19:160–2.
2. **Longstreth GF.** Epidemiology of hospitalization for acute upper gastrointestinal hemmorrhage: a population-based study. *American Journal of Gastroenterology* 1995;90:206–10.
3. **Laine L.** Acute and chronic gastrointestinal bleeding. In: Feldman M; Scharschmidt B; Sleisenger M. editors. *Gastrointestinal and Liver Disease.* Philadelphia: WB Saunders, 1993; pp. 198–217.
4. **Van Dam J; Brugge W.** Endoscopy of the upper gastrointestinal tract. *New England Journal of Medicine* 1999;341:1738–48.
5. **Burnett DA; Rikkers LF.** Nonoperative emergency treatment of variceal hemorrhage. *Surgical Clinics of North America* 1990;70:291–306.
6. **Fleischer D.** Etiology and prevalence of severe persistent upper gastrointestinal bleeding. *Gastroenterology* 1983;84:538.
7. **Gilbert DA.** Epidemiology of upper gastrointestinal bleeding. *Gastrointestinal Endoscopy* 1990;36:8–13.
8. **Savides TJ; Jensen DM; Cohen J; Randal GM; Kovacs OG; Pelayo E; Cheng S; Jensen ME; Hsieh HY.** Severe upper gastrointestinal tumor bleeding: endoscopic findings, treatment, and outcome. *Endoscopy* 1996;28:244–8.
9. **Allum WH; Brearley S; Wheatley KE; Dykes W; Keighley MRB.** Acute haemorrhage from gastric malignancy. *British Journal Surgery* 1990;77:19–20.
10. **Cathcart PM; Cathcart RS; Rambo WM.** Management of massive lower GI bleeding. *American Journal of Surgery* 1977;43:217–27.
11. **Behringer GE; Albright N.** Diverticular disease of the colon: A frequent cause of massive rectal bleeding. *American Journal of Surgery* 1973;125:419.
12. **Elta GH.** Approach to the patient with gross gastrointestinal bleeding. In: Yamada T; Alpers DH; Owyana C. editors. *The Textbook of Gastroenterology.* Philadelphia: Lippincott-Raven, 1995;2:685.
13. **James JF; Friedman LS.** Gastrointestinal bleeding in older people. *Gastroenterology Clinics of North America* 2000;29:1–36.
14. **Bona MJ.** Lower gastrointestinal tract bleeding. *Emergency Medicine Clinics of North America* 1996;14:547–56.
15. **Boley J; Dibiase A; Brandt LJ; Sammartano RJ.** Lower intestinal bleeding in the elderly. *American Journal of Surgery* 1979;137:57–64.
16. **Hasegawa DK; Bloomfield CD.** Thrombotic and hemorrhagic manifestations of malignancy. *Oncology Emergencies* 1981;1:281–95.
17. **Hawkins C; Hanks GW.** The Gastroduodenal toxicity of nonsteroidal anti-inflammatory drugs. A review of literature. *Journal of Pain and Symptom Management* 2000;20:140–51.
18. **Maltz GS; Siegel JE; Carson JL.** Hematological management of gastrointestinal bleeding. *Gastroenterology Clinics of North America* 2000;29:169–85.
19. **College of America Pathologists.** Practice parameters for the use of fresh-frozen plasma, cryoprecipitate, and platelets. *Journal of the American Medical Association* 1994;271:777–81.
20. **Jutabha R; Jensen DM.** Management of upper gastrointestinal bleeding in the patient with chronic liver disease. *Medical Clinics of North America* 1996;80:1035.
21. **Pace V.** Use of nonsteroidal anti-inflammatory drugs in cancer. *Palliative Medicine* 1995;9:273–86.
22. **McCarthy DM.** Nonsteroidal anti-inflammatory drugs-induced ulcers: management by traditional therapies. *Gastroenterology* 1989;96:662–74.

23. **Kim JG; Graham DY.** The misoprostal study group: Helicobacter pylori infection and the development of the gastric or duodenal ulcers in arthritic patients receiving chronic NSAIDS therapy. *American Journal of Gastroenterology* 1994;9:203–7.
24. **Walsh J; Peterson W.** The treatment of Helicobacter pylori infection in the management of peptic ulcer disease. *New England Journal of Medicine* 1995;333:984–91.
25. **Hawkins C.** Audit and use of NSAIDs. *The Lancet* 1998;352:658.
26. **Roth SH; Bennett RE; Mitchell CS; Hartman RJ.** Cimetidine therapy in nonsteroidal anti-inflammatory drugs gastropathy: double-blind longterm evaluation. *Archives of Internal Medicine* 1987;147:1798–801.
27. **Ehsanullah RSB; page MC; Tildesly G; Wood JR.** Prevention of gastroduodenal damage induced by nonsteroidal anti-inflammatory drugs: controlled trial of ranitidine. *British Medical Journal* 1988;297:1017–21.
28. **Robinson MG; Griffin JW; Bowers J; Kogan FJ; Kogut DG; Lanza FL; Warner CW.** Effect of ranitidine on gastroduodenal mucosal damage induces by nonsteroidal anti-inflammatory drugs. *Digestive Diseases and Science* 1989;34:423–8.
29. **Raskin JB; White RH; Jaszewki R; Korsten MA; Schubert TT; Fort JG.** Misoprostol and ranitidine in the prevention of NSAID-induced ulcers: a prospective , double blind, multicenter study. *American Journal of Gastroenterology* 1996;91:223–7.
30. **Yeomans ND; Tulassay ZT; Juhasz L; Racz I; Howard JM; Van Rensburg CJ; Swannell AJ; Hawkey CJ.** A comparison of omeprazole with ranitidine for ulcers associated with nonsteroidal anti-inflammatory drugs. *New England Journal of Medicine.* 1998;338:719–26.
31. **Caldwell JR; Roth SH; WWC; Semble EL; Catell DO; Heller MD; Marsh WH.** Sucralfate treatment of nonsteroidal anti-inflammatory drug-induced gastrointestinal symptoms and mucosal. *American Journal of Medicine* 1987;83:74–82.
32. **Hawkey CJ.** Cox-2 inhibitors. *The Lancet* 1999;353:307–14.
33. **Ellershaw JF.** Corticosteroids and peptic ulceration. *Palliative Medicine* 1994;8:313–19.
34. **Wara P; Stodkilde H.** Bleeding pattern before admission as guideline for emergency endoscopy. *Scandinavian Journal of Gastroenterology* 1985;20:72.
35. **Pereira J; Bruera E.** Emergencies in palliative care. In Pereira J; Bruera E. editors. *The Edmonton Aid to Palliative Care.* Edmonton: University of Alberta, 1996; pp.78.
36. **Schnoll-Sussman F; Kurtz R.** Gastrointestinal emergencies in the critically ill cancer patient. *Seminars in Oncology* 2000;27:270–83.
37. **Cotton RB; Hospenthal MT; Waldram RP; Axon AT.** Early endoscopy of oesophagus, stomach and duodenal bulb in patients with hematemesis and melaena. *British Medical Journal* 1973;2:505–9.
38. **Katon RM; Smith FW.** Panendoscopy in the early diagnosis of upper gastrointestinal bleeding. *Gastroenterology* 1973;65:728–34.
39. **Morrisey JF.** Clinical approach to diagnostic endoscopy in patient with upper gastrointestinal bleeding. *Digestive Diseases and Science* 1981;26:6–11.
40. **Keller RT; Logan GM Jr.** Comparison of emergent endoscopy and upper gastrointestinal series radiography in acute upper gastrointestinal hemorrhage. *Gut.* 1976;17:180.
41. **Nusbaum S; Baum S.** Radiographic demonstration of unknown sites of gastrointestinal bleeding. *Surgical Forum* 1963;14:374.
42. **Winzelberg GG; Mc Kuzick KA; Strauss HW; Waltman AC; Greenfield AJ.** Evaluation of gastrointestinal bleeding by red blood cells labelled in vivo with technecium-99m. *Journal of Nuclear Medicine* 1979;20:1080-6.
43. **Bentley DE; Richardson JD.** The role of tagged red blood cell imaging in the localization of gastrointestinal bleeding. *Archives of Surgery* 1991;126:821.

44. **Vernava AM; Moore BA; Longo WE; Johnson FE.** Lower gastrointestinal bleeding. *Diseases of the Colon and Rectum* 1997;40:846–58.
45. **Jensen DM; Machicado GA.** Diagnosis and treatment of severe hematochezia. The role of urgent colonoscopy after purge. *Gastroenterology* 1988;95:1569–74.
46. **Billingham RP.** The conundrum of lower gastrointestinal bleeding. *Surgical Clinics of North America* 1997;77:241–52.
47. **Wright SW; Chudnofsky CR; Dronen SC; Kothari R; Birrer P; Blanton DM; Bruner A.** Comparison of midazolam and diazepam for conscious sedation in the emergency department. *Annals of Emergency Medicine* 1993;22:201–5.
48. **Collins R; Langman M.** Treatment with histamine H2 antagonists in acute upper gastrointestinal hemorrhage. *New England Journal of Medicine* 1985;314:660–6.
49. **Daneshmend TK; Hawken CJ; Langmann MJ; Logan RF; Long RG; Walt RP.** Omeprazole versus placebo for upper gastrointestinal bleeding: randomized double blind controlled trial. *British Medical Journal* 1992;304:143–7.
50. **Lau J; Sung JJ; Lee K; Yung M; Wong S; Wu J; Chang FK; Enders K; You J; Lee CW; Chan A; Chung S.** Effect of intravenous omeprazole on recurrent bleeding after endoscopic treatment on bleeding peptic ulcers. *New England Journal of Medicine* 2000;343:310–16.
51. **Imperiole TF; Terzn LC; Mc Cullough AJ.** A meta-analysis of somatostatin versus vasopressin in the management of acute esophageal variceal hemorrhage. *Gastroenterology* 1995;109:1289–94.
52. **Sung JJ; Chung S; Lai CW; Chang FK; Leung JW; Yung MY; Kassianides C; Li AK.** Octreotide infusion or emergency sclerotherapy for variceal hemorrhage. *The Lancet* 1993;342:637–41.
53. **Besson I; Ingrand P; Person B; Boutroux D; Heresbach D; Bernard P; Hochain P; Larricq J; Gourlaouen A; Ribard D.** Sclerotherapy with or without octreotide for acute vericeal hemorrhage. *New England Journal of Medicine* 1995;333:355–60.
54. **Dagher L; Patch D; Burroughs A.** Management of oesophageal varices. *Hospital Medicine* 2000,61:711–7.
55. **Seto AH; Dunlaps DS.** Tranexamic acid in oncology. *Annals of Pharmacology* 1996;30:868–70.
56. **McElligott E; Quigley C; Hanks GW.** Tranexamic acid and rectal bleeding. *The Lancet* 1991;337:431.
57. **Dean A; Tuffin P.** Fibrinolytic inhibitors for cancer-associated bleeding problems. *Journal of Pain and Symptom Management* 1997;13:20–24.
58. **Rintels PB; Kenney RM; Crowley JP.**Therapeutic support of the patient with thrombocytopenia. *Hematology and Oncology Clinics of North America* 1994;8:1131–57.
59. **Lassauniere JM; Bertolino M; Hunault M; Zittoun R; Verspieren P; Moh-Klaren J; Jaulmes I; Colombat P.** Platelet transfusions in advanced hematological malignancies: a position paper. *Journal of Palliative Care* 1996;12:38–41.
60. **Zimmerman J; Siguencia J; Tsvang E; Beeri R; Arnon.** Predictors of mortality in patients admitted to hospital for acute upper gastrointestinal hemorrhage. *Scandinavian Journal of Gastroenterology* 1995;30:327–31.
61. **Foster DN; Miloszewski KJA; Losowsly MS.** Stigmata of recent hemorrhage in diagnosis and prognosis of upper gastrointestinal bleeding. *British Medical Journal* 1978;1:1173–7.
62. **Griffiths WJ; Neumann DA; Welsh JD.** The visible vessel as an indicator of uncontrolled or recurrent gastrointestinal hemorrhage. *New England Journal of Medicine* 1979;300:1441–3.
63. **Storey DW; Brown SG; Swain CP; Salmon PR; Kirkham JS; Northfield TC.** Endoscopic prediction of recurrent bleeding in peptic ulcers. *New England Journal of Medicine* 1981;305:915–16.
64. **Wara P.** Endoscopic prediction of major rebleeding. A prospective study of stigmata of hemorrhage in bleeding ulcer. *Gastroenterology* 1985;88:1209–14.

65. **Johnson JH.** Endoscopic risk factors for bleeding peptic ulcer. *Gastrointestinal Endoscopy* 1990;36;516–20.

66. **Loftus AV; Alexander GL; Ahlquist DA; Balm RK.** Endoscopic treatment of major bleeding from advanced gastroduodenal malignant lesions. *Mayo Clin Proceedings* 1994;69:736–40.

67. **D'Amico G; Pagliaco L; Bosch J.** The treatment of portal hypertension: A meta-analytic review. *Hepatology* 1995;22:332–54.

68. **Saeed ZA; Steigmann GV; Ramirez FC; Reveille RM; Goff JS; Hepps KS; Cole RA.** Endoscopic variceal ligation is superior to combined ligation and sclerotherapy for esophageal varices: a multicenter prospective randomized trial. *Hepatology* 1997;25:71–4.

69. **Schrock T.** Colonoscopic diagnosis and treatment of lower gastrointestinal bleeding. *Surgical clinics of North America* 1989;69:1309,1325.

70. **Barth KH.** Radiological intervention in upper and lower gastrointestinal bleeding. *Bailliere's Clinical Gastroenterology* 1995;9:53–69.

71. **Hoskin PJ. Radiotherapy in symptom management.** In: Doyle D; Hank GWC. editors. *The Oxford Textbook of Palliative Medicine*, Oxford: Oxford University Press. 1993; pp. 117–27.

72. **Hussain H; Lapin S; Cappel MS.** Clinical scoring systems for determining the prognosis of gastrointestinal bleeding. *Gastroenterology Clinics of North America* 2000;29:445–50.

73. **Silverstein FE; Gilbert DA; Tedesco FJ.**The national ASGE survey on upper gastrointestinal bleeding. *Gastrointestinal Endoscopy* 1981;27:73–93.

Chapter 15

Malignant ascites

Jeremy Keen and Marie Fallon

Introduction

A recently reported survey of physicians involved in the management of malignant ascites produced comments such as 'generally impossible to manage', 'it is a frustrating clinical situation', and 'a practical and effective solution is needed' (1).

This chapter aims to review briefly the pathophysiology of ascites formation in malignant disease and then to examine the prevalence, associated symptoms and, in more detail, the reported methods of clinical management.

The main frustrations in the management of ascites relate to questions such as the role of diuretic therapy, imaging, and the method of paracentesis, each of which remains poorly tested in formal trials. However, new work in the pathophysiology of ascites formation may lead to more individualized and novel methods of management.

Incidence/Prevalence

Statistics for patients receiving specialist palliative care show that problems secondary to the accumulation of malignant ascites are regularly but not frequently encountered. A review of 1000 consecutive admissions to St Columba's Hospice in Edinburgh showed that 3.6% of patients reported symptoms associated with ascites. The characteristics of this group are further examined in Table 15.1.

An alternative method of estimating the significance of the problems associated with ascites in healthcare is to examine incidence rates in the natural history of specific tumour types. The data from St Columba's Hospice are in keeping with other similar reports in that ovarian, breast, and colonic primary tumours are most frequently associated with the accumulation of ascites. The presence of ascites is usually an indicator of advanced disease and, unfortunately, will have been detectable at the time of initial diagnosis in over half of the patients in whom it develops (2). Patients with ovarian cancer, however, have a longer mean survival from the time of development of ascites compared with those with other tumour types (3). This may relate to ascites being a complication of relatively early stage ovarian cancer with an attendant greater likelihood of response to cytotoxic chemotherapy. However, in one study of patients with stage III and IV disease receiving chemotherapy, the presence of ascites at the start of treatment reduced five-year survival from 46% to 5% (4). In another study of debulking surgery for patients with stage IV disease the presence of ascites was the only independent predictive factor for early tumour progression (5).

Table 15.1 Malignant ascites and related symptoms in 1000 consecutive admissions to St Columba's Hospice (1 January 1997–16 October 1999)

Number of admissions with ascites	**36 (3.6%)**
With visceral pain	15 (42% of those with ascites)
With nausea	13 (36%)
With dyspnoea	9 (25%)
With pain, nausea and dyspnoea	3 (8%)

Symptoms

Symptoms requiring palliation relate to increased intra-abdominal pressure, discomfort of the abdominal wall, dyspnoea, anorexia, early satiety, nausea and vomiting, oesophageal reflux, poor mobility, insomnia related to general discomfort, pain in the groins and subcostal regions, and lower limb oedema.

Pathophysiology

The accumulation of ascites is a result of an imbalance in the normal state of influx and efflux of fluid from the peritoneal cavity. The absorption of radio-labelled serum albumin after intra-peritoneal injection has been measured in humans to be 4–5 ml h^{-1} (6). The small volume of fluid normally present in the peritoneal space reflects a slower rate of fluid efflux. Drainage of peritoneal fluid occurs via the lymphatic system with the diaphragmatic lymphatics probably providing the major pathway. A decreased rate of fluid efflux may occur as a result of blockage of the lymphatic system by tumour and this has been shown histologically in association with malignant ascites in animal experiments. In human subjects, one study demonstrated that 32 of 38 patients with malignant ascites showed no lymphatic absorption of radio-labelled sulphur colloid that had been injected into the peritoneum (7). Conversely, 13 of 14 control subjects did demonstrate lymphatic uptake of the colloid.

It is unlikely that a reduced rate of fluid efflux alone is sufficient to cause the accumulation of massive amounts of ascitic fluid. Indeed, the rate of efflux has been shown to increase as ascites accumulates and intra-abdominal pressure increases, possibly up to rates approaching 80 ml h^{-1}.

The rate of fluid influx into the peritoneal space may be increased in malignancy as a result of two distinct mechanisms. Each mechanism will result in ascitic fluid of different biochemical properties which may respond to different modes of treatment.

1. Increased hepatic venous pressure, as an anatomical consequence of multiple hepatic metastases, results in both fluid leakage into the peritoneum from the sinusoids and, via an increased plasma renin concentration, to the retention of salt and water by the kidneys. The ascitic fluid resulting from this mechanism is similar to that seen as a result of cirrhosis and has the properties of a transudate.
2. An exudate, of relatively high protein concentration, may be produced as a result of increased vascular permeability. Tumour neovasculature is thought to be intrinsically leaky allowing extravasation of fluid, which from peritoneal tumour deposits would

contribute to ascites formation. However, it has long been recognized that ascitic fluid also arises from areas of peritoneum unaffected by tumour (8). The permeability of normal microvessels, such as those that line the peritoneal cavity, can be increased by a variety of cytokines including transforming growth factors α and β, vascular permeability factor, and epidermal growth factor (9). These factors may all be secreted by tumour cells and/or inflammatory monocytes and macrophages.

The relative contribution of these two principal mechanisms of ascitic fluid production can be estimated from the calculation of the serum–ascites albumin gradient. This method has proved more accurate in the classification of the underlying cause of ascites than the traditional total protein content with, for example, ascites developing from constrictive pericarditis having a high protein content and bacterial peritonitis producing ascites of low protein content. The serum–ascites gradient is calculated by subtracting the albumin concentration of the ascitic fluid from that within a serum specimen obtained on the same day. The gradient correlates with the portal venous pressure and a value of $\geq 11\,g\,l^{-1}$ is indicative of the presence of portal hypertension (10). This may be of importance in assessing the likelihood of response to diuretic therapy with an aldosterone antagonist.

Several other tests have been proposed to differentiate malignant from other forms of ascites, including ascitic total protein, fibronectin, lactate dehydrogenase, tumour necrosis factor-α, C4, and haptoglobin. However, in a very recent report it is the ascitic fluid : serum ratios of albumin and interleukin-1α that have proved most accurate in distinguishing between malignant (larger ratio) and non-malignant ascites (11). Such diagnostic tests may, of course, be helpful in terms of prognosis and possibly decisions regarding antitumour therapy but not as an aid to decisions about other forms of palliative treatment.

The formation of chylous ascites is a complication of retroperitoneal tumour spread or its treatment and arises either from damage to lymphatic vessels or through obstruction of lymphatic flow through lymph nodes or the pancreas.

Diagnosis

The diagnosis of the presence of ascites in an individual is usually straightforward, relying on relevant clinical history and examination. Where there is doubt, usually with typical symptoms present in a patient with an obese abdomen or with potential bowel obstruction, ultrasound examination can detect as little as 100 ml of free fluid in the peritoneum. Computerized tomography (CT) scanning is equally as accurate but not always as easily available as ultrasound. Plain abdominal X-rays may be helpful not only in excluding signs suggestive of bowel obstruction but also positive signs of ascites such as a 'ground glass' appearance, loss of psoas shadows and organ definition, and increased spacing of intestinal loops.

Clearly, the presence of ascites in a patient with known malignancy cannot always be assumed to be secondary to the presence of intra-abdominal tumour, and other causes, which necessitate specific modalities of treatment, must be excluded.

Treatment

The palliation of all symptoms related to malignant disease follows the same broad principles of totally individualized care based on the best evidence available from larger populations. It is sometimes tempting to manipulate patients into particular protocols or guidelines and lose sight of the individual risk–benefit analyses for certain management plans.

For the relief of symptoms resulting from complications, such as ascites, which reflect tumour activity, specific antitumour therapy should always be considered if only to discount it in most instances. The development of ascites often complicates ovarian carcinoma relatively early in the course of the disease and is, in fact, a presenting feature in a third of all cases. Malik *et al.* (12) demonstrated complete clearance or significant reduction of ascites in 46% of patients with ovarian cancer treated with systemic cytotoxic chemotherapy. Chylous ascites, when associated with retroperitoneal lymphoma and a consequent disruption of normal lymphatic drainage pathways, may be expected to show some response to chemotherapy if it is the first or second line of treatment. Radiotherapy may also have a role in the relief of symptoms of lymphoma.

The success of the intracavitary instillation of a variety of agents in the control of malignant pleural effusions has encouraged a similar approach to the treatment of malignant ascites. There have been numerous small trials and case series reporting the use of radioisotopes, cytotoxics and, more recently, biological agents and response modifiers to reduce ascitic fluid formation (Table 15.2). A recently reported phase II study found that intraperitoneal instillation of the corticosteroid, triamcinolone hexacetonide, resulted in a significant slowing of ascites accumulation (13). The effect was noted particularly in patients with a serum–ascites albumin gradient of $< 11\,g\,l^{-1}$. The authors postulated the effect to have been mediated through a steroid-induced reduction of the secretion

Table 15.2 Intraperitoneal instillation of agents for treatment of peritoneal malignancy and ascites (44,45)

^{198}Au
$^{32}CrPO_4$
^{32}P
Thiotepa
Fluorouracil
Mustine
Bleomycin
Cisplatinum
Carboplatin
Etoposide
Mitomycin C
Quinacrine
Interferon-α
Interferon-β
Tumour necrosis factor
Interleukin-2
Radiolabelled monoclonal antibodies
Metalloproteinase inhibitor (46)
Corynebacterium parvum
OK-432 (extract from *Streptococcus pyogenes*)

of vascular endothelial growth factor (VEGF). VEGF and its role in the control of tumour growth and ascites production has been the subject of several recently published studies. VEGF has been detected in relatively high concentration in malignant ascites and is known to be one of the factors that can increase capillary permeability and thus potentially facilitate ascites production (14,15). Indeed, peritoneal vascular hyperpermeability was markedly reduced in animal experiments by inhibition of VEGF receptor tyrosine kinase activity by a novel oral agent (16).

Octreotide, the somatostatin analogue, has been suggested to have therapeutic potential for a myriad of different disorders, and indeed there has been a small case series demonstrating a reduction in malignant ascites in two of three patients treated (17). The physiological mechanism remains unclear although one other report suggests a benefit to patients with hepatic cirrhosis and ascites (18).

Diuretics

Diuretic therapy remains the mainstay of the treatment of patients with ascites of non-malignant origin, but the role of diuretics in the management of malignant ascites remains controversial. A recent Canadian survey of the management of malignant ascites reported that whilst 98% of physicians used paracentesis only 61% prescribed diuretics and of these one-quarter felt them to be ineffective (1). The rates of response to diuretics in reported studies range from 38% (19) to 86% (20). Theoretically it would be expected that those patients who demonstrate raised plasma renin activity and hence increased sodium and water retention would have a greater likelihood of response to diuretics. These patients are those who tend to demonstrate a serum–ascites albumin gradient of $\geq 11\,g\,l^{-1}$, where ascites is formed exclusively or principally as a result of intrahepatic metastases. A small study of the use of diuretics in patients with ascites and either massive hepatic metastases, 'peritoneal carcinomatosis', or chylous ascites only demonstrated a reduction in estimated ascitic volume in the group with hepatic metastases (21). Each of the three patients in the group with hepatic metastases had raised plasma renin levels, a high serum–ascites albumin gradient, and responded to the aldosterone antagonist, spironolactone. In another small series, 13 of 15 patients with malignant ascites responded to spironolactone therapy (20). Plasma renin levels were measured in only five patients but were raised in each case. There is a significant body of evidence relating to the optimum use of diuretics in ascites secondary to cirrhosis where 90% of patients would be expected to respond to treatment (10). The majority of trials report the use of spironolactone, but given the long half-life of the active metabolites there may be a delay of up to two weeks before the onset of a significant diuresis. The alternative potassium-sparing diuretic, amiloride, has a much faster onset of action which, in combination with a loop diuretic, has shown to be very useful in the treatment of ascites due to hepatic cirrhosis (22). It therefore may be a more appropriate choice for patients with a relatively short prognoses or in whom early prevention of reaccumulation of ascites after paracentesis is desired. The use of a loading dose of spironolactone has not been reported and the usual regime comprises a starting dose of 100 mg as a single daily dose increasing at two to three day intervals to 400 mg if needed and tolerated. Regular girth measurement may be a more appropriate method of monitoring response to treatment than daily weights and accurate fluid balance recordings. The response to diuretics is thought to occur, in part, as a result of a redistribution of fluid within body compartments rather than wholly dependent on a diuresis (23). A faster onset of diuresis can be obtained by the addition of a loop diuretic such as frusemide (40–160 mg) or bumetanide (1–4 mg). One study has reported a rapid initial response to the use of an intravenous infusion of frusemide during the accumulation period of spironolactone therapy (24).

The initiation of spironolactone therapy is not infrequently associated with nausea unrelated to electrolyte imbalance. The most debilitating side-effects, however, relate to intravascular volume depletion and include postural hypotension, uraemia and, in some cases, renal failure. A proportion of patients with advanced cancer have a paraneoplastic autonomic neuropathy and resultant postural hypotension that can be augmented by aggressive diuretic therapy. Hepatic encephalopathy is an additional potential complication of aggressive diuresis in patients with limited residual hepatic function. It is important to monitor the response to diuretics, particularly as treatment may occur in a community setting. If a reduction in abdominal girth is observed, then the dose should be decreased and titrated to a maintenance level to lessen the chance of side-effects.

Paracentesis

Abdominal paracentesis remains the most commonly employed modality of treatment for malignant ascites (1). It affords quick symptomatic relief in a population that often has a relatively short prognosis and for whom diuretic therapy, if effective, may include a significant lag period. The reported techniques and equipment used for the procedure are numerous and, particularly amongst palliative care physicians, appear to allow full expression of their creativity. A recent exchange on an internet site (palliative-medicine@mailbase.as.uk) provided evidence of the individualized approach to paracentesis. The most significant differences related to the cannula or catheter used for puncturing the peritoneum, the rate of ascitic fluid drainage, and the necessity or not of maintenance of intravascular volume with albumin, colloid, or crystalloid infusions.

A study of 35 patients with ascites and ovarian cancer demonstrated a direct correlation between the measured value of intraperitoneal pressure and the severity of symptoms reported (25). Another recent study helps to confirm that raised intra-abdominal pressure and related symptoms can be significantly relieved after drainage of just a 'few litres' over 2 hours (26). The group of patients reported had a mean of 5.3 litres drained over 24 hours but no significant improvement in symptom relief (of those assessed) after 24 hours than after only 2 hours of drainage. Indeed, only dyspnoea (and not discomfort, nausea, or vomiting) was improved significantly more at 72 hours than at 2 hours of ascitic drainage.

Since symptoms can often be relieved by the removal of relatively small volumes of ascites over a short time period this is to be recommended, particularly in the very frail with a limited prognosis. One to two litres of fluid can be removed simply over 30 minutes via a plastic intravenous cannula. The insertion of the cannula is simple and, if used in conjunction with local infiltration of local anaesthetic, is a relatively comfortable procedure. The removal of such a modest volume is unlikely to cause symptomatic hypovolaemia and the use of a small cannula for a short time is highly unlikely to cause local complications.

Clearly, however, ascites will reaccumulate and should a prognosis be more than a few days, then frequent recurrent small volume paracenteses will be required. One case series and two case reports suggest that this can be achieved by a permanent indwelling catheter that allows frequent small volume drainage without the risks of large volume fluid shifts and repeated peritoneal puncture (27–29). However, most clinicians in this situation would give consideration to the less frequent drainage of larger volumes of ascites through some form of catheter. Peritoneal dialysis, suprapubic urinary bladder, and self-retaining nephrostomy catheters have all been described as useful drainage devices.

The catheter or cannula is introduced into the peritoneum after local infiltration with local anaesthetic. The preferred site is at a point one-third of the way along a line drawn from the anterior superior iliac spine to the umbilicus. Care should be taken if there is a history of abdominal surgery, radiation therapy, intra-abdominal tumour masses, or intestinal obstruction, and if there is any doubt as to the localization of fluid an ultrasound scan should be performed. During anaesthetic infiltration the peritoneal cavity is entered and the needle aspirated to confirm the presence of fluid at the chosen location. Care should be taken not to inject any further local anaesthetic/ascites mixture as the needle is withdrawn since this may 'seed' tumour cells into the subcutaneous tissues. If larger catheters are used, premedication with a benzodiazepine, if liver function is adequate, is a kindness. All catheters and cannulae appear prone to blocking and their use is often complicated by pericatheter leakage of ascitic fluid, particularly if this is under high pressure. Ascitic fluid is usually drained into a collection bag, although some report the use of vacuum bottles (30) which effect a rapid but reportedly 'safe' method of drainage.

The rate at which clinicians choose to drain ascitic fluid is very variable. Guidelines that are often followed are those that have been developed for the drainage of ascites arising as a complication of hepatic cirrhosis and portal venous hypertension. Reports of fatal hypotension complicating the rapid removal of large volumes of ascites led to protocols of conservative methods limiting drainage to 500 ml every 4 hours. However, the use of vacuum bottles allows several litres to be removed in a matter of minutes, with apparently few complications, and is reported to be particularly useful in the out-patient clinic or even the patient's home (30). This technique has not been subjected to detailed scrutiny. Most would favour the immediate drainage of approximately 2 litres of fluid to produce rapid relief of symptoms and a reduction in ascitic pressure to lessen the chances of peri-drain leakage. The rate can then be slowed so that a further 5 litres drains over the next 12–24 hours. Blood pressure should be monitored and the intravascular volume replenished by intravenous infusion of either colloid or plasma protein solution should hypotension develop. Patients without peripheral oedema may be particularly prone to hypovolaemia. Patients with cirrhosis who do not respond to diuretics and are treated with paracentesis are often routinely given intravenous albumin or plasma protein solution (6–8 g albumin per litre of ascites drained). After withdrawal of the drain there is a tendency for a continued leakage of fluid from the drain site. Some operators tie a purse string suture around the site, others place a stoma bag over the site until leakage stops, and one group has suggested the application of enbucrilate adhesive to seal the skin (31).

Complications of paracentesis relate mainly to the potential for a relatively rapid shift of fluid between body compartments. One study reported two deaths from hypotension in a series of 109 consecutive paracenteses performed on 43 patients (6). However, procedural complications include bowel perforation, peritonitis, and localized cellulitis surrounding the drain site. One study reported two deaths from peritonitis in a series of 127 paracenteses in 100 patients (6). Infection was a particular problem in a reported case series of patients with permanent implanted drains (27). A recent series of 10 patients treated with tunneled Pleurx catheters recorded no catheter-related infections with a mean catheter survival of 70 days (32). In this series serial serum albumin measurements demonstrated a progressive decline. However, one case report of the use of an implanted peritoneal dialysis catheter reported only one superficial infection in 17 months during which time the patient drained 1000–1500 ml of ascites twice a week (28). Interestingly, this same patient maintained serum albumin levels despite such prolonged and frequent drainage. However, anecdotal experience would suggest that many patients feel extremely tired for several days following paracentesis and both hyponatraemia and a progressive fall in plasma albumin concentration with repeated paracenteses has been recorded in some series. Patients with severely compromised hepatic function are at particular risk of hepatic failure and encephalopathy over the first 24 hours after ascitic drainage.

Peritoneovenous shunting

Potential problems of repeated paracentesis, such as intravascular hypovolaemia, hypoalbuminaemia, infection, and visceral damage, and the expense, discomfort, and inconvenience of repeated hospital admissions, have prompted the development of alternative drainage procedures. Peritoneovenous shunting was established in the mid-1970s (33) and remains the most common procedure performed. However, no randomized controlled trials have been performed comparing peritoneovenous shunting with repeated abdominal paracentesis. Shunting of ascitic fluid into the stomach (34) and urinary bladder (35) have also been reported, but have presented too many technical difficulties to be useful at present.

Two forms of shunt are commonly used, the original Le Veen and the Denver shunt. Both are designed to allow drainage of ascites into the central venous system, usually via the internal jugular or femoral veins. Drainage occurs principally during inspiration when intrathoracic pressure is lowered allowing ascitic flow along a pressure gradient through a one-way valve. The most common reason for shunt failure is lumen occlusion, which appears to occur more frequently during drainage of malignant ascites than cirrhotic ascites (for the control of which these shunts were first described). The Denver shunt has the theoretical advantage of a manual pumping mechanism to facilitate ascitic flow and clearance of debris. However, no statistical difference in the performance of the two shunts could be found in one comparative study (36).

Successful resolution of ascites and symptom relief with the use of peritoneovenous shunts has been reported in between 62% and 77% of patients (19,37,38). One non-controlled study showed, in addition, a maintenance of serum albumin levels in comparison with a progressive decrease in patients treated with repeated paracenteses (19). This same study measured 'quality of life' by a single question and visual analogue scale (VAS) and found a non-significant trend to an improvement with either paracenteses or shunts and no difference between the two methods of drainage. In the previously quoted survey of physicians' practice only 12 of 44 respondents had used peritoneovenous shunts and 7 found them to be useful (1). The apparent reluctance to use this method is probably a result of the significant complication rate of both the operative procedure and the ongoing operation of the shunt. There is a significant operative mortality in patients with malignant ascites quoted as 13% in one of the larger studies (37), although this is less than that associated with the procedure for ascites associated with cirrhosis. Whilst this high mortality rate is in part to be expected in a frail population undergoing a general anaesthetic or even local anaesthetic and sedation, specific procedure-related mortality is more commonly a result of pulmonary oedema. This complication of a sudden increase in fluid volume within the central venous system can be avoided, in part, by removing a proportion of the ascites

[50%–70% quoted in one study (39)] at operation to reduce pressure and hence flow through the shunt. Many centres would still advocate 'intensive' monitoring with central venous pressure lines for the first 24 hours after surgery.

Overall, complication rates of peritoneovenous shunts of between 25% and 50% are reported (19,37,38). The most common complication is shunt occlusion, either, more commonly, from thrombosis of the venous terminal or alternatively from debris in the peritoneal end. Two studies reported alterations in laboratory measurements of coagulation parameters (increased concentration of fibrinogen degradation products) consistent with subclinical disseminated intravascular coagulation (DIC) in all patients with patent shunts (36,40). Indeed, while such findings may be used as surrogate evidence of shunt patency, frank DIC remains a rare complication. The incidence of DIC is greater in patients with shunts and cirrhotic ascites, a difference that may be explained by a higher concentration of plasminogen–activator–inhibitor in malignant ascites with consequently less potential for fibrinolyitic activity (41). The incidence of post-operative DIC can be reduced by removal of a significant proportion of the ascitic volume intraoperatively (40). Other complications include thromboembolism, vena caval thrombosis, hepatic encephalopathy, peritonitis, and tumour seeding to the subcutaneous tissues of the anterior abdominal wall.

The potential effects of the introduction of tumour cells from the peritoneal cavity into the circulation via the shunt has been examined in a small series of *post mortem* examinations (42). The study reported a variety of observations but concluded that metastases, although occurring in some patients as a direct result of shunt placement, are not clinically significant and do not alter prognosis. This is likely to be related to the short prognosis of the majority of patients who develop malignant ascites.

Peritoneovenous shunts are clearly unsuitable for patients with loculated ascites and are not advised if the ascites is haemorrhagic or the patient has poor renal function or a tendency to hepatic encephalopathy. A recently reported series of patients with ascites and non-gynaecological primary tumours showed the best outcomes of peritoneovenous shunts to occur in patients with normal renal function and tumours of non-gastrointestinal primary origin (43). The relatively long survival of patients with ascites and gynaecological malignancies and the potential savings in terms of repeated hospitalizations for paracentesis makes peritoneovenous shunting an option to be at least considered in all cases.

Summary

New studies into the pathophysiology of ascites production in intra-abdominal malignancy hold some promise for the creation of new and specific ways to slow or halt ascitic fluid production. The investigation of the functions of vascular endothelial growth factor and ways in which this may be inhibited are particularly interesting. At present, however, the management of malignant ascites relies upon the use of diuretics, abdominal paracentesis and peritoneovenous shunts (see Table 15.3).

Studies of the intraperitoneal administration of various cytotoxic agents, radioisotopes, and immune/biological response modifiers continue to be reported. Although it is true to say that these trials have mostly been produced from single centres and involve small numbers of patients, this accusation could also be levelled at much of the evidence for the mainstream approaches to ascites management described above. Whilst not wishing to stifle

Table 15.3 Management of malignant ascites

Diuretics
◆ Most effective if serum–ascites albumin gradient is $<11\,g\,l^{-1}$ (correlating with portal hypertension from extensive liver metastases)
◆ Spironolactone is the drug of first choice but often requires high doses and does have a significant lag-time. Loop diuretics will often speed the response and amiloride, as a potentially faster acting aldosterone antagonist, has not been tested in formal trials.
Paracentesis
◆ Most widely used method of managing malignant ascites
◆ Symptomatic relief may be afforded with the removal of a relatively small volume of ascites. This can be performed for patients with a prognosis measured in days with minimal discomfort employing an intravenous cannula and a collection device
◆ For patients with a longer prognosis, recent studies support the safety of larger volumes of ascites drained relatively quickly. There is no consensus as to whether intravenous fluid replacement should be administered and if so whether this should be albumin, colloid, or crystalloid. Additionally, there is no evidence to suggest that the use of albumin can replace losses in the ascitic fluid drained
◆ Recent studies have demonstrated the use of implanted/tunnelled catheters with regular drainage performed by the patient at home. This is an interesting development which, if its safety and acceptability are confirmed in larger studies, should be recommended, avoiding repeated procedures and hospital admissions
Peritoneovenous shunts
◆ Associated with significant morbidity but can potentially reduce the requirement for repeated hospital admissions, particularly if ascites is rapidly recurrent after paracentesis and is diuretic-resistant
◆ Most useful for patients with gynaecological (principally ovarian) malignancies who have a potentially longer prognosis from the time of the development of ascites. Should also be considered for patients with non-gastrointestinal primary tumours and normal renal function
◆ Complications can be significantly reduced if the majority of the ascitic volume is removed at the time of shunt insertion.

creative approaches to the palliation of symptoms associated with malignant ascites, there is an obvious need for multicentre audits and research to identify the safest and most acceptable approaches to management.

References

1. **Lee CW; Bociek G; Faught W.** A survey of practice in management of malignant ascites. *Journal of Pain and Symptom Management* 1998;16(2):96–101.
2. **Garrison RN; Kaelin LD; Galloway RH; Heuser LS.** Malignant ascites. Clinical and experimental observations. *Annals of Surgery* 1986;203(6):644–51.
3. **Parsons SL; Lang MW; Steele RJ.** Malignant ascites: a 2-year review from a teaching hospital. *European Journal of Surgery and Oncology* 1996;22(3):237–9.
4. **Puls LE; Duniho T; Hunter JE; Kryscio R; Blackhurst D; Gallion H.** The prognostic implication of ascites in advanced-stage ovarian cancer. *Gynecologic Oncology* 1996;61:109–12.

5. **Zang RY; Zhang ZY; Cai SM; Li ZT; Chen J; Tang MQ., *et al.*** Cytoreductive surgery for stage IV epithelial ovarian cancer. *Journal of Experimental and Clinical Cancer Research* 1999;18:449–54.
6. **Parsons SL; Watson SA; Steele RJ.** Malignant ascites. *British Journal of Surgery* 1996;83(1):6–14.
7. **Coates G; Bush RS; Aspin N.** A study of ascites using lymphoscintography with 99m Tc-sulphur colloid. *Radiology* 1973;107:577–83.
8. **Hirabayashi KI; Graham J.** Genesis of ascites in ovarian cancer. *American Journal of Obstetrics and Gynecology* 1970;106:492–7.
9. **De Simone GG.** Treatment of malignant ascites. *Progress in Palliative Care* 1999;7(1):10–16.
10. **Runyon BA.** Care of patients with ascites. *New England Journal of Medicine* 1994;330:337–42.
11. **Alexandrakis MG; Moschandrea J; Kyriakou DS; Alexandraki R; Kouroumalis E.** Use of a variety of biological parameters in distinguishing cirrhotic from malignant ascites. *International Journal of Biological Markers* 2001;16(1):45–9.
12. **Malik I; Abubaker S; Rizwana I; Alam F; Rizvi J; Khan A.** Clinical features and management of malignant ascites. *Journal of the Pakistan Medical Association* 1991;41(2):38–40.
13. **Mackey JR; Wood L; Nabholtz J; Jensen J; Venner P.** A phase II trial of triamcinolone hexacetanide for symptomatic recurrent malignant ascites. *Journal of Pain and Symptom management* 2000;19(3):193–9.
14. **Zebrowski BK; Liu W; Ramirez K; Akagi Y; Mills GB; Ellis LM.** Markedly elevated levels of vascular endothelial growth factor in malignant ascites. *Annals of Surgery and Oncology* 1999;6(4):373–8.
15. **Verhuel HM; Hoekman K; Jorna AS; Smit EF; Pinedo HM.** Targeting vascular endothelial growth factor blockade: ascites and pleural effusion formation. *Oncologist* 2000;(5 Suppl. 1):45–50.
16. **Xu L; Yoneda J; Herrera C; Wood J; Killion JJ; Fidler IJ.** Inhibition of malignant ascites and growth of human ovarian carcinoma by oral administration of a potent inhibitor of the vascular endothelial growth factor receptor tyrosine kinases. *International Journal of Oncology* 2000;16(3):445–54.
17. **Cairns W; Malone R.** Octreotide as an agent for the relief of malignant ascites in palliative care patients. *Palliative Medicine* 1999;13(5):429–30.
18. **McCormick PA; Chin J; Greenslade L; Karatapanis S.** Cardiovascular effects of octreotide in patients with hepatic cirrhosis. *Hepatology* 1995;21:1255–60.
19. **Gough IR; Balderson GA.** Malignant ascites. A comparison of peritoneovenous shunting and nonoperative management. *Cancer* 1993;71(7):2377–82.
20. **Greenway B; Johnson PJ; Williams R.** Control of malignant ascites with spironolactone. *British Journal of Surgery* 1982;69(8):441–2.
21. **Pockros PJ; Esrason KT; Nguyen C; Duque J; Woods S.** Mobilization of malignant ascites with diuretics is dependent on ascitic fluid characteristics. *Gastroenterology* 1992;103(4):1302–6.
22. **Senewiratne B; Sherlock S.** Amiloride ('MK 870') in patients with ascites due to cirrhosis of the liver. *The Lancet* 1968;1:120–2.
23. **Twycross RG; Lack SA.** Ascites. In: *Control of Alimentary Symptoms in Far advanced Cancer.* Edinburgh: Churchill Livingstone, 1986: pp. 282–99.
24. **Amiel SA; Blackburn AM; Rubens RD.** Intravenous infusion of frusemide as treatment for ascites in malignant disease. *British Medical Journal* 1984;288:1041.
25. **Gotleib WH; Feldman B; Feldman-Moran O; Zmira N; Kreizer D; Segal Y., *et al.*** Intraperitoneal pressures and clinical parameters of total paracentesis for palliation of symptomatic ascites in ovarian cancer. *Gynecologic Oncology* 1998;71(3):381–5.
26. **McNamara P.** Paracentesis—an effective method of symptom control in the palliative care setting? *Palliative Medicine* 2000;14:62–4.

27. **Belfort MA; Stevens PJ; DeHaek K; Soeters R; Krige JE.** A new approach to the management of malignant ascites; a permanently implanted abdominal drain. *European Journal of Surgery and Oncology* 1990;16(1):47–53.
28. **Bui CDH; Martin CJ; Currow DC.** Effective community palliation of intractable malignant ascites with a permanently implanted abdominal drain. *Journal of Palliative Medicine* 1999;2(3):319–21.
29. **Sabatelli FW; Glassman ML; Kerns SR; Hawkins IF Jr.** Permanent indwelling peritoneal access device for the management of malignant ascites. *Cardiovascular Intervention Radiology* 1994;17(5):292–4.
30. **Moorsom D.** Paracentesis in a home care setting. *Palliative Medicine* 2001;15:169–70.
31. **Blackwell N; Burrows M.** A sticky tip. *Palliative Medicine* 1994;8:256–7.
32. **Richard HM III; Coldwell DM; Boyd-Kranis RL; Murthy R; Van Echo DA.** Pleurx tunneled catheter in the management of malignant ascites. *Journal of Vascular Intervention Radiology* 2001;12(3):373–5.
33. **Le Veen HH; Christoudias G; Moon IP; Luft R; Falk G; Grosberg S.** Peritoneovenous shunting for ascites. *Annals of Surgery* 1974;180:580–90.
34. **Lorentzen T; Sengelov L; Nolsoe CP; Khattar SC; Karstrup S; von der MH.** Ultrasonically guided insertion of a peritoneo-gastric shunt in patients with malignant ascites. *Acta Radiologica* 1995;36(5):481–4.
35. **Stehman FB; Ehrlich CE.** Peritoneo-cystic shunt for malignant ascites. *Gynecologic Oncology* 1984;18(3):402–7.
36. **Edney JA; Hill A; Armstrong D.** Peritoneovenous shunts palliate malignant ascites. *American Journal of Surgery* 1989;158(6):598–601.
37. **Schumacher DL; Saclarides TJ; Staren ED.** Peritoneovenous shunts for palliation of the patient with malignant ascites. *Annals of Surgery and Oncology* 1994;1(5):378–81.
38. **Helzberg JH; Greenberger NJ.** Peritoneovenous shunts in malignant ascites. *Digestive Diseases and Science* 1985;30(11):1104–7.
39. **Holm A; Halpern NB; Aldrete JS.** Peritoneovenous shunt for intractable ascites of hepatic, nephrogenic, and malignant causes. *American Journal of Surgery* 1989;158(2):162–6.
40. **Reinhold RB; Lokich JJ; Tomashefski J; Costtelo P.** Management of malignant ascites with peritoneovenous shunting. *American Journal of Surgery* 1983;145(4):455–7.
41. **Scott-Coombes DM; Whawell SA; Vipond MN; Crnojevic L; Thompson JN.** Fibrinolytic activity of ascites caused by alcoholic cirrhosis and peritoneal malignancy. *Gut* 1993;34(8):1120–2.
42. **Tarin D; Price JE; Kettlewell MG; Souter RG; Vass AC; Crossley B.** Mechanisms of human tumor metastasis studied in patients with peritoneovenous shunts. *Cancer Research* 1984;44(8):3584–92.
43. **Bieligk SC; Calvo BF; Coit DG.** Peritoneovenous shunting for nongynecologic malignant ascites. *Cancer* 2001;91(7):1247–55.
44. **Marincola FM; Schwartzentruber DJ.** Malignant ascites. In: DeVita VT; Hellman S; Rosenburg SA., editors. *Cancer: Principles and Practice of Oncology*. Philadelphia: Lippincott Williams & Wilkins, 2001; pp. 2745–52.
45. **Fentiman I.** Serous infusions. In: *The Oxford Textbook of Oncology*. New York: Oxford University Press, 1995: pp. 2264–76.
46. **Beattie GJ; Smyth JF.** Phase I study of intraperitoneal metalloproteinase inhibitor BB94 in patients with malignant ascites. *Clinical Cancer Research* 1998;4(8):1899–1902.

Chapter 16

Jaundice in gastrointestinal malignancy

Nathan I. Cherny

Introduction

Jaundice among patients with advanced gastrointestinal malignancy is generally caused by obstruction of biliary drainage, extensive hepatocellular failure due to liver infiltration by metastases, or a combination of both. Uncommonly it may be due to co-morbid conditions such as infectious or drug-induced hepatitis.

Liver infiltration by tumor

Jaundice is a common feature of generalized hepatic dysfunction. Jaundice caused by primary liver cancer or intrahepatic metastases, in the absence of evidence of intrahepatic or extrahepatic cholestasis, is a sign of very extensive dysfunction and it is usually accompanied by other features of liver failure. Patients commonly display signs of incipient encephalopathy, ascites, and have evidence of hypoalbuminemia, and laboratory findings of coagulopathy. Ultrasonic or computerized tomography (CT) imaging of the liver usually demonstrates extensive involvement of the liver by metastases.

Gastrointestinal malignancies are especially prone to spread to the liver because of its portal venous drainage. Extra-abdominal tumors such as bronchogenic carcinoma, breast cancer, and malignant melanoma often spread hematogenously to the liver.

Irrespective of the site of origin of the tumor, jaundice associated with extensive tumor infiltration of the liver is a sign of far advanced disease and is an adverse prognostic factor associated with a relatively short anticipated survival (1–5).

The role of antitumor therapies in this setting depends on the likelihood of anticipated response, the performance status of the patient, and the goals of care. Among patients with tumors that are sensitive to systemic therapies (chemotherapy, hormonal therapy, or immunotherapy) occasional patients will achieve a remission with adequate restoration of liver function to facilitate the resolution of jaundice. In patients with unresponsive disease, liver failure ensues with progression until death.

Biliary obstruction

Tumors may obstruct biliary flow within the liver parenchyma, at the porta hepatis or at any point along the common bile duct until the ampulla of Vater. High obstruction at the ductal confluence may be caused by cholangiocarcinoma, gall-bladder carcinoma, or adenopathy in the porta hepatis secondary to a variety of metastases. Obstruction of the common bile duct is most commonly caused by cancer of the head of pancreas, ampullary carcinoma, or less commonly cholangiocarcinoma or gall-bladder carcinoma (6,7). Rarely, rupture of a hepatocellular carcinoma into the common bile duct may cause a fluctuating obstruction by floating tumor debris (8). Intrahepatic obstruction is relatively uncommon, but may be caused by large metastases compressing the major intrahepatic bile ducts.

Clinical evaluation

Clinical evaluation often yields substantial information in the assessment of the cancer patient who presents with jaundice. It is important to ascertain the tumor type and history to date, if known. The presence of pale stools is strongly suggestive of cholestasis. The abdomen is examined for evidence of hepatomegally, ascites, and features of portal hypertension. Patients should undergo a brief mental status examination and neurological examination for evidence of asterixis.

Diagnostic evaluation

Blood tests

The diagnosis of jaundice is confirmed by the finding of hyper bilirubinemia. Serum bilirubin concentration in normal adults is less than 1–1.5 mg dl^{-1} and varies directly with bilirubin production and inversely with hepatic bilirubin clearance. A serum bilirubin value of 3 mg dl^{-1} is usually required for jaundice or scleral icterus to be clinically evident.

Other initial studies should include a complete blood cell count as well as liver function tests including the activities of alkaline phosphatase and alanine and aspartate aminotransferases, albumin, and prothrombin time. Both gamma-glutamyl transpeptidase and alkaline phosphatase are typically elevated in patients with cholestasis; the combination of an elevated alkaline phosphatase and normal gamma-glutamyl transpeptidase suggests that the alkaline phosphatase is from bone. Conversely, an isolated elevation of gamma-glutamyl transpeptidase may result from certain drugs (e.g. phenytoin) or alcohol even in the absence of liver disease.

Imaging studies

Imaging studies help to identify the presence or absence of intrahepatic metastases, the presence of intrahepatic or extrahepatic cholestasis, and the site of obstruction if present.

Ultrasound External ultrasound is a non-invasive test that can identify the presence or absence of metastases and determine whether the intrahepatic and/or extrahepatic biliary system is dilated.

Computerized tomography (CT) CT may be preferred when a precise definition of anatomic structure and information about the level of obstruction are desired. Both CT and ultrasound may occasionally fail to identify dilated ducts in obstructed patients with cirrhosis and poorly compliant hepatic parenchyma or in patients with primary sclerosing cholangitis. Conversely, the presence of dilated ducts in a patient who has previously undergone cholecystectomy does not necessarily signify obstruction. CT images should be routinely evaluated by two different window levels in order to maximize lesion detection. A soft tissue window (width of 300–500 Hounsfield units [H]) is used for the initial examination of the liver; this allows for evaluation of the adjacent abdominal architecture. A second setting with a narrow window and a lower width (100–150 H) is then used to evaluate the liver, since this setting increases contrast differences between the normal liver parenchyma and abnormalities.

Endoscopic retrograde cholangiopancreatography (ERCP) or percutaneous transhepatic cholangiography (PTC) If dilated ducts are identified, it is generally appropriate to visualize the biliary tree directly by ERCP or PTC. ERCP involves passing an endoscope into the duodenum, introducing a catheter into the ampulla of Vater, and injecting a contrast medium into the distal common bile duct and/or pancreatic duct.

PTC involves the percutaneous passage of a needle through the hepatic parenchyma and injection of a contrast medium into the proximal biliary tree through a peripheral bile duct. The choice between these two procedures depends on the suspected location of the obstruction (proximal versus distal); the presence of a coagulation disorder or prior gastroduodenal surgery that might preclude, respectively, PTC or ERCP; anticipation of a therapeutic maneuver such as stent placement or endoscopic sphincterotomy; and the availability of skilled personnel.

Management of biliary obstruction

Symptomatic management

Biliary obstruction that is asymptomatic in a patient who has a short life expectancy does not require intervention. In many cases, however, jaundice is associated with symptoms of itch, anorexia, and fatigue. Indeed, studies that have evaluated the quality of life of patients before and after relief of biliary obstruction highlight improvements in itch, anorexia, fatigue, and global well-being (9).

Surgical management

Historically, the approach to obstructive jaundice has been biliary bypass surgery. In an extensive review of the 1965–1980 literature, Sarr and Cameron explored the role of surgical palliation for patients with unresectable pancreas cancer (10). In this collected series of over 8000 patients, in comparison with those who underwent abdominal exploration alone, patients who underwent biliary bypass had a lower operative mortality (19% versus 26%) and longer survival (5.4 months versus 3.5 months). Whether these results reflect therapeutic benefit or simply the selection of better-risk patients for the bigger operation, remains speculative. Nonetheless, in this review, 56%–85% of patients who underwent biliary bypass surgery had some degree of clinical benefit, most notably relief of pruritus, improvement in hepatic function, and return of appetite. In modern studies, the mortality associated with bypass surgery is approximately 2.5% (11–14).

The preferred surgical bypass procedure remains a matter of debate. Bypass procedures include cholecystojejunostomy, choledochoduodenostomy, and a choledocho/hepaticoduodenostomy with jejunal Roux-en-Y reconstruction. Some surgeons have advocated cholecystoenterostomy because it can be performed quickly; however, recurrent jaundice is more common due to obstruction at the cystic duct.

Percutaneous drainage

Percutaneous drainage can be achieved with an internal–external catheter that can drain either externally or internally (15–17). These transhepatic catheters are designed with side holes both above and below the level of obstruction in the biliary tree; the tip of the catheter resides within the bowel, so that bile drains through the catheter across the obstruction and out of the side holes into the duodenum. Even when biliary obstructions are complete, in many instances an interventional radiologist can negotiate through a stricture with a combination of guidewires and catheters under fluoroscopic guidance. With placement of an internally draining catheter, nutrition is improved, and metabolic imbalance no longer becomes an issue. Transhepatic catheters are associated with complications of obstruction, leakage, and infection (18). Usually, transhepatic biliary catheters are routinely changed every 2 months to avoid any chance of obstruction.

Endoscopic biliary stent

Endoscopic placement of biliary endoprostheses overcomes the stigma and care requirement of an external drain. A review in 1990 of the extensive literature describing the results of this technique found that stent placement was successful in 91% of attempts (19). Procedure-related mortality was 1.3%, and the overall incidence of cholangitis, fever, or hemorrhage 20%. The median time before occlusion was 4.6 months. Median survival for stented patients was 4.9 months. Percutaneous insertion can be employed successfully in the majority of the 10%–15% of patients who fail attempts at endoscopic stenting.

There are data to suggest that this is a safer approach than the percutaneous route. In a small, randomized trial that included patients with distal as well as proximal malignant biliary obstruction, endoscopic stent insertion was associated with a lower frequency of complications than percutaneous insertion (20). Although both techniques resulted in cholangitis in approximately 20% of patients, the percutaneous technique was associated with a higher 30-day mortality, attributed to complications resulting from hemorrhage or leakage of bile into the peritoneal cavity or pleural space. In addition, the percutaneous technique resulted in discomfort at the insertion site, not experienced by patients who had endoscopic insertion.

Combined percutaneous–endoscopic procedures have been described for patients in whom endoscopic insertion is unsuccessful (21,22). In this approach, a guidewire and fine-bore catheter are introduced percutaneously, and the biliary tree is decompressed. The guidewire is advanced through the obstruction and into the duodenum. An endoscopist then introduces a stent over the guidewire. Once adequate internal drainage as been achieved, the percutaneously placed guidewire and catheter may be withdrawn.

Multiple prospective controlled trials have compared endoscopic polyethylene or Teflon stent placement with surgical bypass in patients with malignant extrahepatic biliary obstruction (23). The overwhelming majority of patients in these trials had pancreas cancer, although some included patients with bile duct cancer as well. The results of all three studies are quite consistent. The two methods were equally successful in alleviating jaundice, and there was no difference in overall survival. Patients who underwent endoscopic stent placement had a shorter initial hospital stay, but a greater frequency of late complications.

The occlusion of plastic endoprostheses generally is managed with repeat endoscopy and stent replacement. The exchange of endoprostheses may be done as long as duodenal intubation with an adequate endoscope remains possible, but does require a second endoscopy. Early prophylactic stent exchange at 3–6 months has been advocated, but an optimal time has not been defined. In patients whose stents have occluded but who are not candidates for endoscopic replacement, percutaneous stenting may be palliative.

Stent blockage is a major problem with Teflon catheters. Obstruction has been attributed to adherence of bacteria to the wall of the stent, resulting in the production of a biofilm that traps debris and ultimately occludes the lumen (24). Self-expanding metal prostheses were introduced to overcome the problem of occlusion. The most commonly used device, the Wallstent®, consists of a stainless steel mesh that is mounted on a 9 Fr delivery catheter. These metal stents have a larger diameter (8–10 mm) and are not removable. They are introduced into the bile duct enclosed in a sheath which is then retracted enabling the stent to expand against the wall of the bile duct. However, metal stents are also permanent, and much more expensive than plastic.

There are four prospective trials in which patients with biliary obstruction were randomized to stenting with either polyethylene or metal stents (24–27) and one trial in which patients were randomized to percutaneous transhepatic stenting with either plastic or metal stents (28). The results are quite consistent. Successful stent placement is seen in at least 95% of patients, and is independent of stent material. There is no impact of type of stent on survival, but the duration of patency is greater for metal stents, resulting in fewer episodes of cholangitis, and fewer total days in hospital. In contrast to plastic stents, when metal stents become occluded, the occlusion is usually the result of tumor growth invading into the lumen around the wire that makes up the wall of the stent. These occlusions are best managed by insertion of a plastic stent through the occluded metal stent (29).

Special case: obstruction at the bifurcation of the hepatic ducts

Patients with biliary obstruction at the bifurcation of the hepatic ducts present a difficult challenge and there is much controversy as to the importance of establishing drainage of both liver lobes in malignant hilar obstruction. Data from a recent retrospective review of 141 patients indicated that the longest survival was achieved with bilateral drainage, and the worst survival in those with obstruction of both lobes but drainage of only one (30).

Symptomatic management of holestatic pruritus

Pruritus is the major symptom of obstructive jaundice. Pruritus may occur with any type of liver disease but is primarily associated with acute or chronic cholestasis. It has been estimated to occur in 20%–50% of jaundiced patients. The intensity of the pruritus varies from mild to severe. It can be persistent or intermittent, and it may be generalized or localized to specific parts of the body; commonly the soles of the feet and palms of the hands.

The pathogenesis of cholestatic jaundice is complex and multifactorial (31). Indirect evidence suggests that it may be caused, at least in part, by dermal itch receptor stimulation by a bile acid, a bile acid derivative, or some other substance that undergoes enterohepatic circulation. A central mechanism, associated with altered neurotransmission in the brain, has also been imputed based on observations that opioids and serotonin antagonists reduce scratching activity in cholestatic patients.

The management of pruritus in this setting is often difficult and it should involve specific antipruritic therapies along with general supportive measures.

- *Anion exchange resins.* Anion exchange resins, which are given by mouth, bind bile acids and other anionic compounds in the intestine, resulting in increased fecal excretion of bound substances. Thus, they decrease the enterohepatic circulation of bile acids. The most widely administered treatment for the pruritus of cholestasis has been the basic anion exchange resin cholestyramine, but another resin, colestipol, is also available (32,33). The maximum recommended dose of cholestyramine is 16 g per 24 h. The resins should be taken at least 2 hours apart from other medications to ensure adequate absorption of the latter.

- *Antihistamines.* Despite common application in this setting, antihistamines are rarely effective.
- *Phenobarbital.* Phenobarbital may relieve pruritus in individual patients, but its utility has not been supported in controlled trials (34). The barbiturate phenobarbital has sedative effects as well as effects on the liver. This drug non-specifically increases the activity of the hepatic microsomal enzyme system by enzyme induction and it is hypothesized that it may act by enhancing the excretion of pruritogens.
- *Rifampicin.* Rifampicin is another microsomal enzyme inducer. There is conflicting data regarding the efficacy of rifampicin. When effective, the onset of effect is relatively rapid. The usual dose is 300–600 mg day^{-1} in divided oral doses (35). In a double-blind, crossover, randomized, short-term study that included nine patients with primary biliary cirrhosis, rifampicin therapy at doses of 150 mg orally twice a day or 150 mg three times a day in patients with serum bilirubin less than or higher than 3 mg dl^{-1}, respectively, was reported to be associated with amelioration of the pruritus of cholestasis as assessed by a visual analogue scale (VAS) of the perception of pruritus (36).
- *Opioid antagonists.* The observation that intravenous naloxone can reduce cholestsic pruritus (37,38) prompted trials of therapy with orally administered antagonists nalmefene and naltexone. In an open label study of nalmefene 2 mg orally twice a day was associated with a significant subjective amelioration of pruritus, as measured by a VAS of pruritus, and a significant decrease in scratching activity (39). Naltrexone at doses of 50 mg day^{-1} has been studied in a placebo-controlled study of patients with the pruritus of cholestasis without apparent toxicity and with subjective relief of their pruritus as assessed subjectively (40). In a small study, some patients achieved relief with buprenorphine (41).
- *5-HT3 antagonists.* Very limited data from a small placebo-controlled study supports a trial of the 5-HT3 antagonist ondansetrone in the management of cholestatic pruritus (42).
- *Other measures.* In addition to these specific therapies, simple measures have been recommended. Such measures include the use of emollients and mild fragrance-free soaps (e.g. fragrance-free Dove, Basis, Aveeno), less frequent bathing, wearing light clothing, and frequent cutting of fingernails.

References

1. **Jaffe BM; Donegan WL; Watson F; Spratt JS Jr.** Factors influencing survival in patients with untreated hepatic metastases. *Surgery, Gynecology and Obstetrics* 1968;127(1):1–11. (The above reports in MacintoshPCUNIX TextHTML format.)
2. **Fischerman K; Petersen CF; Jensen SL; Christensen KC; Efsen F.** Survival among patients with liver metastases from cancer of the colon and rectum. *Scandinavian Journal of Gastroenterology.* Supplement. 1976;37:111–15.
3. **Bengmark S; Domellof L; Hafstrom L.** The natural history of primary and secondary malignant tumours of the liver. 3. The prognosis for patients with hepatic metastases from pancreatic carcinoma verified by laparotomy. *Digestion* 1970;3(1):56–61.

4. **O'Reilly SM; Richards MA; Rubens RD.** Liver metastases from breast cancer: the relationship between clinical, biochemical and pathological features and survival. *European Journal of Cancer* 1990;26(5):574–7.
5. **Hoe AL; Royle GT; Taylor I.** Breast liver metastases—incidence, diagnosis and outcome. Comments. *Journal of the Royal Society of Medicine* 1991;84(12):714–16.
6. **Holzinger F; Schilling M; Z'Graggen K; Stain S; Baer HU.** Carcinoma of the cystic duct leading to obstructive jaundice. A case report and review of the literature. Comments. *Digestive Surgery* 1998;15(3):273–8.
7. **Hu J; Pi Z; Yu MY; Li Y; Xiong S.** Obstructive jaundice caused by tumor emboli from hepato-cellular carcinoma. *American Surgeon* 1999;65(5):406–10.
8. **Chen MF; Jan YY; Jeng LB; Hwang TL; Wang CS; Chen SC.** Obstructive jaundice secondary to ruptured hepatocellular carcinoma into the common bile duct. Surgical experiences of 20 cases. *Cancer* 1994;73(5):1335–40.
9. **Luman W; Cull A; Palmer KR.** Quality of life in patients stented for malignant biliary obstructions. *European Journal of Gastroenterology and Hepatology* 1997;9(5):481–4.
10. **Sarr MG; Cameron JL.** Surgical management of unresectable carcinoma of the pancreas. *Surgery* 1982;91(2):123–33.
11. **Proposito D; Santoro R; Mancini B; Gallina S; Carboni M.** Palliative procedures in the treatment of non-resectable pancreatic tumors. Retrospective study of 294 cases and review of the literature. *Annali Italiani di Chirurgia* 1998;69(2):185–93.
12. **van Wagensveld BA; Coene PP; van Gulik TM; Rauws EA; Obertop H; Gouma DJ.** Outcome of palliative biliary and gastric bypass surgery for pancreatic head carcinoma in 126 patients. Comments. *British Journal of Surgery* 1997;84(10):1402–6.
13. **Shirahatti RG; Alphonso N; Joshi RM; Prasad KV; Wagle PK.** Palliative surgery in malignant obstructive jaundice: prognostic indicators of early mortality. Comments. *Journal of the Royal College of Surgeons of Edinburgh* 1997;42(4):238–43.
14. **Lillemoe KD.** Palliative therapy for pancreatic cancer. *Surgical Oncology Clinics of North America* 1998;7(1):199–216.
15. **Born P; Rosch T; Triptrap A; Frimberger E; Allescher HD; Ott R., *et al.*** Long-term results of percutaneous transhepatic biliary drainage for benign and malignant bile duct strictures. *Scandinavian Journal of Gastroenterology* 1998;33(5):544–9.
16. **Tipaldi L.** A simplified percutaneous hepatogastric drainage technique for malignant biliary obstruction. *Cardiovascular Intervention Radiology* 1995;18(5):333–6.
17. **Gunther RW; Schild H; Thelen M.** Percutaneous transhepatic biliary drainage: experience with 311 procedures. *Cardiovascular Intervention Radiology* 1988;11(2):65–71.
18. **Nomura T; Shirai Y; Hatakeyama K.** Bacteribilia and cholangitis after percutaneous transhepatic biliary drainage for malignant biliary obstruction. *Digestive Diseases and Science* 1999;44(3):542–6.
19. **Naggar E; Krag E; Matzen P.** Endoscopically inserted biliary endoprosthesis in malignant obstructive jaundice. A survey of the literature. *Liver* 1990;10(6):321–4.
20. **Speer AG; Cotton PB; Russell RC; Mason RR; Hatfield AR; Leung JW., *et al.*** Randomised trial of endoscopic versus percutaneous stent insertion in malignant obstructive jaundice. *The Lancet* 1987;2(8550):57–62.
21. **Hall RI; Denyer ME; Chapman AH.** Percutaneous–endoscopic placement of endoprostheses for relief of jaundice caused by inoperable bile duct strictures. *Surgery* 1990;107(2):224–7.
22. **Tsang TK; Crampton AR; Bernstein JR; Ramos SR; Wieland JM.** Percutaneous–endoscopic biliary stent placement. A preliminary report. *Annals of Internal Medicine* 1987;106(3):389–92.
23. **Taylor MC; McLeod RS; Langer B.** Biliary stenting versus bypass surgery for the palliation of malignant distal bile duct obstruction: a meta-analysis. *Liver Transplant* 2000;6(3):302–8.

24. **Huibregtse K; Carr-Locke DL; Cremer M; Domschke W; Fockens P; Foerster E., *et al.*** Biliary stent occlusion—a problem solved with self-expanding metal stents? European Wallstent Study Group. *Endoscopy* 1992;24(5):391–4.

25. **Prat F; Chapat O; Ducot B; Ponchon T; Pelletier G; Fritsch J., *et al.*** A randomized trial of endoscopic drainage methods for inoperable malignant strictures of the common bile duct. Comments. *Gastrointestinal Endoscopy* 1998;47(1):1–7.

26. **Knyrim K; Wagner HJ; Pausch J; Vakil N.** A prospective, randomized, controlled trial of metal stents for malignant obstruction of the common bile duct. *Endoscopy* 1993;25(3):207–12.

27. **Davids PH; Groen AK; Rauws EA; Tytgat GN; Huibregtse K.** Randomised trial of self-expanding metal stents versus polyethylene stents for distal malignant biliary obstruction. Comments. *The Lancet* 1992;340(8834–5):1488–92.

28. **Lammer J; Hausegger KA; Fluckiger F; Winkelbauer FW; Wildling R; Klein GE., *et al.*** Common bile duct obstruction due to malignancy: treatment with plastic versus metal stents. *Radiology* 1996;201(1):167–72.

29. **Kaskarelis IS; Papadaki MG; Papageorgiou GN; Limniati MD; Malliaraki NE; Piperopoulos PN.** Long-term follow-up in patients with malignant biliary obstruction after percutaneous placement of uncovered wallstent endoprostheses. *Acta Radiologica* 1999;40(5):528–33.

30. **Chang WH; Kortan P; Haber GB.** Outcome in patients with bifurcation tumors who undergo unilateral versus bilateral hepatic duct drainage. *Gastrointestinal Endoscopy* 1998;47(5):354–62.

31. **Jones EA; Bergasa NV.** Evolving concepts of the pathogenesis and treatment of the pruritus of cholestasis. *Canadian Journal of Gastroenterology* 2000;14(1):33–40.

32. **Bergasa NV.** The pruritus of cholestasis. *Seminars in Dermatology* 1995;14(4):302–12.

33. **Garden JM; Ostrow JD; Roenigk HH Jr.** Pruritus in hepatic cholestasis. Pathogenesis and therapy. *Archives of Dermatology* 1985;121(11):1415–20.

34. **Laatikainen T.** Effect of cholestyramine and phenobarbital on pruritus and serum bile acid levels in cholestasis of pregnancy. *American Journal of Obstetrics and Gynecology* 1978;132(5):501–6.

35. **Price TJ; Patterson WK; Olver IN.** Rifampicin as treatment for pruritus in malignant cholestasis. *Supportive Care in Cancer* 1998;6(6):533–5.

36. **Ghent CN; Carruthers SG.** Treatment of pruritus in primary biliary cirrhosis with rifampin. Results of a double-blind, crossover, randomized trial. *Gastroenterology* 1988;94(2):488–93.

37. **Terra SG; Tsunoda SM.** Opioid antagonists in the treatment of pruritus from cholestatic liver disease. *Annals of Pharmacotherapeutics* 1998;32(11):1228–30.

38. **Bergasa NV; Talbot TL; Alling DW; Schmitt JM; Walker EC; Baker BL., *et al.*** A controlled trial of naloxone infusions for the pruritus of chronic cholestasis. *Gastroenterology* 1992;102(2):544–9.

39. **Bergasa NV; Schmitt JM; Talbot TL; Alling DW; Swain MG; Turner ML., *et al.*** Open-label trial of oral nalmefene therapy for the pruritus of cholestasis. *Hepatology* 1998;27(3):679–84.

40. **Wolfhagen FH; Sternieri E; Hop WC; Vitale G; Bertolotti M; Van Buuren HR.** Oral naltrexone treatment for cholestatic pruritus: a double-blind, placebo-controlled study. *Gastroenterology* 1997;113(4):1264–9.

41. **Juby LD; Wong VS; Losowsky MS.** Buprenorphine and hepatic pruritus. *British Journal of Clinical Practice* 1994;48(6):331.

42. **Schworer H; Hartmann H; Ramadori G.** Relief of cholestatic pruritus by a novel class of drugs: 5-hydroxytryptamine type 3 (5-HT3) receptor antagonists: effectiveness of ondansetron. *Pain* 1995;61(1):33–7.

Chapter 17

Endoscopic approach in treating gastrointestinal symptoms

Pasquale Spinelli

Introduction

The treatment of the symptoms of a disease has to be done when it is impossible to treat the causes, and is synonymous with the term 'palliation'. Palliation can be divided into (a) *palliative care*, including the general principles of treatment required by the majority of patients with advanced solid tumors and bridging the patient from a specific disease status to the terminal events, and (b) the *control of symptoms*, concerning a former phase in the natural history of the disease, when an acceptable *disease-related quality of life* is at hand.

Following these concepts, the time of palliation should be lengthened, starting the control of symptoms as soon as the disease is classified as an incurable one, and reducing the time of unnecessary anticancer treatments.

When a solid cancer is diagnosed, the disease must be staged, because therapeutic options and prognosis are related to the stage. Since the staging is performed with precise diagnostic procedures, we should be able to separate localized from diffused, and curable from not curable diseases in most cases. We should use all the prognostic possibilities supplied by the most sophisticated diagnostic procedures to single out curable patients as early as possible, avoiding giving anticancer treatments to incurable patients, but treating them for the symptoms they identify.

Before deciding to treat symptoms by themselves we should consider the different curative potents of surgery, radio-, chemo-, immunotherapy, as well as the risk conditions of a particular patient, the side-effects of a particular treatment, the quality of the remaining life, and weigh up the therapeutic procedures with regard to the expected benefits.

Digestive cancers account for about 20% of all diagnosed cancers, and most of them, when advanced, are respond poorly to curative treatments; consequently, patients who do not respond to a cure will need symptomatic, palliative treatments. Gastrointestinal symptoms may be caused by digestive or extradigestive tumors. Most of them affect the digestive cavities and grow into them, occupying space required for digestive functions. The gastrointestinal tract has cavities that function as containers or as canals (the stomach, esophagus, intestine, and biliary and pancreatic tracts). Tumors reduce the spaces and impair the functions of containing and flowing; moreover, by infiltrating and ulcerating the walls of these cavities, tumors generate symptoms and, in particular, they cause hemorrhages, obstructions, perforations, and fistulas.

The most important symptoms of digestive tumors are dysphagia, salivation, vomiting, jaundice, pain, and hemorrhage.

Dysphagia

Dysphagia is defined as an abnormal swallowing; it is the initial symptom of esophageal cancer in 90% of cases, but it may also be caused by compression or infiltration by thyroid or lung tumors, mediastinal lymphomas, or by metastatic involvement of the mediastinum.

Beyond these most common causes, dysphagia in oncologic patients may be due to:

- neurologic reasons, like in cricopharingeal dysphagia due to recurrent nerve palsy by perineural and neural infiltration by tumor tissue; neurological dysphagia may be due also to vagal or sympathetic tumoral infiltration, involvement of the skull base, or brain metastases;
- mucositis by candidosis, bacterial infection, herpes, radiotherapy, or chemotherapy;
- astenia/cachexia.

A patient becomes dysphagic when the diameter of the esophageal lumen is shorter than 14 mm, and often complains of difficulty in swallowing some weeks or months before the diagnosis of esophageal cancer.

When a patient complains of dysphagia, endoscopy is indicated. Esophagoscopy allows us to characterize and to locate a tumor exactly, to measure its length, to appreciate the circular extent and of the residual esophageal lumen (Figure 17.2(a)), and to obtain the histologic confirmation of the clinical diagnosis. Echoendoscopy is extremely useful in determining the level of infiltration of the lesion across the esophageal wall and the eventual presence of metastatic lymph nodes. Infiltration of the wall interrupts the progression of the peristaltic contraction and stops, temporarily or permanently, the progression of food. This interruption is related to the extent of the obstruction and causes different symptoms if it is partial or total: partial obstruction can stop solid food, but allows the passage of liquids; total obstruction, which also stops the flow of liquids, causes liquids to collect above the obstruction and thus the *regurgitation* of undigested material. The capacity of this collection is related with the level of the obstruction, being much larger the closer the lesion is close to the cardia; moreover, total obstruction stops the passage of saliva and causes the onset of another invalidating symptom, namely *salivation*. The patient complaining of salivation is obliged to spit or dribble continuously. These patients are forced to carry large quantities of paper tissues and are deprived of a complete social life. Dysphagia is strictly connected to odynophagia (pain on swallowing), generally caused by inflammation of the esophageal wall or by candidiasis or herpes virus; odynophagia may also cause salivation.

The endoscopic treatment of dysphagia and its consequences has to be done by passing the obstacle that prevents the passage of food: this can be obtained by a nasogastric tube (NGT), by restoring the esophageal lumen by dilation, laser treatment, photodynamic treatment, insertion of a prostheses, or performing a gastrostomy (1). These various options have different indications. The purpose of inserting an NGT is that of feeding with liquid food and is an alternative to a gastrostomy. The indication is restricted to cases in which the stenotic obstacle cannot be dilated more than 4–5 mm; this mainly happens when there is a post-operative or post-radiotherapy fibrotic stenosis that makes a forced dilation dangerous for perforation. The disadvantages of the NGT are of different kinds: the first is esthetic, because the patient is obliged to live with a tube in his nose; the second is functional, because the external surface of the tube adheres strictly to the inner surface of the stenotic tract, and that prevents saliva from being swallowed which causes salivation; the third is sensuous, because introducing food through the tube, the patient is unable to enjoy the taste of food, one of the few pleasant sensations remaining at this stage of life. These disadvantages have to be considered also when planning to perform a gastrostomy, because, apart from the presence of the nasal tube, they are the things most complained about after gastrostomy (2).

Dilation can be performed by pneumatic balloon dilators or by plastic bougies: both can slide along a guide-wire and enlarge the esophageal lumen up to 20 mm, but balloons can also be introduced through the operative channel of the endoscope and guided into the stenotic tract under direct vision. The drawback of dilation is that the stenosis will recur in 1–3 weeks and dilations must be frequently repeated.

Laser treatment aims to reopen the esophageal lumen through the thermal coagulation–destruction of the cancer tissue: power-laser radiation increases the local temperature of the irradiated tissues; the treatment is very precise and safe in appropriate hands and the esophageal lumen can be fully restored to a satisfactory eating function for 4–8 weeks (3).

Photodynamic therapy (PDT), using photosensitizing drugs belonging to the group of porphyrins, activated by light to produce singlet oxygen, and toxic to biological tissue, produces a necrotic effect. Unlike the other procedures performed to allow the passage of food, the necrotic effect of PDT needs 4–8 days to become apparent and the removal of the obstruction lasts for 5–10 weeks (4). Moreover, patients submitted to PDT must avoid direct sunlight for 4–6 weeks because of skin photosensitization (5).

The fate of all these procedures is the recurrence of the obstruction due to the regrowth of the tumor, unless a ***prosthesis*** is inserted after dilating the stenotic tract (6). Plastic and metallic prostheses are available. The plastic ones require a full dilation of the lumen (17 mm to insert a 15 mm prosthesis), unlike the metallic ones that, being expandable, can be introduced through a narrow (7–9 mm) passage, to reach, at the end of the expansion, an internal diameter of 20–22 mm, allowing an optimal and immediate transit for any kind of food (Figure 17.2(b–c)). The insertion of an expandable prosthesis is no more traumatic than a flexible esophagoscopy. The differences between plastic and expandable prostheses are that the plastic ones give rise to a larger number of complications (migration, perforation, obstruction by food impact) whereas the expandable ones are much more expensive, cannot be removed and, being woven as meshes, cannot be used to close fistulas. Recently, covered stents have been manufactured to be used in cases with fistulas, but the possibility of migration is higher than with non-covered stents, particularly when inserted through the cardia.

Prostheses can be obstructed by large morsels or by regrowth of the tumor. The best results are obtained when the prosthesis does not interfere with the mechanism of a sphincter (the pharingo-esophageal or the cardiac sphincter) (7). When the cardiac sphincter is infiltrated by the tumor, and the prosthesis keeps it open, the valvular antireflux mechanism is impaired and the gastric content flows back into the esophagus: the acidic gastric secretion can be responsible of a supraprosthetic esophagitis and this condition causes dysphagia, although the esophagus is still open. However, in patients submitted to gastrectomy or operated on with techniques including vagotomy, in which the gastric environment is alcaline, the reflux through the prosthesis may give rise to an alkaline esophagitis. While in the first group of patients drugs that increase the pH, like proton-pump inhibitors (PPIs), are indicated, in the second group, suffering from an alkaline esophagitis, these drugs worsen the dysphagic symptoms. Consequently, special attention must be paid to the medical treatment of patients with a rebel dysphagia with a patent prosthesis. Special prostheses with antireflux mechanisms have been recently manufactured, but definite results are not yet available. When the pharingo-esophageal sphincter is involved and the insertion of the prosthesis keeps it open, the patient must adapt his swallowing mechanism to this new condition, and that may need some days or weeks to be perfected.

Prostheses are equally used in patients with esophago-cutaneous, esophago-tracheal, esophago-mediastinal, or esophago-pleural *fistulas*. Fistulas can be a result of tumor infiltation or to previous surgery or radiotherapy. Inserting a prosthesis to bypass a fistula allows the restoration of oral feeding and also cures concomitant dermatitis (in cervical fistulas), broncho-pneumonia (in tracheo- and broncho-esophageal fistulas), mediastinitis (in mediastinal fistulas), and pleural effusions (in esophago-pleural fistulas). Obviously, only plastic stents or covered mesh stents can be used with the intention of closing a fistulous passage, because a simple mesh stent would allow the filtration of liquids through the meshes. Covered stents tend to migrate and their application must be carefully evaluated, because an eventual removal may be extremely difficult. If an esophago-tracheal or an esophago-bronchial fistula cannot be treated by inserting a stent into the esophagus (no concomitant stenosis to avoid migration of the stent), the prosthesis can be inserted into the respiratory tract to close the tracheal or the bronchial opening thus avoiding aspiration pneumonia, a frequent cause of death in these patients. Generally, plastic stents are used. The most widely marketed are the Dumon stents, introduced with a rigid tracheo-bronchoscope under general anesthesia. These stents have the advantage of being easily repositioned in the case of migration or can be removed if the fistula closes, as can happen in post-surgical cases.

Bleeding and vomiting

Bleeding and vomiting result mainly from intragastric tumors (8). Polypoid or ulcerated, they may be treated because they produce symptoms linked to the bleeding or to food progression. Malignant ulcerations bleed and produce anemic conditions that speed up the onset of cachexia. To stop the bleeding, endoscopic laser photocoagulation, uni- or multipolar electrocoagulation, cryotherapy, or the injection of sclerosing drugs can be used both for cytoreductive as well as for hemostatic purposes. These treatments are very effective, but the duration of the effect is limited and bleeding usually recurs. The progression of the infiltration of the gastric wall and the presence of polypoid intragastric masses, mainly in the antrum, obstructs the gastric passage and causes gastric distention, nausea and, finally, vomiting. Because all these symptoms are produced by gastric obstruction, they disappear when the obstruction in the stomach is removed after an endoscopic treatment. Duodenal, as well as gastric obstructions can also be treated by performing a translaparoscopic bypass between the gastric body and the first jejunal loop, although expandable prostheses are usable also into the duodenum and into the gastric antrum. The duodenum and the gastric antrum can be obstructed by primary or metastatic tumors. Malignant lymph nodes, pancreatic and ampullary cancers are the most frequent causes of duodenal obstruction. Together with biliary tumors, these conditions are responsible for biliary obstruction and cause malignant jaundice. After the first cannulation of the papilla of Vater performed by Classen *et al.* in 1972 (9) and the resulting operative procedures, jaundice became one of the most important fields of application of the endoscopic techniques.

Malignant jaundice

Malignant jaundice is caused by biliary, pancreatic, or metastatic cancer or by lymphomas obstructing the common bile duct or the hepatic ducts. It is generally concomitant with whitish stools, brown urine, and diffuse itchiness. Pancreatic cancer is the most common cause of malignant biliary obstruction, followed by cholangiocarcinoma, carcinoma of the papilla of Vater, and metastatic tumors. Frequently, when jaundice occurs, the patient has a very advanced disease and palliation of the jaundice is the real purpose of the treatment. The clinical approach and some aspects of endoscopic biliary stenting are addressed in depth in Chapter 16 by Nathan Cherny.

The endoscopic approach has become the palliative treatment of choice, particularly for distal stenoses located at the choledochal level (Figure 17.1(a)). When the obstruction is located into the hepatic hilum, the endoscopic approach is more difficult, but nevertheless palliative treatments other than endoscopic ones (surgical and percutaneous) have a lower success rate and are indicated in the case of failure of the endoscopic procedure (10). Moreover, the endoscopic approach allows a careful inspection of the alimentary tract and particularly of the antro-pyloric and duodenal area: this inspection is useful because of the frequent association of biliary and duodenal obstruction. The insertion of gastro-duodenal prostheses can palliate a concomitant obstruction of the gastric outlet and of the gastro-duodenal passage. To obtain an endoscopic biliary drainage, the obstructed biliary tract must be crossed with a guide-wire introduced through the papilla under endoscopic guidance; a guide-catheter is then passed over it and, lastly, a plastic prosthesis is pushed through the stenotic tract which then allows bile to flow (Figure 17.1(b)).

Plastic stents present the main late complication, consisting of occlusion with biliary sludge; in this case they must be removed and replaced with new ones. This generally happens within 6 months of the introduction. Metallic expandable prostheses, similar to those used in the coronary vessels, in the urethra, and in the tracheo-bronchial tree, have been proposed for the biliary tract. They have a low occlusion and complication rate, are easy to place and can be considered as a permanent procedure in malignant jaundice. The main advantages of the endoscopic approach are the low traumaticity and the immediate effect. In fact, whitish stools become well stained 24–48 hours after the procedure, urine progressively loses its intensive brown color, and itchiness disappears. When endoscopic drainage is impossible, the percutaneous or videolaparoscopic route can be used: the first one allows the insertion of a transhepatic tube, while the second allows a wide exploration of the peritoneal cavity and the performance of a biliodigestive bypass (11). See Figure 17.1.

Constipation

If unexplained, constipation should be clarified. When caused by anticancer chemotherapeutic drugs (mainly vincristine), opioids, metabolic problems like hypokalemia, or global electrolyte imbalances, it is mostly of the adynamic ileus type and is frequently accompanied by generalized abdominal pain. An intestinal obstruction by endoluminal masses or by extraintestinal compressions is more frequently accompanied by colicky pain. A long-standing constipation resistant to common treatments must be managed in an effective way, but the safety of the treatment is compulsory. Endoscopy can help to confirm the diagnosis as well as in treating the distention. These patients are generally submitted to nasogastric

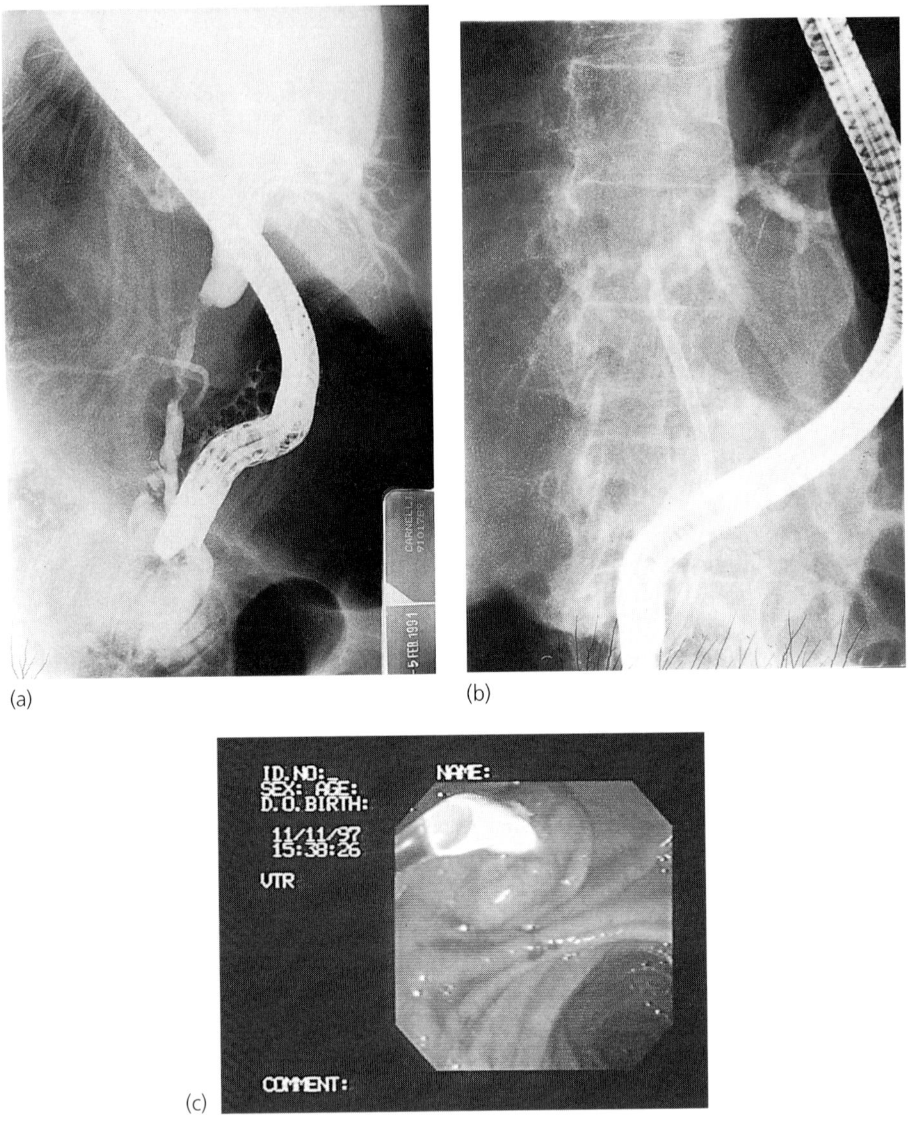

Figure 17.1 Palliation of malignant jaundice. (a) Stenosis of the common bile duct by pancreatic cancer demonstrated by retrograde cholangiography; (b) Biliary endoprothesis; (c) Biliary stent (duodenal view).

intubation for gastroduodenal decompression. A transanal approach might be necessary, so that, after cleaning enemas performed at low pressure, colonoscopy with large-channel endoscopes allows gas and liquids aspiration and deflation of the bowel wall. Colonoscopy must be performed carefully, injecting small quantities of warm water to clean the lumen, taking into consideration that the bowel wall is often very fragile because of concomitant ischemic lesions.

Obstruction

About 10% of intestinal obstructions are caused by malignancies; up to 30% of obstructions result in resolution. More than 60% of malignant obstructions are caused by recurrent cancers. Investigation and treatment in each case is tailored to the individual patient. If a patient, already treated for an intestinal tumor, presents with abdominal distention, vomiting, constipation, and crampy pain, and a plain X-ray of the abdomen shows air–fluid levels and bowel distention, the first choice is endoscopy to locate precisely the cause of the obstruction and to perform, when possible, the first palliative treatment. Indications for surgery are consequent to the endoscopic examination. Surgical procedures can be classified as bowel resections, construction of stomas, or bypass operations. Endoscopic procedures to be considered in the case of obstruction are: dilation, electrocoagulation, laser coagulation, cryotherapy and, lastly, insertion of endoprostheses, all of which are associated with low mortality and morbidity (12). Any treatment has to be performed only in those cases presenting symptoms (obstruction, pain, bleeding) clearly attributable to the tumor. In asymptomatic cases any palliative treatment must be deferred. Patients to be submitted to palliation are those with very advanced and non-removable cancer. They generally present with cachexia and weight loss, and surgical operations carry a high mortality, ±10%, and a survival rate of around 5% at 5 years. Listing the advantages and disadvantages of the different surgical procedures, we must consider, on the one hand, that bypass operations and diverting stomas do not remove the tumor and, consequently, do not alleviate the related symptoms, such as bleeding and pain due to the infiltration of painful structures (peritoneum or periosteum) although surgical procedures will overcome symptoms due to obstruction. On the other hand, morbidity and mortality rates are higher in patients who undergo palliative versus curative surgery.

When only the palliation of symptoms is possible, the purpose of surgery is to bypass the stenotic tract and remove the malignancy, if possible (Figure 17.2). Before acting, some points must be resolved, such as the location of the lesion, its unicity or multiplicity, the degree of the stenosis, the viability of the bowel wall, the real and ultimate cause of symptoms (malignancy, adherences, bands), and the likelihood of spontaneous resolution. The persistance of bowel obstruction has a strong influence on prognostic outcome, and in a multivariate analysis it was the only symptom that had an independent effect. Consequently, it must be managed, and possibly interrupted as soon as possible. After a conventional medical treatment has been established with nasogastric or nasojejunal intubation and intravenous fluids and electrolytes given, and the patient has been monitored with serial physical examinations performed by the same physician, enemas should be performed to clean the colon and a colonoscopy should be made with the purpose of localizing and possibly treating the obstructing lesion. This type of examination must be performed carefully by an experienced endoscopist because of the fragility of the patient and of his intestine, of his hypersensitivity to pain, and of the risk of perforation.

Various endoscopic possibilities of treatment are available, related to the type of obstructing lesion, and in particular its shape, and the bulk occupying the lumen or infiltrating the bowel wall. In the first case, the presence of an obstructing mass, we need first to destroy the mass to re-open the intestinal lumen, and that can be obtained through an endoscopic laser treatment. In the second case, a lesion infiltrating the bowel wall, we can pass a transtenotic guide-wire and slide a dilator on it; once the dilation has been achieved, the emergency

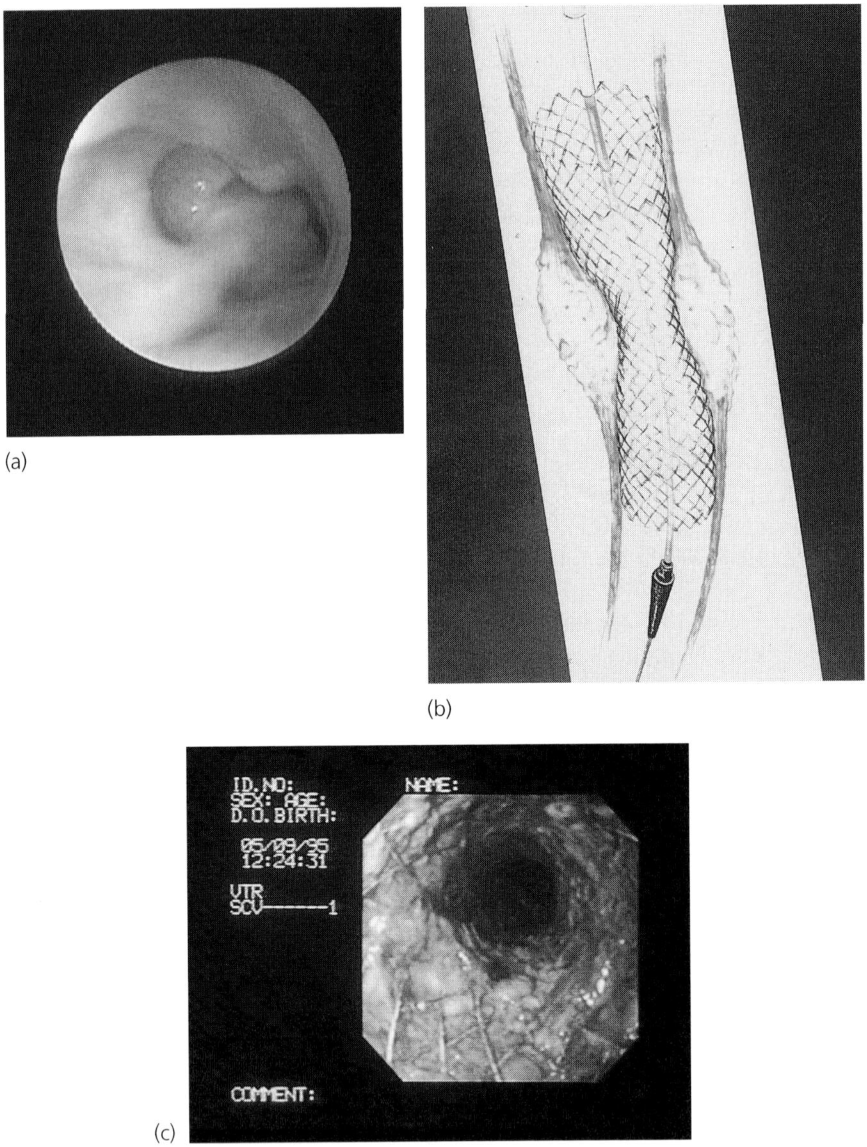

Figure 17.2 Palliation of esophageal cancer. (a) Esophageal stenosis; (b) Expandable prosthesis insertion (scheme); (c) Expandable prosthesis inserted.

problem has been overcome. If the patient is operable, the lesion can be resected or a bypass operation performed through a surgical laparotomic or a laparoscopic procedure to be planned in the following days. If the patient is inoperable for high-risk conditions or because the lesion is not removable, then the endoscopic alternative is the only practicable one. To keep open the intestinal lumen and maintain the bowel functions, an expandable prosthesis must be inserted.

Table 17.1 Symptoms, procedures, and complications in the palliation of GI cancer

Symptoms	Possible endoscopic procedures	Possible complications	%
Dysphagia	Nasogastric tube, gastrostomy	Peritoneal leakage	
	Balloon dilation	Perforation	5
	Laser removal of obstruction	Perforation	1
	Protheses insertion	Perforation	5
	Photodynamic therapy	Photosensitization*	10
Jaundice	Nasobiliary tube	Obstruction–Infection	
	(external drain)		20
	Protheses insertion	Obstruction–Infection	
Constipation/	Transendoscopic lavage		
obstruction	Dilation		
	Electrocoagulation	Perforation	
	Laser coagulation		12
	Cryotherapy	Obstruction/migration	
	Prostheses		

*Can be prevented by avoiding direct sunlight.

The results of the endoscopic treatments can be summarized as follows: dilation by inflatable balloons has a very high percentage of success, ±90%, but stenosis recurs in 1–2 weeks; a similar percentage of success is obtained with a neodimium: YAG laser, but the duration of the results is longer. Inserting a prosthesis with a correct technique and indication allows the large bowel to remain open in more than 80% of treated patients. We started to insert stents in primary rectal tumors and in recurrences of rectal anastomoses about 10 years ago with a success rate of more than 90%. In most of our cases the benefits of the stent last until death (13).

Conclusion

The advantages of endoscopic palliation are:

1 the achievement of an immediate result in the control of symptoms and in the restoration of normal function, whilst other options of palliation, such as radio- and chemotherapy and surgery, are generally more risky and need incomparably longer times to become effective;

2 the absence of contraindications and side-effects, and the possibility of combining endoscopic treatments with other forms of treatment. See Table 17.1.

Palliative treatment in each case should be tailored to the individual patient and some sort of clinical benefit, subject first to the patient's sensitivity and consisting of the removal of symptoms and of an improvement in performance status, should be the primary endpoint.

References

1. **Boyce HW Jr.** Editorial. Stents for palliation of dysphagia due to esophageal cancer. *New England Journal of Medicine* 1993;329:1345–6.
2. **Goodwin WJ; Byers PM.** Nutritional management of head and neck cancer patients. *Medical Clinics of North America* 1993;77:597.
3. **Spinelli P; Dal Fante M; Mancini A.** Endoscopic palliation of malignancies of the upper gastro-intestinal tract using Nd:YAG laser: results and survival in 308 treated patients. *Lasers in Surgery and Medicine* 1991;11:550–5.
4. **Lightdale CJ; Heier SK; Marcon NE., *et al.*** Photodynamic therapy with porfimer sodium versus thermal ablation therapy with Nd:YAG laser for palliation of esophageal cancer: a multicenter randomized trial. *Gastrointestinal Endoscopy* 1995;42:507–12.
5. **Lightdale CJ.** Role of photodynamic therapy in the management of advanced esophageal cancer. *Gastrointestinal Endoscopy Clinics of North America* 2000;10:397–408.
6. **Boyce HW Jr.** Palliation of dysphagia of esophageal cancer by endoscopic lumen restoration techniques. *Cancer Control* 1999;6:73–83.
7. **Spinelli P; Cerrai FG; Meroni E.** Pharingo–esophageal prostheses in malignancies of the cervical esophagus. *Endoscopy* 1991;23:213–14.
8. **Baines MJ.** Symptom control in advanced gastrointestinal cancer. *European Journal of Gastroenterology and Hepatology* 2000;12:375–9.
9. **Classen M; Koch H; Demling L.** Diagnostische Bedeutung des endoscopischen Kontrastdarstellung des Pankreasgangsystems. *Leber Magen Darm* 1972;2:79–81.
10. **Bismuth H; Casting D; Traynor O.** Resection or palliation: priority of surgery in the treatment of hilar cancer. *World Journal of Surgery* 1988;12:39–47.
11. **Costamagna G.** Therapeutic biliary endoscopy. *Endoscopy* 2000;32:209–16.
12. **Spinelli P; Mancini A; Dal Fante M.** Endoscopic treatment of gastrointestinal tumors: Indications and results of laser photocoagulation and photodynamic therapy. *Seminars in Surgical Oncology* 1995;11:307–18.
13. **Spinelli P; Mancini A.** Use of self-expanding metal stents for palliation of rectosigmoid cancer. *Gastrointestinal Endoscopy* 2001;53:203–6.

Chapter 18

Radiotherapy in treating gastrointestinal symptoms

Nora Janjan, Marc Delclos, Matthew Ballo, and Christopher Crane

Introduction

Within this decade 11 million cases of cancer were diagnosed and 5 million people have died from cancer. Over 70% of all cancer patients develop symptoms from either their primary or metastatic disease (1–4). Approximately half the patients diagnosed with cancer will develop metastatic disease. Cancer of the lung, prostate, breast, and rectum constitute more than 50% of all cancer deaths. There is a profound need for expertise in palliative care in oncology. Quality of life is now recognized as an endpoint of secondary importance only to survival (5,6).

The physical symptoms among 350 hospice inpatients with cancer were found to correlate with patient characteristics, general condition, tumor location, and medications. The mean number of symptoms was six on admission and 10 during the course of hospice care (7). The mean number of symptoms correlated directly with the performance status; the performance status was 10–20 with seven symptoms, 30–50 with six symptoms, and ≥60 with four symptoms. Among patients with a performance status of 10–20, anorexia was present in 94%, 47% had edema, and 50% had dyspnea. This is in contrast to patients with a performance status of ≥60 where these symptoms occurred in 29%, 16%, and 10% of cases, respectively. Pain was treated in 65% on admission and in 88% at the time of death.

Barriers to effective pain treatment include lack of assessment, patient reluctance to report pain and to use analgesics, and physician reluctance to prescribe opioids (8–11). The mean pain score, using a Visual Analogue Scale, where 10 is the worst pain imaginable, was 5.2 among 45 inpatients referred for consulation to the pain service; 56% of patients had pain scores ≥5, and 20% had pain scores ≥8 on presentation. All patients had used opioids previously and 41 were receiving opioids at the time of consultation (8). Within 24 hours of using medical management, the mean pain intensity was 2.7 [$P < 0.05$].

Quality of life measurements have been shown to predict for survival and add to the prognostic information derived from the Karnofsky Performance Status (KPS) and extent of disease. Physical symptoms that include pain, dry mouth, constipation, change in taste, lack of appetite and energy, feeling bloated, nausea, vomiting, weight loss, feeling drowsy or dizzy portend a poorer prognosis (12). Among 208 patients with terminal cancer, the overall median survival was 15 weeks. Shorter survival times were independently associated with the following factors: primary site (lung cancer versus breast and gastrointestinal cancers), liver metastases, co-morbidities, weight loss of greater than 8 kg in the previous 6 months, and clinical estimation of a less than 2 month survival by the treating physician. Laboratory assessments including serum albumin levels of less than $3.5\,\mathrm{dg\,l^{-1}}$, lymphocyte counts of less than 1×10^9 per liter, LDH levels of more than 618 units per liter also were associated with a poor prognosis (13). After these independent factors were accounted for in the analysis, other factors, such as the performance status, symptoms other than nausea and vomiting, tumor burden, and socioeconomic characteristics, did not independently impact on prognosis.

Issues regarding the estimation of prognosis are important to the development of a palliative care plan, and they impact on pain control. A significant proportion of physicians will not prescribe opiate analgesics until it is estimated that patients have less than 6 months to live or if patients fail to respond to palliative radiation therapy (11,14). This results in significant under-treatment of cancer-related pain. First, physicians are often unable correctly to predict prognosis. A review of five studies involving a total of 468 patients who were considered to have less than 6 months to live demonstrated that physicians correctly predicted prognosis about half of the time (range, 22%–70%). In these studies the actual median survival was 3.5 weeks (range 2–5 weeks) as compared with the estimated median survival of 6 weeks (4.5 to 8 weeks) by physicians (15). Secondly, patients should not have to suffer with the symptoms of cancer just because they are considered by their physicians to have more than 6 months to live.

Some of the uncertainties in predicting prognosis were overcome in a project, the Study to Understand Prognoses and Preferences for Outcomes and Risks of Treatments (SUPPORT). This study first retrospectively evaluated and developed a model to predict prognosis based on the outcomes of 4301 patients. The model was then prospectively tested on 4028 patients (16). Once developed, the model to predict prognosis was applied by physicians in 1757 cases to estimate the likelihood that a patient would survive 2 and 6 months. Among the cases analyzed were 406 patients with advanced colon cancer, 764 lung cancer patients, and 594 patients with multiple-organ system failure with malignancy. Using this model, the physician estimates were within 7.5% of the model estimates, the model was always within 3% of the actual survival, and the physicians were within 9% of the actual survival. Although physicians were generally accurate in predicting prognosis, patients with metastatic cancer generally overestimated their survival in this study. However, once patients acknowledged that they had a 10% chance of dying within 6 months, they were much more likely to prefer comfort care to life extension. Despite this and efforts to educate physicians and patients about palliative care options and about end-of-life issues, many patients in this recent study continued to receive ineffective cancer treatments and they died in the hospital.

The four most common cancers—lung, breast, prostate, and colorectal—often present with locally advanced tumors and have high rates of metastatic spread to bone and visceral structures (17–19). When metastases are found also in the lung, liver, and/or central nervous system, the prognosis is especially poor. Prognosis is generally dependent on the site(s) and extent of metastatic disease. After bone metastases are diagnosed, the median survivals are 12 months for breast cancer, 6 months with prostate cancer, and 3 months with lung cancer.

In breast cancer, the median survival rate is 48 months when metastases are confined to the skeletal system, but it decreases to only 9 months if visceral metastases are also present (18,19). In prostate cancer, the distribution of bone metastases has prognostic significance. The rate of survival is significantly longer when the metastases are restricted to the pelvis and lumbar spine, and among patients who respond to salvage hormone therapy (20–22). Any metastatic involvement outside the pelvis and lumbar spine results in lower rates of survival irrespective of response to salvage hormone therapy. A bone scan index (BSI) has been formulated based on the degree of tumor involvement in individual bones. The BSI was then related to known prognostic factors and survival in androgen-independent prostate cancer patients (23). In multiple-variable proportional hazards analyses, only the BSI, age, hemoglobin level, and lactate dehydrogenase level were associated with survival. Survival rates were 18.3 months for a BSI of <1.4%, 15.5 months for a BSI of 1.4%–5.1% and 8.1 months for a BSI >5.1%. The site of the primary disease and the presence of a solitary metastatic site are predictive of a more prolonged survival (12,24–27). The presence and the extent of bone metastases predict for progression of disease to other sites (17–22,28,29). The median length of survival is critical to evaluating response to and determining the appropriate recommendations for palliative therapy.

In this context, palliative cancer treatment usually does not impact on overall survival and it is given to maintain comfort. With palliative care, cancer is treated like a chronic disease in which medical efforts try to prevent or manage the symptoms of the disease. Keeping the goals of palliative care in mind, palliative therapy targets symptomatic areas or areas at risk for incurring morbidity with progressive disease. Therapeutic approaches should be used to provide durable control of symptoms and maintain functional integrity such as surgical stabilization of a pathologic fracture. Cancer symptoms are controlled through the direct treatment of the symptoms (e.g. opioids for pain), and by treating the cancer that is the cause of the symptoms. Curative treatment attempts to render the patient disease-free. Palliative therapy controls symptoms. With palliative cancer therapy the goal is to shrink the tumor as much as possible to reduce symptoms. Ineffective therapies that incur morbidity and cost, and provide little to no palliative benefit, should not be administered.

Most cancer patients present with symptoms. Symptoms must be controlled whether treatment is administered with curative or palliative intent. Control of pain facilitates the administration of palliative therapy. The Joint Commission on Accreditation of Healthcare Organizations (JCAHO) issued a new set of standards for the assessment and management of pain that went into effect on January 1, 2001. These standards include that all patients have the right to appropriate assessment and management of pain, and that patients be taught that pain management is an integral part of their cancer treatment.

Analgesics are critical to the relief of symptoms due to cancer. Palliative treatment that targets the cause of symptoms also provides significant relief of cancer-related symptoms. Radiotherapy is cost-effective when compared with analgesic therapy as the only treatment of cancer-related symptoms. The costs for radiotherapy were evaluated among 66 patients who underwent palliative radiation totaling 30 Gy in 10 fractions (72%) or 20 Gy in 5 fractions. Pain scores decreased about 4 points (0–10 scale) after radiotherapy from a median level of 5.58 before radiation to 1.55 after treatment (30). Likewise, pain with movement decreased 5 points from 7.32 before treatment to 1.94 after treatment. The estimated cost of radiotherapy ranged from $1200 to $2500 per patient. With durable pain relief for 9 months, the estimated cost of analgesics over the same time period would have totaled \$9000–\$36 000. In this study, a brief course of radiation therapy proved to reduce pain significantly and was cost-effective when compared with the continued need for analgesics.

Single fraction radiation has been applied extensively in Europe and is the subject of an Radiation Therapy Oncology Group (RTOG) Bone Metastases trial. Because of convenience, cost-effectiveness, and the ability to re-irradiate it is of significant interest in palliative care. The benefit of cost and convenience with a shorter course of radiation may be lost through the continued need for analgesics if pain relief is incomplete. A cost-effectiveness comparison was conducted among 1171 patients who were randomized to receive either 8 Gy in 1 fraction or 24 Gy × 6 fractions. The two treatment arms were equivalent in terms of palliation including analgesic use (31). However, 25% of the 8 Gy arm required retreatment as compared with 7% in the 24 Gy multifraction arm. A cost analysis showed that the 8 Gy arm cost \$1734 (Euro) as compared with \$2305 (Euro) for the multifraction arm, representing a 25% cost difference. However, when the costs of retreatment were included in the analysis, this cost difference was reduced to only 8%, but an economic advantage continued to exist because of the need for decreased radiotherapy capacity. Many issues must be evaluated before single fraction radiation is advocated, and its use must be considered in the context of multidisciplinary treatment. Close follow-up is needed to determine which patients will require retreatment (32).

In most cases radiation therapy can be given efficiently, with few side-effects, and at low relative cost. Despite documented efficacy and cost-effectiveness, palliative radiation therapy is generally considered to be under-utilized (33,34). Unlike other aspects of cancer therapy, tumor control and survival are not the endpoints of therapeutic success in palliative care. The goal of palliative care is to relieve symptoms effectively and efficiently, with the fewest treatment-related symptoms, and to maintain the maximum quality of life for the duration of the patient's life (2–4,25,35–39). The factors that determine the effectiveness of palliative therapy include the percentage of patients who experience persistent/recurrent symptoms, and if these symptoms can be relieved with other therapeutic modalities (38,40,41).

Radiotherapeutic treatment schedules are influenced by the location of the symptomatic tumor site and prognosis. Palliation constitutes a large part of radiotherapeutic practice. At the M.D. Anderson Cancer Center, about 25% of all radiation treatments were administered with palliative intent. This pattern of practice has been stable over 40 years (42).

Radiation can be used alone, or in combination with other antineoplastic therapies. The symptoms most commonly relieved by radiation are pain, bleeding, and obstruction. A number of clinical, prognostic, and therapeutic factors must be considered to determine the optimal treatment regimen for a course of palliative radiotherapy. The clinical status is accounted for in the treatment set-up and in the number of treatments prescribed. The radiation dose–fractionation schedule and technique also should consider the site and volume irradiated, and the integration of other therapies. Many radiotherapeutic options exist for tumors that cause localized symptoms. Brachytherapy and the application of conformal and intensity modulated radiation therapy can better localize radiation dose and reduce side-effects, especially in a previously irradiated area (43–47).

Issues regarding re-irradiation are especially important in palliative therapy. Experimental data suggest that acute responding tissues recover radiation injury in a few months and can tolerate another full course of radiation therapy. However, there is considerable variability in recovery from radiation among late reacting tissues (48). The heart, bladder, and kidney do not exhibit recovery of any late radiation effects. But the skin, mucosa, lung, and spinal cord do recover subclinical radiation injury. This recovery depends on the organ irradiated, the size of the initial dose of radiation, and the interval between doses of radiation. Clinical correlates exist and limited toxicities have generally been reported with re-irradiation (47).

Radiotherapeutic techniques that localize the radiation dose to the recurrent tumor and limit the dose to the surrounding normal tissues allow the re-irradiation of recurrent tumors. These techniques include brachytherapy, conformal external beam radiation, and intensity modulated radiation therapy. Brachytherapy places radioactive sources adjacent to or into tumor masses. The advantage of brachytherapy is based on the inverse-square law. In this, the radiation dose rapidly decreases as the distance increases from the radiation source. For example, only one-fourth the radiation dose is given to tissues that are located 2 cm away from the radiation source. Brachytherapy sources can be placed either temporarily or permanently within the tumor (49). There is a wide variety of brachytherapy sources and strengths that can be used (see Table 18.1). High-dose-rate brachytherapy places an intense radioactive radiation source adjacent to a tumor for a few minutes. This type of brachytherapy is often used to treat tumors involving the biliary tract, cervix, esophagus, and bronchus. Relief of dysphagia ranges between 70% and 85% in a number of published reports when brachytherapy was used in the treatment of esophageal cancer. A combination of a short course of external beam radiation (30 Gy in 10 fractions) plus high-dose-rate brachytherapy used as a localized radiation boost relieves dysphagia for 3–6 months. Relative contraindications include a tumor length of 10 cm or more, extension to the gastroesophageal junction or cardia, skip lesions, extensive extraesophageal spread, macroscopic regional adenopathy, tracheoesophageal fistula, cervical esophageal involvement, or stenosis that cannot be bypassed (46). Low-dose-rate brachytherapy places a lower energy radiation source either adjacent to (temporary implant) or inside tumors (permanent implant). Temporary implants site within a site, much like a drain, generally for 2–5 days and can deliver 20–50 Gy over that time frame. Sources commonly used for low-dose-rate brachytherapy include iridium-192 for temporary implants, and iodine-125 and gold-198 for permanent implants.

Conformal radiation techniques localize the radiation dose using external beam radiation. Because very low doses of radiation are given through a number of beams, no one area of normal tissues receives a significant dose of radiation. The tumor, though, is given the sum of the radiation from the beams and receives a high dose of radiation. This technique has allowed high doses of radiation to be given to areas like the prostate and has allowed for the re-irradiation of normal tissues. Intensity modulated radiation therapy (IMRT) is a form of conformal external beam radiation that administers radiation even more precisely. For example, with IMRT the center of the tumor may receive 2.20 Gy with each radiation treatment to a total dose of 66 Gy over 30 fractions in 6 weeks. In the plan, the periphery of the tumor may receive 2.00 Gy with each radiation treatment to a total dose of 60 Gy. The normal tissues within 2 cm of the tumor (clinical tumor volume to account for possible microscopic tumor extension) may receive 1.8 Gy with each radiation treatment to a total dose of 54 Gy. Any shape or configuration of radiation dose can be designed with IMRT (Figure 18.1). Because of these factors, this radiotherapeutic tool is extremely helpful for unresectable tumors or tumors that recur in a previously irradiated field.

The symptomatic site becomes more important to the palliative approach than whether it results from locally advanced or metastatic tumor. In general, similar radiation portals are

Table 18.1 Physical properties of radionuclides historically and current used in therapy

Element	Isotope	E_β (spectra or range)* (MeV max)	E_γ(MeV)†	$\bar{E}_\gamma$(MeV)	Exposure Rate Constant‡ (R cm²/b/mCi)
Radium and decay products	^{226}Ra	0.017–3.26	0.047–2.44	0.83	10.27
Radon and decay products	^{222}Rn	0.017–3.26	0.047–2.44	0.83	10.27
Cobalt	^{60}Co	0.313	1.17,1.33	1.25	13.07
Cesium	^{137}Cs	0.514,1.17	0.662	0.662	3.275
Gold	^{198}Au	0.96	0.412-1.0888	0.416	2.376
Tantalum	^{182}Ta	0.18–0.514	0.043-1.453	0.67	6.87
Iridium	^{192}Ir	0.24–0.67	0.136-1.062	0.38	4.69
Iodine	^{131}I	0.35–0.61	0.08–0.637	0.364	–
Iodine	^{125}I	None	0.0355	0.028**	1.403
Strontium	^{90}Sr, ^{90}Y	0.54, 2.27	None	None	–
Phosphorus	^{32}P	1.71	None	None	–

I R cm²/h/mCi = 1.9371×10^{-19} cm²/kg/second/Bq.

* A dash separates the minimum and maximum energies of the β-particles in the spectra. All energies listed are the maximum energy of each particle.

† A dash separates the minimum and maximum energies of the γ-rays in the spectra.

‡‡ For an unfiltered point source with $\delta \geq 11.3$ keV.

§ Assumes narrow beam geometry, a condition usually not found in practical brachytherapy applications.

|| For a filtered source with a wall thickness equivalent to 05 mm 90% Pt-10% Ir.[88]

\# For an unfiltered point source with $\delta \geq 11.3$ keV.[32,33]

** Includes X-rays.

†† Includes filtration and anisotropy inherent in commercially available seeds.[7]

‡‡ Approximate values.

Specific$_\gamma$ Ray Constant‡ (R cm^2/b/mCi)	$T_{1/2}$	HVL§ (water) (cm)	HVL§ (lead) (cm)	Current clinical use	Source form
8.25	1622 y	10.6	1.4	Temporary intracavitary and interstitial for gynecologic disease; other sites	Tubes, Needles
8.25	3.82 d	10.6	1.4	Permanent implants, many sites	Seed
13.07	5.26 y	10.8	1.1	Temporary implant to treat melanomas; other eye disease	Plaque
3.226	30 y	8.2	0.65	Temporary intracavitary and interstitial to treat cervical, uterine, vaginal cancer	Tubes, Needles
2.327	2.7 d	7.0	0.33	Permanent implants, prostate, other sites	Seed
6.71#	115 d	10.0	1.2	Temporary interstitial implants	Wire
4.62#	74.2 d	6.3	0.30	Temporary interstitial implants of head, neck, breast, and other sites	Wire, Seeds
2.2	8.06 d	5.8	0.30	'Swallow' for thyroid therapy	Liquid, Capsule
1.208††	60.25 d	2.0	0.04‡‡	Permanent interstitial implants of prostate, lung, other sites	Seed
–	28.9 y, 64 h	0.15	0.014‡‡	Temporary application for shallow lesions (outpatient treatments)	Plaque
	14.3 d	0.1	0.01‡‡	Injection; sodium-bone, blood diseases; chromic-pleural effusions	Liquid

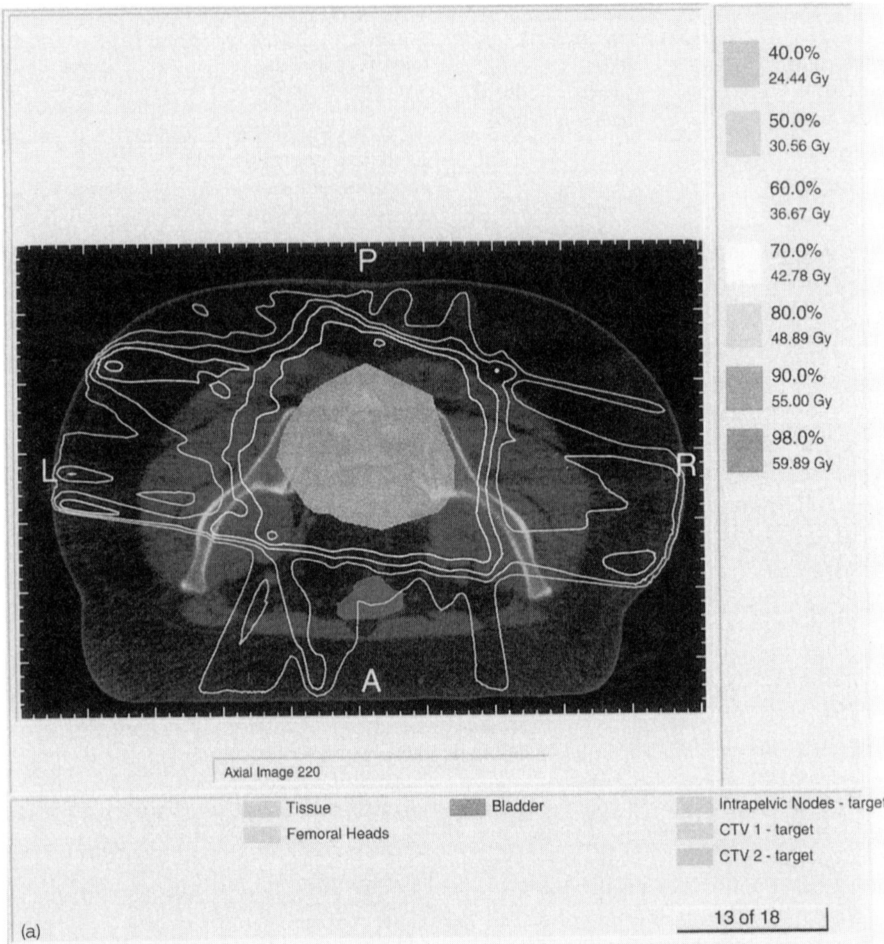

Figure 18.1 (a) IMRT radiation plan that gives 45 Gy/1.8 Gy per fraction over 5 weeks to treat areas at risk for microscopic tumor extension in the pelvis. (b) At the same time a total dose of 55 Gy/2.2 Gy per fraction will be given to the tumor invading the sacral plexus. The dose-volume histogram 9c) shows the distribution of the radiation dose to the tumor or clinical target volume (CTV) and adjacent normal structures.

used to palliate bronchial obstruction due to a primary lung cancer, recurrent breast cancer, or metastatic melenoma. The number of radiation fractions prescribed for treatment with palliative intent depends more on prognosis than primary histology. Common sites palliated by radiation, either alone or in combination with other treatments, include tumor involvement of the lung, pelvis, skin and subcutaneous tissues, brain, and bone. Symptoms resulting from cancer in these sites include pain, bleeding, visceral obstruction, and lymph-vascular obstruction.

The limited radiation tolerance of the normal tissues, like the spinal cord, that are adjacent to a bone metastasis make it impossible to administer a large enough dose of

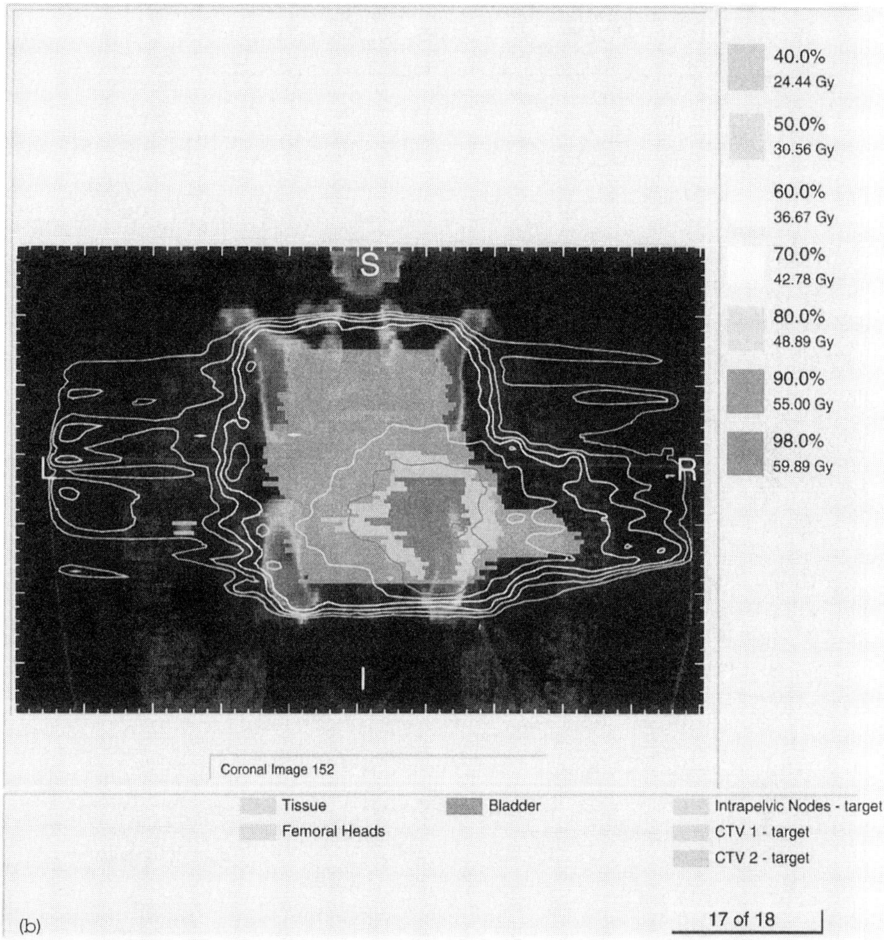

Figure 18.1 (Continued)

radiation to eradicate a measurable volume of tumor. Palliative radiation should result in sufficient tumor regression off critical structures to relieve symptoms for the duration of the patient's life. Control of cancer-related pain with the use of analogesics is imperative to allow comfort during and while awaiting response to therapeutic interventions. Pain represents a sensitive measure of disease activity. Symptoms that recur after palliative radiation most commonly result from localized re-growth of tumor. Close follow-up should be performed after any palliative therapeutic intervention to insure control of cancer and treatment-related pain, and to initiate diagnostic studies to identify progressive or recurrent disease.

Effective palliation of gastrointestinal symptoms requires a clear evaluation of the resectability of the tumor, and of other prognostic factors like the presence and the volume of metastatic disease. Like other aspects of cancer care, a multidisciplinary approach is generally needed for effective palliative care (8,9). Part of the difficulty in determining the best

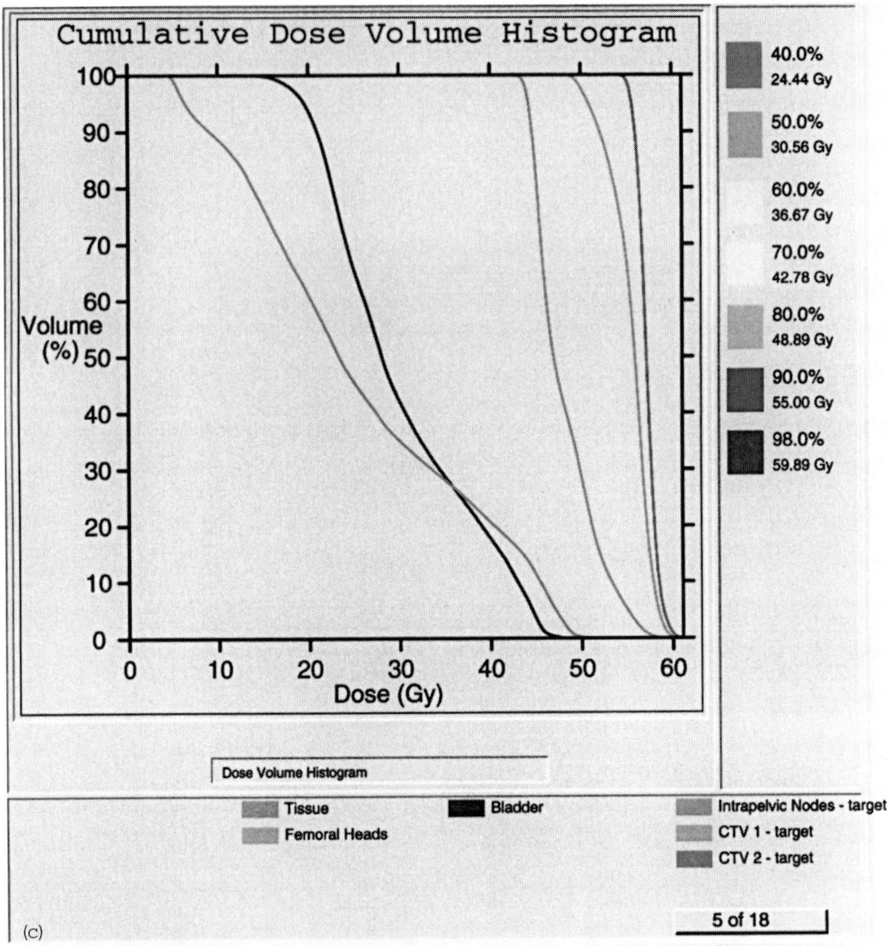

Figure 18.1 (Continued)

multidisciplinary approach relates to the various types of clinical problems that require palliative care. The goal of palliative therapy is the prompt and cost-effective relief of symptoms with little treatment-related morbidity. Symptoms may be caused either from locally advanced tumor involvement or metastatic disease (9). Accounting for these factors allows clinical decisions appropriate to the clinical status and relief of symptoms for the duration of the patient's life.

Palliative radiation treatment schedules

When cure is possible, a high total dose of radiation is administered over 5–7 weeks using a conventional radiation schedule. Conventional radiation schedules administer a radiation dose each day that equals 1.8–2.0 Gy to a total dose of 50 Gy to more than 70 Gy. Conventional radiation can be given with chemotherapy (definitive radiation), pre-operatively, or post-operatively. An example of definitive chemoradiation is the approach used to treat anal cancer. Because chemoradiation is so effective in controlling even locally advanced tumors, surgery is now used only among patients who fail to respond to therapy. Pre-operative radiation is used to shrink a locally advanced primary tumor and often to make an inoperable tumor resectable. The primary role of post-operative radiation therapy is to eradicate residual microscopic tumor cells in the operative bed.

Because patients with inoperable primary disease and/or metastatic disease have a limited life expectancy, palliative radiation is generally given over a shorter period of time. With palliative radiation, a low total dose is given with palliative radiation over 1 to 2 weeks (hypofractionated radiaiton schedule). In contrast to the low daily radiation doses (1.8–2 Gy) given with each treatment during conventional radiation schedules, large daily radiation fractions are given with hypofractionated radiation schedules. There is an inverse relationship between the dose per fraction and the total dose of radiation that can be given. Because of normal tissue tolerance to radiation, the total radiation dose is low when high doses of radiation are given with each fraction. Hypofractionated radiation schedules give high doses of radiation with each fraction and lower total doses of radiation, and they can range from 2.5 Gy per fraction administered over 3 weeks for a total dose of 35 Gy to a single 8 Gy dose of radiation. Most frequently, 30 Gy is administered in 10 fractions over 2 weeks (33,38,50–54). Especially among patients with short life expectancies, many centers administer 20 Gy in 1 week because the rates of pain relief, mobility, and frequency of pathologic fractures are similar to more protracted radiation schedules.

Mathematical relationships exist between the different radiation schedules based on their radiobiological effects on normal tissues. Radiobiologically, a single 8 Gy fraction would give the same side-effects to late reacting tissues as if 18 Gy were given over 9 treatments at 2 Gy per fraction (Bennett). The radiobiologically equivalent dose to the tumor for a single 8 Gy fraction would be 12 Gy if 2 Gy fractions were used. The most common dose fractionation schedule used for palliative radiation in the United States is 30 Gy over 10 fractions. Radiobiologically this is equivalent to 36 Gy at 2 Gy per fraction for late reacting tissues and 32.5 Gy to the tumor.

A shorter radiation schedule is advantageous for patients with poor prognostic factors. Shorter radiation schedules generally administer a higher radiation dose with each radiation fraction. Tumor cell kill is proportional to the radiation dose that is administered. Therefore, symptomatic relief is more quickly achieved because of the large number of tumor cells that are killed in a short period of time. A shorter course of therapy also has a significant impact on quality of life. This short course of treatment not only provides more prompt relief of tumor-related symptoms, but it limits the amount of time needed to come back and forth for radiation treatments. This is particularly important because the median survival is less than 6 months among patients with poor prognostic factors. However, higher radiation doses, which provide more durable pain relief, are considered warranted for patients with good prognostic factors who require treatment over the spine and other critical sites (12,15,16,25,27,38–40,52–59).

The projected length of survival is the critical issue to determine the optimal radiation dose and schedule for palliative radiation. Loosely defined, any course of radiation that relieves symptoms is palliative treatment. More commonly, palliative radiation is designated for patients with incurable disease due to extensive local tumor infiltration and/or metastatic disease. However, symptomatic patients with an extensive primary tumor, but who do not have distant metastases, may still be curable if the tumor is resectable at presentation or after preoperative radiation. Therefore, the radiation schedule that is used to relieve symptoms must be indexed to the potential for tumor resection and overall prognosis.

In one study among patients with bone metastases, only 12 of 245 patients were alive at the time of analysis with approximately 50% alive at 6 months, 25% at 1 year, 8% at 2 years and 3% at 3 years after palliative radiation. For breast cancer patients the survival rates at these time points after palliative radiation were 60%, 44%, 20%, and 7%, respectively. For prostate cancer, the survival rates were 60% at 6 months, 24% at 1 year and there were no patients who survived 2 years (55). In the RTOG trial the median survival for solitary bone metastases was 36 weeks and was 24 weeks for multiple bone metastases (60,61). Significant consideration must be given to patient accessibility, convenience, and cost effectiveness. It is clear that a durable and significant response from radiation, not the schedule of administration, is the key issue in palliative radiation.

Radiation therapy and the treatment of gastrointestinal symptoms

Radiation therapy has three general roles to prevent and to palliate gastrointestinal symptoms. Gastrointestinal symptoms may be caused by a locally advanced tumor or by metastatic disease. First, radiation therapy is used to prevent local recurrence of disease and symptoms by eliminating microscopic residual disease around the primary tumor and in the draining lymphatics. Second, significant tumor regression can result when radiation is administered to locally advanced primary tumors. In these cases, an inoperable symptomatic lesion can become resectable or amenable to a more conservative surgical approach like sphincter preservation for tumors that infiltrate the rectum. Third, radiation therapy can be used to palliate symptoms due to infiltration of visceral structures or metastatic disease to other sites like bone and nerves.

Radiation field arrangement and management of treatment-related side-effects

Careful attention to the technique is important to minimize treatment-related side-effects. Whenever possible, the small bowel should be displaced from the treatment portal. The volume of small bowel in the radiation portal has been shown to directly correlate with radiation toxicity (62). Radiation techniques such as the use of a belly board to displace the small bowel from the radiation portal help to reduce gastrointestinal side-effects (Figure 18.2). Based on computerized tomography (CT) treatment planning in the supine position and in the prone position with the belly board, the median volume of small bowel was reduced by 54% (63). The median dose to the small bowel was 15 Gy with the belly board technique and 24 Gy in the supine position. The median volume of the bladder was also reduced 62% with the belly board technique. When it is not possible to use a belly board because of patient size or due to extension of the tumor to anterior structures, treatment in the prone position is preferred. Another study showed a 70% reduction of small bowel in the radiation field that was independent of patient weight, age, gender, or whether pre- or post-operative radiation was administered (64).

The exclusion of small bowel is particularly important because of the risk for treatment-related diarrhea which resulted from both radiation and chemotherapy. Both of the chemotherapeutic agents used in the treatment of rectal cancer, 5-fluorouracil (5FU)

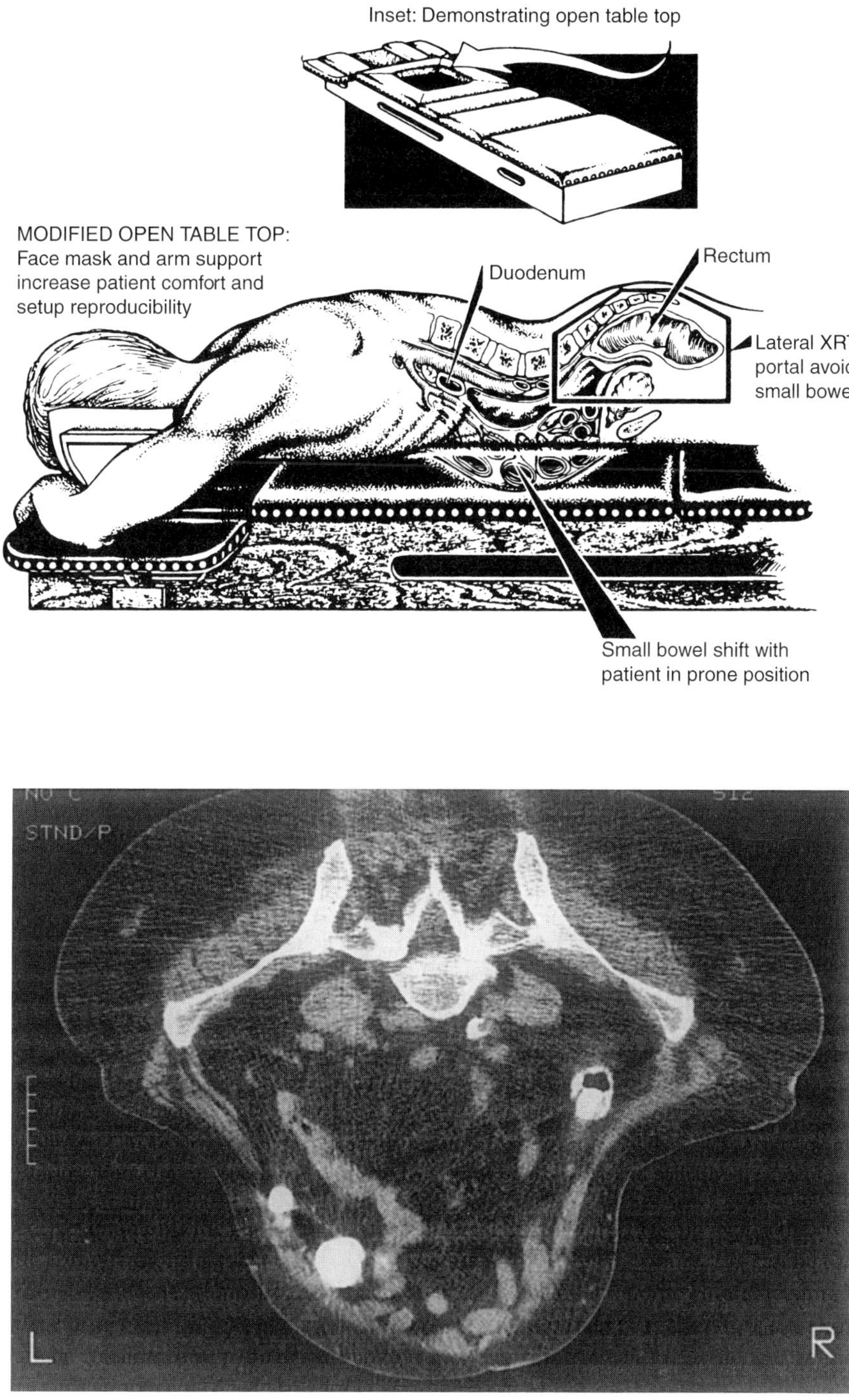

Figure 18.2 The belly board technique places the patient in the prone position and allows the small bowel to fall outside the radiation fields.

and irinotecan (CPT-11) cause diarrhea. In order to administer maximum doses of radiation and chemotherapy without interruption, radiation techniques must exclude as much small bowel as possible and an aggressive supportive care approach is needed during treatment.

When the disease involves the structures in the pelvis, the radiation treatment portals generally encompass the entire pelvis. High-energy photons, like 18 mvX, should be used to reduce integral dose. When the disease is confined to the presacral region and rectum, the external iliac lymph node chain does not need routinely to be included in the treatment portal (65). In these cases a posterior field, and right and left lateral fields are used. Anterior fields should be considered when there is anterior extension of disease to the urogenital regions. In some cases, anterior–posterior fields or a four-field arrangement may prove necessary based on tumor extension and/or anatomical constraints (Figure 18.3). Adequate coverage of the tumor volume should be confirmed with treatment planning imaging. The volume of small bowel in the field can be determined either with contrast used at the time of simulation and/or CT-based treatment planning.

Even with distal rectal involvement, including infiltration of the anal canal, the risk for inguinal node involvement is limited and radiation treatment portals do not need to include the inguinal region. The risk for recurrence in the inguinal region among distal rectal tumors is less than 5% (66). However, radiation techniques should be modified if inguinal lymph nodes are clinically evident and pathologically confirmed to be involved with metastatic disease. Metastatic involvement in the inguinal nodes portends an especially poor prognosis for dissemination of disease (67). Treatment of the inguinal region generally results in localized moist desquamation if the region is included in the radiation portal and a more prolonged radiation schedule is used.

The superior border of a pelvic radiation field, in general, should be placed at the L5–S1 interspace. However, tumor involvement may dictate that the superior border be placed at another location. The inferior border of the field is dictated by the inferior extent of the tumor; generally the inferior aspect of the field should be placed 2 cm inferior to the lowest aspect of the tumor. The anus may need to be included in the treatment field in some cases when the tumor is located in the distal rectum. Whenever possible, however, the anus should be blocked from the radiation portal to reduce treatment-related morbidity such as moist desquamation in the perianal region. For tumors located in the mid- and proximal rectum, the perianal region inferior border of the radiation field is placed at the bottom of the obturator foramen in order that side-effects to the perianal region are avoided. Every effort should be made to exclude small bowel, and to block the genetalia from the lateral treatment portals. Posteriorly, the entire sacrum should be included to adequately treat the nerve roots; this is important to avoid the penumbra (edge and low dose region) of the radiation beam and to ensure adequate radiation dose to the radial margin of resection in the presacral region.

Radiation technique impacts significantly on complications and mortality. Complications due to small bowel toxicity were higher in the Swedish Rectal Cancer Trial because the superior border was placed at L2 in many of the studies, rather than at the L5–S1 interspace (68–70). Higher mortality rates were observed among patients treated with anterior–posterior opposed portals as compared with three- or four-field techniques (15% vs. 3%; $P < 0.001$). Because of these complications, the overall mortality rates were the same for surgery alone and the pre-operative radiation groups. Although the addition of radiation therapy

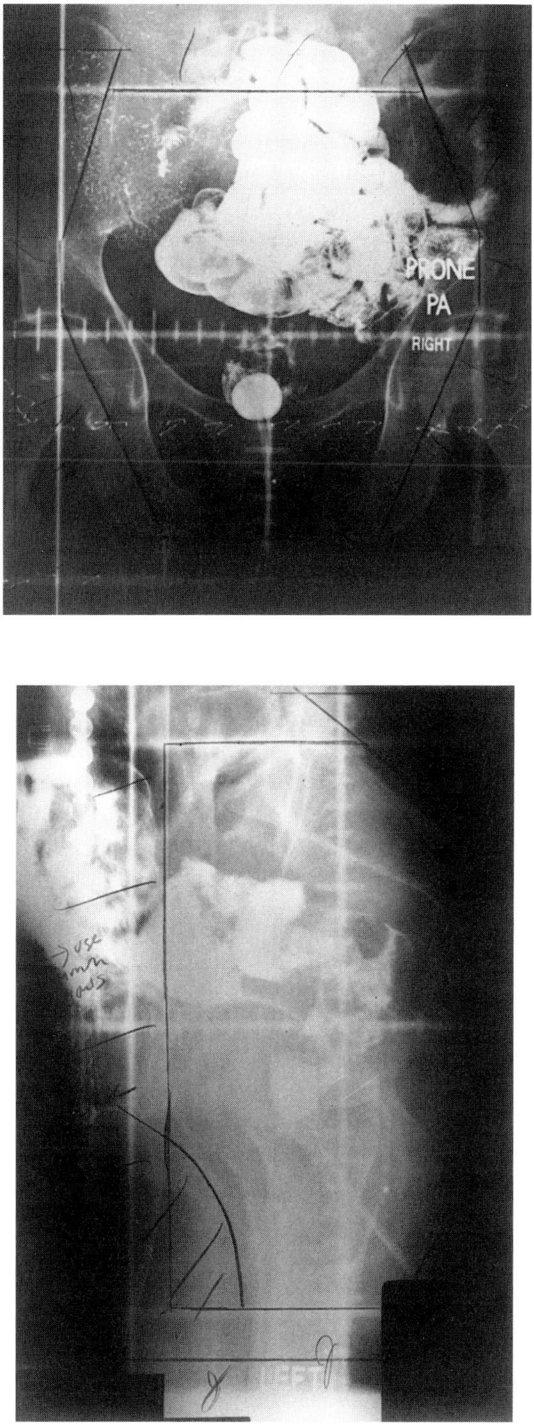

Figure 18.3 Routine radiation portals for rectal cancer.

significantly improved the local control and disease-specific survival rates, the morbidity of radiation therapy was substantial enough to negate the impact of these results. Lumbosacral plexopathy occurred with the pre-operative radiation regimen used in this trial even though peripheral nerves are resistant to the late effects of radiation. Other late adverse effects of this pre-operative radiation regimen included thromboembolism ($P=0.01$), femoral neck and pelvic fractures ($P=0.03$), intestinal obstruction ($P=0.02$), and post-operative fistulae ($P=0.01$). No difference in genitourinary complications was observed.

The importance of radiation technique is demonstrated in another trial that used hypofractionated pre-operative radiation. Among this trial that included 83 patients there was no significant treatment-related morbidity. Like the Swedish Rectal Trial, 25 Gy was given in 5 fractions over 1 week followed by surgery (71,72). However, anterior–posterior portals were avoided and the superior border of the radiation field was limited to the L5–S1 interspace. With a mean follow-up of about 5 years, the actuarial local control rate is reported to be 95% with a disease-specific survival rate of 77%. Only 13% of cases experienced a ≥Grade 3 perioperative or late toxicity; there was a 3.5% incidence of bowel obstruction. No significant difference in the toxicity profile was seen among the 16 patients who also received chemotherapy during radiation.

Approaches have also been taken to minimize side-effects related to chemotherapy, such as hematological and gastrointestinal toxicities during a course of radiation. Using a protracted infusion of 5FU, a higher total dose of chemotherapy can be administered with fewer hematological side-effects (73). A protracted infusion of 5FU decreased hematological side-effects and allowed a higher total dose of chemotherapy. In the post-operative setting, this resulted in improved rates of disease-free and overall survival, although gastrointestinal side-effects, such as diarrhea, increased. Other chemotherapy agents, such as CPT-11, also can result in profound diarrhea (74).

Besides gastrointestinal and hematological side-effects, other toxicities of chemotherapy must also be monitored during a course of chemoradiation. Specifically, mucositis, and hand–foot syndrome can occur. Superinfection, especially with *Candida*, must be closely monitored. Generally, the treatment is symptomatic with the use of salt and soda rinses, and emollients. Occasionally mild nausea can occur, so nutritional and fluid balance must be evaluated.

Because radiation effects are well defined, gastrointestinal toxicities that occur in the first 2 weeks of radiation generally are attributable to chemotherapy. No matter whether it is related to the radiation, the chemotherapy or both, the management of treatment-related diarrhea is generally the same. However, possible infection with *C. difficile* should always be considered. Clinical signs, like fever and blood in the stool, may suggest underlying sepsis and should initiate prompt evaluation (74). Patients should be closely monitored. Other etiologies, such as infection, should be considered if the symptoms are not typical or if they are refractory to usual supportive care strategies.

The symptoms of tumor-related bowel obstruction and neuropathic pain, however, are often relieved in the first few weeks of chemoradiation. Patients will note evidence of tumor sloughing and a small amount of blood with defecation. Symptoms of obstruction will abate during or at the end of radiation as the stools become softer, and the stool caliber increases. Symptom control remains important as the symptoms of bowel obstruction resolve. It is equally important that diarrhea is avoided during the course of radiation to prevent skin irritation, and fluid and electrolyte imbalances.

Management of treatment-related symptoms

A three-step bowel management program has been instituted at the University of Texas M.D. Anderson Cancer Center (75). Results of this bowel management program were prospectively evaluated using a validated bowel assessment survey. With a 95% compliance rate for completion of the survey each week during the course of chemoradiation, no significant differences were documented between the presenting symptoms and the symptoms that were reported at the completion of chemoradiation.

When the treatment portals are outlined, all patients receive written instructions in bowel management, and a prescription for antidiarrheal (loperamide) and an antiemetic agent to be used if necessary. The three-step program anticipates the development of treatment-related toxicity (Table 18.2). The strategy is proactive; at the first sign of symptoms, the patient should proceed to the next step of management (75). Under this program the patient should not have more than three bowel movements in a day; it is important to recognize that the patient does not need to have watery or loose stools to follow the bowel management guidelines. The goal is to prevent, rather than treat, symptoms like frequent stooling, fluid and electrolyte imbalance, and skin irritation.

In this bowel management program, Step 1 uses loperamide as needed, and Step 2 begins a scheduled administration of loperamide to prevent, rather than treat, symptoms of frequent stooling. In Step 3, opioid analgesics are added to the loperamide to relieve the symptoms of abdominal cramping and to exploit the constipating effects of opioid analgesics. Established principles for pain management, which titrate the dose to effect, are used. Unlike loperamide, there is no dose limit with opioid analgesics, and usually the doses

Table 18.2 The University of Texas, M.D. Anderson Cancer Center Three-Step Bowel Management Program. If one step is ineffective, the next step is used. Medications are titrated to effect. The goal is to maintain three or fewer stools per day

	Strategy
Step 1	Loperamide prn; (1–2 tablets)
Step 2	Loperamide (1–2 tablets) qid on a scheduled basis 1/2 hour before meals and before bedtime
Step 3	• Continue loperamide (1–2 tablets) qid and begin opioid analgesics. • Imodium (1–2 tablets) prn • Add a sustained release analgesic [like morphine or oxycodone] and an immediate release analgesic for breakthrough abdominal cramping/stooling. The analgesics are titrated to effect using the same principles that are used in pain management • Because of difficulties in titration and changing needs over the course of radiation, refrain from the use of a fentanyl patch unless used for primary pain management The goal is to give sufficient medications to consistently control frequent stooling + abdominal cramping

of opioids that are required in Step 3 are modest. Because the treatment-related changes in the bowel do not resolve during therapy, a sustained-release analgesic is preferred in Step 3 to avoid the need for multiple doses of medications during the day (75). Medications that have a 3-hour duration of effect, such as tincture of opium or short-acting analgesics, can result in cycles of symptoms as the medication is metabolized and if a strict schedule of administration is not followed; because of this, sleep is often also disrupted. Fentanyl patches are often avoided because of the difficulty in titration, and because analgesic needs are not always stable as the patient undergoes radiation.

Generally skin care is restricted to the perianal region because of the bolus effect in this area. With the first signs of dry desquamation, an emollient that also acts as a barrier for the skin, such as lantiseptic, is constantly placed on the skin except during the time of radiation. When the skin is compromised, routine use of tissues can still result in irritation. In addition to the discomfort, small regions of moist desquamation in the perianal area can place the patient at risk for a secondary infection due to bacteria in the stool. This is of particular concern when chemotherapy is also administered. An emollient with a barrier helps to prevent infection. Among patients who develop a *Candida* infection in the perianal region, a compound with nystatin, desitin, and xylocaine is often of significant benefit. Among patients who develop localized moist desquamation in the perianal area due to treatment of distal rectal tumors, maintain hygiene and derive symptomatic relief with sitz baths or warm compresses and domboro's powder.

Similar approaches have been used for the treatment of chemotherapy-induced diarrhea. Alternative strategies for the control of diarrhea include the use of loperamide with enkephalinase inhibitors, such as acetorphan, to treat the secretory diarrhea induced by CPT-11. The synthetic octapeptide octreotide also is effective with secretory diarrhea. Octerotide prolongs intestinal transit time, promotes absorption of electrolytes in the intestine, decreases mesenteric blood flow, and decreases the secretion of fluids and electrolytes. Octreotide has primarily been used in the treatment of other conditions such as carcinoid syndrome, vasoactive intestinal polypeptide (VIP)-secreting tumors, short-bowel (ileostomy) syndrome, and dumping syndrome. Also, octreoide has been used to treat diarrhea associated with the use of 5FU and in the bone marrow transplant setting (74,76). Complete response rates of more than 90% were observed after 3 days of treatment in two pilot trials with 5FU-based chemotherapy regimens. Given subcutaneously, 100 μg bid to 500 μg tid of octreotide is injected. In other studies, octreotide has been given as a continuous intravenous infusion. The optimal dose and route of administration of octreotide is currently unknown and has been indexed to the clinical presentation (74). The cost effectiveness of the use of octreotide or alternative strategies is indexed to the cost of preventing hospitalization or infusional therapies for treatment-related complications.

Treatment-related symptoms include symptoms that persist or develop after radiation. Late radiation effects become an issue among patients who will live with cancer for many years, and among patients who present with symptomatic disease and undergo potentially curative therapy. Radiation proctitis may represent a continuum of symptoms. Although there is a radiobiological dissociation between acute and late toxicities, one clinical trial linked acute proctitis to three late symptoms (tenesmus, frequency, and diarrhea) and the late EORTC/RTOG score. There appeared to be five subgroups of patients with different levels of rectal symptoms. One group had minimal symptoms; the second group only had an increased number of bowel movements in a day. Group 3 had tenesmus and bleeding, group 4 had tenesmus and increased frequency, and group 5 had all symptoms. Although rectal bleeding and discharge impacted greatly on the EORTC/RTOG scores, tenesmus and bleeding had the most impact on daily living (77). However, a low concordance was found between the patient's assessment of their symptoms and the EORTC/RTOG score.

Another study that involved 386 patients showed a relationship between the development of acute or treatment-related enteritis and chronic bowel injury. Only 13 patients developed symptoms of radiation-induced enteritis; three of these cases also experienced chronic bowel injury. A total of 18 patients developed chronic treatment-related symptoms (78). The risk for reoperation was 5% but chronic proctitis developed in 19% at 5 years. Factors related to an increased risk for complications included transanal excision, increased radiation dose, and increased age.

Pelvic tumors

Most commonly gastrointestinal symptoms that involve the rectum result from primary colorectal, cervical, or urinary tract cancers although metastases from any primary tumor site can occur in this region. Extrinsic tumor compression of the rectum by metastatic disease can also cause obstructive symptoms. Other symptoms can develop from metastatic involvement of the pelvic bones and lumbosacral plexus. Urinary symptoms can occur from ureteral or bladder obstruction, and hematuria. Lymphatic obstruction can result in edema of the genetalia and lower extremities.

Therapeutic approaches for tumors arising in or involving the pelvis account for the significant morbidity of uncontrolled disease. Since most gastrointestinal symptoms in the pelvis arise from rectal involvement, the treatment of rectal cancer will serve as a therapeutic paradigm. The treatment of locally advanced rectal cancer depends on the following factors. First, the presenting symptoms are a key determinant. Among operable patients, surgery may be undertaken first to stop significant bleeding. Second, whether it is possible to resect the tumor. Inoperable patients may benefit from radiation that relieves symptoms and may allow resection of the tumor. Third, whether metastases are present and, if so, the volume of metastatic disease. Significant metastatic disease portends a poor prognosis and more abbreviated courses of radiation would relieve symptoms. If the metastases are resectable and the prognosis is prolonged, then a more aggressive radiation approach is appropriate to prevent possible local tumor recurrence.

Several therapeutic options then exist for locally advanced tumors that involve the rectum. Among these are post-operative, pre-operative, and palliative radiation. Therapeutic techniques such as intraoperative radiation therapy, brachytherapy, and conformal external beam radiation therapy, offer a wide variety of options for tumor regression and control while attempting to minimize treatment-related side-effects.

Post-operative radiation

The advantages of administering radiation post-operatively include the ability to plan treatment based on complete pathological staging of the primary tumor and a theoretical reduction in perioperative morbidity since surgery is performed in an unirradiated field. Pathological tumor staging ensures that adjuvant radiation is indicated and allows more precision in defining the regions that are to be included in the radiation portal (79). For rectal cancer, tumors that are located in the mid to proximal rectum, post-operative radiation is often used because sphincter-preserving surgery can routinely be performed in these cases without the need for tumor down-staging. In addition, prompt surgical intervention and post-operative radiation are indicated in cases in which there is significant bleeding or risk of obstruction.

While CT and magnetic resonance imaging (MRI) are more than 90% accurate in determining metastatic spread prior to treatment, limitations exist with the evaluation of local disease extension. The ability to detect the primary tumor is variable and depends on the size and location of the tumor. Accurate evaluation of pelvic lymph node involvement is about 60%–85% for CT and MRI (80). In a study of 158 rectal cancer patients, CT identified the primary tumor in only 75% of cases (81). The sensitivity and specificity of CT in detecting perirectal fat involvement is about 50%–75%; low-lying rectal tumors are more difficult to evaluate with CT because of the paucity of fat in this region (80–82). The accuracy in detecting tumor involvement of the perirectal fat with transrectal MRI is over 85% in a number of series (82).

The disadvantages of post-operative radiation include relative hypoxia within the operative bed, and potential growth of microscopic residual disease during post-operative healing. Hypoxia enhances resistance to radiation; approximately three times the radiation dose is required to kill hypoxic tumor cells as to kill the same number of well-oxygenated cells. Therefore, higher total doses of radiation are generally administered post-operatively than pre-operatively. In comparison with the 45–50 Gy generally prescribed with pre-operative radiation, 53–55 Gy is usually administered post-operatively. However, the risk of radiation-related short- and long-term gastrointestinal toxicity increases precipitously as the total dose of radiation increases (62). The potential risk of radiation morbidity also increases with post-operative radiation because the small bowel is less mobile due to adhesions.

Although it does not represent a prospective randomized trial, the Patterns of Care Study evaluated survival on the basis of whether radiation was given pre-operatively or post-operatively, and whether chemotherapy was given during radiation. Local failure rates were approximately 10% for all stages and treatment arms. The patterns of Care Study also found a significantly higher survival rate with pre-operative radiation and with post-operative chemoradiation when compared with post-operative radiation. At 5 years, the overall survival rate with post-operative radiation was 50%, and it was 85% with pre-operative radiation, and 69% with post-operative chemoradiation (83).

These studies demonstrated the benefit of radiation therapy in reducing risk for local failure with possible impact on overall survival. Variations in radiation techniques and administered chemotherapy impact significantly on morbidity and outcomes. Although treatment interruptions improve tolerance to therapy, they are generally associated with poorer rates of tumor regression and control of disease. This is due to repopulation of tumor cells during the treatment interruption. It is much like discontinuing an antibiotic midway through a prescribed course.

The routes and schedules of administration of chemotherapy also have a significant impact on patterns of failure and treatment-related side-effects. Some trials included chemotherapy agents that provided no benefit but may have contributed to overall toxicity of therapy. No direct comparison has been performed between pre-operative and post-operative conventional radiation schedules performed with standardized chemotherapy. Therefore, any comparison of the relative advantages and disadvantages of pre-operative and post-operative chemoradiation remain theoretical.

Pre-operative radiation

Pre-operative radiation capitalizes on the disadvantages of post-operative radiation. The key advantage of pre-operative radiation is the potential reduction in tumor size, allowing a greater chance for tumor resection. For rectal cancers, tumor reduction allows resection with a sphincter-preserving surgical procedure; this is especially important for lesions located in the distal rectum. Response to pre-operative radiation also results in sterilization of potential sites of microscopic residual disease, such as the presacral region, the remainder of the pelvic brim, and the regional lymphatics (84–88).

Because the blood supply has not been disrupted by surgery, the effects of both radiation and chemotherapy are potentially enhanced. This allows the administration of a lower dose of radiation, which also reduces the risk for radiation morbidity. The risk of radiation morbidity also decreases with pre-operative radiation because the small bowel is more mobile before surgery and can be displaced from the radiation field (62,89). The ability to assess response to chemotherapy and radiation also may have prognostic importance.

The disadvantages of pre-operative radiation include the lack of pathological tumor staging (84,85). Surgical expertise is needed to minimize perioperative morbidity because surgical resection is performed in an irradiated field (72,90).

For patients with locally advanced rectal cancer, sphincter preservation is a major goal of pre-operative radiation therapy. This is a significant quality of life issue among patients with symptomatic localized disease and among patients who have limited metastatic disease and the potential for prolonged survival. Tumors located <6 cm from the anal verge would generally require an abdominoperineal resection (APR). However, variation exists in surgical practices, whether or not pre-operative radiation is used.

The results with pre-operative chemoradiation for rectal cancer are dependent on the radiation dose and the manner that the chemotherapy is administered. The results of these reports are summarized in Table 6. With pre-operative radiation alone, the pathological complete response rate is about 15%. With bolus or infusional 5FU during the first and last week of radiation, the pathologic complete response rates are about 20%. Using a continuous infusion of 5FU throughout the course of pre-operative radiation, the pathological complete response rate increased to 27% (91). Tumor regression or 'down-staging' is evident in about 65% of cases. Sphincter preservation after pre-operative chemoradiation is possible in more than two-thirds of patients with low rectal cancers.

The concurrent administration of chemotherapy during radiation for rectal cancers demonstrated that chemotherapy improves the therapeutic ratio of administered radiation. These sentinel studies provided a model for combined modality therapy that is used in the treatment of gastrointestinal and nearly every other type of tumors. Chemoradiation is not limited to curative treatment strategies and is used to enhance response during palliative radiation as well. Although the most experience exists with intravenous administration, either bolus or infusional, oral chemotherapeutic agents are now available that are more convenient for patient use.

Radiosensitization by 5FU is thought to occur by affecting the G1–S phase of the cell cycle through the inhibition of thymidylate synthetase. Another metobolite of 5FU, fluorodeoxyuridine monophosphate, is incorporated into ribonucleic acid (RNA) and affects RNA synthesis. When 5FU is given, the early S phase population in the tumor expands and results in enhanced radiosensitivity that is more than that seen with cell synchronization alone (92–94).

Correlated with this are the relationships between radiation repair and the molecular sensors at the G1–S checkpoint, like p53 and cyclin-dependent kinases. In general, radiosensitization is accomplished by limiting tumor repopulation and reducing the efficiency of radiation repair during treatment. When combined with radiation, the effects of 5FU are additive or supra-additive. The potentiation of radiation response is greatest when 5FU is present for about 1 day prior to radiation.

Oral administration of 5FU analogs

A wide variety of oral fluoropyrimidine analogs are becoming available and they offer significant advantages especially for patient convenience. Most of the data relate to their use as chemotherapeutic agents alone. Data remain limited at this point regarding their administration during either pre-operative or post-operative radiation, but preliminary results indicate comparable efficacy.

Objective response rates with oral 5FU analogs are about 40% among the clinical trials in over 580 patients. Response rates were lower, equaling 25%, when oral fluoropyrimidines were administered alone or with lower doses of leucovorin. The highest dose intensities were achieved with 28-day schedules of the drug. Early experience during pre-operative radiation involved a dose escalation trial to establish the maximum tolerated dose (MTD). It was determined that the MTD of oral uracil and tegafur was 350 mg m^{-2} day^{-1} with 90 mg day^{-1} of leucovorin when given 5 days a week concurrent with radiation (95,96). Results were comparable with those with infusional 5FU with a sphincter-preserving surgery performed in 12 of 14 patients and a pathologic complete response in three cases.

Several advantages exist for the use of an oral route for chemotherapy administration. Among these are the ease of administration and avoidance of the inconvenience, discomfort, and cost associated with either bolus or continuous infusion of 5FU (96–98). With this come some concerns regarding compliance in taking the medications. The pharmacokinetics of drug administration must be assurred, especially when taken in lower doses during radiation. It is also unknown if the oral 5FU analog should be taken at a specific time relative to the administration of radiation.

A variety of oral fluoropyrimidines have been developed and each has its own metabolic characteristics that will affect response and toxicity profiles (99,100). Some of the newer agents also may concentrate to a greater degree within tumor cells as compared with infusional 5FU resulting from complete inactivation of dihydropyrimidine dehydrogenase (DPD), which is responsible for the metabolism of 5FU (101). Severe diarrhea is the dose-limiting toxicity in most of these oral agents (102,103). However, in comparison with infusional 5FU, chemotherapy-related side-effects such as mucositis, neutropenia, and hand–foot syndrome are rare with some of the oral 5FU analogs (104).

Many issues need to be resolved before oral fluoropyrimidines become the new standard of care during radiation therapy. Because of the differences among the agents, each will require clinical assessment with radiation therapy. The activity of other agents, such as CPT-11 and oxaliplatin, will need to be considered relative to the use of oral fluoropyrimides as well.

Endocavitary radiation and brachytherapy

Brachytherapy and endocavitary radiation can be used alone or, more commonly, in conjunction with external beam radiation. Administering highly localized doses of radiation can provide high doses of radiation directly to well-defined volumes to achieve local control with definitive radiation. Most often these approaches are used among patients who are unable or unwilling to undergo surgical resection.

Contact or endocavitary radiation is another approach in the conservative management of rectal tumors. Soft 50-kV X-rays are produced by a generator that delivers radiation through a tube that contains an anode and ring filament (105). Two aluminum filters can be used and the 0.5-cm filter is used for most applications. With the 0.5-cm aluminum filter and a focal distance of 4 cm, with a 20 cGy per minute output, and a 3-cm circular field, the percentage depth dose is 100% at 0 mm, 44% at 5 mm, 23% at 10 mm, and 9% at 20 mm depth. Because of this, highly infiltrative tumors are not amenable to contact therapy. The tumor must be within 12 cm of the anal verge and accessible; on occasion, posterior wall tumors are difficult to localize with the cone.

The dose of the first contact treatment is between 30 Gy and 40 Gy in 2 to 4 minutes with a 0.5 mm aluminum filter. One to two weeks later a second application of contact radiation is administered. Three weeks after the initiation of therapy, the third contact application is performed; at this time a smaller (2-cm) cone is generally used to account for tumor regression. For 3-cm tumors, 90–120 Gy is given in 4 to 5 fractions over 5 to 8 weeks. For tumors less than 2 cm that regress completely after two sessions, a total dose of 80 Gy in 4 fractions (30 Gy on day 1; 20 Gy on day 7; 15 Gy on day 21 and 15 Gy on day 36) is sufficient (105). The normal mucosa of the rectal wall should not receive more than 15–20 Gy.

Patient selection is critical to the success of contact therapy. For the same reasons, any patient with lymph node involvement is not a candidate for contact therapy (105). Factors that increase the risk for lymph node involvement, such as high histologic grade, perineural or lymphvascular invasion, or ulceration, generally are contraindications for contact therapy. The response to contact therapy also is predictive of therapeutic success. The chance for local control is good if the tumor regresses by more than 80% of its original volume by 2 weeks after the second contact session.

Complete response is achieved in over 90% of patients with endocavitary therapy. Local failure is reported to be 28%, but the addition of external beam radiation in cases with poor prognostic factors improved local control. Tumor size (>3 cm) and partially fixed tumors significantly influenced local control rates. Accounting for salvage therapy, sphincter preservation was accomplished in 84% and local control was accomplished in 82% (106). Severe late effects occurred in 4% of those treated.

The techniques used for brachytherapy depend on anatomic constraints. Four techniques have been described and include the use of metallic needles through a perineal template, an iridium 'fork', a plastic loop technique, and the use of a remote after-loading device (107). In order to localize the radiation dose to the lesion and avoid treatment of the opposite rectal wall, obturators are often used in conjuction with the implant to distend the rectum.

Patients with lesions <3 cm in size can be treated with brachytherapy alone, but external beam radiation should be added for larger size tumors. Using this approach, 90% rates of local control are obtained without significant complication (107). Although continuous low dose rate brachytherapy is usually used, a pulsed low dose rate can give similar late effects and be considered as an alternative approach (108).

Both endocavitary therapy and brachytherapy offer alternative and effective means of administering localized radiation, especially among patients with limited treatment options. Further integration of these techniques should be considered as therapy is optimized to use more conservative surgical approaches to the treatment of rectal cancer.

Recurrent rectal cancer

Recurrent rectal cancer can vary significantly in its clinical presentation, and it requires a broad range of therapeutic approaches. When the recurrence is identified early and the patient is usually asymptomatic, resection is possible. Regretably, many patients are diagnosed with recurrent rectal cancer once diagnostic evaluations are done to evaluate progressive symptoms, and they are often found to be inoperable. Because the morbidity of recurrent disease is so profound, aggressive therapeutic attempts are frequently undertaken to secure local–regional control.

Recurrent disease among patients who have previously been treated with radiation poses significant challenges. Approaches have included re-irradiation with external beam therapy and intraoperative radiation therapy (IORT). The dose of external beam radiation has varied when given to patients who have previously been treated with radiation, especially when given in conjunction with IORT. Bleeding, pain, and mass effect were palliated with re-irradiation among 100%, 65%, and 24% of cases, respectively; 80%, 33%, and 20%, respectively, were palliated until the time of death (109,110). The acute Grade 3 toxicity rate was 31%, and the late Grade 3 and 4 toxicity rates were 23% and 10%, respectively, including a 17% rate of small bowel obstruction. The only factor that reduced the toxicity rates was hyperfractionation. However, the factors that influenced median survival were KPS, the initial stage of disease, and the radiation dose given at the time of re-irradiation (≤30.6 Gy=22 months vs. >30.6 Gy=9.5 months median survival).

The risk for and outcomes after the diagnosis of recurrent rectal cancer is the same among patients initially treated with an APR or low-anterior resection (18% and 24%, respectively). Of the 175 patients evaluated in one study of recurrent rectal cancer, 25 had an isolated pelvic recurrence (111). The survival rate among the patients with an isolated pelvic recurrence of disease who received radiotherapy was significantly greater (16 months) as compared with those who were treated with palliative operations or analgesics (2.4 months).

One study evaluated 519 patients with locally recurrent rectal cancer at the Princess Margaret Hospital. Relapse of disease occurred after an APR among 326 patients, after a low anterior resection among 151 patients, and in 42 after a local excision. No patients had previously been treated with radiation (112). The mean time between the initial surgery and radiation therapy was 18 months (3–138 months). The relapse was confined to the pelvis among 355 cases, but distant metastases were found in 32% (164 cases) at the time that the local recurrence was also discovered. A total dose of ≥35 Gy was given to 214 patients with 1.8–2.5 Gy fractions. The median survival was 14 months and the median time to local disease progression was 5 months. The pelvic disease progression-free rate was 7% and the 5-year survival was 5%. Multivariate analysis showed that overall survival was correlated to the ECOG performance status, absence of extrapelvic metastases, long intervals between the initial surgery and radiotherapy, total radiation dose, and absence of obstructive uropathy.

No dose–response relationship was found to exist for recurrent rectal cancer on a review of the available retrospective series in the literature. No significant differences were observed in the initial response or the durability of the response to therapy (113). However, a dose–response relationship was suggested when patients with primary untreated cancers and post-operative residual disease were evaluated alone.

Three dose regimens were used at the Peter MacCallum Cancer Institute for incompletely resected, locally recurrent rectal cancer. These regimens included 50–60 Gy (designated as radical radiation) or 45 Gy (high-dose radiation) with conventional fractionation; palliative radiation of <45 Gy was given to others. No significant difference was observed between the radical or high-dose radiation groups with regard to symptomatic relief (about 80%); only 33% of those receiving palliative therapy, however, achieved partial symptomatic relief (114). The estimated median survival was 16 months for all patients; for patients with radical radiation the median survival was 26 months compared with 16 months with high-dose radiation. Survival was compromised when macroscopic residual disease was present with a median survival of 14 months vs. 31 months with only microscopic residual tumor.

Intraoperative radiation has been used as a supplement to external beam radiation or as the only therapy when further external beam radiation is not possible. The outcomes were evaluated among 73 patients with recurrent rectal cancer; 86% of the patients studied had locally recurrent disease without metastases (115). External beam radiation had been previously administered in 52% and the recurrences were located in the presacral region (radial margin) in 55% of cases. Surgical resection allowed for complete macroscopic resection of disease in 57%, partial resection with gross residual disease in 29%, and no resection in 14% of the recurrences. Intraoperative radiation was given ranging from 10 Gy to 25 Gy; 30 patients received either pre-operative or post-operative external beam radiation. Actuarial overall survival equaled 72% at 1 year, 45% at 2 years and 31% at 3 years; the actuarial local control rate was 71%, 48%, and 31%, respectively. The actuarial disease-free survival was 58%, 27%, and 18%. Therefore, controlling symptoms of recurrent disease was a critical factor for quality of life given the relatively extended survival among these patients. Actuarial survival was improved with complete or partial resection. Among the 21 cases of local failure, 8 were in the IORT field, 8 were in the external beam radiation field, and 3 occurred in areas that received both IORT and external beam radiation. In the IORT field, local control was 87% at 1 year, 72% at 2 years, and 65% at 3 years. Actuarial local control in the IORT field was better without rather than with gross residual disease (77% vs. 51% at 3 years). Among patients with an isolated local recurrence and with a partial or complete resection, the local control rates with IORT + external beam radiation was 61% at 3 years and 0% with IORT alone. Four patients had long-term morbidity. These included one case of sciatic plexopathy that resolved with further follow-up (12 Gy IORT + 45 Gy post-operatively). Two cases of sacral necrosis occurred at 6 months (39 Gy pre-operatively + 25 Gy IORT) and at 13 months (40 Gy pre-operatively + 20 Gy IORT). There was one case of necrosis of L5 (28 Gy pre-operatively + 15 Gy IORT) after 51 months of follow-up.

The previous study showed an advantage when external beam radiation was added over IORT alone (115). A phase I/II study of IORT for locally advanced or recurrent rectal cancer that was performed by the RTOG showed an advantage when IORT was added over external beam radiation alone (116). Again, local control was dependent on the amount of residual disease; for all patients, the 2-year actuarial local control rates were 77% (64% among the recurrent disease group) if no gross disease remained vs. 10% if there was gross residual disease after surgery. For all patients and among the recurrent group, the overall survival was improved (88%) if there was no gross residual disease after surgery vs. a 46% survival if gross residual disease was present. The 2-year actuarial risk for major complications attributable to IORT was 16%. In all clinical settings, IORT is feasible and adds less than 1 hour to the surgical procedure (117).

Combined modality therapy, which includes chemoradiation and surgical resection, improved resectability, local control, and survival. In one study of 47 patients who received a pre-operative dose of 45 Gy with concomitant 5FU and mitomycin chemotherapy (118). An objective response to therapy occurred in over 50% of cases and 45% underwent a radical resection. Pain relief was accomplished in 86% and higher radiation doses correlated with better pain control. Radical resection resulted in better local control and survival. The overall 5-year survival and local control rates were 22% and 32%, respectively; when IORT was given, the 5-year rates were 79% and 41%, respectively. The modified Suzuki classification was found to be prognostic. In this classification, F0 indicates that the recurrent tumor has no contact with the pelvic sidewall. In the F1 group, less than one-quarter of the pelvic sidewall is involved, and between one-quarter and one-half of the circumference of the pelvic sidewall is involved in F2 disease. More than one-half of the circumference of the pelvic sidewall is involved in F3 disease. Infiltration of the bone or small bowel occurs in F4 disease. This classification correlated closely with the level of pain, disease-free survival, and overall survival.

No significant difference was seen among three different intraoperative radiation approaches for recurrent colorectal cancer that included IORT, high-dose-rate brachytherapy, and intraoperative placement of iodine-125 seeds. The overall 5-year local control rate was 26% (119). Tumors in the para-aortic region had better rates of local control than tumors located in the pelvis (65% vs. 19% at 5 years), but this did not translate into an improvement in overall survival rates. The 5-year overall survival rate was 4%; only the presence of residual disease (30% for microscopic and 7% for macroscopic at 3 years) and administration of post-operative external beam radiation (48% vs. 12% at 3 years and 24% and 0% at 5 years) influenced overall survival rates. Identifying residual disease may also be difficult. Radioimmuno-guided surgery has been advocated to identify occult tumor deposits that may result in failure to completely resect the disease (120).

Combined modality therapy that includes IORT for recurrent colorectal cancer can result in significant wound-healing problems. With primary closure there is a 46%–65% rate of wound-healing problems. However, introduction of unirradiated tissue via myocutaneous flap reconstruction reduces the risk for major complications to 12% (121,122).

Irrespective of the use of IORT, resection of recurrent disease often requires an extensive surgical procedure for tumor clearance. This is often complicated by a prior history of radiation or re-irradiation. Resection of recurrent disease was possible among 79% of patients (103 of 131 cases) and this resulted in a 31% 5-year survival rate. Favorable prognostic factors included a normal pre-operative CEA level and recurrent tumor that is limited to the bowel wall (123). Aggressive surgical resection, including abdominosacral resection for fixed tumors, also can result in a 31% long-term survival rate (124). These aggressive surgical approaches are possible with reconstruction procedures that include placement of a myocutaneous graft.

In summary, long-term survival is possible among patients with recurrent disease if it is found early and total surgical resection is possible. Radiation therapy is needed to clear potential nests of residual microscopic tumor. Because of prior therapies, such as surgery and radiation, these tumor cells may be in hypoxic regions that require higher radiation doses. Re-irradiation, especially with hyperfractionated treatment schedules, is well tolerated.

Palliative radiation

Achieving local–regional control is important in the management of rectal cancer. Local–regional failure occurs in approximately 75% of all patients who die from rectal cancer. Local failure often results in significant symptoms, such as pain, bleeding, and obstruction, which are difficult to control (125,126). Palliative radiation can relieve the symptoms of pain and bleeding in about 70% of cases. However, high-grade obstructive symptoms may require a diverting colostomy. Occasionally, urinary diversion may also be necessary. Palliative radiation relieves symptoms by causing partial regression of the tumor. The goal is to provide palliation of symptoms for the duration of the patient's life.

At the Princess Margaret Hospital, the most frequent radiation schedule administers 50 Gy in 20 fractions in 4 weeks using a four-field technique. The 5-year survival is dependent on the extent of the tumor; 48% with mobile, 27% with partially fixed, and only 4% of patients with fixed tumors are alive at 5 years (127,128). Tumor extent also predicted for response to radiation; 50% of mobile, 30% of partially fixed, and only 9% of fixed tumors achieved a complete clinical response to radiation. The rate of tumor regression was slow; only 60% achieved a complete response by 4 months and 9 months was required by 90% of those who had a complete response. Of the complete responders, approximately half of the mobile and partially fixed and over 70% of the fixed tumors developed progressive disease. Salvage surgery to relieve symptoms was accomplished without significant complication in over 90% of patients who developed progressive or recurrent disease.

Among 80 patients at the M.D. Anderson Cancer Center with locally advanced rectal cancer presenting with synchronous metastases, hypofractionated radiation with concurrent chemotherapy achieved symptomatic relief in 94% of cases. Hypofractionated regimens included 35 Gy/2.5 Gy per fraction when the tumor extended anteriorly necessitating an anterior–posterior treatment portal. When a belly board technique could be used, 30 Gy in 6 fractions over 3 weeks were given. Endoscopic complete clinical response was achieved in 36% (129,130). Twenty-five patients underwent primary tumor resection. Although the 2-year survival was greater in the group that underwent resection (46% vs. 11%), the colostomy-free survival was greater in the unresected group (79% vs. 51%). Predictors for a worse prognosis included pelvic pain at presentation, biologic equivalent dose at 2 Gy in fractions of < 35 Gy, and poor tumor differentiation. Among patients with locally advanced rectal cancer who also had liver metastases at presentation the median survival was 17 months when treated with palliative radiation and/or chemotherapy (131).

Radiation is often given in cases that are inoperable because of extensive tumor infiltration. Administration of radiation may allow sufficient tumor regression to render a patient operable and offer a chance to be free of disease. Pre-operative radiation totaling 54 Gy and continuous infusion of 5FU was administered to 29 inoperable patients. Resection was undertaken in 23 cases and 18 were resected with curative intent (132). An APR was performed in 13 cases, 3 underwent a low anterior resection and 2 had a local excision. Pathologic findings included a complete response in 13%, and 90% were down-staged. With a median follow-up of 28-months, 15 patients were free of disease. An aggressive surgical approach can render a patient disease-free and may improve overall survival. Multivisceral resection resulted in approximately a 50% survival rate at 5 years among patients with locally advanced rectal cancer (133).

When surgical resection is undertaken among patients who have extensive tumor infiltration, radiation therapy must be administered given the high risk for microscopic residual disease. Prognostic factors are critical to the therapeutic decision process in locally advanced disease. The risk for recurrence exceeds 80% after pelvic exenteration if radiation therapy is not administered (134). This is substantially higher than the risk for local recurrence after locally advanced, but operable, rectal cancer. Because of this, radiotherapeutic approaches have also included the use of IORT in conjuction with external beam therapy.

The use of IORT had significant impact on tumor control and overall survival in the Mayo Clinic experience. Factors that related to improvements in overall survival included the use of pre-operative external beam radiation with chemotherapy plus IORT, and no gross residual tumor after resection (135). The presence of gross residual disease after maximum tumor resection resulted in a 25% risk for progressive disease; this compares with a 5% risk of local tumor recurrence with gross tumor excision. Administration of pre-operative chemoradiation and gross total excision also decreased the risk for distant metastases.

Local control rates are adversely affected without the use of IORT among patients initially presenting with inoperable rectal cancer. Without IORT the local control rate in one series was only 33% as compared with the 92% local control rate achieved when IORT was added to external beam therapy (136). Others have used pre-operative and post-operative radiation with concurrent chemotherapy. With the 'sandwich' technique, the 4-year local failure rate decreased from 23% to 0% and the distant failure rate decreases from 47% to 28% corresponding to an overall survival rate of 41% and 72%, respectively (137).

Pelvis

Hemorrhage, and visceral, lymphvascular, and nerve root obstruction present most commonly with locally advanced or metastatic disease in the pelvis. Treatment may require emergent radiotherapeutic and/or surgical interventions. Hemorrhage is commonly associated with tumors involving the rectum and genitourinary tracts. As with tumors in the lung, radiation is an effective means of stopping active bleeding. Colorectal cancers are often diagnosed among patients with unexplained bleeding.

Colorectal tumor involvement may also result in obstruction requiring stent placement to maintain the integrity of the visceral lumen while administering radiation (126,138–141). Occasionally a diverting colostomy will be required to bypass intestinal obstruction or fistula formation. If these procedures are not performed, intestinal colic can be palliated quickly with opioids but anticholinergics, such as scopolamine, atropine, and loperamide, decrease peristalsis in the smooth muscle of the intestinal tract (126,141). Intestinal obstruction can also result in nausea and vomiting which can be palliated with nasogastric decompression and pharmacologic agents. Octreotide, an analog of somatostatin, reduces gastrointestinal secretions, motility, splanchnic blood flow, has a proabsorptive effect on water and ions, and may inhibit the secretion of vasoactive intestinal peptide. These actions help to disrupt the distention–intestinal secretion–peristalsis cycle and bleeding (141).

Because these tumors are generally locally advanced, preoperative radiation is given with conventional fractionation if no or limited metastatic disease is evident; this is intended to stop bleeding, render the patient operable, and provide a chance for cure. With extensive metastatic disease, 30–35 Gy can be given over 2 to 3 weeks to palliate symptoms of bleeding and obstruction. Fractionation included 35 Gy in 14 fractions, 30 Gy in 10 fractions and 30 Gy in 6 fractions given twice weekly for 3 weeks (129,130). Diverting colostomy was required by 16% of patients prior to radiation. No significant treatment-related toxicities were observed. Whether administered as conventional or hypofractionated radiation with infusional 5-fluorouracil, symptoms from the primary tumor resolved in 94% of cases and the endoscopic complete response rate was 36%. The colostomy-free survival rate was 87% among patients who underwent palliative chemoradiation, and 51% among patients who received pre-operative chemoradiation. When surgery was performed, the 2-year survival was 46% as compared with 11% with palliative chemoradiation. Symptomatic pelvic control was not significantly different and was 81% for palliative chemoradiation and 91% for pre-operative chemoradiation (129). Predictors for the control of pelvic disease included pelvic pain at presentation, a biologically equivalent dose <35 Gy at 2 Gy per fraction, and poor pathologic differentiation. Poor pathologic differentiation and selection for palliative chemoradiation predicted for a worse overall survival.

The pelvic lymph nodes and major blood vessels may become obstructed by tumor. This most frequently is seen when the tumor arises in pelvic structures but can also occur with pelvic metastases from breast and other cancers. Lymphvascular obstruction results in painful edema that is refractory to diuretic and other therapies. When severe, fluid and electrolyte imbalances can occur. Pelvic radiation can relieve lymphvascular obstruction through tumor regression.

Pelvic tumors can also invade the sacral plexus and result in intractable pain. Tumor can tract along nerve roots and can be associated with bony invasion of the sacrum. Pain due to visceral and/or lymphvascular obstruction often responds more rapidly to palliative radiation than the neuropathic pain seen with sacral plexus involvement. Other radiotherapeutic approaches, like brachytherapy, are extremely limited when the cancer persists or recurs after external beam radiation. Interventional pain management techniques are frequently required to control pain associated with sacral plexus involvement.

Reirradiation of the pelvis for symptomatic recurrence has generally been well tolerated, although data are limited. Care must be taken to exclude the intestines from the radiation portals given a 3.9 increased risk for late small bowel toxicity. The data are limited with regard to treatment volume, but the cumulative radiation dose, re-irradiation dose, and the time interval between courses were not found to be related to late radiation toxicity (48).

Skin and subcutaneous tissues

Tumors can cause ulceration of the skin and subcutaneous tissues that are often painful and distressing due to constant drainage. Representing a source for the development of sepsis in immunocompromised patients, localized radiation can be applied to destroy tumor and allow re-epithelialization of the skin. Radiation that treats only the skin and subcutaneous tissues (electron beam therapy) is generally used to avoid radiation side-effects underlying uninvolved normal structures. Although usually 10 radiation treatments are given, the course of radiation can be abbreviated further ranging from 1 to 5 days. Occasionally these lesions are treated with brachytherapy. The radioactive sources can be placed in a mold that sits on top of the tumor and delivers treatment over a few minutes (high dose rate) or a few days (low dose rate).

Gastric tumors

Both primary and metastatic tumors can result in significant upper gastrointestinal symptoms. As in other tumors, radiation therapy can be used as an adjuvant to surgery or as a primary palliative treatment. Anatomical constraints and the intrinsic sensitivity of the normal small bowel to radiation limit the role of radiotherapy as a regional modality. Unlike rectal cancer where much of the small bowel can be displaced from the radiation field, the radiation tolerance of the small bowel is a more significant issue. Localized segments of the small bowel can tolerate doses of 45–50 Gy with convention fractionation of 1.8–2.0 Gy per fraction; however, tolerance to radiation is significantly less when large volumes of bowel are in the radiation field or if high radiation doses are used with each treatment fraction.

The effects of radiation on the stomach were studied in the past when radiotherapy was used to treat peptic ulcer disease because it reduced gastric acid secretion. Serial biopsies performed among three patients treated with 1600 roentgen in 10 equal fractions to the entire stomach showed a loss of cytoplasmic detail and a disappearance of cytoplasmic granules in the parietal and chief cells as early as 8 days after the initial XRT treatment (142). These changes were termed 'coagulation necrosis' and occurred with a relative sparing of the mucosal surface. About 2 weeks after radiation, the glandular pits deepened, there was sloughing of the parietal and chief cells, and the cells at the glandular neck were proliferating. Three weeks after radiation therapy there was a patchy loss of glandular architecture, and thinning of the mucosa; the surface epithelial cells varied in appearance from flat to columnar. At 5 weeks the mucosal and glandular architecture began to revert towards normal. Six weeks after radiation nearly all radiation changes had resolved, with only focal areas of glandular coagulation necrosis being evident. Even though the same dose was used in each of three patients treated, the time of onset of the earliest changes varied between 5 and 16 days. The severity and duration of the changes also varied. The healing of radiation-induced lesions in the stomach is characterized by re-epithelialization with fibrosis and contraction in 2 to 3 years (143). Another study was performed among 88 patients who were treated with 1800 roentgen in 10 equal fractions for peptic ulcer disease. Achlorhydria was documented in 35 patients and varied in duration from a few days to 6 months. A series of 1500 patients was treated with similar doses in the University of Chicago series, and 40% of patients experienced a 50% reduction in gastric acid secretion for a year or more (•). Treatment-related side-effects, such as gastritis, ulceration, and obstruction, are unusual at doses below 4000 cGy, but they increase in incidence when radiation doses of more than 5000 cGy are used (145–150). Modern radiation techniques allow the safe administration of radiation to the upper abdomen to relieve tumor-related symptoms. Most often, 5FU chemotherapy is combined with radiation when this site is treated. Using these techniques, the risk for treatment-related side-effects is less than 10% when 50–55 Gy is given and about 10%–15% with radiation doses that exceed 60 Gy (143,146, 147,151–160).

Clinically, radiation therapy has been useful in palliating upper gastrointestinal bleeding and pain form gastric cancers. The most common presenting symptoms of gastric cancer are upper abdominal discomfort, weakness from anemia, and weight loss (161). Exophytic tumors can cause significant bleeding. Infiltrative tumors can invade the celiac plexus and cause severe back pain like that observed with pancreatic cancer. Tumor infiltration resulting in linitis plastica is associated with an extremely poor prognosis (155,156,162,163). Epigastric pain from gastric cancer can also result from acid secretion. Early satiety, hematemesis, and melena occur less commonly. Obstructing lesions in either the antrum or cardia can cause vomiting or dysphagia, respectively. Radiotherapy effectively palliates the symptoms of locally advanced gastric cancer. Several series indicate that 50%–75% of patients experience improvement of bleeding, gastric outlet obstruction, and pain (146,164–166).

Treatment-related side-effects are known, and medications should be administered prophylactically. The critical structures in a typical radiation field for gastric cancer or metastases to the stomach include the stomach, small intestine, liver, kidneys, and the spinal cord. Acute reactions that occur with radiation of these structures include gastritis, nausea and vomiting, anorexia, diarrhea, abdominal cramping, fatigue, and suppression of blood counts. These symptoms can occur at any time during the course of radiation. Prophylactic antiemetic therapy, such as that given with administration of systemic therapy, should be given prior to and during the course of radiation as needed. Frequently, the most common antiemetics, such as perchloroperazine, are sufficient to control symptoms, but some patients will require other agents. Prior to initiation of chemoradiation at the University of Texas M.D. Anderson Cancer Center, most patients undergo laparoscopic placement of a jejunostomy-feeding tube to support the needs for nutrition and hydration.

Chemoradiation trials

Studies looking at patients with unresectable or partially resected gastric cancer indicate that chemoradiation can be curable in a small percentage of patients (149,155,156,167). A randomized trial administered 35–40 Gy of radiation with and without bolus 5FU for unresected gastrointestinal malignancies. A small group of gastric cancer patients was found to have a superior 5-year survival (12% vs. 0%). Further evidence of the importance of 5FU administration came from a randomized study conducted by the European Organization for Research and Treatment of Cancer (EORTC) (168) that showed a survival advantage in patients treated with chemoradiation compared with those who were treated with radiation alone to 55.5 Gy.

The Gastrointestinal Tumor Study Group (GITSG) conducted a trial in incompletely resected gastric cancer. Chemotherapy alone using 5FU and methyl CCNU was compared with a split course of radiation to a dose of 50 Gy and bolus 5FU given at the start of each course of radiotherapy (169). The trial was discontinued early due to at least six treatment-related deaths and six disease-related deaths in the combined modality arm with the first 6 months of therapy. In spite of this, a statistically significant survival benefit was seen in the combined arm at 5 years (20% vs. 6%; $p < 0.01$). Modern supportive care, conventional treatment planning, and infusional chemotherapy schedules would only have enhanced the difference in favor of the combined arm.

The importance of aggressive supportive care in the setting of a multidisciplinary care team cannot be over-emphasized. This is illustrated by the GITSG experience (169). Even though the chemoradiation group eventually had a better outcome, 6 of 45 patients in that group died because of sepsis of nutritional inadequacy. The routine use of prophylactic antiemetics, and jejunostomy tube feeding vastly improves treatment tolerance. Feeding tubes can obviate the need for intravenous fluid replacement or hyperalimentation and reduce the incidence of hospitalization for acute reactions. Nutritionists should monitor patients' caloric intake and weight, provide calorie goals, and serve as a resource for other nutrition-related issues.

Patterns of failure

Gastric cancer can spread via direct extension, lymphatic or hematologic invasion, and transperitoneal dissemination. Critical organs such as the pancreas, diaphragm, transverse colon, duodenum, spleen, jejunum, liver, left kidney, left adrenal gland, and the celiac axis are in close proximity and are frequently involved. Lymphatic spread initially occurs to the perigastric nodes along the lesser and greater curvatures, then to lymphatics which accompany all three branches of the celiac axis. Remote lymphatic spread can occur to the hepatoduodenal, peripancreatic, superior mesenteric, and para-aortic nodal chains. Similar to the esophagus and duodenum, clinically occult spread beyond the gross lesion can occur through the abundant subserosal and submucosal lymphatics. Positive peritoneal cytology at the time of tumor resection has been found in 16%–35% of patients (170–172), but not all patients with positive cytology are destined to develop peritoneal carcinomatosis (170–174). However, transperitoneal spread occurs in 23%–43% of post-gastrectomy patients (174–177). Because of this, isolated locoregional failure occurs in 29%, and 88% have a component of locoregional failure within one year of surgery (177). Distant metastasis occurs most commonly via the portal venous drainage to the liver. Less commonly the lungs are involved, but tumors involving the gastroesophageal junction have a stronger tendency to spread to the lungs.

Radiation techniques

Radiation treatment portals are based on the observed patterns of failure. Patients should be simulated with an empty stomach and treated in the morning before eating to minimize the treatment volume and organ motion due to stomach distention. Generally opposed anterior and posterior or oblique portals are used. The use of lateral fields is not advisable among patients with an intact stomach because the gastric fundus frequently extends too far posteriorly. In these instances the kidneys and spinal cord cannot be shielded without blocking the tumor. Customized blocking is used to shield the critical structures in the radiation field including small bowel, liver, spinal cord, and kidneys.

In most cases the radiation field should include the entire stomach or gastric bed and draining lymphatics. Based on the patterns of spread, the radiation fields should include the gastric, gastroepiploic, celiac, porta hepatis, subpyloric, gastroduodenal, splenic-supra pancreatic, and retropancreaticoduodenal nodes. The celiac axis usually arises at the bottom of T12, and the porta hepatis is found 4–5 cm to the right of the T11–L1 vertebral bodies. The remaining nodal tissue can be encompassed by treating the stomach and the medial portion of the duodenal 'C-loop' or the stomach and duodenal bed. The lower border usually extends to the inferior aspect of L3 in order to encompass the entire 'C-loop'. For proximal tumors that involve the cardia or gastroesophageal junction the paraesophageal nodes should be included and a 5-cm margin should be included in the cephalad field margin. For distal lesions at or near the gastroduodenal junction, a 5-cm margin of duodenum should be included.

Radiation fields that treat the stomach generally include the entire left kidney. Conformal radiation techniques that exclude the kidney are not possible because the stomach is a highly mobile structure. When 50% of a single kidney receives radiation doses of more than 26 Gy, the creatinine clearance decreases by 10%. When the entire kidney receives more than 26 Gy of radiation, a 24% decrease in creatinine clearance has been observed (178). However, the development of a clinically relevant compromise of kidney function is rare when one kidney is spared from the radiation field.

Radiation-induced liver disease, often called radiation hepatitis, is characterized by the development of anicteric ascites approximately 2 weeks to 4 months after hepatic irradiation (179). The whole liver has been treated safely to doses >20 Gy, a significant risk for radiation hepatitis exists when doses of more than 35 Gy are given (180,181). The risk of radiation hepatitis, however, is dependent on both the radiation dose and the volume of liver that is treated (182,183). Small volumes of the liver can tolerate high doses of irradiation (184).

Palliative chemotherapy

The most active single agents in gastric cancer are 5FU, mitomycin, and doxorubicin (150,185–187). Although randomized studies have shown an advantage in median survival when multiagent chemotherapy is compared with best supportive care, there has been no advantage in long-term survival (188–190). The advantage of multiagent regimens over single agent treatment also has not been established (191). The median survival is relatively short (5–7 months) in most studies. Due to the high morbidity and cost as well as the lack of an established benefit of multiagent regimens, patients should be offered supportive care, including palliative chemoradiation, or participation in a clinical trial that evaluates new agents and/or combinations.

Small bowel tumors

Since the small bowel and surrounding mesenteric lymphatics are mobile, regional treatment for malignancies of the jejunum and ileum would have to include very large fields. But, the tolerance of the whole abdomen to radiation is less than the dose required to sterilize tumor (192). Because of this, most cancers of the small intestine are treated by surgical resection. However, the fixed region of the duodenum (the C-loop) around the pancreas can be treated, especially if there is local infiltration into adjacent visceral structures. Regional lymphatics are frequently involved and the competing risk of distant failure is modest in duodenal cancer (193–197). The primary site and regional lymphatic drainage can be safely treated to 45–50 Gy, which is a dose that reliably sterilizes microscopic residual disease. Radiotherapy portals should cover the entire duodenum as well as the hepatoduodenal, peripancreatic, superior mesenteric, periportal, sybpyloric, gastroduodenal, and paraaortic nodal chains. At least a 5 cm mucosal margin proximally and distally is recommended due to the potential for submucosal spread. Localized boost doses of at most 10 Gy to areas felt to be a highest risk can be given with external beam radiotherapy or with IORT. The risk of duodenal ulceration and/or perforation increases sharply at total doses higher than 55 Gy (198).

Pancreatic tumors

The initial goals in the evaluation and treatment of the symptomatic patient are to determine resectability, to establish a histologic diagnosis, and to re-establish biliary tract outflow. The most common presenting symptoms of pancreatic cancer are jaundice, weight loss due to anorexia and exocrine insufficiency, and abdominal pain. Jaundice is usually a presenting symptom in pancreatic head lesions. Patients with lesions arising in the body or tail more often present with pain. Pain is a symptom of locally advanced disease. It is typically described as sharp and knife-like located in the mid epigastric region with radiation to the back and is often a clinical indicator of unresectable disease. With surgery alone, 50–80% of cases will develop local recurrence of disease (199–201). The most common distant sites of failure are in the liver and peritoneum (201). The lungs and bone are involved less commonly by distant disease.

The pancreas is drained by an abundant supply of lymphatics. Primary drainage occurs to the pancreaticoduodenal, suprapancreatic, pyloric lymph, and pancreaticoslpenic nodal regions, which all drain to the celiac lymph nodes and to the superior mesenteric nodes. The porta hepatis nodal region can also be involved, especially in advanced disease. The pancreatic duct and common bile are closely related as they travel through the head of the pancreas on their way to the ampulla of Vater. Invasion or compression of the common bile duct and main pancreatic duct are responsible for the presenting symptoms of jaundice and pancreatic exocrine insufficiency.

The divisions of the vagus and splanchnic nerves form the celiac and superior mesenteric plexuses. Nerve fibers reach the pancreas and other abdominal organs by traveling along the celiac and superior mesenteric artery and their branches. Direct extension of tumor to the first and second celiac ganglia posteriorly leads to characteristic sharp pain, which is perceived as back pain.

Radiation therapy

The acute effects of radiotherapy to the upper abdomen are outlined above in the section on gastric cancer. Nausea commonly occurs. With severe acute reactions, ulceration of the stomach or duodenum can occur. The routine use of prophylactic antiemetics and either a proton pump inhibitor or H-2 blocker is recommended. Diarrhea is less common due to the relatively small volume of jejunum that is typically in the field because the radiation fields that are used to treat the pancreas are generally smaller than those used to treat the stomach.

The dose-limiting structures surrounding the pancreas include the stomach, duodenum, small bowel, kidneys, spinal cord, and liver. The dose of conventional external beam radiotherapy that can safely be used in the upper abdomen is based on the tolerance doses of surrounding organs, and has been established in patients receiving radiotherapy alone (142,143,145,202–205), and in combination with 5FU (198,206,207). With conventional fractionation, given at 2 Gy per fraction, 50 Gy is well tolerated. If large volumes are radiated, the risk for radiation injury of the gastric and duodenal mucosa increases between 50 Gy and 60 Gy. But, radiation doses up to 68 Gy are well tolerated, with or without 5FU-based chemotherapy, if only a limited volume of mucosa is radiated (208).

A four-field technique using anterior, posterior, and opposed lateral fields allows sparing of critical tissues such as the liver, kidneys, stomach, spinal cord, and small bowel. The anterior–posterior (AP–PA) portals exclude a significant volume of liver and the kidneys. Because of the limited spinal cord tolerance, lateral fields are also used with post-operative treatment that totals 50.4 Gy. A radiation dose contribution is generally restricted to 20 Gy to limit the radiation dose to the liver and kidney tissue in the lateral fields.

For lesions located in the pancreatic head, the AP–PA fields typically cover T11–L3. The celiac trunk, which is typically located at T12, should be covered with a 2 cm margin superiorly. The inferior margin includes the C-loop of the duodenum. The left border is generally located 2 cm to the left of the vertebral body edge, and the right field border is defined by the C-loop and the porta hepatis. When a biliary stent has been placed this facilitates coverage of the porta hepatis. This usually means that the upper right border of the field is located 4–5 cm to the right of the vertebral body edge and the anterior aspect of the lateral field is 5–6 cm from the anterior vertebral body edge. Similar fields are used for tumors of the pancreatic body and tail, except that the splenic hilum is covered. The right field border is typically located 2 cm from the right vertebral body edge. Because of observed toxicities, there is a trend to reduce the radiation volume when potent radiosensitizers, such as gemcitabine, are administered with radiation. In these cases the radiation volume is restricted to a 1 cm area around the tumor (209).

The role of conformal radiation therapy in pancreatic cancer is currently undefined. There are no published clinical data analyzing the clinical impact of this technique. Conformal radiation therapy may allow escalation of the radiotherapy dose and/or a reduction in toxicity with chemotherapeutic agents such as gemcitabine.

Nearly 20 years ago, external-beam radiation therapy and concomitant 5FU chemotherapy was shown to prolong survival in patients with locally advanced adenocarcinoma of the pancreas in a landmark randomized trial conducted by the Gastrointestinal Tumor Study Group (GITSG) (206,210). This study showed that concurrent 5FU prolonged the median survival over treatment with radiation alone. In spite of this, local disease was a component of the first clinical site of failure in more patients who were treated with 40 Gy than were treated with 60 Gy. This suggestion of improved local control with 60 Gy vs. 40 Gy was offset by the problem of competing risk from distant failure. Additional randomized studies from the Mayo clinic and the GITSG support the superiority of combined modality therapy (149,211–214) over either radiation or chemotherapy alone.

Despite the generally poor overall prognosis with pancreatic cancer, most treatment programs for pancreatic cancer administer radiation over 4–6 weeks to deliver 45–60 Gy. In response to this, a program of rapid-fractionation radiation, totaling 30 Gy in 10 radiation fractions over 2 weeks, was initiated for resectable and unresectable patients at the University of Texas M.D. Anderson Cancer Center (207). The subset of 41 patients who completed protocol-based pre-operative chemoradiation and pancreaticoduodenectomy (27 patients who received standard-fractionation chemoradiation totaling 50.4 Gy and 14 patients who received rapid-fractionation chemoradiation totaling 30 Gy) was compared with 19 patients who received pancreaticoduodenectomy and post-operative adjuvant chemoradiation totaling 50.4 Gy with 5FU. The overall median follow-up for these 60 patients was 19 months. No patient who received pre-operative chemoradiation experienced a delay in surgery because of chemoradiation toxicity, but 6 (24%) of 25 eligible patients did not receive intended post-operative chemoradiation because of delayed recovery following pancreaticoduodenectomy. In contrast to the rapid fractionation group treated to 30 Gy over 2 weeks, hospitalization, due to acute gastrointestinal toxicity, was required by one-third of the pre-operative patients who received 50.4 Gy over 5.5 weeks (215). Local control of disease was achieved in every patient who received pre-operative chemoradiation and pancreaticoduodenectomy, but peritoneal (regional) recurrence occurred in 10% of these patients. Local or regional recurrence occurred in 21% of patients who received post-operative chemoradiation after pancreaticoduodenectomy.

More recently, our data from 132 consecutive patients who received pre-operative chemoradiation and pancreaticoduodenectomy for adenocarcinoma of the pancreas also supported the use of rapid-fractionation chemoradiation (216). Forty-four patients received 45–50 Gy in 25–28 fractions, and 88 patients received 30 Gy in 10 fractions. Concurrent chemotherapy consisted either of 5FU, paclitaxel, or gemcitabine. IORT was delivered to 74 of the 105 patients. The first site of failure occurred in the tumor bed in 8% in the 129 patients evaluable for local failure. There was no significant difference between the groups that received 30 Gy (9%) and the group that received 45–50.4 Gy (11%). None of the 25 patients that received 45 or 50.4 Gy and IORT experienced a local recurrence as the first site of recurrence. The overall median survival from the time of tissue diagnosis was 21 months. Neither the dose of pre-operative EBRT, the chemotherapy agent used, nor the delivery of IORT influenced survival duration. Univariate and multivariate analyses revealed superior survival times among patients who had no pathologic evidence of lymph node metastasis ($P=0.03$).

When disease was found to be unresectable at laparotomy, other studies have also shown substantial improvements in local control when IORT or brachytherapy was used, but this has resulted in only modest improvements in median survival (217–223). Although improvement in local control appears to produce some improvement in median survival, high rates of intra-abdominal failure in unirradiated areas continue to prevent a significant improvement in long-term survival.

Because the risk of systemic failure is so high, novel radiosensitizers such as paclitaxel and gemcitabine have recently been investigated for their role in the treatment of pancreatic cancer. A randomized trial of gemcitabine vs. 5FU as first-line therapy among patients with advanced pancreatic adenocarcinoma demonstrated a modest median survival benefit (4.41 months vs. 5.65 months, $P=0.0025$) for those patients who received gemcitabine (•). Gemcitabine was approved for use among patients with inoperable or metastatic pancreatic cancer based on quality of life improvements compared with supportive care; however, no improvements in overall survival were seen in this group of patients (224–227). Because gemcitabine is a potent radiation sensitizer, a significant increase in toxicity has been observed when gemcitabine was combined with palliative radiation without long-term impact in survival or quality of life (228–234). The palliative benefit of chemoradiation with gemcitabine remains investigational.

A recently completed phase I dose escalation study performed at the M.D. Anderson Cancer Center highlights the limitations of the use of concurrent gemcitabine and radiation. Profound normal tissue effects arising within the field of irradiation included nausea, anorexia, abdominal pain, gastrointestinal bleeding, dehydration, and profound fatigue. Hospital admission was required for management of nausea/vomiting and dehydration among 44% of the patients. The risk of hospitalization appeared to be gemcitabine dose-related. Similar chemoradiation-related toxicities have been reported in unresectable pancreatic cancer with paclitaxel, another potent radiosensitizer (235).

The available pre-clinical data indicate that optimizing the combination of gemcitabine with radiation is dependent on both timing and schedule. *In vitro* studies conducted at the M.D. Anderson Cancer Center indicate that inhibition of the repair of radiation-induced DNA damage by gemcitabine is dose-dependent, and that this effect is still apparent at 24–48 hours after removal of gemcitabine (236). Studies of the kinetics of cellular recovery have shown that normal tissues appear to recover more quickly from gemcitabine treatment than tumor tissues. Radiation sensitization of the tumor was best when gemcitabine was administered 24 hours before radiation (dose modification factor of 1.54). A time-dependent inhibition of DNA synthesis has been shown with gemcitabine ($50\,mg\,kg^{-1}$) when it was delivered at various times before and after radiation (228). It was found that the best tumor response occurred when gemcitabine was given 24–72 hours before radiation. Weekly, rather than biweekly or daily doses of gemcitabine maintained the tumor response but decreased toxicities in the jejunum (229). The normal tissue toxicities with gemcitabine may be tissue-specific. One study that evaluated the oral mucosa showed better response, and less radiation toxicity was seen with twice-weekly gemcitabine when it was compared with once-weekly gemcitabine (237). Determining the optimal time for gemcitabine administration during radiation to a specific site may greatly impact treatment response and toxicities (234).

The response to gemcitabine is also dependent on the rate of infusion. A randomized, phase II trial was conducted among patients with metastatic pancreatic cancer in which the infusion rates of gemcitabine were compared (227). An improved objective response (16.6% vs. 2.3%) was confirmed on CT when $1500\,mg\,m^{-2}$ at 10 mg per minute was given compared with administration of a higher dose of $2200\,mg\,m^{-2}$ over a 30-minute infusion. There was also a benefit in median and overall survival benefit (23% vs. 0% at 1 year) among patients treated with a more rapid infusion rate. Although most of the clinical studies that have been conducted have used a 30-minute gemcitabine infusion, these data would indicate that higher doses administered over 30 minutes may limit efficient intracellular utilization of the chemotherapy.

Because the gemcitabine dose limitation is predominantly attributable to gastrointestinal toxicity within the radiation field, it is reasonable to conclude that the radiation field size is a critical variable. Weekly doses of gemcitabine, in the range of $200–400\,mg\,m^{-2}$, are tolerated when the radiation fields that encompass the primary tumor and regional lymphatics. Doses in the range of $700–1000\,mg\,m^{-2}$ have been given with similar fields. From these preliminary prospective clinical data the tolerated dose of gemcitabine with radiation appears to be inversely related to the radiotherapy dose and field size that is used.

Protecting normal tissues from the effects of chemoradiation can also theoretically be accomplished by adding a pharmacologic radioprotector. The addition of amifostine to twice-weekly gemcitabine has recently been reported to enable dose escalation of a twice-weekly gemcitabine-based chemoradiation schedule from $60–120\,mg\,m^{-2}$ in a phase I dose-escalation study (238).

Because surgical resection of the primary tumor remains the only potentially curative treatment for pancreatic cancer, pre-operative chemoradiation has been studied for its ability to convert locally unresectable pancreatic cancer to resectable disease. Only 10% of clinically unresectable patients treated with 5FU or paclitaxel-based chemoradiation are able to eventually undergo margin-negative resection. Preliminary reports indicate that the margin negative resectability rate could be as high as 40%–50% among selected unresectable patients treated with gemcitabine-based chemoradiation.

Locally advanced pancreatic cancer is associated with significant symptoms. Radiation therapy is effective in relieving pain and biliary obstruction. Prognosis, however, remains poor due to regional disease. Strategies that target these patterns of failure are aimed to improve rates of resectability and response to systemic therapy. However, significant toxicities have been observed with newer systemic agents. This experience underscores the need to understand fully the site-specific normal tissue toxicities when a systemic agent is combined with radiation. Advances in care must adequately address the palliative benefit and minimize treatment-related toxicity.

Conclusions

Radiation therapy is an effective modality to palliate symptoms due to cancer involvement of the gastrointestinal tract. Although the gastrointestinal tract can be the site of metastatic disease, locally advanced disease from a gastrointestinal malignancy is the most common cause of symptoms. Goals of therapy include palliation of presenting symptoms and an attempt to allow resection of the primary disease. Resection of the primary disease allows the opportunity for curative therapy among some patients, and durable control of symptoms from the primary tumor among incurable patients.

For all sites of gastrointestinal malignancies, curative and palliative radiation therapy is now combined with systemic chemotherapy. Palliative therapy must address the known toxicities observed with the radiation to that site. Newer techniques, such as conformal radiation therapy, help to localize the radiation dose, minimize toxicities, and allow re-irradiation of recurrent tumors. Attempts to improve response to therapy, especially palliative therapy, must also account for the toxicities of systemic therapies. Beyond the systemic toxicities of chemotherapy, the enhancement of radiation toxicities must be considered.

Significant improvements have been achieved with chemoradiation for gastrointestinal cancers. These trials have served as paradigms for the use of chemoradiation in other sites. Future strategies, especially for palliative therapy, involve enhancement of tumor response, while minimizing treatment-related normal tissue effects.

References

1. **Cleeland CS; Gonin R; Hatfield AK; Edmonson JH; Blum RH; Stewart JA; Pandya KJ.** Pain and its treatment in outpatients with metastatic cancer. *N Engl J Med* 1994;330:592–596.
2. **Jacox AK; Carr DB; Payne R.**, eds. Management of cancer pain. Clinical practice guideline no. 9, Rockville, MD: Agency for Health Care Policy and Research; 1994 (AHCPR publication no. 94-0592).
3. **Jacox A; Carr DB; Payne R.** New Clinical Practice Guidelines for the management of pain in patients with cancer. *N Engl J Med* 1994;330:651–655.
4. **Brescia FJ; Portenoy RK; Ryan M; Krasnoff L; Gray G.** Pain, opioid use, and survival in hospitalized patients with advanced cancer. *J Clin Oncol* 1992;10:149–155.
5. Anonymous. Outcomes of cancer treatment for technology assessment and cancer treatment guidelines. *J Clin Oncol* 1996;14:671–679.
6. **Cassel EJ.** The nature of suffering and the goals of medicine. *N Engl J Med* 1982;306:639–645.
7. **Morita T; Tsunoda J; Inoue S; Chihara S.** Contributing factors to physical symptoms in terminally-ill cancer patients. *J Pain Symptom Manage* 1999;18:338–346.
8. **Manfredi PL; Chandler S; Pigazzi A; Payne R.** Outcomes of cancer pain consultations. *Cancer* 2000;89:920–924.
9. **Janjan NA; Payne R; Gillis T; Podoloff D; Libshitz HI; Lenzi R; Theriault R; Martin C; Yasko A.** Presenting symptoms in patients referred to a multidisciplinary clinic for bone metastases. *J Pain Symptom Manage* 1998;16:171–178.
10. **Pargeon KL; Hailey BJ.** Barriers to effective cancer pain management: a review of the literature. *J Pain Symptom Manage* 1999;18:358–368.
11. **Von Roenn JH; Cleeland CS; Gonin R., *et al.*** Physicians attitudes and practice in cancer pain management: a survey from the Eastern Cooperative Oncology Group. *Ann Intern Med* 1993;119:121–126.
12. **Chang VT; Thaler HT; Polyak TA; Kornblith AB; Lepore JM; Portenoy RK.** Quality of life and survival—the role of multidimensional symptom assessment. *Cancer* 1998;83:173–179.
13. **Vigano A; Bruera E; Jhangri GS; Newman SC; Fields AL; Suarez-Almazor ME.** Clinical survival predictors in patients with advanced cancer. *Arch Intern Med* 2000;160:861–868.
14. **Cleeland CS; Janjan NA; Scott CB; Seiferheld WF; Curran WJ.** Cancer pain management by radiotherapists: a survey of Radiation Oncology Group physicians. *Int J Radiation Oncology Biol Phys* 2000;47:203–208.
15. **Lamont EB; Christakis NA.** Some elements of prognosis in terminal cancer. *Oncology* 1999;13:1165–1170.
16. **Zhong Z; Lynn J.** Review of the Lamont/Christakis Article. *Oncology* 1999;13:1172–1173.

17. **Greenwald HP; Bonica JJ; Bergner M.** The prevalence of pain in four cancers. *Cancer* 1987;60:2563–2569.
18. **Sherry MM; Greco FA; Johnson DH; Hainsworth JD.** Breast cancer with skeletal metastases at initial diagnosis—distinctive clinical characteristics and favorable prognosis. *Cancer* 1986;58:178–182.
19. **Sherry MM; Greco FA; Johnson DH; Hainsworth JD.** Metastatic breast cancer confined to the skeletal system. *Am J Med* 1986;81:381–386.
20. **Lai PP; Perez CA; Lockett MA.** Prognostic significance of pelvic recurrence and distant metastases in prostate carcinoma following definitive radiotherapy. *Int J Radiat Oncol Biol Phys* 1992;24:423–430.
21. **Yamashita K; Denno K; Ueda T; Komatsubara K; Kotake T; Usami M; Maeda O; Nakano S; Hasegawa Y.** Prognostic significance of bone metastases in patients with metastatic prostate cancer. *Cancer* 1993;71:1297–1302.
22. **Knudson G; Grinis G; Lopez-Majano V; Sansi P; Targonski P; Rubenstein M; Sharifi R; Gruinan P.** Bone scan as a stratification variable in advanced prostate cancer. *Cancer* 1991;68:316–320.
23. **Sabbatini P; Larson SM; Kremer A; Zhang ZF; Sun M; Yeung H; Imbriaco; Horak I; Conolly M; Ding C; Ouyang P; Kelly WK; Scher HI.** Prognostic significance of extent of disease in bone in patients with androgen-independent prostate cancer. *J Clin Oncol* 1999;17:948–957.
24. **Grabowski CM; Unger JA; Potish RA.** Factors predictive of completion of treatment and survival after palliative radiation therapy. *Radiology* 1992;184:329–332.
25. **Reuben DB; Mor V; Hiris J.** Clinical symptoms and length of survival in patients with terminal cancer. *Arch Int Med* 1988;148:1586–1591.
26. **Fielding LP; Henson DE.** Multiple prognostic factors and outcome analysis in patients with cancer-communication from the American Joint Committee on Cancer. *Cancer* 1993;71:2426–2429.
27. **Portenoy RK; Miransky J; Thaler HT; Hornung J; Bianchi C; Cibas-Kong I; Feldhamer E; Lewis F; Matamoros I; Sugar MZ; Olivieri AP; Kemeny NE; Foley KM.** Pain in ambulatory patients with lung or colon cancer. *Cancer* 1992;70:1616–1624.
28. **Borre M; Nerstrom B; Overgaard J.** The natural history of prostate carcinoma based on a Danish population treated with no intent to cure. *Cancer* 1997;80:917–928.
29. **Perez CA; Cosmatos D; Garcia DM; Eisbruch A; Poulter CA.** Irradiation in relapsing carcinoma of the prostate. *Cancer* 1993;71:1110–1122.
30. **Macklis RM; Cornelli H; Lasher J.** Brief courses of palliative radiotherapy for metastatic bone pain. *Am J Clin Oncol* 1998;21:617–622.
31. **Steenland E; Leer J; van Houselingen H; Post WJ; van den Hout WB; Kievit J; de Haes H; Martijn H; Oei B; Vonk E; van der Steen-Banasik E; Wiggenraad RGJ; Hoogenhout J; Warlam-Rodenhuis C; van Tienhoven G; Wanders R; Pomp J; van Reijn M; van Mierlo T; Rutten E.** The effect of a single fraction compared to multiple fractions on painful bone metastases: a global analysis of the Dutch Bone Metastasis Study. *Radiotherapy and Oncology* 1999;52:101–109.
32. **Chandler SS; Sarin R.** Single fraction radiotherapy for bone metastases: are all questions answered? Radiotherapy and *Oncology* 1999;52:191–193.
33. SBU—The Swedish Council on Technology Assessment in Health Care. *Acta Oncologica* 1997;35[Suppl 6; Vol 1]:89–97.
34. **Hanks GE.** The crisis in health care costs in the United States: some implications for radiation oncology. *Int J Radiat Oncol Biol Phys* 1992;23:203–206.
35. **Porzsolt F.** Goals of palliative cancer therapy: scope of the problem. *Cancer Treat Rev* 1993;19(Suppl A):3–14.
36. **Porzsolt F; Tannock I.** Goals of Palliative Cancer Therapy. *J Clin Oncol* 1993;11(2):378–381.

37. **Cella DF; Tulsky DS.** Quality of life in cancer: definition, purpose, and method of measurement. *Cancer Invest* 1993;11:327–336.
38. **Janjan NA.** Radiation for bone metastases—conventional techniques and the role of systemic radiopharmaceuticals. *Cancer* 1997;80:1628–1645.
39. **Liu L; Meers K; Capurso A; Engebretson TO; Glicksman AS.** The impact of radiation therapy on quality of life in patients with cancer. *Cancer Practice* 1998;6:237–242.
40. **Arcangeli G; Micheli A; Arcangeli F; Giannarelli D; Pasta O; Tollis A; Vitullo A; Ghera S; Benassi M.** The responsiveness of bone metastases to radiotherapy: the effect of site, histology and radiation dose on pain relief. *Radiotherapy and Oncology* 1989;14:95–101.
41. **Mithal NP; Needham PR; Hoskin PJ.** Retreatment with radiotherapy for painful bone metastases. *Int J Radiation Oncology Biol Phys* 1994;29:1011–1014.
42. **Janjan NA.** An emerging respect for palliative care in radiation oncology. *J Palliative Med* 1998;1:83–88.
43. **Janjan NA; Waugh KA; Skibber JM; Curley SA; Carrasco CH; Lawrence D; Richli WR; Thomas J; Berner P; Lawyer A; Horton JL.** Control of unresectable recurrent anorectal cancer with Au198 seed implantation. *J Brachytherapy Int* 1999;15:115–129.
44. **Thames HD; Buchholz TA; Smith CD.** Frequency of first metastatic events in breast cancer: implications for sequencing of systemic and local-regional treatment. *J Clin Oncol* 1999;17:2649–2658.
45. **Pearlstone DB; Janjan NA; Feig BW; Yasko A; Hunt KK; Pollock RE; Lawyer A; Horton J; Pisters PWT.** Re-resection with brachytherapy for locally recurrent soft tissue sarcoma arising in a previously irradiated field. *The Cancer Journal from Scientific American* 1999;5:31–38.
46. **Shasha D; Harrison LB.** The role of brachytherapy for palliation. *Semin in Radiation Oncol* 2000;10:221–239.
47. **Morris DE.** Clinical experience with retreatment for palliation. *Semin in Radiation Oncol* 2000;10:210–221.
48. **Nieder C; Milas L; Ang KK.** Tissue tolerance to reirradiation. *Semin in Radiation Oncol* 2000;10:200–209.
49. **Erickson B; Janjan N; Wilson JF.** Brachytherapy: more versatile, more important for local control. *Internal Medicine* 1993;14(5):33–46.
50. **Powers WE; Ratanatharathorn V.** Palliation of bone metastases. Chapter 82:2199–2219. In: Principles and Practice of Radiation Oncology, 3rd edition; CA Perez & LW Brady, eds.; Lippincott Raven, Publishers; 1998.
51. **Rose CM. Kagan AR.** The final report of the expert panel for the Radiation Oncology Bone Metastasis Work Group of the American College of Radiology. *Int J Radiation Oncology Biol Phys* 1998;40:1117–1124.
52. **Bates T; Yarnold JR; Blitzer P; Nelson OS; Rubin P; Maher J.** Bone metastases consensus statement: *Int J Radiation Oncology Biol Phys* 1992;23:215–216.
53. **Niewald M; Tkocz HJ; Abel U; Scheib T; Walter K; Nieder C; Schnabel K; Berberich W; Kubale R; Fuchs M.** Rapid course radiation therapy vs. more standard treatment: a randomized trial for bone metastases. *Int J Radiation Oncology Biol Phys* 1996;36:1085–1089.
54. **Ben-Josef E; Shamsa F; Williams AO; Porter AT.** Radiotherapeutic management of osseous metastases: a survey of current patterns of care. *Int J Radiation Oncology Biol Phys* 1998;40:915–921.
55. **Gaze MN; Kelly CG; Kerr GR; Cull A; Cowie VJ; Gregor A; Howard GCW; Rodger A.** Pain relief and quality of life following radiotherapy for bone metastases: a randomised trial of two fractionation schedules. *Radiotherapy and Oncology* 1997;45:109–116.
56. **Barton M.** Tables of equivalent dose in 2 Gy fractions: a simple application of the linear quadratic formula. *Int J Radiation Oncology Biol Phys* 1995;31:371–378.

57. **Bates T.** A review of local radiotherapy in the treatment of bone metastases and cord compression. *Int J Radiation Oncology Biol Phys* 1992;23:217–221.
58. **Awan AM; Weichselbaum RR.** Palliative radiotherapy. *Hematology/Oncology Clinics of North America* 1990;4:1169–1181.
59. **Ratanatharathorn V; Powers WE; Moss WT; Perez CA.** Bone metastases: review and critical analysis of random allocation trials of local field treatment. *Int. J Radiation Oncology Biol Phys* 1999;44:1–18.
60. **Tong D; Gillick L; Hendrickson FR.** The palliation of symptomatic ossesous metastases-final results of the study by the Radiation Therapy Oncology Group. *Cancer* 1982;50:893-899.
61. **Blitzer PH.** Reanalysis of the RTOG study of the palliation of symptomatic osseous metastasis. *Cancer* 1985;55:1468–1472.
62. **Minsky BD; Conti JA; Huang Y; Knopf K.** Relationship of acute gastrointestinal toxicity and the volume of irradiated small bowel in patients receiving combined modality therapy for rectal cancer. *J Clin Oncol* 1995;13:1409–1416.
63. **Koelbl O; Richter S; Flentje M.** Influence of patient positioning on dose-volume histogram and normal tissue complication probability for small bowel and bladder in patients receiving pelvic irradiation: a prospective study using a 3D planning system and a radiobiological model. *Int J Radiation Oncology Biol Physics* 1999;45:1193–1198.
64. **Das IJ; Lanciano RM; Movsas B; Kagawa K; Barnes SJ.** Efficacy of a belly board device with CT-simulation in reducing small bowel volume within pelvic irradiation fields. *Int J Radiation Oncology Biol Physics* 1997;39:67–76.
65. **Chun M; Timmerman RD; Mayer R; Ling MN; Sheldon J; Fishman EK.** Radiation therapy of external iliac lymph nodes with lateral pelvic portals: identification of patients at risk for inadequate regional coverage. *Radiology* 1995;194:147–150.
66. **Taylor N; Crane C; Skibber J; Feig B; Ellis L; Vauthey JN; Hunt K; Curley S; Hamilton S; Cleary K; Dubrow R; Allen P; Sanfilippo N; Brown T; Wolff R; Sinicrope F; Hoff P; Janjan N.** Elective groin irradiation is not indicated among patients with adenocarcinoma of the rectum extending to the anal canal. Radiology [Suppl] Abstract 628; page 352; 2000.
67. **Tocchi A; Lepre L; Costa G; Liotta G; Mazzoni G; Agostini N; Miccini M.** Rectal cancer and inguinal metastases – prognostic role and therapeutic indications. *Dis Colon Rectum* 1999;42:1464–1466.
68. **Frykholm GJ; Glimelius B; Pahlman L.** Preoperative or postoperative irradiation in adenocarcinoma of the rectum: final treatment results of a randomized trial and an evaluation of late secondary effects. *Dis Colon Rectum* 1993;36:564–572.
69. **Frykholm GJ; Isacsson U; Nygard K; Montelius A; Jung B; Pahlman L; Glimelius B.** Preoperative radiotherapy in rectal carcinoma-aspects of acute adverse effects and radiation technique. *Int J Radiation Oncol Biol Phys* 1996;35:1039–1048.
70. **Pahlman L; Glimelius B.** Pre- or postoperative radiotherapy in rectal and rectosigmoid carcinoma: a report from a randomized multicenter trial- Ann Surg 1990; 211:187–195.
71. **Myerson RJ; Genovesi D; Lockett MA; Birnbaum E; Fleshman J; Fry R; Kodner I; Menteer J; Picus J; Read T; Walz B.** Five fractions of preoperative radiotherapy for selected cases of rectal carcinoma: long-term tumor control and tolerance to treatment. *Int J Radiation Oncology Biol Physics* 1999;43:537–543.
72. **Swedish Rectal Cancer Trial.** Improved survival with preoperative radiotherapy in resectable rectal cancer. *N Engl J Med* 1997;336:980–987.
73. **O'Connell MJ; Martenson JA; Wieand HS; Krook JE; Macdonald JS; Haller DG; Mayer RJ; Gunderson LL; Rich TA.** Improving adjuvant therapy for rectal cancer by combining protracted-infusion fluorouracil with radiation therapy after curative surgery. *N Engl J Med* 1994;331:502–507.

74. **Wadler S; Benson AB; Engelking C; Catalano R; Field M; Kornblau SM; Mitchell E; Rubin J; Trotta P; Vokes E.** Recommended guidelines for the treatment of chemotherapy-induced diarrhea. *J Clin Oncol* 1998;16:3169–3178.

75. **Callister M; Janjan N; Crane C; Bisanz A; Evetts P; Allen P; Cleeland; C.** Effective Management of Symptoms during Preoperative Chemoradiation for Locally Advanced Rectal Cancer. *Int J Radiation Oncology Biol Physics* 48 [Suppl]: Abstract 60, p. 177; 2000.

76. **Kornblau S; Benson AB; Catalano R; Champlin RE; Engelking C; Field M; Ippoliti C; Lazarus HM; Mitchell E; Rubin J; Stiff PJ; Vokes E; Wadler S.** Management of cancer treatment related diarrhea: issues and therapeutic strategies. *J Pain Symptom Manage* 2000;19:118–129.

77. **Denham JW; O'Brien PC; Dunstan RH; Johansen J; See A; Hamilton CS; Bydder S; Wright S.** Is there more than one late radiation proctitis syndrome? *Radiotherapy and Oncology* 1999;51:43–53.

78. **Miller AR; Martenson JA; Nelson H; Schleck CD; Ilstrup DM; Gunderson LL; Donohue JH.** The incidence and clinical consequences of treatment-related bowel injury. *Int J Radiation Oncology Biol Phys* 1999;43:817–825.

79. **Minsky BD.** Multidisciplinary management of resectable rectal cancer. *Oncology* 1996;10:1701–1714.

80. **Zerhouni EA; Rutter C; Hamilton SR; Balfe DM; Megibow AJ; Francis IR; Moss AA; Heiken JP; Tempany CMC; Aisen AM; Weinreb JC; Gatsonis C; McNeil BJ.** CT and MR imaging in the staging of colorectal carcinoma: report of the Radiology Diagnostic Oncology Group II. *Radiology* 1996;200:443–451.

81. **Horton KM; Abrams RA; Fishman EK.** Spiral CT of colon cancer: imaging features and role in management. *RadioGraphics* 2000;20:419–430.

82. **Vogl TJ; Pegios W; Mack MG; Hunerbein M; Hintze R; Adler A; Lobbeck H; Hammerstingl R; Wust P; Schlag P; Felix R.** Accuracy of staging rectal tumors with contrast-enhanced transrectal MR imaging. *AJR* 1997;168:1427–1434.

83. **Coia LR; Gunderson LL; Haller D; Hoffman J; Mohiuddin M; Tepper JE; Berkey B; Owen JB; Hanks GE.** Outcomes of patients receiving radiation for carcinoma of the rectum. *Cancer* 1999;86:1952–1958.

84. **Minsky BD.** Adjuvant therapy of rectal cancer. *Semin Oncol* 1999;26:540–544.

85. **Minsky BD.** Preoperative radiation therapy followed by low anterior resection with coloanal anastomosis. *Semin Radiation Oncol* 1998;8:30–35.

86. **Bosset JF; Pelissier EP; Manion G; Pavy JJ; Horiot JC; Hamers HP; Bartelink H.** Plea for a preoperative adjuvant approach in the management of rectal cancer. *Int. J Radiation Oncology Biol Phys* 1994;29:205–208.

87. **Rich TA; Skibber JM; Ajani JA; Buchholz DJ; Cleary KR; Dubrow RA; Levin B; Lynch PM; Meterissian SH; Roubein LD; Ota DM.** Preoperative infusional chemoradiation therapy for stage T3 rectal cancer. *Int J Radiat Oncol Biol Phys* 1995;32:1025–1029.

88. **Rich TA.** Adjuvant radiotherapy for rectal cancer: more on pre- or postoperative therapy. *Int J Radiat Oncol Biol Phys* 1995;32:547–548.

89. **Coucke PA; Sartorelli B; Cuttat JF; Jeanneret W; Gillet M; Mirimanoff RO.** The rationale to switch from postoperative hyperfractionated accelerated radiotherapy to preoperative hyperfractionated accelerated radiotherapy in rectal cancer. *Int J Radiation Oncology Biol Phys* 1995;32:181–188.

90. **Janjan NA; Khoo VS; Rich TA; Evetts PA; Goswitz MS; Allen PK; Skibber JM.** Locally advanced rectal cancer: surgical complications after infusional chemotherapy and radiation therapy. *Radiology* 1998;206:131–136.

91. **Janjan NA; Khoo VS; Abbruzzese J; Pazdur R; Dubrow R; Cleary KR; Allen; PK; Lynch PM; Glober G; Wolff R; Rich TA; Skibber J.** Tumor downstaging and sphincter preservation with

preoperative chemoradiation in locally advanced rectal cancer: The M.D. Anderson Cancer Center experience. *Int J Radiation Oncology Biol Phys* 1999;44:1027–1038.

92. **Kinsella TJ**. An approach to the radiosensitization of human tumors. *Canc J from Sci American* 1996;2:184–193.
93. **Koutcher JA; Alfieri AA; Thaler H; Matei C; Martin DS**. Radiation enhancement by biochemical modulation and 5-fluorouracil. *Int J Radiation Oncology Biol Physics* 1997;39:1145–1152.
94. **Milas L**. Chemoradiation interactions: potential of newer chemotherapeutic agents. *American Society of Clinical Oncology Educational Handbook*, pp 207–213; 2000.
95. **Hoff PM; Janjan NA; Saad ED; Skibber J; Crane C; Lassere Y; Cleary KR; Benner S; Pazdur R**. Phase I Study of Preoperative Oral UFT/Leucovorin and Radiation Therapy in Rectal Cancer. *J Clin Oncol* 2000.
96. **Hoff PM; Saad ED; Janjan NA; Skibber J; Pazdur R**. Preoperative UFT/Leucovorin and Radiation Therapy in Rectal Cancer. *Oncology* [Suppl 9]; 2000.
97. **Liu; G; Franssen; E; Fitch; MI; Warner; E**. Patient preferences for oral versus intravenous palliative chemotherapy. *J Clin Oncol* 1997;15:110–115.
98. **Hirata; K; Sasaki; K; Yamamitsu; S; Shirasaka; T**. A comparison of 5-fluorouracil concentration of 5-fluorouracil drip infusion versus oral UFT in plasma of same patients [in Japanese]. *Gan To Kagaku Ryoho* [Jpn J Cancer Chemother] 1993;20:1409–1411.
99. **Hoff; PM; Pazdur; R; Benner; SE; Canetta; R**. UFT and leucovorin: a review of its clinical development and therapeutic potential in the oral treatment of cancer. *Anticancer Drugs* 1998;9:479–490.
100. **Ho; DH; Pazdur; R; Covington; W., *et al.*** Comparison of 5-fluorouracil pharmacokinetics in patients receiving continuous infusion and oral uracil plus N1-(2′-tetrahydrofuryl)-5-fluorouracil. *Clin Cancer Res* 1998;4:2085–2088.
101. **Okabe; H; Toko; T; Saito; H., *et al.*** Augmentation of the chemotherapeutic effectiveness of UFT, a combination of tegafur [1-(2-tetrahydrofuryl)-5-fluorouracil] with uracil, by oral l-leucovorin. *Anticancer Res* 1997;17:157–164.
102. **Pazdur; R; Douillard; J-Y; Skillings; JR., *et al.*** Multicenter phase III study of 5-fluorouracil (5-FU) or UFT™ in combination with leucovorin (LV) in patients with metastatic colorectal cancer. *Proc Am Soc Clin Oncol* 18:263a, 1999 (abstract 1009)
103. **Carmichael; J; Popiela; T; Radstone; D., *et al.*** Randomized comparative study of ORZEL® (oral uracil/tegafur (UFT™) plus leucovorin (LV)) versus parenteral 5-fluorouracil (5-FU) in patients with metastatic colorectal cancer. *Proc Am Soc Clin Oncol* 1999;18:264a, (abstract 1015)
104. **Pazdur; R; Lassere; Y; Rhodes; V., *et al.*** Phase II trial of uracil and tegafur plus oral leucovorin: an effective oral regimen in the treatment of metastatic colorectal carcinoma. *J Clin Oncol* 1994;12:2296–2300.
105. **Gerard JP; Romestaing P; Ardiet JM; Mornex F**. Endocavitary radiation therapy. *Semin Radiation Oncol* 1998;8:13–23.
106. **Maingon P; Guerif S; Darsouni R; Salas S; Barillot I; d'Hombres A; Bone-Lepinoy MC; Fraisse J; Horoit JC**. Conservative management of rectal adenocarcinoma by radiotherapy. *Int J Radiation Oncology Biol Phys* 1998;40:1077–1085.
107. **Salembier C; Battermann JJ**. Interstitial brachytherapy in the conservative treatment of anal and rectal cancers. *Endocurietherapy/Hyperthermia Oncology* 1996;12:183–189.
108. **Armour EP; White; JR; Armin AR; Corry PM; Coffey M; DeWitt C; Martinez A**. Pulsed low dose rate brachytherapy in a rat model: dependence of late rectal injury on radiation pulse size. *Int J Radiation Oncology Biol Phys* 1997;38:825–834.
109. **Lingareddy V; Ahmad NR; Mohiuddin M**. Palliative reirradiation for recurrent rectal cancer. *Int J Radiation Oncology Biol Physics* 1997;38:785–790.

110. **Mohiuddin M; Marks GM; Lingareddy V; Marks J.** Curative surgical resection following reirradiation for recurrent rectal cancer. *Int J Radiation Oncology Biol Physics* 1997;39:643–649.

111. **Nymann T; Jess P; Christiansen J.** Rate and treatment of pelvic recurrence after abdominoperineal resection and low anterior resection for rectal cancer. *Dis Colon Rectum* 1995;38:799–802.

112. **Wong CS; Cummings BJ; Brierley JD; Catton CN; McLean M; Catton P; Hao Y.** Treatment of locally recurrent rectal carcinoma-results and prognostic factors. *Int J Radiation Oncology Biol Physics* 1998;40:427–435.

113. **Wong R; Thomas G; Cummings B; Froud P; Shelley W; Withers R; Williams R.** In search of a dose-response relationship with radiotherapy in the management of recurrent rectal carcinoma in the pelvis: a systematic review. *Int J Radiation Oncology Biol Physics* 1998;40:437–446.

114. **Guiney MJ; Smith JG; Worotniuk V; Ngan S.** Results of external beam radiotherapy alone for incompletely resected carcinoma of rectosigmoid or rectum: Peter MacCallum cancer Institute Experience 1981-1990. *Int J Radiation Oncology Biol Phys* 1999;43:531–536.

115. **Bussieres E; Gilly FN; Rouanet P; Mahe MA; Roussel A; Delannes M; Gerard JP; Dubois JB; Richaud P.** Recurrences of rectal cancers: results of a mutlimodal approach with intraoperative radiation therapy. *Int J Radiation Oncology Biol Physics* 1996;34:49–56.

116. **Lanciano RM; Calkins AR; Wolkov HB; Buzydlowski I; Noyes RD; Sause W; Nelson D; Willett C; Owens JC; Hanks GM.** *J Surg Oncol* 1993;53:20–29.

117. **Sofo L; Ratto C; Doglietto GB; Valentini V; Trodella L; Ippoliti M; Nucera P; Merico M; Bellantone R; Bossola M; Cellini N; Crucitti F.** Intraoperative radiation therapy in integrated treatment of rectal cancers-results of a phase II study. *Dis Colon Rectum* 1996;39: 1396–1403.

118. **Valentini V; Morganti AG; De Franco A; Coco C; Ratto C; Doglietto GB; Trodella L; Ziccarelli L; Picciocchi A; Cellini N.** Chemoradiation with or without intraoperative radiation therapy in patients with locally recurrent rectal carcinoma-prognostic factors and long term outcome. *Cancer* 1999;86:2612–2624.

119. **Martinez-Monge R; Nag S; Martin EW.** Three different intraoperative radiation modalities [electron beam, high-dose-rate brachytherapy, and Iodine-125 brachytherapy] in the adjuvant treatment of patients with recurrent colorectal adenocarcinoma. *Cancer* 1999;86:236–247.

120. **Schneebaum S; Papo J; Fraif M; Baratz M; Baron J; Skornik Y.** Radioimmunoguided surgery benefits for recurrent colorectal cancer. *Ann Surg Oncol* 1997;4:371–376.

121. **Kim HK; Jessup JM; Beard CJ; Bornstein B; Cady B; Stone MD; Bleday R; Bothe A; Steele G; Busse PM.** Locally advanced rectal carcinoma: pelvic control and morbidity following preoperative radiation therapy, resection, and intraoperative radiation therapy. *Int J Radiation Oncology Biol Physics* 1997;38:777–783.

122. **Shibata D; Hyland W; Busse P; Kim HK; Sentovich SM; Stelle G; Bleday R.** Immediate reconstruction of the perineal wound with gracilis muscle flaps following abdominoperineal resections and intraoperative radiation therapy for recurrent carcinoma of the rectum. *Ann Surg Oncol* 1999;6:33–37.

123. **Salo JC; Paty PB; Guillem J; Minsky BD; Harrison LB; Cohen AM.** Surgical salvage of recurrent rectal carcinoma after curative resection: a 10-year experience. *Ann Surg Oncol* 1999;6:171–177.

124. **Wanebo HJ; Antoniuk P; Koness RJ; Levy A; Vezeridis M; Cohen SI; Wrobleski DE.** Pelvic resection of recurrent rectal cancer-technical considerations and outcomes. *Dis Colon Rectum* 42:1438–1448; 1999.

125. **Wesselmann U; Burnett AL; Heinberg LJ.** The urogenital and rectal pain syndromes. *Pain* 1997;73:269–294.

126. **Mancini I; Bruera E.** Constipation in advanced cancer patients. *Support Care Cancer* 1998;6:356–364.
127. **Wong CS; Brierley JD.** External beam radiation therapy alone. *Semin Radiation Oncol* 1998;8:3–12.
128. **Brierly JD; Cummings BJ; Wong CS; Keane TJ; O'Sullivan B; Catton CN; Goodman P.** Adenocarcinoma of the rectum treated by radical external radiation therapy. *Int J Radiation Oncology Biol Phys* 1995;31:255–259.
129. **Crane CH; Janjan NA; Abbruzzese JL; Curley S; Vauthey JN; Sawaf HB; Dubrow R; Allen P; Ellis LM; Hoff P; Wolff RA; Lenzi R; Brown TD; Lynch P; Cleary K; Rich TA; Skibber J.** Effective pelvic symptom control using initial chemoradiation without colostomy in metastatic rectal cancer. *Int J Radiation Oncology Biol Phys* 2001;49:107–116.
130. **Janjan NA; Breslin T; Lenzi R; Rich TA; Skibber JM**: Avoidance of Colostomy Placement in Advanced Colorectal Cancer with Twice Weekly Hypofractionated Radiation Plus Continuous Infusion 5-Fluorouracil. *J Pain Symptom Manage* 2000;20:266–272.
131. **Scoggins CR; Meszoely IM; Blanke CD; Beauchamp RD; Leach SD.** Nonoperative management of primary colorectal cancer in patients with Stage IV Disease. *Ann Surg Oncol* 1999;6:651–657.
132. **Videtic GMM; Fisher BJ; Perera FE; Bauman GS; Kocha WI; Taylor M; Vincent MD; Plewes EA; Engel CJ; Stitt LW.** Preoperative radiation with concurrent 5-fluorouracil continuous infusion for locally advanced unresectable rectal cancer. *Int J Radiation Oncology Biol Physics* 1998;42:319–324.
133. **Rowe VL; Frost DB; Huang S.** Extended resection for locally advanced colorectal carcinoma. *Ann Surg Oncol* 1997;4:131–136.
134. **Luna-Perez P; Delgado S; Labastida S; Ortiz N; Rodriguez D; Herrera L.** Patterns of recurrence following pelvic exenteration and external radiotherapy for locally advanced primary rectal adenocarcinoma. *Ann Surg Oncol* 1996;3:526–533.
135. **Gunderson LL; Nelson H; Martenson JA; Cha S; Haddock M; Devine R; Fieck JM; Wolff B; Dozois R; O'Connell MJ.** Locally advanced primary colorectal cancer: intraoperative electron beam and external beam irradiation +/– 5-FU. *Int J Radiation Oncology Biol Physics* 1997;37:601–614.
136. **Kim HK; Jessup JM; Beard CJ; Bornstein B; Cady B; Stone MD; Bleday R; Bothe A; Steele G; Busse PM.** Locally advanced rectal carcinoma: pelvic control and morbidity following preoperative radiation therapy, resection, and intraoperative radiation therapy. *Int J Radiation Oncology Biol Physics* 1997;38:777–783.
137. **Chan AKP; Wong AO; Langevin JM; Jenken DA; Khoo R; Heine JA; Buie WD; Johnson DRE.** "Sandwich" preoperative and postoperative combined chemotherapy and radiation in tethered and fixed rectal cancer: impact of treatment intensity on local control and survival. *Int J Radiation Oncology Biol Phys* 1997;37:629–637.
138. **Blinkert CA; Ledermann H; Jost R; Saurenmann P; Decurtins M; Zollikofer CL.** Acute colonic obstruction: clinical aspects and cost-effectiveness of preoperative and palliative treatment with self-expanding metallic stents – a preliminary report. *Radiology* 1998;206:199–204.
139. **Camunez F; Echenagusia A; Simo G; Turegano F; Vazquez J; Barreiro-Meiro I.** Malignant colorectal obstruction treated by means of self-expanding metallic stents: effectiveness before surgery and in palliation. *Radiology* 2000;216:492–497.
140. **Goldberg RM; Fleming TR; Tangen Cm; Moertel CG; Maddonald JS; Haller DG; Laurie JA.** Surgery for recurrent colon cancer: strategies for identifying resectable recurrence and success rates after resection. *Ann Intern Med* 1998;129:27–35.
141. **Rousseau P.** Management of malignant bowel obstruction in advanced cancer: a brief review. *J Palliative Medicine* 1998;1:65–72.

142. **Goldgraber M; Rubin C; Palmer W., *et al.*** The early gastric response to irradiation; a serial biopsy study. *Gastroenterology* 1954;27:1–20.
143. **Roswitt B; Malsky S; Reid C**. Radiation tolerance of the gastrointestinal tract. *Frontier in Radiation Therapy Oncology* 1971;5:160–180.
144. **Hueper W; DeCarvajal-Forero J**. The effects of repeated irradiation of the gastric region with small doses of roentgen rays upon the stomach and blood of dogs. *Am J Roentgenol* 1944;40:1938–1945.
145. **Hamilton F**. Gastric ulcer following radiation. *Archives of Surgery* 1947;55:394–399.
146. **Klaassen DJ; MacIntyre JM; Catton GE; Engstrom PF; Moertel CG**. Treatment of locally unresectable cancer of the stomach and pancreas: a randomized comparisonn of 5-fluorouracil alone with radiation plus concurrent and maintainance 5-fluorouracil – an Eastern Cooperative Oncology Group study. *J Clin Oncol* 1985;3:373–378.
147. **Caudry M; Escarmant P; Maire JP; Demeaux H; Guichard F; Azaloux H**. Radiotherapy of gastric cancer with a three field combination: feasibility, tolerance, and survival. *Int J Radiation Oncology Biol Physics* 1987;13:1821–1827.
148. **Haas CD; Mansfield CM; Leichman LP; Considine B; Bukowski RM**. Combined "nonsimultaneous radiation therapy and chemotherapy with 5-FU, doxorubicin, and mitomycin for residual localized gastric adenocarcinoma: a Southwest Oncology Group pilot study. *Cancer Treatment Reports* 1983;67:421–424.
149. **Moertel CG; Childs DS; Jr.; Reitemeier RJ; Colby MY; Jr.; Holbrook MA**. Combined 5-fluorouracil and supervoltage radiation therapy of locally unresectable gastrointestinal cancer. *Lancet* 1969;2: 865–867.
150. **Schein PS; Smith FP; Woolley PV; Ahlgren JD**. Current management of advanced and locally unresectable gastric carcinoma. *Cancer* 1982;50:2590–2596.
151. **Brookland RK; Rubin S; Danoff BF**. Extended field irradiation in the treatment of patients with cervical carcinoma involving biopsy proven para-aortic nodes. *Int J Radiation Oncol Biol Phys* 1984;10:1875–1879.
152. **Ballon SC; Berman ML; Lagasse LD; Petrilli ES; Castaldo TW**. Survival after extraperitoneal pelvic and paraaortic lymphadenectomy and radiation therapy in cervical carcinoma. *Obstetrics and Gynecology* 1981;57:90–95.
153. **Hughes RR; Brewington KC; Hanjani P., *et al.*** Extended field irradiation for cervical cancer based on surgical staging. *Gynecologic Oncology* 1980;9:153–161.
154. **Fletcher GH; Rutledge FN**. Extended field technique in the management of the cancers of the uterine cervix. *Am J Roentgenology, Radium Therapy, and Nuclear Med* 1972;114:116–122.
155. **Asakawa H; Otawa H; Yamada S; Matsumoto K**. Combined therapy of gastric carcinoma with radiation and chemotherapy. *Tohoku Journal of Experimental Medicine* 1982;137:445–452.
156. **Asakawa H; Takeda T**. High energy x-ray therapy of gastric carcinoma. *Nippon Gan Chiryo Gakkai Shi-Journal of the Japanese Society for Cancer Therapy* 1973;8:362–371.
157. **Emami B; Watring WG; Tak W; Anderson B; Piro AJ**. Para-aortic lymph node radiation in advanced cervical cancer. *Int J Radiation Oncology Biol Phys* 1980;6:1237–1241.
158. **Macdonald JS; Schnall SF**. Adjuvant treatment of gastric cancer. *World J Surg* 1995;19:221–225.
159. **Roswit B; Malsky SJ; Reid CB**. Severe radiation injuries of the stomach, small intestine, colon and rectum. *Am J Roentgenology, Radium Therapy and Nuclear Med* 1972;114:460–475.
160. **Rubin SC; Brookland R; Mikuta JJ; Mangan C; Sutton G; Danoff B**. Para-aortic nodal metastases in early cervical carcinoma: long-term survival following extended-field radiotherapy. *Gynecologic Oncol* 1984;18:213–217.

161. **Wanebo HJ; Kennedy BJ; Chmiel J; Steele G; Jr.; Winchester D; Osteen R.** Cancer of the stomach. A patient care study by the American College of Surgeons. *Ann of Surg* 1993;218:583–592.

162. **Teramoto T; Onda M; Tokunaga A., *et al.*** Prognostic evaluation of peritoneal lavage smears and gastric wall brushing smears in gastric cancer surgery. *Gan to Kagaku Ryoho* [Japanese J Canc Chemotherapy] 1995;22:1606–1609.

163. **Maruta K; Shida H.** Some factors which influence prognosis after surgery for advanced gastric cancer. *Ann Surg* 1968;167:313–318.

164. **Buffet C; Turner K; Pelletier G; Etienne JP.** Palliative radiotherapy [letter]. *Br J Surg* 1983;70:131.

165. **Falkson G; van Eden EB.** A controlled clinical trial of fluorouracil plus imidazole carboxamide dimethyl triazeno plus vincristine plus bischloroethyl nitrosourea plus radiotherapy in stomach cancer. *Med and Ped Oncol* 1976;2:111–117.

166. **Gunderson LL; Hoskins RB; Cohen AC; Kaufman S; Wood WC; Carey RW.** Combined modality treatment of gastric cancer. *Int J Radiation Oncol Biol Phys* 1983;9:965–975.

167. **Wieland C; Hymmen U.** Mega-volt therapy of malignant stomach neoplasms. *Strahlentherapie* 1970;140:20–26.

168. **Bleiberg H; Goffin JC; Dalesio O., *et al.*** Adjuvant radiotherapy and chemotherapy in resectable gastric cancer. A randomized trial of the gastro-intestinal tract cancer cooperative group of the EORTC. *Eur J of Surg Oncol* 1989;15:535–543.

169. **Gastrointestinal Tumor Study Group.** A comparison of combination chemotherapy and combined modality therapy for locally advanced gastric carcinoma. *Cancer* 1982;49:1771–1777.

170. **Hayes N; Wayman J; Wadehra V; Scott DJ; Raimes SA; Griffin SM.** Peritoneal cytology in the surgical evaluation of gastric carcinoma. *Br J Cancer* 1999;79:520–524.

171. **Benevolo M; Mottolese M; Cosimelli M., *et al.*** Diagnostic and prognostic value of peritoneal immunocytology in gastric cancer. *J Clin Oncol* 1998;16:3406–3411.

172. **Nakajima T; Harashima S; Hirata M; Kajitani T.** Prognostic and therapeutic values of peritoneal cytology in gastric cancer. *Acta Cytologica* 1978;22:225–229.

173. **Koga S; Kaibara N; Iitsuka Y; Kudo H; Kimura A; Hiraoka H.** Prognostic significance of intraperitoneal free cancer cells in gastric cancer patients. *J Canc Research and Clin Oncol* 1984;108:236–238.

174. **Papachristou DN; Fortner JG.** Local recurrence of gastric adenocarcinomas after gastrectomy. *J Surg Oncol* 1981;18:47–53.

175. **McNeer G; Vandenberg H; Donn F., *et al.*** A critical evaluation of subtotal gastrectomy for cure in cancer of the stomach. *Ann Surg* 1951;134:2–7.

176. **Landry J; Tepper JE; Wood WC; Moulton EO; Koerner F; Sullinger J.** Patterns of failure following curative resection of gastric carcinoma. *Int J Radiation Oncol Biol Phys* 1990;19:1357–1362.

177. **Gunderson LL; Sosin H.** Adenocarcinoma of the stomach: areas of failure in a reoperation series [second or symptomatic look] clinicopathologic correlation and implications for adjuvant therapy. *Int J Radiation Oncol Biol Phys* 1982;8:1–11.

178. **Willett CG; Tepper JE; Orlow EL; Shipley WU.** Renal complications secondary to radiation treatment of upper abdominal malignancies. *Int J Radiation Oncol Biol Phys* 1986;12:1601–1604.

179. **Lawrence TS; Robertson JM; Anscher MS; Jirtle RL; Ensminger WD; Fajardo LF.** Hepatic toxicity resulting from cancer treatment. *Int J Radiation Oncol Biol Phys* 1995;31:1237–1248.

180. **Komaki R; Wadler S; Peters T., *et al.*** High-dose local irradiation plus prophylactic hepatic irradiation and chemotherapy for inoperable adenocarcinoma of the pancreas. A preliminary report of a multi-institutional trial [Radiation Therapy Oncology Group Protocol 8801]. *Cancer* 1992;69:2807–2812.

181. **Ingold J; Reed G; Kaplan H; Bagshaw M.** Radiation hepatitis. *Am J Roentgenol* 1965;93:200–208.
182. **Lawrence TS; Ten Haken RK; Kessler ML., *et al.*** The use of 3-D dose volume analysis to predict radiation hepatitis. *Int J Radiation Oncol Biol Phys* 1992;23:781–788.
183. **McGinn CJ; Ten Haken RK; Ensminger WD; Walker S; Wang S; Lawrence TS.** Treatment of intrahepatic cancers with radiation doses based on a normal tissue complication probability model. *J Clin Oncol* 1998;16:2246–2252.
184. **Dawson LA; McGinn CJ; Normolle D., *et al.*** Escalated focal liver radiation and concurrent hepatic artery fluorodeoxyuridine for unresectable intrahepatic malignancies. *J Clin Oncol* 2000;18:2210–2218.
185. **Gastrointestinal Tumor Study Group.** Phase I-II chemotherapy studies in advanced gastric cancer. *Cancer Treatment Reports.* 1979;63:1871–1876.
186. **Comis RL; Carter SK.** A review of chemotherapy in gastric cancer. *Cancer* 1974;34:1576–1586.
187. **Moertel CG.** Chemotherapy of gastrointestinal cancer. *Clinics in Gastroenterology* 1976;5:777–793.
188. **Pyrhonen S; Kuitunen T; Nyandoto P; Kouri M.** Randomised comparison of fluorouracil, epidoxorubicin and methotrexate [FEMTX] plus supportive care versus supportive care alone in patients with non-resectable gastric cancer. *Br J Cancer* 1995;71:587–591.
189. **Glimelius B; Ekstrom K; Hoffman K., *et al.*** Randomized comparison between chemotherapy plus best supportive care with best supportive care in advanced gastric cancer. *Ann Oncol* 1997;8:163–168.
190. **Murad AM; Santiago FF; Petroianu A; Rocha PR; Rodrigues MA; Rausch M.** Modified therapy with 5-fluorouracil, doxorubicin, and methotrexate in advanced gastric cancer. *Cancer* 1993;72:37–41.
191. **Cullinan SA; Moertel CG; Fleming TR., *et al.*** A comparison of three chemotherapeutic regimens in the treatment of advanced pancreatic and gastric carcinoma. Fluorouracil vs. fluorouracil and doxorubicin vs. fluorouracil, doxorubicin, and mitomycin. *JAMA* 1985;253:2061–2067.
192. **Whelan TJ; Dembo AJ; Bush RS., *et al.*** Complications of whole abdominal and pelvic radio-therapy following chemotherapy for advanced ovarian cancer. *Int J Radiation Oncol Biol Phys* 1992;22:853–858.
193. **Lai EC; Doty JE; Irving C; Tompkins RK.** Primary adenocarcinoma of the duodenum: analysis of survival. *World J Surg* 1988;12:695–699.
194. **Kerremans RP; Lerut J; Pennick FM.** Primary malignant duodenal tumors. *Ann Surg* 1979;190:179–182.
195. **Spira IA; Ghazi A; Wolff WI.** Primary adenocarcinoma of the duodenum. *Cancer* 1977;39:1721–1726.
196. **Joesting DR; Beart RW; Jr.; van Heerden JA; Weiland LH.** Improving survival in adenocarcinoma of the duodenum. *Am J Surg* 1981;141:228–231.
197. **Almark A; Andersson A; Larson A.** Primary carcinoma of the duodenum. *Ann Surg* 1980;191:13–18.
198. **Spitz FR; Abbruzzese JL; Lee JE; Pisters PWT; Lowy AM; Fenoglio CJ; Cleary KR; Janjan NA; Goswitz MS; Rich TA; Evans DB.** Preoperative and postoperative chemoradiation strategies in patients treated with pancreaticoduodenectomy for adenocarcinoma of the pancreas. *J Clin Oncol* 1997;15:928–937.
199. **Willett CG; Lewandrowski K; Warshaw AL; Efird J; Compton CC.** Resection margins in carcinoma of the head of the pancreas. Implications for radiation therapy. *Ann Surg* 1993;217:144–148.

200. **Westerdahl J; Andren-Sandberg A; Ihse I.** Recurrence of exocrine pancreatic cancer-local or hepatic? *Hepato-Gastroenterology* 1993;40:384–387.

201. **Griffin JF; Smalley SR; Jewell W; Paradelo JC; Reymond RD; Hassanein RE; Evans RG.** Patterns of failure after curative resection of pancreatic carcinoma. *Cancer* 1990;66:56–61.

202. **Coia LR; Myerson RJ; Tepper JE.** Late effects of radiation therapy on the gastrointestinal tract. *Int J Radiation Oncol Biol Phys* 1995;31:1213–1236.

203. **Bowers R; Brick I.** Surgery in radiation injury of the stomach. *Surgery* 1947;22:20–40.

204. **Hoshi H.** Histologic study on the effect of preoperative irradiation of gastric cancer. *Tohoku J of Experimental Med* 1968;96:293–311.

205. **Evans DB; Abbruzzese JL; Cleary KR., *et al.*** Preoperative chemoradiation for adenocarcinoma of the pancreas: excessive toxicity of prophylactic hepatic irradiation. *Int J Radiation Oncol Biol Phys* 1995;33:913–918.

206. **Moertel CG; Frytak S; Hahn RG; O'Connell MJ; Reitemeier RJ; Rubin J; Schutt AJ; Weiland LH; Childs DS; Holbrook MA; Lavin PT; Livstone E; Spiro H; Knowlton A; Kalser M; Barkin J; Lessner H; Mann-Kaplan R; Ramming K; Douglas HO; Jr.; Thomas P; Nave H; Bateman J; Lokich J; Brooks J; Chaffey J; Corson JM; Zamcheck N; Novack JW.** Therapy of locally unresectable pancreatic carcinoma: a randomized comparison of high dose [6000 rads radiation alone, moderate dose radiation [4000 rads] plus 5-fluorouracil, and high dose radiation plus 5-fluorouracil: The Gastrointestinal Tumor Study Group. *Cancer* 1981;48:1705–1710.

207. **Klinkenbijl JH; Jeekel J; Sahmoud T; van Pel R; Couvreur ML; Veenhof CH; Arnaud JP; Gonzalez DG; de Wit LT; Hennipman A; Wils J.** Adjuvant radiotherapy and 5-fluorouracil after curative resection of cancer of the pancreas and periampullary region: phase III trial of the EORTC gastrointestinal tract cancer cooperative group. *Ann Surg* 1999;230:776–782.

208. **Dawson LA; McGinn CJ; Normolle D; Ten Haken RK; Walker S; Ensminger W; Lawrence TS.** Escalated focal liver radiation and concurrent hepatic artery fluorodeoxyuridine for unresectable intrahepatic malignancies. *J Clin Oncol* 2000;18:2210–2218.

209. **McGinn C; Shureiqui J; Robertson J; Eckhauser F; Smith D; Decker D; Neumann B; Keller B; Brown D; Strawderman M; Lawrence T.** A phase I trial of radiation dose escalation with full dose gemcitabine in patients with pancreatic cancer. *J Clin Oncol* [ASCO Proc]:abstract 1999;18:274a.

210. **Gastrointestinal Tumor Study Group.** A multi-institutional comparative trial of radiation therapy alone and in combination with 5-fluorouracil for locally unresectable pancreatic carcinoma. *Ann Surg* 1979;189:205–208.

211. **Mohiuddin M; Cantor RJ; Biermann W; Weiss SM; Barbot D; Rosato FE.** Combined modality treatment of localized unresectable adenocarcinoma of the pancreas. *Int J Radiation Oncol Biol Phys* 1988;14:79–84.

212. **Gastrointestinal Tumor Study Group.** Radiation therapy combined with adriamycin or 5-fluorouracil for the treatment of locally unresectable pancreatic carcinoma. *Cancer* 1985;56:2563–2568.

213. **Gastrointestinal Tumor Study Group.** Treatment of locally unresectable carcinoma of the pancreas: comparison of combined-modality therapy [chemotherapy plus radiotherapy] to chemotherapy alone. *J National Cancer Institute* 1988;80:751–755.

214. **Klaassen DJ; MacIntyre JM; Catton GE; Engstrom PF; Moertel CG.** Treatment of locally unresectable cancer of the stomach and pancreas: a randomized comparison of 5-fluorouracil alone with radiation plus concurrent and maintainance 5-fluorouracil-an Eastern Cooperative Oncology Group study. *J Clin Oncol* 1985;3:373–378.

215. **Evans DB; Rich TA; Byrd DR; Cleary KR; Connelly JH; Levin B; Charnsangavey C; Fenoglio CJ; Ames FC.** Preoperative chemoradiation and pancreaticoduodenectomy for adenocarcinoma of the pancreas. *Arch of Surg* 1992;127:1335–1339.

216. **Todd KE; Gloor B; Lane JS; Isacoff WH; Reber HA.** Resection of locally advanced pancreatic cancer after down-staging with continuous infusion 5-fluorouracil, mitomycin-C, leucovorin, and dipyridamole. *J Gastrointestinal Surg* 1998;2:159–166.

217. **Roldan GE; Gunderson LL; Nagorney DM; Martin JK; Ilstrup DM; Holbrook MA; Kvols LK; McIlrath DC.** External beam versus intraoperative and external beam irradiation for locally advanced pancreatic cancer. *Cancer* 1988;61:1110–1116.

218. **Gunderson LL; Martin JK; Kvols LK; Nagorney DM; Fieck JM; Wieand HS; Martinez A; O'Connell MJ; Earle JD; McIlrath DC.** Intraoperative and external beam irradiation +/– 5-FU for locally advanced pancreatic cancer. *Int J Radiation Oncology Biol Phys* 1987;13:319–329.

219. **Mohiuddin M; Regine WF; Stevens J; Rosato F; Barbot D; Biermann W; Cantor R.** Combined intraoperative radiation and perioperative chemotherapy for unresectable cancers of the pancreas. *J Clin Oncol* 1995;13:2764–2768.

220. **Garton GR; Gunderson LL; Nagorney DM; Donohue JH; Martin JK; McIlrath DC; Cha SS.** High-dose preoperative external beam and intraoperative irradiation for locally advanced pancreatic cancer. *Int J Radiation Oncology Biol Phys* 1993;27:1153–1157.

221. **Shipley WU; Tepper JE; Warshaw AL; Orlow EL.** Intraoperative radiation therapy for patients with pancreatic carcinoma. *World J Surg* 1984;8:929–934.

222. **Mohiuddin M; Rosato F; Barbot D; Schuricht A; Biermann W; Cantor R.** Long-term results of combined modality treatment with I-125 implantation for carcinoma of the pancreas. *Int J Radiation Oncology Biol Phys* 1992;23:305–311.

223. **Shipley WU; Nardi GL; Cohen AM; Ling CC.** Iodine-125 implant and external beam irradiation in patients with localized pancreatic carcinoma: a comparative study to surgical resection. *Cancer* 1980;45:709–714.

224. **Burris HA; III; Moore MJ; Andersen J; Green MR; Rothenberg ML; Modiano MR; Cripps MC; Portenoy RK; Storniolo AM; Tarassoff P; Nelson R; Dorr FA; Stephens CD; Von Hoff DD.** Improvements in survival and clinical benefit with gemcitabine as first-line therapy for patients with advanced pancreas cancer: a randomized trial. *J Clin Oncol* 1997;15:2403–2413.

225. **Casper ES; Green MR; Kelsen DP; Heelan RT; Brown TD; Flombaum CD; Trochanowski B; Tarassoff PG.** Phase II trial of gemcitabine [2,2′-difluorodeoxycytidine] in patients with adenocarcinoma of the pancreas. *Investigational New Drugs* 1994;12:29–34.

226. **Rothenberg ML; Burris HA; III; Anderson JS; Moore M; Green MR; Portenoy RK; Casper ES; Tarassof PG; Storniolo AM; Von Hoff DD.** Gemcitabine: effective palliative therapy for pancreas cancer patients failing 5-FU. *J Clin Oncol* [ASCO Proc] 1995;14:198.

227. **Tempero M; Plunkett W; Ruiz V; van Haperen J; Hainsworth H; Hochster R; Lenzi R; Abbruzzese J.** Randomized phase II trial of dose intense gemcitabine by standard infusion vs. fixed dose rate in metastatic pancreatic adenocarcinoma. *J Clin Onc* [Proc ASCO] 1999;18:Abstr 1048.

228. **Milas L; Fujii T; Hunter N; Elshaikh M; Mason K; Plunkett W; Ang KK; Hittelman W.** Enhancement of tumor radioresponse in vivo by gemcitabine. *Cancer Res* 1999;59:107–114.

229. **Mason KA; Milas L; Hunter NR; Elshaikh M; Buchmiller L; Kishi K; Hittelman K; Ang KK.** Maximizing therapeutic gain with gemcitabine and fractionated radiation. *Int J Radiation Oncology Biol Phys* 1999;44:1125–1135.

230. **Joschko M; Webster L; Groves., *et al.*** Radioenhancement by gemcitabine with accelerated fractionated radiotherapy in a human tumor xenograft model. *Radiation Oncology Investigation* 1997;5:62–71.

231. **Lawrence TS; Chang EY; Hertel L; Shewach D.** Gemcitabine radiosensitizes human pancreas cancer cells. *Proc American Assoc Clinical Research* 1994;35:A3855.

232. **Lawrence T; Eisbruch A; Shewach D.** Gemcitabine-mediated radiosensitization. *Semin in Oncol* 1997;24[2,S7]:S724-S728.

233. **Wolff R; Janjan NA; Lenzi R; Abbruzzese JL; Goswitz M; Charsangavej C; Pisters PWT; Lee J; Evans DB.** Treatment related toxicities with rapid-fractionation external beam radiation and concomitant gemcitabine for locally advanced nonmetastatic adenocarcinoma of the pancreas. *Int J Radiation Oncology Biol Phys* [Suppl 1; ASTRO Proc] 1998;42:201; abstract #153.

234. **Hittelman W; Fujii T; Hunter N; Konishi H; Mason K; Gregoire V; Plunkett W; Milas L.** Identification of a window of therapeutic opportunity for the combination of gemcitabine and radiation. *Proc Am Assoc for Cancer Res* 1996;37:A1973.

235. **Safran H; Cioffi W; Iannitti D; Mega A; Akerman P.** Paclitaxel and concurrent radiation for locally advanced pancreatic carcinoma. *Frontiers in Bioscience* 1998;3:E204–206.

236. **Huang N; Hittelman W.** Transient inhibition of chromosome damage repair after ionizing radiation by gemcitabine. *Proc Amer Assoc for Cancer Res* 36:612; abstract A3643; 1995.

237. **Fields MT; Eisbruch A; Normolle D; Orfali A; Davis MA; Pu AT; Lawrence TS.** Radiosensitization produced in vivo by once vs. twice-weekly 2′2′-difluoro-2′-deoxycytidine [gemcitabine]. *Int J Radiation Oncology Biol Phys* 2000;47:785–791.

238. **Yavuz A; Aydin F; Yavuz M; Lis E; Yaris N.** A Phase I trial of radiation therapy plus concurrent fixed dose of Amifostine with escalating doses of twice-weekly gemcitabine in advanced pancreatic cancer. *J Clin Oncol* [Proc ASCO] 2000;19:Abstract 1105.

Chapter 19

Drug therapy for cancer-associated anorexia

Aminah Jatoi and Charles L. Loprinzi

The impact of cancer-associated anorexia

Anorexia is a distressing symptom for patients with advanced cancer. In *The Death of Ivan Ilych*, Tolstoy alludes to the anguish and global sense of loss that accompanies loss of appetite (1):

> ... all foods became increasingly distasteful and disgusting to him ... his mind went back to the raw... plums of his childhood, their peculiar flavor and the flow of saliva when he sucked their stones, and along with that taste came a whole series of memories of those days....

Equally eloquent and equally troubling are observations from family members who served as care-givers during the later stages of their loved one's illness. In a series of interviews among cancer patients and their care-givers, Holden quotes a husband as he cares for his wife who is losing both her appetite as well as her battle with cancer (2):

> It is so frightening for me to see her lose weight. I knew something was drastically wrong. I blamed myself for not feeding her the right things.

The scope of this psychological toll is broad and severe. Formal studies among patients with advanced cancer underscore the pervasive impact of this symptom. In a comprehensive prospective analysis of 1000 patients with advanced cancer, Walsh and others found that anorexia was tied for third as the most noxious symptom reported by patients (3). As many as 66% of patients in this series were experiencing it. Thus, not only is anorexia a profound source of distress for cancer patients and their families, but it is also highly prevalent.

The negative prognostic impact of this pervasive and distressing symptom is well established. In a North Central Cancer Treatment Group (NCCTG) study, Loprinzi *et al.* found that among 1115 patients with advanced lung or colorectal cancer, anorexia, as diagnosed by a patient-completed questionnaire, predicted a limited survival (4). Even in a multivariate analysis that included physicians' and patients' assessment of performance status and psychological parameters, anorexia stood as a powerful, independent predictor of patient outcome. Complementing data from the Eastern Cooperative Oncology Group (ECOG) demonstrating a direct association between weight loss and poor prognosis (5), the NCCTG study, as well as subsequent confirmatory studies, substantiates concerns from healthcare providers and family care-givers that this adverse symptom predicts an early demise for patients with cancer.

If all discussions on the palliation of cancer-associated anorexia must be prefaced with justification for undertaking them, the foregoing provides it. The above data clearly demonstrate that cancer-associated anorexia creates anguish for patients and their families, is prevalent, and carries an adverse prognostic impact. This chapter reviews the etiology and treatment of this noxious symptom.

An overview of cancer-associated anorexia and wasting

Anorexia is only one facet of a complex syndrome that includes loss of appetite, alterations in taste, aberrant body composition changes, fluctuations in resting energy expenditure and other metabolic perturbations, and at times mechanical impairments within the alimentary tract. The terms 'cancer-associated wasting and anorexia', 'cachexia', or 'the cancer anorexia/cachexia syndrome' are commonly used to refer to this syndrome. Weight loss is a marker of its severity, but weight measurements alone belie a complex underlying pathophysiology. Anorexia is difficult to separate from other manifestations of this syndrome, and mediators of anorexia, such as tumor necrosis factor-alpha (TNFα), interleukin-1 (IL-1), and interleukin-6 (IL-6), appear to contribute to tissue wasting and anorexia concurrently. For example, a recent study by Torelli *et al.* demonstrated that tumor-bearing mice given a soluble pegylated 55-kDa tumor necrosis factor (TNF) receptor construct significantly improved their food intake compared with a vehicle-treated group and at the same time gained more weight (although no body composition studies were undertaken) (6). As another example of this interrelationship, Chance *et al.* have hypothesized that tissue wasting may have direct effects on anorexia severity. These investigators observed a 113% increase in blood ammonia levels at approximately the same time that anorexia began to develop in tumor-bearing rodents (7), illustrating how various aspects of this syndrome might be linked. The role of lean tissue breakdown, the generation of nitrogen waste and ammonia, and the exacerbation of anorexia has not yet been well defined in clinical studies, however.

Yet if the hypothesis by Chance *et al.* is correct and if the generation of nitrogenous waste and ammonia from lean tissue breakdown leads to anorexia, then the dramatic body composition changes observed in cancer patients might explain the severity of this symptom. These body composition changes include a disproportionate and excessive loss of lean tissue. Cohn *et al.* studied 50 weight-losing cancer patients with a battery of body composition assessment techniques, including tritiated water, total body potassium measurement, and prompt neutron activation (8). Results were compared with those from individuals of comparable age and gender. Cancer patients manifested wasting within all body compartments, but there appeared to be a dramatic reduction of lean tissue, and most notably of muscle mass. Although the mechanisms behind this lean tissue wasting have not yet been fully elucidated, recent studies have implicated the ubiquitin–proteasome pathway (9), the direct effects of proteolysis-inducing factor (10), and NF-kappaB-induced loss of MyoD messenger RNA (11). At the same time, many weight-losing cancer patients manifest a constellation of hyperglycemia, hypertriglyceridemia, and an exaggerated insulin response to glucose loads. The findings seen in adipose tissue wasting appear to be mediated by lipid-mobilizing factor from the tumor (12). Such body composition changes stand in stark contrast to those seen in the starving host where lean tissue is initially well-preserved, and hunger, not anorexia, prevails.

As mentioned above, alterations in resting energy expenditure (REE) as well as other metabolic aberrations also appear to contribute to cancer-associated anorexia wasting and anorexia. Although it is unclear whether such alterations directly impact on anorexia severity, both anorexia and increases in REE appear to share common mediators. Increased REE has been observed in patients with hematologic malignancies, sarcomas, and lung cancer (13–15). This hypermetabolism tips the energy balance in favor of weight loss. As an example of the effects of tumor necrosis factor-alpha, a well-described mediator of anorexia, Starnes *et al.* administered a recombinant form of this cytokine to a group of cancer patients (16). They observed increased REE and an increase in whole body protein metabolism. In a more recent study, Staal-van den Brekel examined the relationship between REE and factors such as soluble tumor necrosis factor receptor 55 (STNF-R55) (17). Among 87 patients with non-small-cell lung cancer, 67 were deemed hypermetabolic on the basis of a ≥110% increase in the ratio of measured to predicted values based on gender- and age-specific regression equations. Hypermetabolic patients manifested increased levels of STNF-R55 compared with other patients. As alluded to above in the study by Torelli *et al.*, TNFα and its soluble receptors also appear to mediate anorexia (6). Hence, these mediators effect different aspects of this syndrome: they appear both to increase metabolic rate and to decrease appetite.

In addition to alterations in metabolism and body composition, a diminished caloric intake also contributes to weight loss. Theologides *et al.* formally evaluated dietary intake among patients with advanced cancer (18). Among the 39 patients evaluated in this trial, 18 had lost more than 10% of their premorbid weight. At the same time, over half of these weight-losing patients reported a greater than 300 kcal drop in their daily dietary intake prior to study participation. Although this study included a relatively small sample size, it was one of the first to evaluate the eating habits of patients with advanced cancer, and it suggests that weight-losing cancer patients do, in fact, eat less. What foods are they eating and avoiding? This question is difficult to answer because many factors, including the initiation of antineoplastic treatment, intermittent hospitalization, and increasing debility converge to alter eating habits and impair patients' ability to make and act upon free-thinking food selections. The majority of studies suggests, however, that cancer patients acquire aversions to certain foods, most notably those that are protein-rich (19), such as meat products.

Causes of cancer-associated anorexia

Several factors might explain why cancer patients eat less. First, depression is pervasive and often manifests as decreased food intake. As many as 50% of lung cancer patients suffer from it (20). Moreover, functional impairment is a risk factor for depression (20). Because depression, decreased appetite, and functional impairment appear to intertwine to configure a downward spiral among many cancer patients, it becomes difficult to clearly delineate depression's impact on cancer-associated anorexia. Nonetheless, based on the prevalence of depression within this patient population and based on the fact that anorexia is a common manifestation of depression, it appears plausible that depression worsens anorexia in this setting.

Secondly, mechanical reasons also contribute to poor oral intake, although prevalence rates to gauge the impact of this factor have not been well studied. Odynophagia from tumor, from mucositis or from another etiology; obstruction of the alimentary tract; or malabsorption contribute to caloric deficits. Many patients and healthcare providers also cite nausea and vomiting from antineoplastic treatment as another cause of poor oral intake. It is important to point out, however, that several studies suggest that chemotherapy leads to weight gain in the adjuvant setting and, at times, in the setting of metastatic disease for reasons that remain to be fully elucidated (21).

Thirdly, altered taste may also contribute to poor oral intake. Some researchers have argued that altered taste does not exist among cancer patients and that what patients describe as altered taste represents nothing more than taste aversions which result from eating after emetogenic antineoplastic treatment. As recently reviewed by Bartoshuk, the field suffered a notable set back when some of the original data that described a heightened sensitivity to bitter foods was unable to be replicated, and a misplaced decimal point in one of the original publications resulted in an erroneously significant *P*-value (22). This area of research continues to suffer from a lack of methodical investigations among chemotherapy-treated cancer patients. However, as also reviewed by Bartoshuk, observations from individuals exposed to radiation suggest that there is taste alteration among this subset of cancer patients. A telling account of such radiation-induced effects comes from MacCarthy-Leventhal, a physician who received radiation for head and neck cancer (23):

> It is difficult to explain to other people this 'blindness of the mouth'. They can bandage their eyes, but they find it hard to imagine the disgust and suspicion engendered by a 'cindery bolus' in the blind mouth. Those faithful sentries, the taste buds are dead.

Dr MacCarthy-Leventhal died in 1959, prior to the publication of her case report, which instructs us so well on the suffering associated with altered taste.

Finally, and as alluded to earlier, cytokines, and hormones are other factors that might explain further the etiology of cancer-associated anorexia. TNFα, IL-1, and IL-6 have been studied the most extensively, but there are others. Prior studies, mostly in animal models, have demonstrated that the administration of these cytokines is associated with loss of appetite, up-regulation of these cytokines is associated with anorexia in cancer, and blocking these cytokines attenuates anorexia (6,24,25). Such data suggest these cytokines might be important therapeutic targets in future clinical trials aimed at palliating cancer-associated anorexia.

Recent studies have also suggested that perhaps by means of their effects on the hypothalamus, certain hormones might play a role in mediating cancer-associated anorexia. Again, most of these studies have occurred in animal models. However, our group recently acquired preliminary data on 73 patients with advanced cancer. Over 90% of these patients reported at least a 50% decline in baseline appetite in the preceding 2 months. Although we found no significant correlations between anorexia severity and circulating concentrations of neuropeptide y, leptin, or cholecystokinin 8, we did find that concentrations of neuropeptide y were slightly lower among these anorectic cancer patients compared with historical healthy controls (manuscript submitted). These results require further confirmation, but nonetheless suggest that further study of these hormones is warranted.

The palliation of cancer-associated anorexia

Among patients with advanced cancer, drug therapy occasionally plays a role in the palliation of anorexia. In choosing to attempt pharmacologic manipulation of appetite, three factors must be considered. The first involves selecting the appropriate patient. Prior studies have demonstrated that increased caloric intake benefits some cancer patients and not others. Under specific circumstances in the perioperative setting, in the setting of stem cell or bone marrow transplantation, and during treatment for head and neck cancer, studies suggest that patients might derive benefit from caloric supplementation (26–30). For these patients pharmacologic manipulation of appetite is too indirect an approach to guarantee adequate caloric intake and instead either enteral or parenteral feeding should be considered. In contrast, among patients with advanced, incurable cancers and anorexia, data are sparse to justify direct, aggressive efforts to increase caloric intake. In fact, several studies suggest that nutritional support can be detrimental and that nutritional counseling does little to impact patients favorably. For example, McGeer *et al.* published a meta-analysis that showed that parenteral nutrition resulted in no benefits but rather an increased rate of infectious complications in cancer patients who were receiving chemotherapy (31). Ovesen *et al.* found that among cancer patients receiving chemotherapy, dietary counseling led to increased caloric intake but did not result in improved survival, response rates, or quality of life compared with a control group (32). Therefore, among these patients the aim of therapy is to assuage the discomfort associated with anorexia, not to increase caloric intake. The second consideration involves a search for co-morbidities. In our anecdotal experience, treatment of pain, depression, and altered taste (see below), for example, sometimes improves appetite. Consideration of treatable, related co-morbidity should be undertaken before resorting to appetite stimulants. Finally, the third factor to consider is whether pharmacologic manipulation of appetite is in fact necessary. A frank discussion with patients and family members about the reasons for and implications of anorexia often relieves the guilt derived from patients' inability to meet eating goals. It provides reassurance that the patient is not starving. An important point we often underscore to patients and family members is that the starving patient feels hunger whereas the patient with cancer-associated wasting does not. After such discussions, it is our experience that some cancer patients choose to forgo drug therapy.

When patients and healthcare providers opt for appetite stimulants, megestrol acetate and corticosteroids are reasonable choices to consider. To date, these two agents are the only ones that have proven successful in stimulating appetite in multiple, randomized, placebo-controlled trials in this setting. Because, these agents are equivalent in their orexigenic effects, megestrol acetate might be preferable among patients with a longer life expectancy because its long-term side-effect profile is preferable. On the other hand, if patients have had problems with thrombophlebitis (a side-effect and contraindication for megestrol acetate), if cost is an issue (megestrol acetate is more expensive), or if life expectancy is viewed in terms of weeks instead of months, then dexamethasone might be the better option. The studies cited below provide justification for this approach.

Multiple studies suggest that progestational agents improve appetite in patients with advanced cancer and anorexia. These agents, presumably and in part, appear to exert these orexigenic effects by means of down-regulation of IL-6 (33). While both megestrol acetate and medroxyprogesterone have been studied, the former has been studied most extensively. Initial data from Tchekmedyian *et al.* suggested that megestrol acetate may play a role in the palliation of cancer-associated anorexia. All together, however, at least 15 published placebo-controlled trials in cancer patients have evaluated megestrol acetate's appetite-stimulatory effects (34). Thirteen demonstrate that megestrol acetate improves appetite.

In a North Central Cancer Treatment Group (NCCTG) study, Loprinzi *et al.* published one of the first randomized, placebo-controlled trials to test the orexigenic effects of this agent (35). These investigators randomly administered megestrol acetate 800 mg day^{-1} versus placebo to 133 evaluable weight-losing and/or anorexic patients with advanced cancer. When patients completed questionnaires measuring appetite, it became clear that megestrol acetate was promoting it. Sixty per cent of patients in the megestrol acetate group stated that the study medication was improving their appetite in contrast to 42% in the placebo-treated group (P=0.009). In response to similar appetite-related questions, a significantly greater percentage of patients who received the megestrol acetate continued to describe favorable orexigenic effects with this hormone. Moreover, over 15% of these patients demonstrated a ≥10% increase in weight over baseline in contrast to none in the placebo-treated group. Because patient data were censored in the setting of edema, these results are particularly noteworthy insofar as they suggest this weight gain is not the result of fluid retention. Finally, as an unexpected benefit, patients who received megestrol acetate demonstrated significantly lower rates of nausea and vomiting. At the same time, this drug is reasonably well tolerated. Use of this agent entails a slight increase in the risk of thrombophlebitis, particularly in patients receiving concomitant chemotherapy. Megestrol acetate might also cause transient adrenal insufficiency, a potentially life-threatening complication if not anticipated and treated in the presence of serious infection, surgery, or trauma. In summary, the above data demonstrate that megestrol acetate improves appetite in patients with advanced cancer, leads to non-fluid weight gain in a small subgroup of patients, improves nausea and vomiting, and is well tolerated for the most part.

The foregoing 15 placebo-controlled trials with megestrol acetate spawned other questions. What accounts for the weight gain observed in this trial: augmentation of lean tissue or fat? Is there an optimal dose of megestrol acetate in this setting? Is there a prophylactic role for megestrol acetate in patients with advanced cancer where it might benefit patients prior to the development of cancer-associated anorexia and weight loss? To answer the first question, Loprinzi *et al.* evaluated 12 women who were receiving megestrol acetate for breast cancer with body composition assessment which included dual X-ray absorptiometry and tritiated water (36). Seven of these women subsequently gained weight. When these 7 women underwent reassessment of their body composition, it became clear that it was fat mass —not lean tissue—that accounted for the weight gain attributed to this hormone. Thus, megestrol acetate appears to augment the fat compartment, not lean tissue. The implications of this finding should be underscored: despite the effects of megestrol acetate on appetite, it does not reverse the underlying pathophysiology of cancer-associated anorexia and wasting, and a crucial aspect of this syndrome—namely wasting of lean tissue—continues to run rampant.

With regard to the second question, in another NCCTG trial, Loprinzi *et al.* examined the optimal dose of megestrol acetate for the palliation of cancer-associated anorexia (37). These investigators compared the doses of this hormone that had been used successfully in earlier trials. A total of 342 evaluable patients were randomized to one of four doses: 160 mg day^{-1}, 480 mg day^{-1}, 800 mg day^{-1}, or 1280 mg day^{-1}. Although there appeared to be an initial dose–response effect with megestrol acetate, this effect did not persist beyond the 800 mg dose. Based on these data as well as on the cost of this agent, it appears reasonable to initiate treatment with megestrol acetate at a dose of 160–400 mg day^{-1} and escalate to 800 mg over a 2-week period if no improvement in appetite is observed. Recently, the oral suspension form of megestrol acetate has gained popularity and is thought to be more bioavailable. With the use of the oral suspension form, a reasonable maximal target dose is 600 mg day^{-1}.

In answer to the third question as to whether megestrol acetate should be used prophylactically in patients who are not yet experiencing anorexia, another NCCTG study provided the answer. This question arose not only from data that demonstrated megestrol acetate promotes appetite but also from studies that suggest anorexia predicts a poor prognosis for cancer patients. A logical and clinically relevant next step was to see whether an intervention to improve anorexia also improved prognosis. Rowland *et al.* randomized 243 evaluable patients with extensive stage small-cell lung cancer to receive either megestrol acetate 800 mg day^{-1} versus placebo (38). Patients received concurrent antineoplastic treatment, which consisted of etoposide, cisplatin, and thoracic radiation. Although patients who received the megestrol actetate experienced significantly lower rates of nausea and vomiting compared with the placebo-treated group, there was no statistically significant difference in survival between the two groups. Somewhat concerning, however, was the finding that the group treated with megestrol acetate manifested a lower response rate to chemotherapy (68% versus 80%) in megestrol acetate versus placebo-treated patients, respectively ($P=0.03$), an observation that might be explained by an inadvertent and perhaps unavoidable prognostic imbalance between groups. Taken together, these results suggest that megestrol acetate should be restricted to the palliation of anorexia and that there is no prophylactic role prior to the development of anorexia.

In addition to megestrol acetate, corticosteroids are well-tested orexigenic agents that play a role in the palliation of cancer-associated anorexia. These agents are thought to promote appetite by means of their suppression of inflammatory mediators; they might also have orexigenic effects exerted directly on appetite centers within the hypothalamus. In the first placebo-controlled trial ever published in this field, Moertel *et al.* examined 116 patients with advanced gastrointestinal malignancies (39). None of these patients was receiving antineoplastic treatment. All had a life expectancy of 2 months or less, and all had a 'poor nutritional intake'. Patients received either placebo versus dexamethasone 0.75 mg four times a day versus dexamethasoe 1.5 mg four times a day. At 4 weeks, 26% of the patients in the placebo-treated group reported an improvement in appetite in contrast to 55% in the dexamethasone-treated group ($P<0.05$). Although dropout rates were high in this trial, the three survival curves were superimposed upon one another. Thus, the differences in appetite detected at 1 month likely reflected the beneficial effects of dexamethasone, not selection bias from high premature dropout rates in a particular study arm. The results from Moertel *et al.* have been replicated in subsequent studies, thus clearly demonstrating that corticosteroids have orexigenic effects in patients with advanced cancer.

Both megestrol acetate and dexamethasone, when prescribed in the doses mentioned above, are fairly equivalent in their orexigenic potency. A recent study published by the NCCTG provides some guidance as to when to use which agent (40). Loprinzi *et al.* evaluated 475 weight-losing or anorexic cancer patients who were randomized to one of three arms: megestrol acetate 800 mg day^{-1} versus dexamethasone 0.75 mg four times a day versus the androgen fluoxymesterone. Although the third arm of this trial, the fluoxymesterone arm, did not appear promising, the other two study arms demonstrated that both megestrol acetate and dexamethasone were equivalent in their orexigenic effects. When asked in a questionnaire to rate their appetite at 1 month to what it was before starting the study medication, 74% versus 66% reported improvement in the megestrol acetate versus dexamethasone arms, respectively ($P = 0.8$). Other questions aimed at evaluating appetite demonstrated similar equivalent effects. However, toxicity rates were different between the two groups. Myopathy rates were higher in the dexamethasone-treated arm: 6% versus 18% in the megestrol acetate-treated versus dexamethasone-treated arms, respectively. Similarly, rates of Cushingoid changes were also higher among patients who received dexamethasone: 1% versus 6%, respectively, as were rates of peptic ulcer disease: 0% versus 3%, respectively. In addition, it appeared that these rates of toxicity influenced patients' continued study participation. Study removal rates for patient refusal or toxicity was 25% in the megestrol acetate-treated arm and 36% in the dexamethasone arm, although some of these patients likely stopped therapy for disease-related toxicity that they inaccurately attributed to drug therapy. Based on these data, we recommend that dexamethasone be reserved for patients (a) who have a contraindication to megestrol acetate (for example, a history of thrombophlebitis), (b) who choose this agent because of its cheaper cost, or (c) who are likely to receive only short-term treatment because of a limited life expectancy.

Other promising appetite stimulants

Besides progestational agents and corticosteroids, there are other agents that look interesting for the palliation of cancer-associated anorexia but require further study. First, Lissoni *et al.* recently completed a randomized placebo-controlled trial to test melatonin (41). Studying 100 patients with metastatic cancer, these investigators found a lower rate of weight loss was in the group that received melatonin at a dose of $20\,\mathrm{mg\,day^{-1}}$. While these results appear promising, further confirmatory Phase III studies are necessary. Second, another placebo-controlled trial found that the agent cyproheptadine, a histamine and serotonin antagonist, led to modest orexigenic effects (42). No significant weight increases were observed between the two study groups. Although the investigators in this trial thought that cyproheptadine's minimal orexigenic effects appeared to be 'too little too late' in this group of wasting patients, this agent might be useful in carcinoid patients with anorexia because of its role as a serotonin antagonist. Third, preliminary data from Boasberg *et al.* suggest that thalidomide at a dose of $100–200\,\mathrm{mg\,day^{-1}}$ may stabilize weight loss among patients with advanced cancer (43). Presumably working by means of shortening the half-life of mRNA TNFα, this agent appeared to stabilize weight in this Phase II trial. Other clinical trials have also noted increases in appetite as secondary endpoints. Placebo-controlled trials are necessary to confirm these findings. Fourth, Agteresch *et al.* recently evaluated the potential role of adenosine triphosphate (ATP) in 58 patients with cancer-associated weight loss. ATP, an energy source, might compensate for the metabolic changes that lead to energy deficits and weight loss in patients with advanced cancer (44). In this trial, patients were randomized to receive either ATP or no ATP. This trial was not double blinded, but a modest increase in weight was noted in the group that received the ATP, while a drop in weight was observed in the group that did not receive it. Although these investigators did not specifically evaluate appetite, their results appear promising enough to warrant further investigation in a study where appetite might perhaps be another endpoint. Finally, eicosapentaenoic acid (EPA), an omega-3 fatty acid, has led to weight gain in recent Phase II studies (45) and has also led to a survival advantage in a small placebo-controlled trial in patients with advanced cancer (46). Laboratory studies suggest that EPA might suppress proteolysis-inducing factor (PIF) as well as IL-6. An ongoing study being conducted by the NCCTG is evaluating this agent's potential role in treating cancer-associated wasting in a direct comparison with megestrol acetate, with anorexia being a major endpoint in this trial.

A special note should be made on zinc sulfate. As mentioned earlier, many cancer patients who have received radiation to the head and neck area experience alterations in their ability to taste food. Several Phase II trials have suggested that zinc sulfate improves taste in this setting. Recently, Ripamonti *et al.* examined the use of this mineral in a randomized, placebo-controlled trial (47). Eighteen patients with head and neck cancer were studied. Patients received either zinc sulfate 45 mg or placebo three times a day starting from the time they began to experience altered taste up to 1 month after completion of radiation. Using detailed taste acuity assessment, these investigators found that 1 month after completion of radiation, the zinc-sulfate-treated group manifested a faster recovery of taste compared to the placebo-treated group. These results require confirmation but suggest that zinc sulfate may play an important role among patients with altered taste after radiation treatment.

Less promising agents

Finally, a brief comment should be made of other drugs that have been studied in cancer-associated anorexia and weight loss but have not proven to be efficacious. Dronabinol is the active ingredient in marijuana and several anecdotal reports and Phase II studies suggested that it might have a role in the treatment of cancer-associated anorexia. However, the NCCTG conducted a large Phase III trial which included over 400 patients and found that megestrol acetate was superior to dronabinol as an orexigenic agent and that combination therapy added nothing over and above the favorable orexigenic effects obtained from megestrol acetate alone (manuscript in preparation). Secondly, metoclopramide has been proposed as a helpful agent for patients with cancer-associated anorexia. The underlying hypothesis behind testing this agent centers on its ability to increase gastric motility. In a recent trial by Bruera *et al.*, 26 cancer patients with dyspepsia were randomized to receive either metoclopramide 40 mg twice a day or placebo (48). The study included a cross-over to the alternate arm after 4 days. Although there was a trend toward improvement in nausea and dyspepsia, patients did not report an improvement in anorexia, a secondary endpoint. Admittedly, this trial was small, duration of treatment was short, and anorexia was not the primary endpoint. Nonetheless, these data suggest that metoclopramide is not a useful agent for cancer-associated anorexia. Thirdly, pentoxifylline, a methylxanthine derivative which inhibits TNFα production, has also been evaluated (49). A randomized, placebo-controlled clinical trial was conducted by the NCCTG. This study found no favorable effects on appetite or body weight. Fourthly, hydrazine sulfate inhibits phosphoenolpyruvate kinase, an enzyme involved in gluconeogenesis. Large placebo-controlled clinical trials have failed to demonstrate that this agent provides benefit to patients with advanced cancer (50). Finally, anabolic agents have also proved disappointing. Although several studies have been performed in cancer patients, a recent Phase III NCCTG trial among patients with advanced cancer and weight loss and/or anorexia found that the androgen, fluoxymesterone, had less effect on weight gain or appetite than either megestrol acetate or dexamethasone (40).

Conclusions

Anorexia is severe and pervasive among patients with advanced cancer. Accurate recognition of this symptom and appropriate counseling of patients and family members is an important aspect of oncologic care. As illustrated by Holden, guilt is a common reaction on the part of family members. 'It is so frightening for me to see her lose weight… I blamed myself for not feeding her the right things.' In some circumstances, pharmacologic manipulation of appetite is indicated. Under such circumstances progestational agents and corticosteroids might be of help.

References

1. **Tolstoy L.** *The Death of Ivan Illych.* New York: Harper & Row, 1967: pp. 282,297.
2. **Holden CM.** Anorexia in the terminally ill cancer patient: the emotional impact on the patient and the family. *Hospice Journal* 1991;24:73.
3. **Walsh D; Donnelly S; Rybicki L.** The symptoms of advanced cancer: relationship to age, gender, and performance status in 1000 patients. *Supportive Care in Cancer* 2000;8:175.
4. **Loprinzi CL; Laurie JA; Wieand HS., *et al.*** Prospective evaluation of prognostic variables from patient-completed questionnaires. North Central Cancer Treatment Group. *Journal of Clinical Oncology* 1994;12:601.
5. **Dewys WD; Begg C; Lavin PT., *et al.*** Prognostic effect of weight loss prior to chemotherapy in cancer patients. Eastern Cooperative Oncology Group. *American Journal of Medicine* 1980;69:491.
6. **Torelli GF; Meguid MM; Moldawer LL., *et al.*** Use of recombinant human soluble TNF receptor in anorectic tumor-bearing rats. *American Journal of Physiology* 1999;277:R850.
7. **Chance WT; Zhang FH; Foley-Nelson T; Fischer JE.** Hyperammonemia and anorexia in Morris hepatoma-bearing rats. *Physiology and Behavior* 1991;50:397.
8. **Cohn SH; Gartenhaus W; Sawitsky A; Rai K., *et al.*** Compartmental body composition of cancer patients by measurement of total body nitrogen, potassium, and water. *Metabolism* 1981;30:222.
9. **Williams A; Sun X; Fischer JE; Hasselgren PO.** The expression of genes in the ubiquitin–proteasome proteolytic pathway is increased in skeletal muscle from patients with cancer. *Surgery* 1999;126:744.
10. **Todorov P; Cariuk P; McDevitt R; Coles B., *et al.*** Characterization of a cancer cachectic factor. *Nature* 1996;379:739.
11. **Guttridge DC; Mayo MW; Madrid LV; Wang CY; Baldwin AS.** NF-kappaB-induced loss of MyoD messenger RNA: possible role in muscle decay and cachexia. *Science* 2000;289:2363.
12. **Todorov PT; McDevitt TM; Meyer DJ., *et al.*** Purification and characterization of a tumor lipid-mobilizing factor. *Cancer Research* 1998;58:2353.
13. **Staal-van den Brekel AJ; Schols AMW; ten Velde GP., *et al.*** Analysis of energy balance in lung cancer patients. *Cancer Research* 1994;54:6430.
14. **Stallings VA; Vaisman N; Chan HS., *et al.*** Energy metabolism in children with newly diagnosed acute lymphoblastic leukemia. *Pediatric Research* 1989;26:154.
15. **Peacock JL; Inculet RI; Corsey R., *et al.*** Resting energy expenditure and body cell mass alterations in noncachectic patients with sarcomas. *Surgery* 1987;102:465.
16. **Starnes HF; Warren RS; Jeevanandam M; Gabrilove JL., *et al.*** Tumor necrosis factor and the acute metabolic response to tissue injury in man. *Journal of Clinical Investigation* 1988;82:1321.

17. **Staal-van den Brekel AJ; Dentener MA; Schols AM., *et al.*** The increased resting energy expenditure and weight loss are related to a systemic inflammatory response in lung cancer patients. *Journal of Clinical Oncology* 1995;13:2600.
18. **Theologides A; Ehlert J; Kennedy BJ.** The calorie intake of patients with advanced cancer. *Minnesota Medicine* 1976;59:526.
19. **Holmes S.** Food avoidance in patients undergoing cancer chemotherapy. *Supportive Care in Cancer* 1993;6:326.
20. **Hopwood P; Stephens RJ.** Depression in patients with lung cancer: prevalence and risk factors derived from quality of life data. *Journal of Clinical Oncology* 2000;18:893.
21. **Demark-Wahnefried W; Winer EP; Rimer BK.** Why women gain weight with adjuvant chemotherapy for breast cancer. *Journal of Clinical Oncology* 1993;11:1418.
22. **Bartoshuk LM.** Chemosensory alterations and cancer therapies. *National Cancer Institute, Monograph* 1990;9:179.
23. **MacCarthy-Leventhal EM.** Post-radiation mouth blindness. *The Lancet* 1959;2:1138.
24. **Fong Y; Moldawer LL; Marano M., *et al.*** Cachectin/TNF or IL-1 alpha induces cachexia and redistribution of body proteins. *American Journal of Physiology* 1989;256:R659.
25. **Gelin J; Moldawer LL; Lonnroth C., *et al.*** Role of endogenous tumor necrosis factor alpha and interleukin 1 for experimental tumor growth and the development of cancer cachexia. *Cancer Research* 1991;51:415.
26. Anonymous. Perioperative total parenteral nutrition in surgical patients. *New England Journal of Medicine* 1991;321:525.
27. **Fan ST; Lo M; Lai ECS., *et al.*** Perioperative nutritional support in patients undergoing hepatectomy for hepatocellular carcinoma. *New England Journal of Medicine* 1994;331:1547.
28. **Weisdorf SA; Lysne J; Wind D., *et al.*** Positive effect of prophylactic total parenteral nutrition on long-term outcome of bone marrow transplantation. *Transplantation* 1987;43:833.
29. **Daly JM; Hearne B; Dunaj J., *et al.*** Nutritional rehabilitation in patients with advanced head and neck cancer receiving radiation therapy. *American Journal of Surgery* 1984;148:514.
30. **Nayel H; el-Ghoneimy E; el-Haddad S.** Impact of nutritional supplementation on treatment delay and morbidity in patients with head and neck tumors treated with irradiation. *Nutrition* 1992;8:13.
31. **McGeer AJ; Detsky AS; O'Rourke K.** Parenteral nutrition in cancer patients undergoing chemotherapy: a meta-analysis. *Nutrition* 1990;6:233.
32. **Ovesen L; Allingstrup L; Hannibal J., *et al.*** Effect of dietary counseling on food intake, body weight, response rate, survival, and quality of life in cancer patients undergoing chemotherapy: a prospective randomised study. *Journal of Clinical Oncology* 1993;11:2043.
33. **Nishimura R; Nagao K; Miyayama H., *et al.*** An analysis of serum interleukin-6 levels to predict benefits of medroxyprogesterone acetate in advanced or recurrent breast cancer. *Oncology* 2000;59:166.
34. **Jatoi A; Kumar S; Sloan J; Nguyen PL.** On appetite and its loss. *Journal of Clinical Oncology* 2000;18:2930.
35. **Loprinzi CL; Ellison NM; Schaid DJ., *et al.*** Controlled trial of megestrol acetate for the treatment of cancer anorexia and cachexia. *Journal of the National Cancer Institute* 1990;82:1127.
36. **Loprinzi CL; Schaid DJ; Dose AM., *et al.*** Body composition changes in patients who gain weight while receiving megestrol acetate. *Journal of Clinical Oncology* 1993;11:152.
37. **Loprinzi CL; Michalak JC; Schaid DJ., *et al.*** Phase III evaluation of four doses of megestrol acetate as therapy for patients with cancer anorexia and/or cachexia. *Journal of Clinical Oncology* 1993;11:762.

38. **Rowland KM; Loprinzi CL; Shaw EG., *et al.*** Randomized placebo-controlled trial of cisplatin and etoposide plus megestrol acetate/placebo in extensive stage small-cell lung cancer: a North Central Cancer Treatment Group study. *Journal of Clinical Oncology* 1996;14:135.
39. **Moertel CG; Schutt AJ; Reitemeier RJ; Hahn RG.** Corticosteroid therapy of preterminal gastrointestinal cancer. *Cancer* 1974;33:1607.
40. **Loprinzi CL; Kugler JW; Sloan JA., *et al.*** Randomized comparison of megestrol acetate versus dexamethasone versus fluoxymesterone for the treatment of cancer anorexia/ cachexia. *Journal of Clinical Oncology* 1999;17:3299.
41. **Lissoni P; Paolorossi F; Tancini G., *et al.*** Is there a role for melatonin in the treatment of neoplastic cachexia? *European Journal of Cancer* 1996;32A:1340.
42. **Kardinal CG; Loprinzi CL; Scahid DJ., *et al.*** A controlled trial of cyproheptadine in cancer patients with anorexia and/or cachexia. *Cancer* 1990;65:2567.
43. **Boasberg PD; O'Day SJ; Weisberg M., *et al.*** Thalidomide induced cessation of weight loss and improved sleep in advanced cancer patients with cachexia. *Proceedings of the American Society of Clinical Oncology* 2000: 2396A.
44. **Agteresch HJ; Dagnelie PC; van der Gaast A., *et al.*** Randomized clinical trial of adenosine 5′-triphosphate in patients with advanced non-small cell lung cancer. *Journal of the National Cancer Institute* 2000;92:321.
45. **Wigmore SJ; Barber MD; Ross JA., *et al.*** Effect of oral eicosapentaenoic acid on weight loss in patients with pancreatic cancer. *Nutrition and Cancer* 2000;36:177.
46. **Gogos CA; Ginopoulos P; Salsa B., *et al.*** Dietary omega-3 polyunsaturated fatty acids plus vitamin E restore immunodeficiency and prolong survival for severely ill patients with generalized malignancy: a randomized controlled trial. *Cancer* 1998;82:395.
47. **Ripamonti C; Zecca E; Brunelli C., *et al.*** A randomized, controlled trial to evaluate the effects of zinc sulfate on cancer patients with taste alterations caused by head and neck irradiation. *Cancer* 1998;82:1938.
48. **Bruera E; Belzile M; Neumann C., *et al.*** A double blind, crossover study of controlled-release metoclopramide and placebo for the chronic nausea and dyspepsia for advanced cancer. *Journal of Pain and Symptom management* 2000;19:427.
49. **Goldberg RM; Loprinzi CL; Mailliard JA., *et al.*** Pentoxyfylline for treatment of cancer anorexia and cachexia? A randomized, double-blind, placebo-controlled trial. *Journal of Clinical Oncology* 1995;13:2856.
50. **Loprinzi CL; Goldberg RM; Su JQ., *et al.*** Placebo-controlled trial of hydrazine sulfate in patients with newly diagnosed non-small cell lung cancer. *Journal of Clinical Oncology* 1994;12:1126.

Chapter 20

Artificial nutrition I: General approach and parenteral nutrition

Federico Bozzetti

Introduction

For over 30 years artificial nutrition (AN) has had a major impact in many fields of medicine, including surgery, oncology, intensive care, gastroenterology, and transplantation.

Except in patients with primary undernutrition, who account for a small percentage in Western countries and are usually elderly individuals unable to provide themselves with adequate oral intake, AN has been used in clinical conditions in which, for a variety of reasons, the normal intake of food was impossible or contraindicated, while maintenance of nutritional status was essential for the patient to allow the primary therapy to control the disease and eventually to achieve full recovery.

AN has played an ancillary role in the therapy of many severe diseases, although recently the discovery that some nutrients are indispensable in some conditions and have a pharmacologic effect at certain doses has led AN to resemble a 'therapy' more than a simply supportive treatment. This chapter examines the main indications and the use of AN and the specific issues associated with parenteral nutrition.

Rationale for nutritional support

Patients with advanced cancer are candidates for nutritional support if they are unable to eat, severely malnourished, or both. However, an effort should always be made to define the priority of nutritional support and of nutritional status within the context of symptoms complained of by patients and the complexity of the treatments planned by the oncologist and nutritionist.

AN nutrition includes both the more sophisticated total parenteral nutrition (TPN) as well as the simplest administration of sip feeding. It is evident that the more demanding, expensive, and complex a treatment is, the more appropriate must the recommendation for its use be.

From a practical point of view, the clinician should consider the following issues with regard to individual cases:

1 What would change for this patient, who is currently unable to eat and clearly malnourished or with an incipient malnuitrition, should his/her nutrition be provided artificially and his/her nutritional status maintained or improved by means of AN?

2 If a nutritional support is indicated, what would the best way of administering it be, and the best nutritional regimen?

The first point requires an approximate estimate of the life expectancy of the patient, which depends on the state of the disease and nutritional status and the possible benefits of AN.

Life expectancy

When dealing with a cachectic or mortal disease, such as an advanced malignancy which is no longer amenable to treatment, nutritional support may be appropriate only if patients are expected to die from starvation rather than from the progression of their disease. In such a case, it may be reasonable to delay the final outcome.

It is well known that exhaustion of the protein mass is the major determinant in mortality from starvation (14,20). The release of proteins may be reduced to a certain extent thanks to the availability of adequate fat stores, which enable obese subjects to survive starvation for several months and even for periods as long as up to one year (12,31). As starvation progresses, however, the continuous nitrogen loss, despite the presence of adequate adipose reserves (29,30), may cause death from myofibrils fragmentation (20) and other lean mass organ depletion (14).

In healthy adult subjects, a nitrogen loss critical for survival occurs after a loss of 33%–37% of usual/ideal weight (23), i.e. after 60–75 days of starvation, as demonstrated by the tragic experience of the Leningrad siege (9), the Warsaw Ghetto (18,39), and the Irish hunger strike (24).

Tony Bland, the 21-year-old English soccer fan who was crushed in the Hillsborough disaster on 15 April 1985 and remained in a persistent vegetative state (PVS) for several years while on enteral nutrition, died after 11 days following authorization for removal of the feeding tube (2).

Table 20.1 reports the correlation between nitrogen loss and the time necessary to reach a 30%–35% depletion crucial for survival. The net nitrogen loss estimated in cancer patients is included between condition A and condition C. However,it must be considered that several cancer patients candidated to home artificial nutrition (HAN) are already depleted at the initial evaluation.

Several authors (1,11,16,25–27,32,36,40) have tried to assess the length of survival in advanced cancer patients based on clinical and/or biochemical evaluations. Such assessments are of interest not only for physicians involved in palliative care but also for oncologists and nutritionists. The former will, in fact, dose therapy based on expected survival, without running the risk of being extremist; the latter must decide whether to undertake a program as demanding and expensive as home parenteral nutrition.

Table 20.1 Lean mass depletion in relation to some pathological conditions

Clinical condition	Nitrogen loss (g day^{-1})	Times (days) necessary to lose 30% of	
		Muscular mass	Body cell mass
A. Chronic starvation	3	82	139
B. Severe sepsis or trauma	20	13	20
C. Infection coupled with starvation	15	10	21

Table 20.2 Studies that have investigated the accuracy of the estimation of survival in advanced cancer patients

Reference	Method	Conclusions
Parkes (32)	Clinical	Insufficiently accurate
Addington-Hall *et al.* (1)	Spitzer quality of life	Inaccurate
Bruera *et al.* (11)	Weight loss of 10 kg in addition to cognitive failure and dysphagia	Predicts one-month survival with 74% accuracy
Yates *et al.* (39)	Karnofsky Index	Low score (50) predicts short-term survival. High score inaccurate
Mor *et al.* (27)	Karnofsky Index	Insufficiently accurate
Evans and McCarthy (16)	Karnofsky Index	Wide confidence limits
Rueben et al. (36)	Karnofsky Index	Valuable when associated with symptom profile

Some of the most significant studies are listed in Table 20.2. Almost no predictive indices are generally exempt from criticism since, as the authors themselves admit, they are not—but for a few exceptions (13,25,26,33)—very accurate.

In a recent paper, Caraceni *et al.* (13) showed in a study involving a large number of patients that subjects with a favorable palliative prognostic score (<5.5) have a >70% probability of surviving 2 or 3 months, depending on the presence or absence of delirium. However, in a prospective cohort study in which 343 physicians estimated the length of survival of 468 patients (15), median observed survival was 24 days, and physicians overestimated survival by a factor of 5.3. Overall, 20% of the predictions were accurate, i.e. within 33% of the number of days that the patient actually survived, while 17% were pessimistic. Accuracy is higher when predicting a short-term exitus; it is definitely worse when patients who are not actually moribund are considered.

A recent systematic review of the literature on survival prediction in terminal cancer patients (38) has identified eight variables definitely associated with a decreased survival (that is, their independent predictive value appeared to be consistent across well-designed studies), namely low performance status, clinical estimation of survival, congnitive impairment, anorexia, dyspnoea, xerostomia, weight loss, and dysphagia. It is noteworthy that some of these variables are not simply predictive (i.e. anorexia, dysphagia, weight loss) but they may be involved in the progressive clinical deterioration of the patient; they or their effects may be to some extent counteracted by appropriate nutritional support and consequently have a limited application in all patients who are potential candidates for nutritional support.

Effects of AN on nutritional status

The nutritional and metabolic effects of TPN and ienteral nutrition (EN) have been reviewed elsewhere (4,5) and are summarized below:

1 TPN and EN usually achieve similar nutritional and metabolic results. Some reports suggest a better preservation of the visceral protein status with glutamine-free TPN and of the immune function with standard EN (Table 20.3).

Table 20.3 Effects of TPN and EN on nutrition variables

Variable	Response	
	TPN	EN
Weight	↑	↑
Body fat	↑	↑
Muscle mass[a]	=	=
Lean body mass		
N balance	+	+
Total body K	↑	↑ (=)
Total body N	= ↑	= ?
Serum proteins		
Total protein	=	=
Albumin	=	= o ↓
TIBC, CHE	=	= ↑
Ceruloplasmin	=	=
TBPA	↑ or =	= or ↑
RBP	↑	–
Protein flux	↑ or =	=
Synthesis, catabolism	=	=
Immune humoral response		
IgG, IgA, IgM	=	=
C3, C4	=	↑
C3PA	–	↑
CH50	–	=
Immune cellular response		
Neutrophils	=	
Lymphocytes (total/subpopulation)	=	↑ or =
Chemotaxis/phagocytosis	=	

(a) 3-Methylhistidine, amino acid efflux, anthropometry, creatinine-height index
TIBC: total iron-binding capacity
CHE: cholinesterase
TBPA: thyroxin-binding prealbumin
RBP: retinol-binding protein

2 The common response to nutritional support is a decline in the progressive deterioration of the nutritional status. If the malignancy is not too aggressive and enables the patient to be fed for several weeks, it is possible to recover some nutritional indices. In contrast, if the tumor is extremely aggressive or the patient severely emaciated, there may not be enough time to achieve a nutritional benefit from AN.

3 Despite the substantial equivalence of the two types of AN, there are differences between TPN and EN which may be significant from the clinical point of view:

- TPN is 'passive' nutrition: patients do not realize that they are receiving 1000–2000 or more calories per day because the solution may be concentrated in a small volume and administered over a 24-hour period. If patients already have central venous catheters, which are usually very useful for any other type of therapy, palliative–supportive therapy or blood-sampling, they may not be aware that they are receiving therapy, nutrition, or both.

- In contrast, EN is 'forced' nutrition: patients may not tolerate beyond a certain volume of the enteral diet due to the onset of satiety. Since the liquid enteral formula cannot be manipulated and concentrated, there is a critical volume of about 1500 ml per day which the patient must receive to avoid a deficient administration of minerals and vitamins.
- TPN can be delivered under all conditions, whereas EN requires an accessible and working gut (the modalities of accessing the gut will be discussed later). The concept of a working gut is a broad one: it means not only the capability of transfer nutrients in the gut to digest and absorb them, but, generically speaking, also the ability to well tolerate and accept the desired volume in the 24 hours.
- TPN is a more expensive and demanding procedure, and it is associated with potentially more severe complications than EN. However, should a complication occur with TPN (i.e. hyperglycemia), nutrition administration can be corrected without interruption more easily than with EN (i.e. if vomiting or diarrhea occur).

Baseline requirement

If the goal of AN is the attempt to maintain or restore nutritional status because tumor progression is relatively indolent and the patient fairly asymptomatic despite the incumbent threat of malnutrition and hypophagia, then the clinician should consider the requirements of macro and micronutrients.

Water

The normal balance of water in the body is summarized in Table 20.4. However, patients with advanced malignancy frequently have metabolic disturbances that dictate a restriction in water administration:

- Cachexia is often associated with expansion of the extracellular water volume.
- Patients candidated to TPN are often affected by peritoneal carcinomatosis, which can sharply precipitate if there is an overzealous administration of water, glucose, and sodium.
- Since the early pioneering studies of Gamble (19) in 1946, it has been known that glucose reduces renal sodium excretion and, for the same reasons, the loss of extracellular fluid. In subsequent studies Bloom (3) confirmed the inhibition of salt excretion by carbohydrates. Insulin is thought to be the most probable mediator of sodium retention and could do so through an increased sympathetic activity. The effects of a glucose-based TPN on positive water and sodium balance have been demonstrated by Rudman (35) and subsequently described in oncologic patients by Fan (17), Bozzetti (8), and Gray (21).
- In cancer patients there may be excessive production of antidiuretic hormone (ADH) due to the tumor (28), to the presence of nausea which frequently occurs in advanced stages of disease, or to the administration of morphine. Moreover, the wasting syndrome is associated with loss of intracellular water and solutes which affect the hypothalamic osmoreceptor cells to stimulate the ADH release at levels that maintain serum osmolality and serum sodium levels at subnormal values (37). As a consequence, the clearance of free water is decreased, also because the urea load presented to the kidney is reduced secondary to

Table 20.4 Water balance in the healthy adult

Water		**ml**
Intake		
Drinks		1100
Food		500–900
Water from oxidation		400
◆ Protein	0.39–0.41×g	
◆ Carbohydrate	0.56–0.60×g	
◆ Lipid	1.07×g	
	Total	2000–2400
Output		400
Perspiration	(14.4 per kg)	600
Sweat		80–100
Feces		1000–1300
	Total	
		2000–2400

Modified from Alper, C. in: *Modern Nutrition in Health and Disease*. Wahl, M.G. and Goodhart, R.S., eds, Lea and Febiger, Philadelphia, 1968.

protein malnutrition, whereas the synthesis of endogenous water is maintained by the oxidation of carbohydrates and fats (22) and insensible water loss drops due to reduced physical activity (10). Finally, it is a common experience that it is easier to hydrate a patient when the load of fluid is inadequate rather than the opposite condition.

Energy

Many studies have shown that cancer patients may be hypometabolic, normometabolic, or hypermetabolic. When energy expenditure is expressed by unit of body cell mass a consistent percentage of patients are shown to be hypermetabolic. However, since physical activity accounts for about 25% of total energy expenditure, and energy expended in digestion about 5%, and most of these patients are confined to bed or to a chair and are hypophagic, the energy supply cannot be excessive, and a value between 20 and 30 kcal per kg per day seems to be appropriate. A simplified way to estimate the basal energy expenditure for healthy subjects is about 1 kcal per kg per hour. Furthermore, the need to achieve a positive energy balance depends on whether one is aiming for just the maintenance or a recovery of the nutritional status. Since there is evidence from experimental tumors and balances across to human tumors that glucose more than lipids is a preferred fuel for cancer cells, a high lipid/glucose ratio (i.e. 50 : 50) is desirable.

Protein

A supply of 1–2 g per kg per day is usually acceptable, provided that the BUN values are in the normal range.

Micronutrients

These are administered in the usual doses. Concern for correcting potential deficiencies or preventing them should be greater than the fear of stimulating tumor growth or interrupting the balance between tumor and host. In my experience the choice is not between TPN or a hypocaloric regimen, but between whether or not to nutritionally support the patient. If one accepts the first option, the nutritional regimen should be adequate in macro and micronutrients.

Total parenteral nutrition

Regimen

An approximate estimate of the composition of the infusional substrates (micronutrients) to be delivered daily is reported in Table 20.5.

Glucose

At present, glucose is the only carbohydrate energy source for parenteral nutrition (about 3.7 kcal per 1 g) and is used as aqueous solutions of various concentrations, usually from 20% to 60%, depending on the desired total volume load. The central nervous system, red cells, renal medulla, and bone marrow are glucose-dependent tissues: this means that they use only glucose as an energy source. In fact, the central nervous system can use ketone bodies at the time of prolonged starvation, but during parenteral nutrition ketogenesis is blocked and glucose is the primary substrate for this organ. As the central nervous system consumes 100–150 g of glucose per day and this amount is fully oxidized, the provision of 100–150 g of glucose is the minimal supply in order to prevent gluconeogenesis.

Gluconeogenesis, during which amino acids obtained from body protein breakdown are converted in the liver to glucose, leads to the rapid loss of proteins (100 g of protein is necessary to produce 56 g of glucose). Thus, the administration of 100 g glucose has a definitive protein-sparing effect and reduces gluconeogenesis.

The usual daily dose of glucose in parenteral nutrition is 200–400 g.

Essential fatty acid deficiency, fatty liver infiltration, and increased production of CO_2 have been reported when glucose was used as the sole energy source to cover energy requirements.

Table 20.5 Requirements for water and electrolytes during TPN in adults

Substrate	Requirement per kg per day
Water	30 ml
Sodium	1 mmol
Potassium	1–1.5 mmol
Magnesium	0.05–0.2 mmol
Calcium	0.05–0.15 mmol
Chloride	1–3 mmol
Phosphate	0.2–0.5 mmol

To prevent the incidence and severity of metabolic alterations during parenteral nutrition, the infusion rate of glucose should not exceed 5 mg per kg per minute (0.5 g per kg per hour) and a daily dose of 4–5 g per kg.

Lipid emulsion

Lipids are the most dense energy substrates: 1 g yields about 9 kcal. It has been suggested that lipids should provide at least 50% of the total non-protein energy as is done in patients with insulin resistance or pulmonary dysfunction. Fats are administered in the form of lipid emulsion (preferably 20%–30%) containing droplets with a triglyceride core which is surrounded by a phospholipid layer (egg or soya lethicin). Fat emulsions are isotonic and may be given via a peripheral vein. At present LCT and medium chain triglycerides (MCT)/long chain triglycerides (LCT) lipid emulsions are accessible. The maximum dose is up to 2 g per kg per day and the maximal infusion rate is 0.10 g per kg per hour with LCT and 0.15 g per kg per hour with a mixed MCT/LCT emulsion. Other lipids (short-chain fatty acids, omega-3 fatty acids, structured lipids) are now being marketed.

Amino acids

Amino acids provide about 4 kcal per g, but since the main goal of TPN is to maintain or restore body protein status, the rationale is to cover with glucose and lipids energy requirements of the host and provide the amino acids to be incorporated into proteins rather than catabolized for energy. Amino acid solutions are available in concentrations ranging from 5% to 15% and are typically composed of 40%–50% essential amino acids and 50%–60% non-essential ones. The maximum daily dose is up to 2 g per kg per day with an infusion rate up to 0.1 g per kg per hour.

Infusion

The selected substrates should be compounded in a single bag, paying close attention to the stability of calcium and inorganic phosphate and of the lipid emulsion, and ensuring absolute sterility. The advantages of using a single bag are cost savings and reduced risk of contamination during preparation, handling and delivery, improved use of nutrients, reduced cost and risk of contamination of IV tubing, syringes, and connectors, safety and ease of administration, and reduced rate of metabolic complications. The addition of fat emulsions reduces vein irritation by decreasing the osmolarity of the nutrition formula, allowing administration via peripheral veins. Regular administration is made possible by the use of a volumetric pump. Cyclic administration, for instance during the night, is preferable (within the limitations allowed by the metabolic capacity of the body) since both the metabolic use of substrates is better and mobilization of patients, depending on their performance status, is possible too.

Catheter

Many patients will already harbor a central venous catheter (CVC), originally inserted for the delivery of chemotherapy or for blood-sampling. If a nutritional support is planned, we strongly recommend inserting a central venous catheter since the TPN regimen must be designed based on the nutritional requirements of the patient and not on the capacity/

tolerance of the peripheral vein. Percutaneous catheterization of the subclavian vein is probably the best option since the subclavicular region may be adequately dressed (and consequently the CVC well secured) in comparison with the neck or the inguinal regions.

The percutaneous approach allows a sample change over a guidewire, should the need arise for diagnostic confirmation or for replacing a new sterile CVC in place of an infected one.

Subcutaneous tunnelization improves the stability of the CVC, reduces the risk of contamination (not of infection), and makes more diffcult the exchange over a guidewire. Multilumen CVC should be avoided if they are not strictly necessary: the more the lumens the higher the risk of infection and the greater the difficulty in managing the infection through the antibiotic locks.

A totally implanted device (TID) has no role in this condition. If the nutritional support has to be administered every day, or if other drugs are often necessary, the TID acts as an external CVC, where the tube is substituted by a needle: the skin barrier is constantly violated (the advantage of the totally hidden CVC is lost) and connection through a needle is more painful than through the hub of a external CVC.

Catheter after-care

In order to prevent CVC-related infections, and to maintain patency, external CVC and TID must be precisely cared for, preferably according to written protocol.

The CVC exit site must be covered by sterile gauze pads to be changed every 48 hours, or air permeable self-adhesive waterproof foil (op-site) to be changed twice or thrice a week, or when wet or soiled. Surgical sterility must be maintained during the maneuver:

1. The dressing is removed being careful not to dislodge the CVC.
2. The skin around the exit site is scrubbed with ethanol and povidone–iodine or chlorexidine solution, beginning from the exit site and progressing outwards. The procedure is repeated three times.
3. Povidone–iodine ointment is applied and a new dressing fixed.

There is no standard practice for CVC flushing. Usually the CVC should be flushed with 0.9% saline after each use. If the pause between infusions is just a few hours, heparinization is not necessary, but for longer intervals it is advised that the saline flush be followed by heparin lock ($100\,\mathrm{IU\,mL^{-1}}$) given in volume to the filling volume of the CVC.

The CVC should be clamped in the proper place when tubing is connected/disconnected to prevent air embolism or blood back-flow and subsequent CVC thrombosis. Permanent CVCs are produced with a click-clamp which allows CVC closing for a while between flushing and closing with a cap.

Standard CVCs usually have no clamps and the click-clamp is applied to a special extension tube. This tubing is changed once a week and works much better than the three-way stop-cock. The time interval between changes of infusion sets and caps varies from 24 to 72 hours, depending on the guidelines of the producers, type of CVC, and equipment and local policy.

The most important part of the CVC care is to avoid unnecessary manipulation and use of the extension tube, sets, and stop-cock, and to strictly follow the rules of the aseptic prepration of flushing solutions, connections and disconnections of the infusion lines as well as the preparation of the nutritive bag.

Outcome

It is extremely difficult to evaluate the effect of nutritional support due to the ambiguity of AN in these conditions: is AN a medical therapy or a primary basic care? These issues have recently been reviewed in *Clinical Nutrition* (6).

In the attempt to reach a consensus on the controversial topic of whether terminal cancer patients should be fed or simply hydrated, an interdisciplinary meeting was held a few years ago under the auspices of the European Association for Palliative Care (7) which included oncologists from different branches (surgery, chemotherapy, radiotherapy), nutritionists, palliativists, psychologists, bioethicists, nurses, and even a patient receiving home TPN and her relatives. It was impossible to draw rigid guidelines but only to give suggestions about an holistic approach to the problem and the need to consider many other aspects of the difficult and complex care of these patients, without focusing on the nutritional and water metabolism alone.

From a traditional Hippocratic medical point of view, we can expect that if enough time is allowed for AN to work (i.e. if the tumor is not in rapid progress, nutritional support may go on for several weeks), nutritional deterioration is blunted or offset and sometimes a slight replenishment of the host may be achieved.

If the primary cause of death of the patient is starvation, a prolongation of survival may be achieved. This may be a benefit for patients and their families provided that the burden of total care is not excessive, and that other symptoms are successfully managed by palliative care. Obviously, maintaining with AN the life of a patient who is severely dyspnoic or in such pain that he/she requires continuous sedation for relief is not recommended. On the other hand, both patients and their families tend to consider nutrition as an act of love, and to identify the lack of nutritional support as a condemnation to death. In such circumstances the goals of nutritional support should be realistically discussed to lead to the conclusion by all the individuals involved in the decision-making process that nutritional support may have a role, even if limited, until there is no evidence that it does no harm.

References

1. **Addington-Hall JM; MacDonald LD; Anderson HR.** Can the Spitzer Quality of Life Index help to reduce prognostic uncertainty in terminal care? *British Journal of Cancer* 1990;62:695–9.
2. **Airedale NHS Trust v Bland: Judgements of Family Divisions, Court of Appeal (Civil Division) and House of Lords.** In: Fennell P: Harpwood V; Johnson H; Gwena C., editors. London: Butterworth Medico-Legal Reports, Butterworths, 1993;12: pp. 64–143.
3. **Bloom WL.** Inhibition of salt excretion by carbohydrate. *Archives of Internal Medicine* 1962;109:80–6.
4. **Bozzetti F.** Effects of artificial nutrition on the nutritional status of cancer patients. *Journal of Parenteral and Euteral Nutrition* 1989;13:406–20.
5. **Bozzetti F.** Nutritional support in the adult cancer patient. *Clinical Nutrition* 1992;11:167–79.
6. **Bozzetti F; Bozzetti V.** Home artificial nutrition in incurable cancer patients: rationale and ethics. *Clinical Nutrition* 2001:20 (Supplement 2): 23–27.
7. **Bozzetti F; Amadori A; Bruera E; Cozzaglio L; Corli' O; Filiberti A; Rapin CH., *et al.*** Guidelines on artificial nutrition versus hydration in terminal cancer patients. *Nutrition* 1996;12:163–7.

8. **Bozzetti F; Ammatuna M; Migliavacca S; Facchetti G; Cozzaglio L; Morabito A.** Comparison of glucose vs. glucose fat solutions in cancer patients: a controlled cross-over study. *Clinical Nutrition* 1990;9:325–30.
9. **Brozek J; Wells S; Keys A.** Medical aspects of semistarvation in Leningrad (Siege 1941–1942). *American Review of Soviet Medicine* 1946;4:70–86.
10. **Bruera E; Belzile M; Watanabe S; Fainsinger RL.** Volume of hydration in terminal cancer patients. *Supportive Care in Cancer* 1996;4:147–50.
11. **Bruera E; Miller MJ; Kuehn N; MacEachern T; Hanson J.** Estimate of survival of patients admitted to a palliative care unit : a prospective study. *Journal of Pain and Symptom Management* 1992;7:82–6.
12. **Cahill GF Jr.** Starvation in man. *New England Journal of Medicine* 1970;282:668–75.
13. **Caraceni A; Nanni O; Maltoni M; Piva L; Indelli M; Arnoldi E., *et al.*** Impact of delirium on the short term of prognosis of advanced cancer patients. *Cancer* 2000;89:1145–9.
14. **Cherel Y; Robin J.P; Heitz A; Calgari C; LeMaho Y.** Relationship between lipid availability and protein utilization during prolonged fasting. *Journal of Comparative Physiology* 1992;162:305–13.
15. **Christakis NA; Lamont EB.** Extent and determinants of error in doctors' prognosis in terminally ill patients: Prospective cohort study. *British Medical Journal* 2000;320:469–73.
16. **Evans C; McCarthy M.** Prognostic uncertainty in terminal care: can the Karnofsky index help? *The Lancet* 1985;i:1204–6.
17. **Fan ST; Lau WY; Wong KK; Chan PM.** Preoperative parenteral nutrition in patients with esophageal cancer: a prospective, randomised clinical trial. *Clinical Nutrition* 1988;8:23–7.
18. **Fliederbaum J.** Clinical aspects of hunger disease in adults. In: Winick M., editor. *Hunger Disease: Studies by the Jewish Physicians in the Warsaw Ghetto.* New York: John Wiley & Sons, 1979: pp. 11–43.
19. **Gamble JL.** Physiological information gained from studies on life raft ration. *Harvey Lectures* 1946;42:247–73.
20. **Garnett ES; Barnard DL; Ford J; Goodbody RA; Woodehouse MA.** Gross fragmentation of cardiac myofibrils after therapeutic starvation for obesity. *The Lancet* 1969;1:914–16.
21. **Gray GE; Meguid MM.** Can total parenteral nutrition reverse hypoalbuminemia in oncology patients? *Nutrition* 1990;6:225–8.
22. **Kerndt P; Naughton J; Driscoll C; Loxterkamp A.** Fasting: the history, pathophysiology, and complications. *Western Journal of Medicine* 1982;137:379–99.
23. **Kotler DP; Tierney AR; Wang J; Pierson RN Jr.** Magnitude of body-cell-mass depletion and the timing of death from wasting in AIDS. *American Journal of Clinical Nutrition* 1989;50:444–7.
24. **Love G.** Weight loss during hunger strike. In: Allison SP (Editor). The uses and limitations of nutritional support. *Clinical Nutrition* 1992;11:319–30.
25. **Maltoni M; Nanni O; Pirovano M; Scarpi E; Indelli Martini C; Monti M; Arnoldi E; Piva L; Amadori, D.** for the Italian Multicentric Study Group on Palliative Care. Successful validation of the palliative prognostic score in terminally ill cancer patients. *Journal of Pain and Symptom Management* 1999;17(4):240–7.
26. **Maltoni M; Pirovano M; Scarpi E; Marinari M; Indelli M; Arnoldi E; Gallucci E; Frontini L; Piva L; Amadori D.** Prediction of survival of patients terminally ill with cancer. *Cancer* 1995;75(10):2613–22.
27. **Mor V; Laliberte L; Morris L; Morris J; Wiemann M.** The Kanofsky Performance Status Scale. An examination of its reliability and validity in a research setting. *Cancer* 1984;53:2002–7.
28. **Moser AM; Streeten DHP.** Disorders of the neurohypophysis. In: Isselhacher KJ, *et al.*, editors. *Harrison's Principles of Internal Medicine*, 13th edn. New York: McGraw-Hill, 1994: pp. 1921–30.

29. **Owen OE; Felig P; Morgan AP; Wahren J; Cahill GF Jr.** Liver and kidney metabolism during prolonged starvation. *Journal of Clinical Investigation* 1969;48:584–94.

30. **Owen OE; Reichard GA Jr; Patel MS; Boden G.** Energy metabolism in feasting and fasting. In: Koachko DM; Anderson RR; Heimberg M. editor. *Proceedings of the Twelfth Midwest Conference on Endocrinology and Metabolism. Hormones and Energy Metabolism. Advances in Experimental Medicine and Biology.* New York: Plenum Press, 1979:3:169–88.

31. **Owen OE; Smalley KJ; D'Allessio DA; Mozzoli MA; Dawson EK.** Protein, fat and carbohydrate requirements during starvation: anaplerosis and cataplerosis. *American Journal of Nutrition* 1998;68:12–34.

32. **Parkes CM.** Accuracy of predictions of survival in later stages of cancer. *British Medical Journal* 1972;2:29–31.

33. **Pirovano M; Maltoni M; Nanni O; Marinari M; Indelli M; Zaninetta G; Petrella V; Barni S; Zecca E; Luporini G; Labianca R; Amadori D.** for the Italian Multicenter and Study Group on Palliative Care. A new palliative prognostic score: a first step for the staging of terminally ill cancer patients. *Journal of Pain and Symptom Management* 1999;17(4):231–9.

34. **Report of a Meeting of Physicians and Scientists at the Royal Marsden Hospital, Sutton.** Small-cell lung cancer. *The Lancet* 1995;345:1285–9.

35. **Rudman D; Millikan WJ; Richardson TJ; Bixler TJ; Stackhouse J; McGarrity WC.** Elemental balances during intravenous hyperalimentation of underweight adult subjects. *Journal of Clinical Investigation* 1975;55:94–104.

36. **Rueben DB; Mor V; Hiris J.** Clinical symptoms and length of survival in patients with terminal cancer. *Archives of Internal Medicine* 1988;148:1586–91.

37. **Steiner N; Bruera E.** Methods of hydration in palliative care patients. *Journal of Palliative Care* 1998;14(2):6–13.

38. **Viganõ A; Dorgan M; Buckingham J; Bruera E; Suarez-Almazor ME.** *Palliative Medicine* 2000;14:364–74.

39. **Winick M.** editor. *Hunger Disease: Studies by the Jewish Physicians in the Warsaw ghetto.* New York: John Wiley & Sons, 1979.

40. **Yates J; Chalmer B; McKegney P.** Evaluation of patients with advanced cancer using the Karnofsky Performance Status. *Cancer* 1980;45:2220–4.

Chapter 21

Artificial nutrition II: Enteral nutrition

Cecilia Gavazzi

Introduction

Oral nutrition should always be the first choice of feeding patients with advanced cancer (1,2). Every effort should be made to satisfy the patient's requirements in terms of calories, proteins, vitamins, and minerals, utilizing a dietician's counselling and commercially available nutritional supplements. However, patients with a markedly reduced oral intake due to dysphagia, obstruction of the high gastrointestinal tract, or severe anorexia can benefit from enteral nutrition (EN).

Enteral feeding is a physiological method of delivering nutrients to the gastrointestinal tract through a tube that can be placed into the stomach, the duodenum, or the jejunum, bypassing the first portion of the digestive system. Like oral feeding it is based on the absorption of nutrients through the intestinal mucosa and therefore should be used only in patients with functional bowels.

Compared with oral feeding, EN has several advantages (3) which can overcome some of the major problems that limit oral intake in advanced cancer patients.

1. Nutrient solutions can be delivered at a slow and continuous rate allowing an optimal absorptive capacity, reducing the feeling of early satiety and overcoming the problem of delayed gastric emptying.
2. In patients with dysphagia or stenosis of the upper gastrointestinal tract, the distal end of the tube can be positioned below the obstruction, so that nutrients can be delivered at a regular rate.
3. Specific nutrient solutions that may not be tolerated orally, because of taste fatigue or food aversion, can also be administered.

Compared with parenteral nutrition, EN is more physiologic and safer to manage, less expensive, maintains the gut barrier and immunologic functions (4), and avoids the risk of septic complications associated with intravenous feeding. Furthermore, EN can be easily performed at home by most patients and their families; in fact, home enteral feeding has grown rapidly in different European and American countries (5). Therefore EN should always be considered in patients with a functional gastrointestinal tract who need artificial nutritional support (6).

Indications and contraindications

The major indications for EN in advanced neoplastic patients are summarized in Table 21.1 and can be divided into the following subgroups:

1. ***Obstructive malignant lesions of the upper gastrointestinal tract.*** The lesion may be intrinsic, commonly in the cancer of the pharynx, larynx, oesophagus, and stomach, or extrinsic as in neoplasms of the head of the pancreas, determining a stenosis of the duodenum, or such as a mediastinic mass causing a compression of the oesophagus.
2. ***Dysphagia due to neurologic causes.*** This can be related to the tumour itself, such as in a neoplastic lesion of the central nervous system with paralysis of the lower cranial nerves, or other more general neuromuscular causes, such as in cerebrovascular accidents or neurological disorders.
3. ***Dysphagia due to iatrogenic causes.*** This is generally present in head and neck tumours as a consequence of surgical or radiation treatment.
4. ***Marked reduction of oral intake.*** With no evidence of obstruction, this is often associated with severe anorexia, early satiety, delayed emptying, and/or food aversion. Inflammatory conditions such as stomatitis or oesophagitis can also limit oral food assumption.

Intestinal mechanical obstruction is the *only absolute contraindication* to enteral feeding. However, in patients with diffuse peritoneal carcinosis, peritonitis, intractable vomiting, paralytic ileum, severe diarrhoea, and enteric fistulae, EN should be avoided (7).

Table 21.1 Indications for EN

Obstructive malignant lesion

- Intrinsic: cancer of the mouth, pharynx, larynx, oesophagus, and stomach
- Extrinsic: cancer of the head of the pancreas, mediastinic mass

Neurological dysphagia

- Oncological: cancer of the central nervous system
- Other: cerebrovascular accident
  neuromuscolar disorder
  collagen-vascular disorder

Iatrogenic dysphagia

- Damage after surgical intervention on the mouth, pharynx, and oesophagus
- Post-radiotherapy fibrosis in the head and neck
- Osteoradionecrosis of the mandible
- Fistulas

Reduction of oral intake

- Severe anorexia
- Early satiety
- Delayed emptying
- Stomatitis or oesophagitis (mucosal candidiasis)

Planning EN

Once the decision to support the patient with enteral tube feeding has been made, the following points should be considered:

1. The type of enteral access to be positioned, e.g. nasoenteric tube or gastro/jejunostomy, and the site of the most distal part of the tube where the enteral nutrition should be delivered, e.g. stomach, duodenum, or jejunum.
2. The quantity and type of enteral regimen to be administered and the method of delivery.
3. Possible complications and problems associated with short-term or long-term tube feeding.

Choosing the enteral access

The route selected for tube feeding depends upon the estimated duration of the feeding, the condition of the gastrointestinal tract, the presence and site of obstructions, and the risk of pulmonary aspiration.

When EN is planned for a short term (<30 days), a *nasoenteric tube* is recommended; when the patient seems to require a prolonged tube feeding (>30 days) a tube *gastrostomy* or *jejunostomy* should be considered.

Whenever EN is administered into the stomach, this allows a more complete digestion and absorption and makes the management easier. However, in all patients with high risk of aspiration, such as in the presence of gastroparesis, reflux oesophagitis, and altered consciousness, or in patients with unresectable gastric or pancreatic cancer, the distal portion of the tube should be placed in the second portion of the duodenum or in the jejunum.

Nasoenteric tubes technically refer to any feeding tube that is placed nasally into the stomach or beyond. Preferably the tube should be small in calibre (French 8–12), and made of a soft material such as silicone rubber and radiopaque.

The physician or nurse can easily place the tube at the bedside of patients without obstruction of the upper gastrointestinal tract. The passage beyond the pylorus can be obtained by turning the patient on the right position and/or with pharmacological assistance. The use of 10 mg of metoclopramide, a dopamine agonist (8), or $3\,mg\,kg^{-1}$ erythromycin IV, a motilin agonist, before tube placement (9) is associated with an 85%–90% successful passage of the tube into the duodenum. Special tubes, developed by Bengmark, are capable of spontaneously passing through the pylorus (10). In patients with malignant obstruction or neurological dysphagia a fluoroscopic or endoscopic guidance may be necessary (11). Pulmonary intubation should always be excluded before starting EN: the position of the tube tip should be checked after blinded or endoscopic placement by injecting air and auscultating, aspirating gastric acid, or by X-ray (12).

Table 21.2 summarizes the clinical complications that may occur with the use of a nasoenteric tube. The most common complications are local irritation and pain or discomfort and are mostly related to the prolonged use of a large-sized tube, made with a hard material. Mechanical complications such as tube dislodgement, knotting, or obstruction are also common and they account for approximately 60% of the reasons for removal (13).

Gastrostomy should always be considered in patients that require prolonged tube feeding, with no risk of aspiration and normal duodenum transit. Gastrostomy can be placed with

Table 21.2 Clinical nasoenteric tube complications

Discomfort and pain
Nasal mucosal irritation/ulceration
Nasal trauma/pyriform sinus perforation
Epistaxis
Otitis media
Oesophageal perforation/tracheoesophageal fistula
Gastric/duodenal perforation
Pulmonary intubation/tube feeding into pulmonary tree
Gastrointestinal bleeding
Arrhythmia
Myocardial infarction

an endoscopic, radiologic, or surgical procedure; each technique has its own risks, benefits, and complications. Since 1980, percutaneous endoscopic gastrostomy (PEG) has largely replaced operative gastrostomy, being a safe, well-tolerated and cost-effective procedure (14). It does not require general anaesthesia, but only IV sedation, and can be performed in a short-term hospital stay. The limit of this technique in cancer patients is the presence of an voropharynx lesion or oesophageal stricture that precludes the passage of the gastroscope.

The percutaneous fluoroscopic gastrostomy (PFG) procedure was developed later on and it is less diffuse. However, the procedure can also be performed using the Seldinger technique under fluoroscopic guidance in patients with head and neck malignancies with a severe stenosis, and it seldom requires sedation, except in children (15,16). The most serious complications of PEGs and PFGs are related to intra-abdominal leaks from the stomach and deep stromal infections. Morbidity and mortality related to these procedures vary as reported in different studies. In the largest single-centre study PEG placement was successful in 95% of 314 consecutive patients; there was a 1% procedure-related mortality and a 3% major complication rate (17). Most probably the risk of complication is slightly higher in patients with malignancies (18). There are continuous refinements of these procedures and ongoing improvements of commercial kits; a comparison of techniques in terms of mortality and morbidity is difficult because of the lack of randomized studies including the three procedures. However, the patient's underlying disease and local expertise and availability must be considered when deciding between different techniques. Both the endoscopic and fluoroscopic procedures are contraindicated in the presence of severe ascites or when there is interposition of the liver or transverse colon between the stomach and the abdominal wall. Laparoscopy gastrostomies have recently been performed (19), but this procedure, at present, still needs to be performed in an operating room and with general anesthesia.

Jejunostomy should always been considered in patients with a high risk of pulmonary aspiration. The indications for the use of jejunostomy in advanced cancer patients include tracheal aspiration, reflux oesophagitis, gastroparesis, or unresectable gastric or pancreatic cancer. The first surgical jejunostomy was performed in 1878 (20) and since then different procedures have been developed; a minilaparotomic jejunostomy was described by Delany *et al.* (21) in 1973, and in patients without previous abdominal surgery it can now be easily performed with IV sedation and local anaesthesia. Major complications of surgical jejunostomy are early dislodgement and peritoneal leakage. Jejunostomy tubes are all small in size (< 7 French) and therefore they have a high risk of obstruction. Percutaneous endoscopic or radiological jejunstomy and transgastric jejunostomy have also been developed to prevent aspiration (22), but these procedures should be considered as a second choice.

Feeding regimens and enteral formulations

An enteral feeding regimen should be planned taking into consideration the patient's basal energy requirement and the level of physical activity, if any. An estimation of overall intake of calories by oral nutrition should also be calculated and deducted from the total energy requirement. The enteral regimen reported to improve nutritional status in cancer patients is 35 kcal per kg per day (23). However, reaching a total amount of 30 kcal per kg per day can be a reasonable objective considering the major aim of nutritional care in advanced cancer patients is the prevention of continuous deterioration of the nutritional status and the often concomitant gastrointestinal symptoms, such as constipation, diarrhoea, abdominal pain, etc. that might limit the total amount of EN tolerated.

In patients with total aphagia, in addition to the caloric intake, the free water requirement must also be considered: 30–35 ml per kg weight per day. Free water accounts for approximately 80%–90% of enteral formulations; when water requirement is not satisfied by oral or EN, additional free water can be supplied as flushes through the feeding tube. Sterilized water should be used only in patients fed into the jejunum.

Enteral formulations should be differentiated into natural and artificial. Natural formulations are obtained from an extemporaneous or industrial mixture of natural food, while artificial formulations are obtained from a mixture of chemically defined substances. Natural formulations prepared extemporaneously have a high risk of bacterial contamination and/or enzymatic deterioration.

A wide range of artificial formulations have been developed that may satisfy different situations or disease states; however, polymeric, normocaloric, lactose-free diets, with or without fibre, meet most of patients' needs. Other formulations include hypercaloric, hypocaloric, hyperproteic, and elemental diets; their major characteristics are described in Table 21.3.

Table 21.3 Enteral formulations

Polymeric diets	**kcal/100 mv**	**Osmolarity**	**Carbohydrates[b]**	**Proteins[b]**	**Lipids[b]**
Hypocaloric	50–75	130–210	45–50	15–16	35
Normocaloric[a]	100	250–350	50–55	15–17	30–35
Hypercaloric[a]	150–200	300–500	43–60	14–20	30–40
Hyperproteic[a]	120	290–350	40–53	18–23	30–32
Elemental diets	100	350–400	60–75	16–18	9–22

[a]Formula available with or without fibre.

[b]Carbohydrates, proteins and lipids are expressed as percentage of total calories.

Special formulas for renal, pulmonary, or hepatic failure, glucose intolerance and formulas enriched with immunostimulating nutrients are also available. Polymeric formulations contain carbohydrates, fats, and protein in complex forms, which require some degree of digestion and absorption. A standard formulation generally provides 100–120 calories per 100 ml; carbohydrates account for 50%–60% of the total energy, fats for 30%–40%, and protein for 12%–20%; osmolarity ranges from 220 to 350 mOsm per litre. The presence of soluble or insoluble fibre in the formulation is important to maintain the throphic status of the bowel mucosa, particularly in the colon, and might be useful in the presence of constipation or in certain cases of diarrhoea (24,25).

Elemental diets are a mixture of small particles, such as maltodestrines, free aminoacids or dipeptides and easily absorbed fats, such as medium chain triglycerid oil. Elemental diets have a high osmolarity and their use is indicated only in patients with severe reduced digestive and absorptive capacity.

Formulations for specific organ failure or formulations enriched with immunostimulating nutrients are more expensive compared with a normocaloric polymeric diet and should be considered only in the presence of severe organ failure and long-term use.

Enteral products designed for patients with renal failure are highly concentrated, low in protein, phosphorus, magnesium, potassium, and sodium. A special formulation is also available for patients undergoing dialysis (26). The use of enteric formulations fortified with branched chain amino acids and with a low level of aromatic amino acid may be useful in patients with hepatic failure and risk of encephalopathy (27). The pulmonary formula provides the majority of calories as fat (55%), in order to limit the production of CO_2, and is indicated in patients with chronic obstructive pulmonary disease.

Methods of delivering EN

Enteral feeding may be delivered by bolus, gravity, or with the assistance of a pump-controlled technique. The modality of feeding should be decided on the basis of the site of the tip of the enteral access and the patient's compliance. Feeding into the stomach can be easily done by bolus or gravity, while feeding into the jejunum should be performed with the help of a peristaltic pump, in order to control the delivery rate. Intermittent feeding can be planned in patients with a nasogastric tube or gastrostomy, where the stomach can act as a reservoir; it is more physiological and allows the patient to have free intervals for daily activity. Natural formulations can be used in patients with gastrostomy, but should be discouraged in patients with a nasogastric tube because of a high risk of obstruction. In patients with a nasoduodenal tube or jejunostomy, continuous feeding is indicated, and artificial formulations with limited osmolarity (≤350 mOsm) should be used. Jejunal feeding should be started at a rate of 20 ml per hour and progressively increased to a maximum of 80 ml per hour. In all cases the total planned regimen should be reached in 3–4 days, monitoring the patient's compliance and possible complications.

Complications associated with tube feeding

Complications associated with tube feeding can be classified as mechanical and clinical (Table 21.4). The most frequent mechanical complication is tube obstruction, which occurs more often in small-sized nasoenteric tubes or jejunostomy. The best method to overcome this problem is to prevent it, by washing the internal tube with 20 ml of water every

Table 21.4 Complications associated with tube feeding

Mechanical

- Tube obstruction
- Tube dislodgement

Clinical

- Aspiration pneumonia
- Nausea, vomiting
- Abdominal distension
- Diarrhoea: high osmolarity, high rate of delivery, altered intestinal microflora, formula contamination, lactose intolerance
- Constipation
- Peristoma infection
- Metabolic complications: dehydration, electrolyte imbalance

6–8 hours, after discontinuation of enteral feeding, or after the patient's meals. The use of hot water, peroxide water, Coca-Cola, or pancreatic enzymes have been suggested to unclog the tube (28). Later dislodgement of tubes can also occur, and in the case of gastrostomy or jejunostomy they should be replaced as soon as possible in order to avoid closure of the enteral stomy and to allow easy repositioning.

Among clinical complications the most serious and fearful is aspiration pneumonia. As previously reported, aspiration occurs more frequently in patients with altered consciousness or gastroparesis and should be prevented by delivering EN into the second/third portion of the duodenum or into the jejunum. However, when feeding into the stomach, the patient should be kept in a semirecumbent position and the initial delivery rate should be low (40 ml per hour) or the bolus should be small. These precautions can also prevent or limit other side-effects, such as nausea, vomiting, and abdominal distension.

Diarrhoea is the most common clinical complication of tube feeding (29). The aetiology is multifactorial (30) and the overall condition of the patient seems to be the most important factor. Hyperosmolar formulations and high delivery rates are often associated with diarrhoea. An alteration of the intestinal microflora is often present in advanced cancer patients who might have been treated routinely with antibiotics and acid-suppressive medication such as histamine blockers or omeprazolo. Furthermore, the use of drugs that reduce intestinal motility, such as antispastics and morphine, may cause a bacterial overgrowth which can lead to diarrhoea.

Hypoalbuminaemia has been suggested to cause oedema in the intestinal mucosa predisposing patients to diarrhoea, although it is controversial if the low level of albumine is the cause or simply a common feature of more severe patients, being at risk of developing diarrhoea (31). Intolerance to lactose and formula contamination should also be considered as a possible cause of diarrhoea.

The prolonged use of antispastic drugs and morphine may also cause constipation that can be worsened by enteral feeding. The use of formula enriched with soluble and insoluble fibre and the introduction of a high volume of free water may help to overcome this problem. Peristomal infection is a complication that can be easily prevented with regular medication or gastrostomy or jejunostomy.

Metabolic complications can also occur in long-term enteral feeding, but these are rare and generally not severe. Dehydration and electrolyte imbalance can occur as a consequence of diarrhoea and of an inadequate free water requirement adjustment. In long-term EN trace element or vitamin deficiencies have been reported (32).

References

1. **Rivadeneira DE; Evoy D; Fahey TJ; Lieberman MD; Daly JM.** Nutritional support of the cancer patient. *CA a Cancer Journal for Clinicians* 1998;48:69–80.
2. **Mercadante S.** Nutrition in cancer patients. Supportive Care in Cancer 1996;4:10–20.
3. **Shikes M.** Nutrition therapy for the cancer patient. *Hematology/Oncology Clinics of North America* 1996;10:221–34.
4. **Alverdy J; Chi HS; Sheldon GF.** The effect of parenteral nutrition on gastrointestinal immunity: the importance of enteral stimulation. Annals of Surgery 1985;202:681–4.
5. **Elia M.** An international perspective on artificial nutrition support in the community. *The Lancet* 1995;345:1345–9.
6. **ASPEN Board of directors.** *Journal of Parenteral and Enteral Nutrition* 1993;17(Suppl.):7–9.
7. **American Gastroenterological Association Technical Review on Tube Feeding for Enteral Nutrition.** *Gastroenterology* 1995;108:1282–301.
8. **Lord LM; Weiser-Maimone A; Pulhamus M; Sax HC.** Comparison of weighted vs. unweighted enteral feeding tubes for efficacy of transpyloric intubation. *Journal of Parenteral and Enteral Nutrition* 1993;17:271–3.
9. **Di Lorenzo C; Lachman R; Hyman PE.** Intravenous erythromycin for postpyloric intubation. *Journal of Pediatric Gastroenterology and Nutrition* 1990;11:45–47.
10. **Bengmark S; Jeppsson B; Tranberg KG; Andersson R.** Spontaneous passage of feeding tube in the correct position in the upper intestine after 4 hours. *Lakartidningen* 1989;86:2204.
11. **Gutierrez ED; Balfe DM.** Fluoroscopically guided nasoenteric feeding tube placement: results of a 1-year study. *Radiology* 1991;178:759–62.
12. **Raff MH; Cho S; Dale R.** A technique for positioning nasoenteral feeding tubes. *Journal of Parenteral and Enteral Nutrition* 1987;11:210–13.
13. **Ciocon JO; Silverstone FA; Graver LM; Foley CJ.** Tube feedings in elderly patients. Indications, benefits and complications. *Archives of Internal Medicine* 1988;148:429–33.
14. **Faries MB; Rombeau JL.** Use of gastrostomy and combined gastrojejunostomy tubes for enteral feeding. *World Journal of Surgery* 1999;23:603–7.
15. **Ho CS; Yeung EY.** Percutaneus gastrostomy and transgastric jejunostomy. *American Journal of Roentgenology* 1992;158:251–7.
16. **Cozzi G; Gavazzi C; Civelli E; Milella M; Salvetti M; Scaperotta G; Bozzetti F; Severini A.** Percutaneous gastrostomy in oncologic patients: analysis of results and expansion of the indications. *Abdominal Imaging* 2000;25:239–42.
17. **Larson DE; Burton DD; Schroeder KW; DiMagno EP.** Percutaneous endoscopic gastrostomy. Indications, success, complications, and mortality in 314 consecutive patients. *Gastroenterology* 1987;93:48–52.
18. **Clarkston WK; Smith OJ; Walden JM.** Percutaneous endoscopic gastrostomy and early mortality. *Southern Medical Journal* 1990;83(12):1433–6.

19. **Rosser JC Jr; Rodas EB; Blancaflor J; Prosst RL; Rosser LE; Salem RR.** A simplified technique for laparoscopic jejunostomy and gastrostomy tube placement. *American Journal of Surgery* 1999;177:61–5.

20. **Surmay M.** Observation d' enterostomie. *Bulletin Général de Thérapeutique Médicale et Chirurgicale* 1878;65:324–6.

21. **Delany HM; Carnevale NJ; Garvey JW.** Jejunostomy by needle catheter technique. *Surgery* 1973;73:786–90.

22. **Baskin WN.** Advances in enteral nutrition techniques. *American Journal of Gastroenterology* 1992;87(11):1547–53.

23. **Bennegard K; Eden E; Ekman L; Schersten T; Lundholm K.** Metabolic response of whole body and peripheral tissues to enteral nutrition in weight-losing cancer and noncancer patients. *Gastroenterology* 1983;85:92–9.

24. **Bowling TE; Silk DB.** Pathophysiology of diarrhoea and the role of fiber in enteral nutrition. Clinical Nutrition 1994;14(Suppl.):84–96.

25. **Kapadia SA; Raimundo AH; Grimble GK; Aimer P; Silk DB.** Influence of three different fiber-supplemented enteral diets on bowel function and short-chain fatty acid production. *Journal of Parenteral and Enteral Nutrition* 1995;19:63–8.

26. **Ledermann SE; Shaw V; Trompeter RS.** Long-term enteral nutrition in infants and young children with chronic renal failure. *Pediatric Nephrology* 1999;13:870–5.

27. **Cabre E; Gonzalez-Huix F; Abad-Lacruz A; Esteve M; Acero D; Fernandez-Beñares F; Xiol X; Gassul MA.** Effect of total enteral nutrition on the short-term outcome of severly malnourished cirrhotics: a randomized controlled trial. *Gastroenterology* 1990;98:715–20.

28. **Marcuard SP; Stegall KL.** Unclogging feeding tubes with pancreatic enzyme. *Journal of Parenteral and Enteral Nutrition* 1990;14:198–200.

29. **Silk DBA; Payne-Jame JJ.** Complications of enteral nutrition. In: Rombeau & Caldwell, editors. *Clinical Nutrition. Enteral Tube Feeding.* Philadelphia: Saunders, 1990; 510–31.

30. **Edes TE; Walk BE; Austin JL.** Diarrhoea in tube-fed patients: feeding formula not necessarily the cause. *American Journal of Medicine* 1990;88:91–3.

31. **Borlase BC; Bell SJ; Lewis EJ; Swails W; Bistrian BR; Forse RA; Blackburn GL.** Tolerance to enteral tube feeding diets in the hypoalbuminemic critically ill, geriatric patients. *Surgery Gynecology and Obstetrics* 1992;174:181–8.

32. **McWhirten HP; Hambling CE; Pennington CR.** The nutritional status of patients receiving home enteral feeding. *Clinical Nutrition* 1994;13:207–11.

Chapter 22

Hydration

Robin Fainsinger

Introduction

A 65-year-old man presents with a two week history of increasing abdominal discomfort. Up until that point he had been active and in good health, although he had noted a loss of weight of approximately 3 kg over the previous two months. Investigations confirm pancreatic cancer with liver metastases. Approximately one week after diagnosis he presents to the emergency room of his local hospital with nausea and vomiting, and clinical evidence of dehydration. He is admitted with a suspected bowel obstruction for investigation. He is rehydrated with intravenous fluids. Diagnostic imaging does not show any evidence of a bowel obstruction. The patient's symptoms settle and he is able to resume a reasonable oral intake and is discharged home.

Over the course of six weeks increasing abdominal pain requires morphine 10 mg orally every four hours and achieves good pain control. However he also experiences poor appetite and loss of weight of a further 5 kg. He again develops nausea and vomiting. A history reveals he has been very inconsistent in taking his laxatives, bowel movements have been extremely irregular and very hard and difficult. A rectal examination reveals a significant amount of hard stool in the rectum. Oral intake has been minimal, and urine output has also decreased accordingly. The patient expresses a preference to remain at home. The family physician suggests a bowel regime to overcome the constipation, and parenteral hydration at home using hypodermoclysis overnight. The patient and his wife are content to follow the advice of their health care providers, as is there usual approach to health matters. The patient continues to deteriorate over the next six weeks with persistent anorexia and increasing asthenia. Intermittent nausea and vomiting results in the oral morphine being changed to the subcutaneous route, and increasing abdominal pain requires increasing morphine to 120 mg subcutaneously per day. As the patient's oral intake has remained minimal, the family physician has continued with the hypodermoclysis at 1 liter over night. The increasingly bed-ridden patient's cognition also starts to deteriorate as he interacts less and less with his family and spends more time sleeping. A son and daughter arrive in their parent's home to assist and support their mother in caring for their father. The daughter had sought advice on caring for her father from a friend who is a hospice nurse. She questions the value of ongoing hydration at this point, suggesting that her father would have less nausea and vomiting, and perhaps be more comfortable if the hypodermoclysis was to be discontinued. The son is a nephrologist who believes that hydration is necessary to maintain normal renal function, and avoid the accumulation of medications causing side-effects. The patient and his wife have continued to rely on their family physician to provide information and direction on the most appropriate management.

This patient and family situation highlights some of the complexity that surrounds the widely debated and controversial topic of hydration in terminally ill patients. At the center of the discussion is the desire to keep patients as comfortable as possible while avoiding unnecessary management or procedures. Clinicians making these decisions need to sort through expressions of opinion, information on pathophysiology and biochemical changes, research looking at a variety of outcomes, differing family and cultural expectations, and consensus statements on the topic. This diverse information has then to be applied to the specific trajectory of patient's illness.

Pros and cons of hydration

There is no controversy that terminally ill patients should be encouraged to maintain adequate hydration via the oral route. The debate and controversy essentially revolves around the use of supplemental parenteral hydration. There are many reports in the literature illustrating opposing perspectives from both a clinical and ethical viewpoint (1–11). (See also Chapter 23 by MacDonald.) In the past reviews on this subject have referenced a similar collection of clinical anecdotes and opinions of health care workers dealing with terminally ill patients. These arguments for and against hydrating terminally ill patients have been summarized as follows (6–7):

1. Arguments against parenteral hydration:
   - Comatose patients do not experience symptom distress.
   - Parenteral fluids may prolong dying.
   - Dehydration results in less urine and less need to void and use catheters.
   - Dehydration results in less gastrointestinal fluid and less nausea and vomiting.
   - There is less problem with respiratory tract complications such as cough and pulmonary edema.
   - The frequency and severity of edema and ascites are decreased.
   - Dehydration may act as natural anesthetic for the central nervous system.
   - Parenteral hydration is uncomfortable and limits patient mobility.
2. Arguments for parenteral hydration:
   - Dying patients are more comfortable with parenteral hydration.
   - There is no evidence that fluids prolong life.
   - Dehydration can cause confusion, restlessness, and neuromuscular irritability.
   - Oral hydration is given to dying patients complaining of thirst, and therefore parenteral hydration should also be administered.
   - Emphasis on poor quality of life detracts from efforts to improve comfort and life quality.
   - Parenteral hydration is a minimum standard of care.
   - Withholding parenteral fluid from dying patients may result in withholding therapies to other compromised patient groups.

It is usually the 'traditional medical model' that argues for initiating or maintaining parenteral hydration in terminally ill patients. It would seem reasonable to observe that most terminally ill patients dying in hospitals world wide will have an intravenous line in place at the time of death, unless they have undergone a rapid deterioration or experienced an unexpected demise. This is well illustrated by a Canadian report (12) where 73 of 106 cancer patients dying in a tertiary care hospital were noted to have intravenous fluids.

It is not difficult to envisage the problems inflicted on cachetic cancer patients by an unthinking policy of maintaining intravenous hydration with volumes in excess of 3 liters per day. Complications such as increased respiratory and gastrointestinal symptom distress are reflected in the arguments against parenteral hydration. The reports in the literature that argue against parenteral hydration suggest that many health care professionals looking after terminally ill patients have reacted to the generalized use of intravenous fluids and negative effects of this management by concluding that no parenteral hydration is the preferred approach. This has been reinforced by the anecdotal literature reports of palliative care doctors and nurses noting that many terminally ill patients appear to die comfortably without parenteral hydration. However review of this literature (7) indicates that these arguments are essentially based on anecdotal reports that are unsubstantiated by scientific data.

There has been the danger that the harm inflicted on terminally ill patients by an unthinking approach to parenteral hydration could be replaced by the simplistic opposite approach that no parenteral hydration would be best for all of these patients. However, it has been suggested that there are other issues to consider (6,7,13–16).

1 It is well recognized that dehydration causes confusion and restlessness in non-terminal patients. Problems of delirium and agitation are often reported in terminally ill patients.
2 Reduced intravascular volume and glomerular filtration rate caused by dehydration are accepted as a cause of pre-renal failure. Opioid metabolite accumulation in the presence of renal failure, resulting in confusion, myoclonus and seizures, has been well documented.

Reports in regard to agitated delirium and terminal restlessness are frequently reported in the palliative care literature (see Chapter 23). The discussion of these problems has often centered on the need for pharmacological management including sedation. Burke *et al.* (17) reported midazolam use for sedation of 'terminal restlessness' in 20% of hospice in-patients. Back (18) discussed possible causes and management of terminal restlessness in patients with advanced malignant disease. Dehydration was not listed as a possible underlying cause despite acknowledging that opioid metabolites in the presence of renal impairment might cause terminal restlessness. Lichter and Hunt (19) studied the symptoms of terminally ill patients in the last 48 hours of life and reported restlessness in 42% of patients, while noting that 'frequently sedation will be unavoidable.' Myoclonus was reported in 12% of this study group.

Ventafridda *et al.* (20) reported that 9% of patients required sedation for agitated delirium in a study of unendurable symptoms requiring sedation for cancer patients during their last days of life. This prompted our group to report in 1991 (21) that agitated delirium was the most frequent problem requiring sedation in the last week of life in 10% of our patients. However, we later noted that the severity of agitated delirium requiring sedation in our palliative care unit had decreased to 3% (22). We speculated that a change in our practice to include more frequent use of hypodermoclysis for hydration, switching opioids earlier when toxicity developed, and the use of less sedating treatments, such as haloperidol for delirium, was decreasing the prevalence and difficulty of managing agitated delirium in our patients (23).

Palliative care groups have continued to report requiring innovative approaches to the pharmacological management of symptoms associated with agitated delirium, including the use of intravenous propofol (24,25). A Japanese hospice group (26) reported requiring sedation to manage agitated delirium in 23% of their patients. A retrospective chart review of 76 consecutive patients dying at St Christopher's Hospice in Cape Town, South Africa, found that 22 (29%) patients required sedation for agitated delirium. None of these patients was treated with parenteral hydration, and the patients requiring sedation were administered significantly higher doses of opioids during a longer admission to this in-patient setting (27).

More recent reports on the use of sedation have suggested that agitated delirium appears to be less problematic in a number of different settings in Edmonton, Canada (28), where parenteral hydration is more common practice, compared with requirements for sedation in a number of other international settings (29).

As a result it has been suggested that dehydration could be a reversible component of agitated delirium and may be ignored by an approach that focuses on a sedative pharmacological solution to this distressing situation (30). It may be illogical for a patient to receive medications for agitated delirium, myoclonus, and seizures if in some situations these problems could be prevented or corrected by the use of parenteral hydration.

Hydration research

Research into the use of hydration in palliative care settings has tended to focus on three dimensions (31): the association between biochemical findings and hydration status; between biochemical findings and clinical symptoms; and between hydration status and clinical symptoms.

In regard to the first issue of the association between biochemical findings and hydration status, there is no controversy in accepting dehydration as a cause of renal failure (32–34). While parenteral hydration is routinely accepted as standard management in other settings, the impact of dehydration and rehydration on the renal function and electrolyte balance of terminally ill patients is still questioned. Dunphy *et al.* (5) stated that the published blood biochemistry of patients dying in hospice in-patient units suggest a 'greater degree of biochemical normality than might be predicted'. Waller (35) noted that a linear correlation between measurable indices of dehydration and fluid volume provided still needs to be demonstrated.

Oliver (36) has been quoted (5,37) as demonstrating the 'biochemical normality' of terminally ill patients who had not received parenteral hydration. However, closer examination reveals results on 22 patients with advanced cancer who died unexpectedly while being studied for hypercalcemia. These patients dying within 48 hours of venepuncture demonstrated uremia in 5 with a mean urea 24.7 mmol l^{-1} (range: 21–35), 5 patients were uremic and hypercalcemic (mean urea 23.3 mmol l^{-1}, range: 13–58; mean corrected calcium 3.36 mmol l^{-1}, range: 2.84–4.05). The remaining 12 patients had a mean urea of 9.6 mmol l^{-1} (range: 4–14, normal 2.5–6.5).

A study by Burge reported 52 palliative care subjects with a wide range of oral intake alone. It was stated that mean and median of serum sodium, osmolality, and urea were within the normal range of 100% of the subjects. However, closer examination of the reported figures reveals a sodium range of 116–147 mmol l^{-1} (normal range 135–145), and a urea of 2.1–24.6 mmol l^{-1} (normal range 2.1–8.2) (38).

Waller *et al.* (39) reported 68 hospice in-patients whose blood was collected during the final 48 hours of life. A state of dehydration as reflected by blood and urine parameters was reported in 59 of 68 patients. A subgroup of 13 of these 68 patients were receiving intravenous fluids at the rate of 1–2 liters per day. The group not receiving hydration and a mean urea of 141 mg%±84 (normal range 30±15). A surprise finding was that the intravenous group had a mean urea of 151 mg%±105. In the discussion this was explained as possibly due to a selection bias, in that the patients receiving intravenous fluids may have been more dehydrated at the outset. In addition, the intravenous fluids were commenced prior to transfer, as it is not the practice of this hospice to institute parenteral hydration in their patients (35,40).

Ellershaw *et al.* (41) reported 82 hospice patients with advanced cancer that underwent biochemical investigation as part of a dehydration study. Patients deemed to be dying, taking only sips of fluid, and no longer able to tolerate oral medications were entered into the study. In contrast, our group (42) reported a prospective open study of 100 consecutive patients dying in our palliative care unit, 69 of whom received hypodermoclysis for an average of 14±18 days. Hypodermoclysis was well tolerated in most patients with an average volume of 1203±505 ml per day. A comparison of results from these two reports is summarized in Table 22.1 (43).

A report by Morita *et al.* (44) provided further information on the biochemistry of terminally ill cancer patients at the end of life, and concluded that relatively small amounts of parenteral hydration may result in less abnormal biochemistry, particularly with regard to renal function, than patients not receiving parenteral hydration.

Research on the association between biochemical findings and hydration status compared with clinical symptoms has produced often conflicting reports that have looked at a variety of clinical outcomes. Much of the early literature was based on anecdotal opposing view points, as illustrated by two case reports (45,46). Andrews *et al.* (45) reported three patients managed without parenteral hydration. The conclusion was that dehydration had palliative benefits with a reduction in edema, respiratory secretions, congestion, and fluid overload. Yan and Bruera (46) reported three terminally ill patients for whom parenteral hydration was deemed to have helped maintain or recover cognition in two while assisting recovery and discharge in the third.

There have now been an increasing number of attempts to study this issue more carefully. Burge (38) noted that dry mouth is commonly reported as the most distressing symptom for dehydrated terminally ill patients. This study was a quantitative assessment of the experience of dehydration in advanced cancer patients. A cross-sectional survey examined

Table 22.1 A comparison of two studies

	Ellershaw et al.		**Fainsinger et al.**	
	Mean	**Normal range**	**Mean**	**Normal range**
Urea (mmol l^{-1})	15.5	2.5–6.5	8.8	3.2–8.2
Creatinine (μml l^{-1})	177	60–120	101	62–133
Sodium (mmol l^{-1})	140	133–148	136	141–148
Potassium (mmol l^{-1})	4.8	3.5–5.0	4.1	3.5–4.8
Total protein (g l^{-1})	58	60–85	54	68–81

severity and distribution of thirst, dry mouth, bad taste, nausea, pleasure in drinking, fatigue and pain, as well as the association of these symptoms with objective measures of dehydration. All symptoms except pain and nausea were moderately severe, but there was no association between severity and fluid intake. The study concluded that parenteral hydration on the basis of fluid intake and laboratory measures were not helpful if the aim was to reduce thirst. Conclusions were limited by the short study duration, exclusion of sicker patients by the study design, and the use of unreliable methods to assess hydration. McCann *et al.* (47) examined the symptom prevalence and management of hunger and thirst in terminally ill patients not receiving parenteral hydration. Of 48 consecutive patients, 32 were able to participate in the study and indicate their sensations of hunger and thirst for most of the time from initial admission until death. There were 20 patients (63%) who never experienced hunger, while 20 (62%) reported either no or minimal thirst. Symptoms of hunger, thirst, and dry mouth were apparently well managed with sips or mouth care.

Ellershaw *et al.* (41) investigated the relationship between symptoms and dehydration in 82 patients, none of whom was receiving parenteral hydration. Assessments were made of respiratory tract secretions, thirst, and dry mouth. No statistically significant relationship was found between the level of hydration and respiratory tract secretions. Only 28% of patients were able to respond to questions. The mean time from entry on study to death was 2 days. Of those able to respond, 87% reported a dry mouth, while 83% reported thirst. No significant association was demonstrated between the level of hydration and these symptoms. The authors acknowledged that the effect of renal failure and possible consequences of agitation and confusion were not assessed, and that further research was necessary to clarify the importance of this issue for terminally ill patients. Musgrave *et al.* (48) studied the effect of intravenous fluids on a group of terminal cancer patients dying in a hospital oncology unit. More than 90% of patients in this unit usually die while receiving intravenous fluids. Data were collected on 30 patients during the last week of life, receiving intravenous hydration in a range of 500–3000 ml per day. Only 19 of the 30 patients were able to indicate their thirst intensity, with 6 patients reporting mild thirst, 8 moderate thirst, and 4 severe thirst. No relationship was demonstrated between level of thirst, intravenous fluids, and biochemical parameters. In a further report by Musgrave (49) the effects of intravenous hydration on fluid retention signs in terminally ill cancer patients was studied. The presence of crepitations, ascites, and leg edema was studied in 21 patients receiving intravenous hydration on the day of death. There was evidence of crepitations in 81%, ascites in 62%, and leg edema in 52%. No relationship between the prevalence of signs and fluid balance was evident.

Our group had noted that we administer smaller volumes by hypodermoclysis (42), than the larger volumes of intravenous fluids typically given to hospital in-patients. A retrospective review examined the volume and hydration modality of consecutive terminally ill cancer patients in two different settings (50). In a palliative care unit 203 of 290 patients received hypodermoclysis at a daily volume of 1015±1035 ml per day for 12±8 days. No patients required discontinuation of hypodermoclysis for side-effects such as edema, respiratory distress, or congestive heart failure. At the in-patient cancer center, 30 consecutive terminally ill cancer patients received intravenous hydration at a daily volume of 2080±720 ml per day ($P<0.001$), for 11.5±5 days. The retrospective study design could not establish toxicity resulting from intravenous hydration at the cancer hospital setting.

However, these results do suggest that in some situations cancer patients may be receiving excessive hydration that could cause side-effects such as edema, congestive heart failure, or increased respiratory and gastrointestinal symptom distress.

Vullo-Navich *et al.* (37) reported a prospective clinical study evaluating the effect of oral fluid intake alone on serum sodium and comfort levels in 31 terminal patients not provided with hypodermoclysis or intravenous hydration. No statistical differences in comfort scores between pre-dehydration and dehydration phases were noted. The authors concluded that their findings reinforced the belief that fluid depletion in dying patients results in relatively benign symptoms. This report was followed by a correspondence suggesting different interpretations of the significance of the results (40,51,52).

The change of standard practice in the palliative care unit in Edmonton with regard to assessment and management of dehydration and cognitive impairment resulted in a retrospective chart review of 117 and 162 patients admitted in 1988–1989 and 1991–1992, respectively (53). The prevalence of agitated impaired mental status decreased from 26% to 10%. Use of hydration increased from 32% to 73% ($P<0.001$), the mean volume administered per day did not change significantly. The number of patients undergoing opioid rotation increased from 21% to 41% ($P<0.001$), the mean opioid dose per day did not change significantly. The mean prevalence of regular use of haloperidol decreased from 24% to 8% ($P<0.01$), the mean haloperidol dose decreased from 5.6 mg to 3.6 mg per day ($P<0.01$). Use of other psychoactive drugs such as benzodiazepines and neuroleptics also decreased significantly. The authors concluded that the data suggested that routine cognitive assessment, opioid rotation, and hydration may reduce the frequency of agitated confusion in terminally ill cancer patients. However, while suggesting that hydration may have a role in this change, it was not possible to determine the relative contributions of these three factors.

Ashby *et al.* (54) measured plasma concentrations of morphine and its metabolites in 36 hospice patients. The data were analysed in relation to dose, serum creatinine, and presence or absence of opioid induced side-effects. Nineteen patients experienced symptoms attributed to morphine, with 10 experiencing nausea and vomiting and 9 experiencing acute delirium. Serum creatinine was elevated in patients with adverse effects ($P=0.03$), as were the dose-corrected plasma morphine metabolites. The 7 patients with serum creatinine concentrations above the normal range had symptoms attributed to opioid-induced side-effects. The authors concluded that morphine metabolites may be a causal or aggravating factor in nausea and vomiting and cognitive impairment in palliative patients with significant renal impairment.

Wood *et al.* (55) reported 18 patients on a palliative care unit receiving morphine for cancer pain who completed a study employing a range of neuropsychological tests assessing cognitive function. The data were correlated with biochemical tests of renal function as well as concentrations of morphine and its metabolites. Seven patients were reported to have some degree of nausea and vomiting, thought to be an opioid side-effect, and had higher serum creatinine concentrations, worse neuropsychological performance, and significantly higher morphine metabolite concentrations. Although the authors concluded that it was not possible to determine relative causal contribution, renal function and plasma concentrations of morphine and metabolites were thought to be important.

Lawlor *et al.* (56) noted that delirium impedes communication and contributes to symptoms distress in patients with advanced cancer, and attempted to evaluate the occurrence, precipitating factors, and reversibility of delirium in these patients. A prospective serial assessment was completed in a cohort of 113 patients with advanced cancer. Reversal of delirium occurred in 46 (49%) of 94 episodes in 71 patients. Univariate analysis demonstrated reversibility associated with psychoactive medications and dehydration. The authors concluded that while delirium is multifactorial, hydration using hypodermoclysis may be one of the potentially useful measures to consider.

Few reports have examined the role of parenteral hydration in patients presenting with malignant bowel obstruction. Our group (57) reported 15 patients in a consecutive review of 100 patients who required medical management for bowel obstruction. All 15 patients received hydration with hypodermoclysis at a mean volume of 1313±537 ml per day. Measures of symptom distress included visual analogue scales for nausea, and suggested that intensive medical management, including parenteral hydration, could provide good symptom control. A more recent study by Ripamonti *et al.* (58) reported a prospective trial involving 17 patients with inoperable malignant bowel obstruction who were randomized to receive octreotide or scopolamine butylbromide. Compared with the home care patients, the hospitalized patients received significantly more parenteral hydration and drank more fluids. While there was no difference in the daily thirst and dry mouth intensity in relation to the amount of parenteral hydration, independent of antisecretory treatment, the patients receiving less parenteral hydration presented with significantly more nausea and drowsiness. The authors hypothesized that the nausea and drowsiness may have been due to the accumulation of toxins produced in the gastrointestinal tract in these patients, and that intravenous hydration may have played a role in reducing these symptoms.

Viola *et al.* (59) summarized the existing evidence regarding the effects of fluid status and fluid therapy in palliative care situations by performing a systematic review. They examined the existing clinical evidence pertaining to the effect of fluid status and fluid therapy in palliative care patients. Six studies were selected for inclusion (38,39,41,47,48,53). The authors concluded that given the limitations present in these six studies, it was impossible to draw firm conclusions regarding clinical care.

Alternative hydration techniques

Nasogastric tubes and gastrostomy

Nasogastric tubes are uncomfortable and prolonged use in a palliative care setting is avoided where possible (57,58). Percutaneous gastrostomies are more commonly used in the setting of head and neck or esophageal cancer where the patient has increasing dysphagia and may benefit from nutrition as well as hydration (60). As patients deteriorate the need to continue enteral hydration often requires a review of the goals of care. Difficulty in discontinuing management and ease of access can result in the ongoing provision of calories and water in circumstances where this might not otherwise have been instituted. As patients deteriorate there may be an increased risk of aspiration pneumonia if percutaneous gastrostomies continue to be used excessively.

Hypodermoclysis

Many articles critical of parenteral hydration in terminally ill patients have only referred to parenteral hydration by the intravenous route. The safety of hypodermoclysis has been well documented and reported in non-cancer patients (61,62). There have been a number of reports in palliative care populations demonstrating the ease of administration and minimal toxicity (42,63,64).

Most reports (6,7) have recommended the use of solutions with electrolytes, as non-electrolyte solutions have been reported to draw fluid into the interstitial space. Initial recommendations suggested rates of infusion should be limited to the range of 100–120 ml per hour, but later reports suggested patients tolerating boluses of up to 500 ml per hour (61,62). Traditionally it has also been recommended that hyaluronidace should be added to the fluid to promote absorption in a dose ranging from 150–750 units per liter (6,7).

Our group has reported a randomized, double-blind study to compare bolus subcutaneous infusions with either 150 or 300 units of hyaluronidase (65). A group of 25 patients was randomized to receive a local injection of hyaluronidase 300 units or hyaluronidase 150 units immediately before the one hour infusion of 500 ml of a solution made up of two-thirds dextrose 5% and one-third normal saline. The next day the patients were crossed over and each patient received the alternative treatment. Treatments were well tolerated by all patients with minimal problems. Patient and investigator preference for treatment was not significantly different.

A recent shortage of hyaluronidase, as well as anecdotal reports from other centers and observations of our group of patients having good absorption of hypodermoclysis without hyaluronidase, resulted in a report of 24 consecutive patients receiving hypodermoclysis without hyaluronidase (66). Hydration was maintained for a mean of 12 ± 9 days. Rates of infusion were highly variable in a range between 20 and 300 ml per hour. Three patients received twice daily boluses of 500 ml over one hour, 13 patients received overnight hydration, and the remaining 8 patients received continuous subcutaneous hydration. Average site duration of infusion was 3.3 ± 3.6 days. Only two patients required the addition of hyaluronidase in order to maintain hypodermoclysis. Our program has now changed our hydration policy and hyaluronidase is only used in patients where initial attempts at hypodermoclysis result in discomfort or problems with absorption.

Proctoclysis

Intravenous hydration can be uncomfortable and difficult in the home, while hypodermoclysis can increase the expense of parenteral hydration, particularly where hyaluronidase is required. This prompted Bruera *et al.* (67) to attempt the use of rectal hydration in terminally ill cancer patients. In 17 adult patients with dehydration, proctoclysis was offered as an alternative when technical resources were not adequate for the use of hypodermoclysis. Tap water was used, and the rectal infusion was increased from 100 ml to a maximum of 400 ml per hour, unless fluid leakage occurred before the maximum volume was achieved. The mean daily volume, hourly rate, and duration was reported as 1035±150 ml per day, 224±58 ml per hour, and 14±8 days, respectively. Rectal hydration was noted to be well tolerated with minimal side-effects in the majority of patients. The daily cost of supplies was estimated 2.78 Canadian dollars for intravenous fluids, 4.56 dollars for hypodermoclysis, and 0.11 dollars for rectal hydration. A response to this report noted that this was not new, and proctoclysis had been used frequently prior to the 1930s to administer volumes of up to six pints per day (68). A follow-up report by Bruera *et al.* (69) reported on a follow-up experience of rectal hydration in 78 advanced cancer patients. Volumes infused, patient tolerance, and side-effects were similar to the earlier report, suggesting that this is a safe, effective, and low-cost technique for the delivery of hydration in terminally ill cancer patients.

Social and cultural perspectives on hydration

It has been pointed out that there are other important issues to consider in regard to the use of hydration (70). (See also chapter 23.) Patient and family attitudes, level of comfort with the situation, and education can all influence the decision. Health care workers' attitudes, level of education, and biases in presentation can also affect the outcome. Morita *et al.* (71) attempted to clarify patients' and family members' perceptions about rehydration and to identify contributing factors for decision-making. A prospective structured survey was performed on 121 hospice patients in Japan who had insufficient oral intake. The patients' performance status, fluid retention symptoms, denial, the physician's recommendations, the patient's and family members' beliefs about the effect of hydration on the patients' distress, and family members' anxiety about withholding rehydration were significantly associated with decision-making. Multiple regression analysis revealed the patient's denial, the physician's recommendations determined by the patient's performance status and fluid retention symptoms, and family members' belief that rehydration could worsen the patient's distress as independent determinants for rehydration. The main determinants for rehydration therapy were the patient's performance status, fluid retention symptoms, denial, and care receivers' beliefs about the effect of rehydration on the patient's distress.

A Canadian study (72) identified issues that are important to family care-givers when deciding whether or not artificial hydration should be provided to patients with advanced cancer. A qualitative study using semistructured interviews was carried out in a home support and inpatient division of a palliative care program in Halifax, Nova Scotia. Factors influencing care-givers included symptom distress issues, ethical and emotional considerations, information exchanged between health professionals and family, and culture. Perceived benefits of artificial hydration were central to the ethical, emotional, and cultural considerations involved in the care-givers' decision-making. The authors concluded that discussions with care-givers should evaluate the patient's wishes and attitudes, provide as accurate information as is available about the pros and cons, and carefully evaluate any expressed concerns.

A recent article attempting to present the values of the Jewish faith with regard to terminal dehydration (73) illustrates the difficulty of applying cultural and ethnic research and opinion. Letters in response varied from describing this as an 'excellent article' (74) to 'extremely offensive in its references to Jewish people' (75).

It is also worth noting that it has been proposed that terminal dehydration or voluntary cessation of drinking may provide an alternative to physician-assisted suicide. Miller and Meier (76) suggest that terminal dehydration accompanied by standard palliative care management, 'offers patient's a way to escape agonizing, incurable conditions that they consider to be worse than death, without requiring transformation of the law and medical ethics'. Quill *et al.* (77) suggest that voluntary cessation of 'drinking are clinical options that may be acceptable to a patient and physician and do not require fundamental changes in the law'.

Conclusion: Consensus and Future Research

Consider again the case report described at the beginning of this chapter. Discussion of the management in this setting, and the manner in which information should be presented to the family remains open to the interpretation of the literature reviewed above and the biases of the health care providers involved. We could perhaps achieve consensus that dehydration is a cause of renal failure, and that hypodermoclysis is a safe and effective way of providing parenteral hydration. Some would perhaps agree that rehydration of terminally ill patients may result in better biochemical parameters at the end of life, and that there is sufficient evidence to recommend that if terminally ill patients are not rehydrated, medications such as opioids should be gradually decreased to avoid accumulation and toxic side-effects. There is likely to be consensus that the major issue is the benefit or harm that parenteral hydration will cause to terminally ill patients unable to sustain adequate oral fluid intake.

The conflicting conclusions of review and consensus statements in this area highlight the unresolved debate. Slomka (9) concluded that dehydration causes no symptom distress and that parenteral fluids do not add to the comfort of dying patients. Zerwekh (78) reports that 'artificial hydration is a misguided mercy that neither gives comfort nor prolongs life'. Smith (79) states that 'dehydration in terminal illness has not been found to produce distressing symptoms or to shorten life; it may even be beneficial'.

Chadfield-Mohr and Byatt (80) are more cautious in concluding that the decision to institute parenteral hydration in terminally ill patients is a complex one, and that a rule applicable to all circumstances is impossible. An awareness of factors involved in a specific case and relevant research findings will be more likely to provide a considered and appropriate decision.

Consensus statements of larger groups have also tended to be more cautious in their conclusions. The European Association for Palliative Care sponsored an expert committee of clinicians from different specialities to make recommendations on hydration in the terminal phase of disease (81). It was acknowledged that part of the controversy related to the definition of the terminal cancer patient and difficulty in predicting life expectancy. In reaching a decision a three-step process was proposed. Step one involved assessment of a number of issues including clinical condition, symptoms, expected survival, spontaneous oral intake, and psychological profile. Step two involved the assessment of pros and cons, and step three involved periodic re-evaluation.

A joint working party of the National Council for Hospice and Specialist Palliative Care Services and the Ethics Committee of the Association for Palliative Medicine of Great Britain and Ireland prepared a statement on artificial hydration (82). They concluded that:

1 A blanket policy of artificial hydration or no artificial hydration is ethically indefensible.
2 Although evidence is limited, artificial hydration in imminently dying patients influences neither survival nor symptom control.
3 Artificial hydration is unlikely to alleviate symptoms of thirst and dry mouth in people who are terminally ill.
4 Appropriate palliative care will involve consideration of the option of parenteral hydration, where dehydration results from a potentially correctable cause.
5 The clinical team has the responsibility to make assessments concerning the relevance of hydration to the experience of individual patients.
6 The interest of patients cannot be subordinated to the anxieties of relatives.

The need to consider individual circumstances and predictions of life expectancy in evaluating the potential benefit of parenteral hydration is illustrated in Figure 22.1 (6). Despite coming from different perspectives, there is consensus from a number of palliative

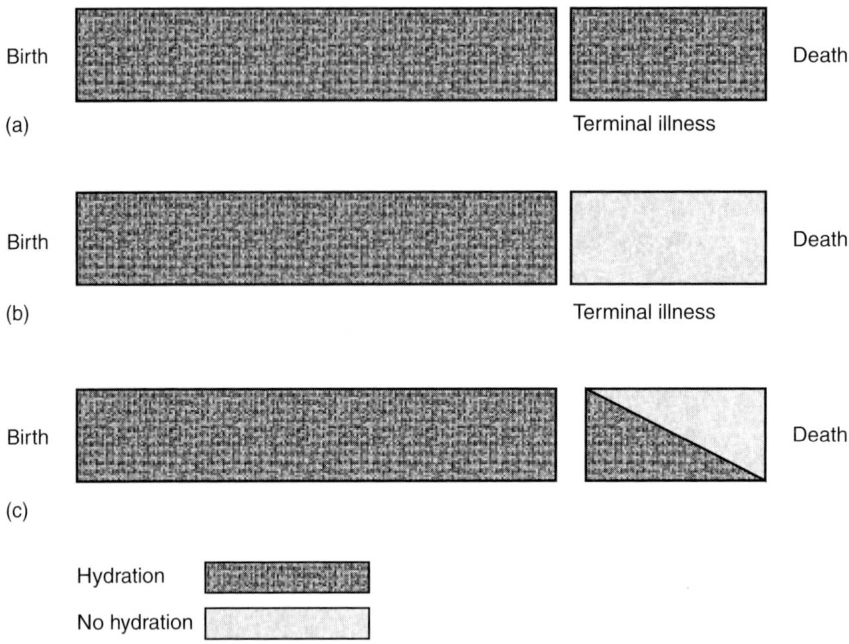

Figure 22.1 Hydration practice. (a) Hospital model; (b) hospice model; (c) individualized model.

care groups (5,30,59) that:

1 The data available are inadequate for any final conclusions to be reached on this issue.

2 Careful individual assessment of the relevance of dehydration to each clinical situation is required.

3 Further definitive research is required.

Where should we proceed with future research? Researchers in this area are confronted with many challenges. It is worth noting that a systematic review attempted to clarify the physical diagnosis of hypovolemia in adults (83). The authors concluded that in patients with vomiting, diarrhea, or decreased oral intake, few findings, with the exception of serum electrolytes, urea, and creatinine levels, have proven value. Viola *et al.* (59) suggested that we need more rigorous designs to test hypotheses regarding the effects of fluid deficiency and fluid therapy on mental status, thirst, and dry mouth. Furthermore, the subpopulation of the terminally ill to whom the controversy of parenteral hydration applies is not that clear. Researchers need to agree on a common set of outcomes and measurement tools for use in palliative care research in order to facilitate comparison and synthesis of data across a variety of studies. The clinical and practical difficulties of doing research in palliative care has often been noted (84,85). These difficulties are only too obvious when speculating on how a randomized, double-blind control study could be applied to aspects of the parenteral hydration debate. Despite the previous research, it seems reasonable to conclude that we have only begun to scratch the surface of possible ways in which we can examine this area further.

References

1. **Craig GM.** On withholding nutrition and hydration in the terminally ill: has palliative medicine gone too far? *Journal of Medical Ethics* 1994;20:139–43.
2. **Ashby M; Stoffell B.** Artificial hydration and alimentation at the end of life: A reply to Craig. *Journal of Medical Ethics* 1995;21:135–40.
3. **Dicks B.** Rehydration or dehydration? *Supportive Care in Cancer* 1994;2:88–90.
4. **Dunlop RJ; Ellershaw JE; Baines MJ; Sykes N; Saunders CM.** On withholding nutrition and hydration in the terminally ill: has palliative medicine gone too far? A reply. *Journal of Medical Ethics* 1995;21:141–3.
5. **Dunphy K; Finlay I; Rathbone G; Gilbert J; Hicks F.** Rehydration in palliative and terminal care: if not—why not? *Palliative Medicine* 1995;9:221–8.
6. **Fainsinger RL; Bruera E.** The management of dehydration in terminally ill patients. *Journal of Palliative Care* 1994;10:55–9.
7. **Fainsinger RL; Bruera E.** Hypodermoclysis for symptom control vs the Edmonton Injector. *Journal of Palliative Care* 1991;7:5–8.
8. **Meares CJ.** Terminal dehydration. A review. *American Journal of Hospice and Palliative Care* 1994;11(3):10–14.
9. **Slomka J.** What do apple pie and motherhood have to do with feeding tubes and caring for the patient? *Archives of Internal Medicine* 1995;155:1258–63.
10. **Smith SA.** Patient induced dehydration—can it ever be therapeutic? *Oncology Nursing Forum* 1995;22:1487–91.
11. **Wilkes E.** On withholding nutrition and hydration in the terminally ill: has palliative medicine gone too far? A commentary. *Journal of Medical Ethics* 1994;20:144–5.
12. **Burge FI; King DB; Wilson D.** Intravenous fluids and the hospitalized dying: a medical last rite? *Canadian Family Physician* 1990;86:883–6.
13. **Fainsinger RL; Bruera E; Watanabe S.** Rehydration in palliative care. *Palliative Medicine* 1996;10:165–6.
14. **Fainsinger RL.** Deshydratation et soins palliatifs. In: Roy DJ; Rapin C., editors *Less Annales de Soins Palliatifs.* Centre de Bioethique. Institut de Recherches Cliniques de Montreal, 1995;3:171–80.
15. **Fainsinger RL.** Nutrition and hydration for the terminally ill. *Journal of the American Medical Association* 1995;273:1736.
16. **MacDonald SM; Fainsinger RL.** Symptom control: the problem areas. *Palliative Medicine* 1994;8:167–8.
17. **Burke AL; Diamond PL; Hulbert J.** Terminal restlessness—its management and the role of midazolam. *Medical Journal of Australia* 1999;155:485–7.
18. **Back IN.** Terminal restlessness in patients with advanced malignant disease. *Palliative Medicine* 1992;6:293–8.
19. **Lichter I, Hunt E.** The last 48 hours of life. *Journal of Palliative Care* 1990;6:7–15.
20. **Ventafridda V; Ripamonti C; DeConno F; Tamburini M; Cassileth BR.** Symptom prevalence and control during cancer patients' last days of life. *Journal of Palliative Care* 1990;6:7–11.
21. **Fainsinger RL; Bruera E; Miller MJ., *et al.*** Symptom control during the last week of life on a palliative unit. *Journal of Palliative Care* 1991;7:5–11.
22. **Fainsinger RL; MacEacheron T; Miller MJ., *et al.*** The use of hypodermoclysis for rehydration in terminally ill cancer patients. *Journal of Palliative Care* 1992;8:70.
23. **Fainsinger RL; Tapper M; Bruera E.** A perspective on the management of delirium in the terminally ill. *Journal of Palliative Care* 1993;9:4–8.

24. **Mercadante S; deConno F; Ribamonti C.** Propofol in terminal care. *Journal of Pain and Symptom Management* 1995;10:639–42.
25. **Moyle J.** Use of propofol in palliative medicine. *Journal of Pain and Symptom Management* 1995;10:643–6.
26. **Morita T; Inoue S; Chihara S.** Sedation for symptom control in Japan: the importance of intermittent use and communication with family members. *Journal of Pain and Symptom Management* 1996;12:32–8.
27. **Fainsinger RL; Landman W; Hoskings M; Bruera E.** Sedation for uncontrolled symptoms in a South African hospice. *Journal of Pain and Symptom Management* 1998;16(3):145–52.
28. **Fainsinger RL; deMoissac D; Mancini I; Oneschuk D.** Sedation for delirium and other symptoms in terminally ill patients in Edmonton. *Journal of Palliative Care* 2000;16(2):5–10.
29. **Fainsinger RL; Waller A; Bercovici M; Bengtson K; Landman W; Hosking M; Nunez-Olarte JM; deMoissac D.** A multi-centre international study of sedation for uncontrolled symptoms in terminally ill patients. *Palliative Medicine* 2000;14:257–65.
30. **Fainsinger RL; Bruera E.** When to treat dehydration in a terminally ill patient? *Supportive Care in Cancer* 1997;5:205–11.
31. **Morita T; Ichiki T; Tsunoda J., *et al.*** Three dimensions of the rehydration—dehydration problem in a palliative care setting. *Journal of Palliative Care* 1999;15(2):60–1.
32. **Badr K; Ichikawa I.** Prerenal failure: a deleterious shift from renal compensation to decompensation. *New England Journal of Medicine* 1988;319:623–9.
33. **Brady HR; Singer GG.** Acute renal failure. *The Lancet* 1995;346:1533–40.
34. **Weinberg A; Minakar KL.** Dehydration. Evaluation and management in older adults. *Journal of the American Medical Association* 1995;274:1552–6.
35. **Waller A.** Letter to the Editor. *American Journal of Hospice Palliative Care* 1995;7:5–6.
36. **Oliver D.** Terminal dehydration. Letter. *The Lancet* 1994;ii:631.
37. **Vullo-Navich K; Smith S; Andrews M., *et al.*** Comfort and incidence of abnormal serum sodium, BUN, creatinine and osmolality in dehydration of terminal illness. *American Journal of Hospice and Palliative Care* 1998;15(2):77–84.
38. **Burge FI.** Dehydration symptoms of palliative care cancer patients. *Journal of Pain and Symptom Management* 1993;8:454–64.
39. **Waller A; Hershkowitz M; Adunsky A.** The effect of intravenous fluid infusion on blood and urine parameters of hydration and on the state of consciousness in terminal cancer patients. *American Journal of Hospice Palliative Care* 1994;11(6):22–7.
40. **Waller A; Adunsky A.** Enigma of terminal dehydration. *American Journal of Hospice and Palliative Care* 1999;16(2):442.
41. **Ellershaw JE; Sutcliffe JM; Saunders CM.** Dehydration and the dying patient. *Journal of Pain and Symptom Management* 1995;10:192–7.
42. **Fainsinger RL; MacEacheron T; Miller MJ., *et al.*** The use of hypodermoclysis for rehydration in terminally ill cancer patients. *Journal of Pain and Symptom Management* 1994;9:298–302.
43. **Fainsinger RL.** Biochemical dehydration in terminally ill cancer patients. *Journal of Palliative Care* 1999;15(2):59–61.
44. **Morita T; Ichika T; Tsunoda J., *et al.*** Biochemical dehydration and fluid retention symptoms in terminally ill cancer patients whose death is impending. *Journal of Palliative Care* 1998;14(4):60–2.
45. **Andrews M; Bell ER; Smith SA., *et al.*** Dehydration in terminally ill patients. Is it appropriate palliative care? *Post Graduate Medicine* 1993;93:201–8.
46. **Yan E; Bruera E.** Parenteral hydration of terminally ill cancer patients. *Journal of Palliative Care* 1991;7:40–3.

47. **McCann RM; Hall WJ; Groth-Juncker A.** Comfort care for the terminally ill patients: the appropriate use of nutrition and hydration. *Journal of the American Medical Association* 1994;272:1263–6.
48. **Musgrave CF; Bartle N; Opstad J.** The sensation of thirst in dying patients receiving IV hydration. *Journal of Palliative Care* 1995;11:17–21.
49. **Musgrave CF.** Fluid retention and intravenous hydration in the dying. *Palliative Medicine* 1996;10:53.
50. **Bruera E; Belzile M; Watanabe S; Fainsinger RL.** Volume of hydration in terminal cancer patients. *Supportive Care in Cancer* 1996;4:147–50.
51. **Fainsinger RL.** Dehydration of the terminally ill. *American Journal of Hospice and Palliative Care* 1998;15(5):255–6.
52. **Smith S.** Defending dehydration study. *American Journal of Hospice and Palliative Care* 1998;15(6):311.
53. **Bruera E; Franco JJ; Maltoni M; Watanabe S., *et al.*** Changing pattern of agitated impaired mental status in patients with advanced cancer: association with cognitive monitoring, hydration, and opioid rotation. *Journal of Pain and Symptom Management* 1995;10:287–91.
54. **Ashby M; Fleming B; Wood M., *et al.*** Plasma morphine and glucuronide (M3G and M6G), concentrations in hospice in-patients. *Journal of Pain and Symptom Management* 1997;14:157–67.
55. **Wood MN; Ashby MA; Somogyi AI., *et al.*** Neuropsychological and pharmacokinetic assessment of hospice in-patients receiving morphine. *Journal of Pain and Symptom Management* 1998;16:112–20.
56. **Lawlor PG; Gagnon B; Mancini IL., *et al.*** Occurrence, causes, and outcome of delirium in patients with advanced cancer. *Archives of Internal Medicine* 2000;160:786–94.
57. **Fainsinger RL; Spachynski K; Hanson J., *et al.*** Symptom control in terminally ill patients with malignant bowel obstruction. *Journal of Pain and Symptom Management* 1994;9:12–18.
58. **Ripamonti C; Mercadante S; Groff L., *et al.*** Role of octreotide, scopolamine butylbromide, and hydration in symptom control of patients with inoperable bowel obstruction and nasogastric tubes: a prospective randomized trial. *Journal of Pain and Symptom Management* 2000;19:23–24.
59. **Viola RA; Wells GA; Peterson J.** The effects of fluid status and fluid therapy on the dying: a systematic review. *Journal of Palliative Care* 1997;13(4):41–52.
60. **Steiner N; Bruera E.** Methods of hydration in palliative care patients. *Journal of Palliative Care* 1998;14(2):6–13.
61. **Constans T; Dutertre J; Froge E.** Hypodermoclysis in dehydrated elderly patients: Local effects with and without hyaluronidase. *Journal of Palliative Care* 1991;7:10–12.
62. **Molloy DJ; Cunje A.** Hypodermoclysis and the care of old adults. An old solution for new problems? *Canadian Family Physician* 1992;38:2038–43.
63. **Hays H.** Hypodermoclysis for symptom control in terminal cancer. *Canadian Family Physician* 1985;31:1253–6.
64. **Bruera E; Legris M; Keuhn N; Miller MJ.** Hypodermoclysis for the administration of fluids and narcotic analgesics in patients with advanced cancer. *Journal of Pain and Symptom Management* 1990;5:218–220.
65. **Bruera E; de Stoutz ND; Fainsinger RL., *et al.*** Comparison of two different concentrations of hyaluronidase in patients receiving one hour infusions of hypodermoclysis. *Journal of Pain and Symptom Management* 1995;10:505–9.
66. **Centeno C; Bruera E.** Subcutaneous hydration with no hyaluronidase in patients with advanced cancer. *Journal of Pain and Symptom Management* 1999;17(5):305–6.
67. **Bruera E; Schoeller T; Pruvost M.** Proctoclysis for hydration of terminal cancer patients. *The Lancet* 1994;344:1699.

68. **Needham D.** Proctoclysis for hydration. *The Lancet* 1995;345:596.
69. **Bruera E; Pruvost M; Schoeller T.** Proctoclysis for hydration of terminally ill cancer patients. *Journal of Pain and Symptom Management* 1998;15:216–9.
70. **Baumrucker S.** Science, hospice, and terminal dehydration. *American Journal of Hospice and Palliative Care* 1999;16(3):502–3.
71. **Morita T; Tsunoda J; Inoue S., *et al.*** Perceptions and decision-making on rehydration of terminally ill cancer patients and family members. *American Journal of Hospice and Palliative Care* 1999;16(3):509–16.
72. **Parkash R; Burge F.** The family's perspective on issues of hydration in terminal care. *Journal of Palliative Care* 1997;13(4):23–7.
73. **Bodell J; Weng MA.** The Jewish patient in terminal dehydration: a hospice ethical dilemma. *American Journal of Hospice and Palliative Care* 2000;17(3):185–8.
74. **Schur TG.** Life and afterlife in Jewish tradition. *American Journal of Hospice and Palliative Care* 2000;17(5):296–7.
75. **Rothstein JM.** Out of context? *American Journal of Hospice and Palliative Care* 2000;17(5):297.
76. **Miller FG; Meier DE.** Voluntary death: a comparison of terminal dehydration and physician-assisted suicide. *Annals of Internal Medicine* 1998;128:559–62.
77. **Quill TE; Meier DE; Block SD., *et al.*** The debate over physician-assisted suicide: empirical data and conversant views. *Annals of Internal Medicine* 1998;128:552–8.
78. **Zerwekh JV.** Do dying patients really need IV fluids? *American Journal of Nutrition* 1997;97(3):226–30.
79. **Smith SA.** Controversies in hydrating the terminally ill patient. *Journal of Intravenous Nursing* 1997;20(4):193–200.
80. **Chadfield-Mohr SM; Byatt CM.** Dehydration in the terminally ill—iatrogenic insult or natural process? *Post Graduate Medicine J* 1997;73:476–80.
81. **Amadori D; Bruera E; Cozagloi L., *et al.*** Guidelines on artificial nutrition versus hydration in terminal cancer patients. *Nutrition* 1996;12(3):163–7.
82. **National Council for Hospice and Specialist Palliative Care Services.** Artificial hydration (AH) for people who are terminally ill. *European Journal of Palliative Care* 1997;4(4):124.
83. **McGee S; Abernethy WB; Simel DL.** Is this patient hypobolemic? *Journal of the American Medicine Association* 1999;281:1022–9.
84. **Jordhoy MS; Kaasa S; Fayers P., *et al.*** Challenges in palliative care research; recruitment, attrition and compliance: experience from a randomized controlled trial. *Palliative Medicine* 1999;13:299–310.
85. **Ling J; Rees E; Hardy J.** What influences participation in clinical trials in palliative care in a cancer centre? *European Journal of Cancer* 2000;36:621–6.

Chapter 23

Ethical considerations in feeding or hydrating advanced cancer patients

Neil MacDonald

Introduction

Medical ethics is not a secular religion where dogma slowly responds to moral issues. Rather, it relates to the specific needs of individual patients and families, while the interpretation of principles is highly dependent upon new knowledge. In turn, albeit slowly in the case of palliative care, knowledge coupled with awareness will ultimately change the attitudes and priorities of health professionals. The changing panorama of the use of assisted hydration and nutrition by patients with advanced chronic illness illustrates this point.

Health professionals are products of their culture and society. Among many distinctive cultural features, all societies place special value on food and drink. Aside from sustenance of life, we meet as families over the table; we celebrate and, in turn, obtain solace on occasion through food and libations; we honour others by inviting them to share our meals; and we universally regard the nourishment of a loved one as a family duty of the highest order. Families often do not talk of nutrition in a biologic sense; they talk of duties and family bonds which they may feel are ruptured if they cannot sustain a family member's ability to eat and drink.

Disagreements between professional staff and families over the use of technical means of feeding or hydrating patients are among the most commonly encountered sources of misunderstanding and angry discourse between families and health professionals. Because of a desire to avoid this unpleasantness and, perhaps, since professionals are creatures of their own culture, decisions may be made to inaugurate or maintain assisted nutrition, even though there is no a priori ethical or biological rationale for these decisions.

This chapter explores the considerations that influence decisions on hydration and nutrition towards the end of life, and offers a series of guidelines which may assist health professionals and families to make decisions that are in the best interests of the patient.

Nutrition

Professional attitudes—education—research

Unlike pain, professionals may regard symptoms related to malnutrition (weight loss, anorexia, fatigue) as inherent aspects of illness, and thus not amenable to correction unless the disease process can be reversed.

Surveys show that many patients in hospitals are malnourished (1), yet identifying under-nutrition and offering patients an attractive, palatable diet is often not recognized as a priority within institutions. This cavalier attitude relates in part to deficient education and research.

Research

While protein–calorie malnutrition is common in patients with advanced cancer, and recent animal work presents many intriguing leads for study, research interest is extremely modest; only four studies out of 2561 abstracted by the American Society of Clinical Oncology in the year 2000 related to cancer cachexia.

Most cancer patients are over 65, and the effects of malnutrition are particularly troublesome in the elderly. Asthenia and cachexia limit patient mobility and create dependence upon others. In most developed countries, families are smaller, children often live at a distance, and fewer people are available to support dependent family members. The pathophysiology of cancer-induced debility is not clearly exposed, but we have sufficient information to proceed with human interventional trials [e.g. recent data on the effects of omega-3 fatty acids on cancer cachexia (2)]. It is important to note that the mechanisms of severe muscle and weight loss in cancer patients are similar (with the exception of the tumour-produced factors) to similar syndromes in patients with other chronic advanced illnesses (e.g. congestive heart failure, renal failure, and rheumatoid arthritis). Therefore, the data from cancer trials may apply to many other disorders where debility is common.

Research priorities should ethically reflect population needs, probability for success, and application of advances, at reasonable cost, in both developed and developing nations. Considering the importance of the wasting disorders, both in terms of human suffering and of costs to family and society, it is ethically problematic that research on the causes of debility in cancer and related disorders is disproportionately low in comparison with costly research on expensive, profitable (at least for the sponsoring firms) cancer chemotherapy.

Education

Studies on the teaching of nutrition within medical schools suggests that it is modest in comparison to its community importance (3,4). An ethical problem arises when the manifest needs of patients are not reflected by the educational priorities of health professional schools. If physicians and nurses are not adequately taught basic principles of nutrition and simple nutritional counselling skills, then they may ignore correctable problems and fail to offer adequate guidance and support to patients and families.

Not only individuals have ethical responsibilities; collectivities such as departments, deans' offices, and hospitals must also demonstrate high ethical standards, setting priorities and allocating resources. We all must die, and many of us will die following a period of profound debility and malnutrition. This period of debility may be shortened if malnutrition were identified at an early moment, followed by the application of preventive and remedial therapies.

It is important to recognize the difference between inequality and inequity (5). Physicians have tended to regard malnutrition as an inequality, i.e. a problem about which little can be done. In the author's view, failures to prioritize nutritional problems actually is an example of an inequity, i.e. an unfair and unjust distinction, the dimensions of which we can change. The lack of emphasis on nutritional problems in both education and research is inequitous and stands as an ethical problem inadequately addressed by the stewards of our collectivities, our granting agency directors, medical leaders, and deans.

Even in palliative care we may regard weight loss as qualitatively different from other symptoms which we would vigorously combat. For example, a prominent palliative care textbook states that 'routine weighting of the patient should be avoided' (6). Later on, it states that 'appetite stimulants are appropriate only in a minority of anorexia patients' (6). Closing a professional eye to the relentless progression of an important symptom is not wise. While, upon weighing, some degree of dismay may be noted by the patient (who is, no doubt, very aware of the problem), professional interest in patient appetite and function, communicated in a humane and sensitive fashion, should more than 'balance' (no pun intended) the presence of weight loss. Are there any other symptoms or signs that a professional is routinely asked to ignore? I think not.

What happens, however, if we regard problems with nutrition as, similar to pain, unique pathophysiologic abnormalities linked to illness, but which may be specifically addressed, with resultant effects on not only the quality of life, but the course of illness?

Adoption of this mindset will result in an emphasis on

- early recognition of nutritional deficiencies;
- early application of drug and nutrient therapies which may enhance appetite and reverse weight loss (7,8);
- advice on simple established measures to improve patient intake (e.g. dietary counselling, a salubrious environment for meals, and nursing assistance for those who need it);
- prioritization of research programmes aimed at translating new findings on the metabolic aspects of disease to the clinical setting;
- constant review of ethical tenets governing hydration and nutrition therapy.

Family support

The sharing of a meal and taking evident pleasure in food and company are inherently strong features of any culture. For example, in a recent qualitative study of ethical issues encountered by family, volunteers, and staff in our palliative care unit, a Portuguese woman stated, 'We are of the Portuguese culture where we don't eat to live, we live to eat. So it is emotionally very difficult to agree with the withholding of food and water, even though I think that the medical logic is right.' In this study, although both patients and families on the unit knew that death was near, issues of nutrition and hydration were commonly raised. While the relentless progress of disease prevented reversal of malnutrition from which many patients suffered, families nevertheless expected that, for as long as possible, health professionals would show skilful attention to nutritional issues.

Throughout history, and today in many hospitals throughout the developing world, because of a paucity of professional staff, families willingly accept the responsibility for providing family members with food and drink, and assisting with its ingestion. Today, in some developed countries, as a result of financial cutbacks, the quality of nutrition offered to patients is problematic, while there may no longer be sufficient numbers of nursing personnel to assist patients. Visiting family members viewing hospital fare consisting of cold, white chicken, white boiled potatoes, and white cauliflower in a glutinous white sauce, all served on a chilly white plate, get the message that they had better attend to nutritional needs and bring in food from the outside. They also become involved in the simple but important issues that determine food intake:

- Can the patient see and reach the food?
- Is the patient in a proper position for eating or drinking?
- Are utensils and cups easily used?
- If utensils are handled with difficulty, is someone available to assist with drinking and feeding?
- Are meal times flexible, as they would be at home?
- Is someone available to offer gentle encouragement?

Family members, particularly with teaching, can fulfil the above roles in hospital, as they would at home. However, it has been said that to withstand the rigours of illness, bring friends, family, and money. Increasingly, we encounter people bereft of all three supports; who shall care for their nutritional needs at home or in an institution?

One may argue that this problem more appropriately relates to the ethics of resource allocation. Medical ethical issues, however, form part of a complex mosaic. Thus, the failure of a health system to provide basic essential services for all people who are forced to enlist its services will lead to a number of patient problems, one of which may be progressive malnutrition.

Technical nutritional support

While early identification and preventive therapy of malnutrition do not appear to be a medical priority, when cachexia is far advanced and the technical means to reverse it are futile, ironically some physicians may then order enteral or parenteral therapy. Although ethicists do not assign a rank order to sustaining medical procedures, among physicians a substantial minority regard the provision of calories as a fundamental aspect of care, somehow different from other technical therapies (9,10). For example, 11% of dying non-small-cell lung cancer patients in the SUPPORT study were receiving tube feedings within 3 days of death (11). Ahronheim and colleagues noted that a similar percentage of advanced cancer patients were receiving tube feedings in their hospital on the last days of life (12).

Currently, enteral or parenteral nutrition would be reserved, outside the setting of a clinical trial, for

- patients with nutritional problems, undergoing major surgery or high dose chemotherapy and/or radiotherapy;
- cancer patients who do not have the cachexia–anorexia syndrome (v.i.), but who are starving because of obstructive lesions;
- patients recovering from therapies that induce severe, prolonged gastrointestinal problems.

Absent from this list are malnourished cancer patients whose weight loss and wasting are secondary to the cachexia–anorexia syndrome. This syndrome remains to be clearly defined, but clinicians will recognize its presence in patients who do not have obstructive problems or specific gastrointestinal disorders and who commonly have an increase in positive acute phase proteins (e.g. C-reactive proteins) and decrease in albumin which is not secondary to wastage. Unfortunately, repeated trials of enteral or parenteral therapy in patients with advanced cancer have not resulted in substantive patient benefit (13). Unless one can reverse the aberrant metabolic state associated with cachexia–anorexia, calories will be wasted, and the adverse effects associated with the technical administration of nutrients may cause great harm (e.g. aspiration pneumonias and systemic infections).

Resource allocation

Enteral and parenteral nutrition are costly. Aside from nutrient expenses, human capital, which may otherwise be more compassionately and effectively employed, is expended. Every health system must consider the proportionate use of limited resources. Commencing artificial means of nutrition with unclear goals or in futile situations is ethically problematic.

Using proportionate care

The above discussion focuses on the biological rationale underpinning decisions to withhold technical nutritional means. What about the age-old consideration that food and drink are not therapies but rather that they represent an absolute final covenant of care?

Earlier, ethicists would talk of 'extraordinary' or 'extra-extraordinary' treatments when talking about the wisdom of starting a treatment or withdrawing it. These terms, however, seem to give a fundamentally different ethical weight to various types of therapy. At the present time, we tend to think of life-sustaining treatments, be it simple hydration, nutrition, or withdrawal of respiratory support, as points on a continuum, whose application is either reasonably proportionate in view of the patient's situation, or disproportionate.

This terminology is helpful, and reflects the view that there is no clear ethical distinction to be made between various categories of life-sustaining measures. Rather, for each of them, the critical question to ask is: 'Is this approach reasonable to apply, or to continue to apply, in view of the patient's circumstances and the family's understanding and concerns?' While this approach is certainly logical, at the bedside, clinicians continue to find it far easier to decide not to commence a treatment than to withdraw it, while they will also often assign a priority to maintenance of hydration and nutrition in patients where other sustaining therapies may be withdrawn (9). Sometimes, disproportionate therapies may be used as a result of family pressure.

The submission of patients to futile procedures that cause suffering is ethically unacceptable. The technical procedures required to provide the patient with enteral or parenteral feeding are ranked as severely uncomfortable by experienced patients. Once in place, varying levels of continuing discomfort may occur, while patients are now at greater risk of a set of complications that are occasionally life-threatening, but always adding to suffering (e.g. aspiration, haemorrhage, infection). Therefore, before undertaking a therapeutic adventure with enteral or parenteral feeding, both biological and psychosocial goals must be clearly defined. A time-frame for assessment must be stated, and the potential benefits must be commensurate with risk. Moreover, as the suffering associated with any technical procedure is directly in proportion to the experience and competence of the operator, those who already bear a high burden of suffering should not be exposed to incompetence. The 'first team' should always be called upon to carry out procedures on those already in pain.

Guidelines—technical nutritional support

In light of the solid evidence that has accumulated on this point, the ethical physician will normally abjure the use of standard enteral or parenteral therapies in patients with advanced cancer and the cachexia–anorexia syndrome.

In the three-dimensional clinical world where complex, seemingly contradictory considerations often arise, stark dictums may not be readily applied.

The following guidelines may be helpful:

1 Preventing family misunderstandings late in the course of illness may be obviated by earlier discussions. For example, newly diagnosed pancreatic cancer patients enrolled in our Integrated Pancreatic Cancer Programme are provided with an information brochure that contains the following passage (14):

> **Will I do better if I force myself to eat or if I take food by artificial means, such as through my veins or a tube in my stomach?**
>
> In almost all circumstances, the answer to this question is a clear and definite 'no'. Indeed, forcing food, or the complications associated with intravenous feeding or tube feeding can cause major problems such as an increased risk of infections, or vomiting with inhaling food into the lungs. The extra calories supplied by artificial means are not effectively available to our muscles or other tissue. Why? Because the inflammatory reaction created by cancer and certain tumour products blocks their use.
>
> This information, while clearly established after numerous medical studies, is often poorly understood by people in the community. It is only natural for family and friends to wish to ensure that a loved one is well fed. They often become distressed when their family member or friend is not eating, and will sometimes overly encourage a person to eat, or ask doctors to order artificial means of nutrition when it is not helpful for the patient.
>
> We know that forced feeding does not make one live longer, may cause one to live for a shorter period of time, and is commonly a source of confusion and distress within families.
>
> This does not mean that it is not important to take part in family meals, as these social occasions are very important for enjoyment of life. The advice contained in this patient brochure is designed to help you enjoy these activities while maintaining a reasonable nutritional state.

2 Patients and families can always refuse to accept technical means of nutrition.

3 The onus is on families, patients, and physicians to provide a rationale for using enteral or parenteral therapy in the setting of advanced cancer.

4 When borderline cases arise (e.g. is the patient starving to death because of an obstruction who otherwise would not die imminently?) nutrition can be provided on a clearly stated time-limited basis to permit analyses of success.

Conclusion

In this section we have categorically stated that, with unusual exceptions, the use of enteral and parenteral therapy in far advanced cancer patients who are not receiving aggressive radio- or chemotherapy is not helpful, and because of the increased suffering associated with these invasions and the illogical use of resources, is contraindicated on ethical grounds.

As discussed earlier, today's ethical standards are not fixed, and may change as the fruits of tomorrow's research are applied. The reader must be aware of current studies using so-called 'immuno-nutrition' for critically ill patients undergoing surgery or recovering from severe trauma or a variety of acute life-threatening illnesses. In contrast to the standard enteral or parenteral therapy of today, immuno-nutrient mixes may include possible immune-enhancing or disease-modifying compounds such as arginine, glutamine, branch chain amino acids, omega-3 fatty acids, among other compounds. Use of these modified diets has been demonstrated to be beneficial in a variety of acute illness settings (15,16). At this time, it is not indicated that these enhanced forms of enteral and parenteral nutrition should be used in a setting of far advanced disease; one could, however, conceive of an ethical clinical trial involving the use of newer approaches to artificial nutrition in selected patients with far advanced cancer who initially present with severe malnutrition. It is possible that the absolute pronouncements of the moment will be more nuanced in the future. Physicians should keep a watching brief on this area of research.

Hydration

No one would argue that it is essential to maintain patients in a reasonable state of hydration until the last days of life. At some poorly defined point in these last days, however, an argument, which is not yet fully resolved, ensues on the value of maintaining hydration. Most palliative care physicians appear to favour allowing patients to become dehydrated for several days before death. They are concerned about the effects of invasive therapies on patient/family dignity and comfort, while on biological grounds many in the palliative care community, albeit on small studies supplemented with anecdotal evidence and personal observation, will argue that hydration not only may meaninglessly prolong life, but may also cause actual harm. Conversely, other physicians believe that the 'antihydration' argument is simplistic, and fear that thoughtless adherence *will* cause harm, particularly in patients continuing on complex drug therapies. The arguments on either side of the issue have been stated by Fainsinger and colleagues in a number of articles and are published in his chapter.

On reviewing these arguments, one notes that Level I evidence is not present for any of the points. Many are simply expressions of common sense (less fluid intake—less urination), while others seem reasonable (less fluid—less vomiting and less pulmonary congestion). In view of altered pathophysiology at the end of life, however, other factors may be more influential than hydration in causing vomiting or pulmonary oedema. We know little about the potential for suffering in comatose people, while the argument that dehydration decreases levels of consciousness, and therefore reduces suffering, is somewhat circular.

With respect to 'arguments for', similarly, many of the arguments are not based on sound ethical or biological principles. As with nutrition, parenteral hydration is certainly not to be regarded as a 'minimum standard of care' and its employment can only be ethically justified if it is carried out at the patient/family request or if professional judgement dictates that hydration will improve the patient's quality of existence. Certainly, arguments to the effect that withholding fluids from dying patients represents the 'thin edge of the wedge' which will negatively impact on the care of other patients should be regarded as an unproven and highly unlikely scenario.

The concern that dehydration and electrolyte imbalance increase the risk of a confusional state, with its penumbra of distress for family members, is worthy of detailed review. While dignity is intact if we are treated in a dignified and respectful fashion, regardless of our physical state, patients do not wish to spend their last hours in a delirious state, completely uncharacteristic of their personality, and which will create anguish amongst family members leaving them with horrible memories.

The 'pro/con' arguments are a mixture of principle, personal opinion, and fact. The gathering of factual data and its interpretation can help us to develop guidelines and refine our principles. The following 'pro/con' debates lend themselves to further analysis based on factual data:

- Alleviation of thirst
- End stage confusion
- Influence on symptoms

Thirst

Osmolality is maintained within a narrow range through the regulatory activity of osmoreceptors in the anterior hypothalamus which influence the production of vasopressin, a hormone modulating the reabsorption of solute-free water in the kidney. An increase in plasma osmolality leads to vasopressin production and the stimulation of thirst osmoreceptors, similarly located, but probably distinct from vasopressin osmoreceptors (17). Unknown cerebral pathways are stimulated, and the patient is led to seek a drink, thus lowering osmolality. Drops in blood volume also stimulate thirst, although this mechanism is probably less significant in everyday life. Reduced volume leads to the release of renin in the kidney and the production of angiotensin-2 and aldosterone. Possibly these agents stimulate thirst, but there may be other mechanisms that directly mediate volume-related thirst. As anyone who has gulped a drink after a game of squash knows, thirst is immediately slaked by drinking, long before fluid can be absorbed to influence body osmolality. Presumably, an oropharyngeal reflex exists which, when stimulated by the presence of fluid in the nasopharynx and/or the act of swallowing, inhibits generation of the sensation of thirst by the hypothalamus and cerebrum. For unknown reasons, older people, who make up the bulk of palliative care patients, have a decreased appreciation of thirst.

Does one need carefully to regulate plasma osmolality and blood volume in order to prevent thirst in dying patients? The answer, based on modest evidence, is, apparently, 'no'. One study suggests that there is no correlation between the use of parenteral hydration and the sensation of thirst (18), while thirst can be readily alleviated through impeccable mouth care and keeping the mouth moist with small amounts of fluid and ice chips (19).

And yet, the dying commonly complain of thirst. As with other symptoms, we may lack sufficient language discrimination to separate centrally mediated thirst from the unpleasant sensation generated by a dry mouth. Among other causes, mouth breathing, candidiasis, and many medications used in palliative care cause the oral mucosa to dry out. As stated above, this sensation may be prevented, in part, by early identification of thrush, judicious use of anticholinergic medication, and can be alleviated by excellent mouth care, including continuous efforts to keep the mucous membranes moist.

Other symptoms

There is no convincing evidence that the state of hydration influences nausea, vomiting, or respiratory tract secretions. Ellershaw and colleagues could not detect a significant relationship between hydration status and respiratory tract secretions (20). The author is not aware of similar studies looking at gastrointestinal symptoms. In the light of current knowledge, control of respiratory or gastrointestinal symptoms should not be used as a rationale for restricting fluids in the last days of life.

Dehydration has been said to increase the risk of bed sores (21) and constipation (22). Again, while the connection seems logical, hard data is scarce.

Confusional states

Few symptoms are more distressing for family members and professional staff than the emergence of a delirious state in a previously sentient patient. An ethical imperative exists to identify prodromal states, and to prevent them, if possible. Dehydration and consequent hypernatraemia can induce confusion. Hypernatraemia is not common in palliative care patients, and serum osmolalities do not tend to be elevated. Rather, hyponatraemia is commonly seen in patients with a variety of advanced chronic illnesses.

A plethora of symptoms bedevil patients towards the end of life, each one of which may lead a physician to offer a pharmacological solution. Therefore, complex drug regimens are common in palliative care, including many agents with psychoactive properties. Opioids are commonly used up until the time of death. If renal perfusion is inadequate, plasma levels of the parent compound and its metabolites will increase, with consequent risk of opioid toxicity, including confusion.

In the early 1990s, the Edmonton Palliative Care Programme changed its policy and began to combat dehydration using parenteral fluids, usually administered by hypodermoclysis (v.i.). A retrospective study suggested that more vigorous use of hydration may have contributed to the decrease in confusion that was observed in comparison with an earlier time period (23). The programme, at that time, however, also used opioid rotation more frequently, and introduced a formal symptom assessment system. Early identification of change in mental status, use of lower dose opioid therapy, and clearance of drug metabolites may all have contributed to the reduced incidence of confusion. Soon thereafter, the continuing controversy on the place of hydration led colleagues in Edmonton and Ottawa to contrast their policies and study outcomes (24). Each programme attempted to recruit comparable patients from consecutively admitted cancer patients. Following their standard practice, the Edmonton patients received hypodermoclysis, while Ottawa patients were treated after the fashion common in palliative care units of the day, i.e. no parenteral fluids were administered. Fluid balance, mini-mental status examination (MMSE), or delirium rating scales (DRS) scores, together with medication practice, were measured. Ultimately, 60 patients (33 in Ottawa and 27 in Edmonton) were available for study. While mental status deteriorated in both groups, the Ottawa group recorded poorer MMSE and DRS scores. Was this outcome secondary to their policy on hydration? We cannot say with certainty, as Ottawa patients, overall, also received more sedating and anticholinergic drugs. Moreover, despite the best efforts of both groups, it may be that the two groups were not sufficiently comparable in important characteristics.

Therefore, based on clinical studies, the weight of evidence suggests that modest hydration may reduce the incidence of confusional states. Some have suggested that further studies attempt to recruit multiple patients in a truly randomized trial in order to determine whether hydration influences confusion. In the author's opinion, the effects of reduced renal output on plasma drug and drug metabolite levels, coupled with the clinical studies available, create a situation where it would be difficult to conclude that clinical equipoise exists. Patients receiving drugs cleared by the kidney which may cause delirium must have their drugs carefully monitored. If reduction or termination are not possible, ensuring a reasonable state of hydration appears to be a wise and ethical course.

Hydration—the symbolism of support

Physicians and families alike appear to share the view that water is essential, not only for life, but stands as a symbolic continuing bond of support. In one study in a teaching hospital, 70% of the patients died with an IV line in place (25). Among other forms of life support, a study by Christakis indicated that parenteral fluids were the least likely to be withdrawn (10).

In contrast, the weight of palliative care literature regards reduced intake of fluids at the end of life as a natural, possibly helpful event (26). The above review of factual data on symptom incidence and prevention suggests that, at least for one critical symptom, namely confusion, this stance is probably not tenable.

Nevertheless, technical means of life support are viewed askance in palliative care for their effects on patient dignity and the concern that they interfere with patient–family interaction.

In contrast to parenteral or enteral nutrition, fluids can be readily administered using a simple and inexpensive technique, hypodermoclysis. An even older and cheaper technique, proctoclysis, has been successfully employed (27). This technique was used in the sixteenth century by Thomas More to save his dehydrated daughter from the 'sweating sickness', contrary to the medical opinion of the day which advocated 'bleeding', with predictably horrendous results. It is worthy of note that some articles critical of the use of parenteral hydration only consider parenteral hydration via the intravenous route.

Hypodermoclysis is safe and adverse events are uncommon (28). In the absence of fluid-losing states, the Edmonton group recommends parenteral fluids in the range of 1000 ml per day. In most people, this amount of fluid administered as an electrolyte solution (normal saline, or two-thirds 5% dextrose and one-third saline) can be readily absorbed in selected interstitial spaces such as the anterior chest wall. Formerly it was thought that fluid would not be absorbed unless hyaluronidase was administered. Recent evidence suggests that this agent is not required, and that infusion rates in the range of 20–100 ml per hour are tolerated by most individuals.

Employing hypodermoclysis precludes the often painful task of seeking an intravenous line; hypodermoclysis may be started by individuals, other than physicians and nurses, who receive a short, simple course of training. Therefore, home therapy can be readily provided.

Physicians should be familiar with the literature on hypodermoclysis. Fainsinger provides specific technical recommendations and references to hypodermoclysis in his chapter (Chapter 22). The ease of using hypodermoclysis has, in the author's opinion, shifted the goalposts towards a more ready acceptance of hydration in previously controversial situations.

Hydration in association with sedation

Not uncommonly, intractable symptoms, notably pain and delirium, may result in a patient spending his or her last hours in a state of pharmacologically-induced sedation. Previously called 'terminal sedation', efforts are under way to change this phrase to 'total sedation' (29) or 'palliative sedation' to convey the view that, while sedation often accompanies patients' last hours, it is not comparable to active euthanasia, as drugs employed do not kill, and the process can be reversed. This is true if sedation is accompanied by minimal hydration.

The patient will surely die of the direct effect of sedation over a few days if hydration is not provided. This observation has led some to refer to sedation practice as 'slow euthanasia' (30). The principal effective counter-argument raised to equating sedation without hydration to euthanasia depends upon the ethical principle that the patient is not obliged to accept any therapy, nor is a patient obliged to eat or drink. Therefore, one may refuse hydration and request sedation. Some may argue that combining the ethical principles of double effect and patient autonomy to justify sedation without hydration is a bit of a stretch; at present this issue remains a topic for continued rational ethical debate.

Based on current factual evidence and ethical thought, the author believes the following guidelines for hydration are reasonable:

1 Competent patients can accept or refuse hydration when given pertinent information.

2 For incompetent patients, the balancing of advantages and disadvantages should be undertaken. Incompetent patients will be represented by legal guardians or trusted family members.

3 Unlike technical nutrition, where the onus lies on the physician and family to justify its use in end-stage cancer, hydration should ordinarily be maintained throughout the last weeks of life. If not employed, the onus lies on the physician and family to justify withdrawal of fluid support.

4 A time-limited trial of hydration is always recommended if there is doubt about the advantages and disadvantages.

5 If patients are receiving drugs where plasma levels and likely pharmacodynamic effects depend upon renal clearance of the drug and its metabolites, hydration should be maintained, unless there is a contraindication.

6 Unless an intravenous line is already in place for other reasons, technical hydration should be attempted via the subcutaneous route (hypodermoclysis).

These guidelines, modelled upon guidelines on enteral feeding published by the Bioethics Centre at the University of Alberta, relate to the last *days and weeks* of life. Hydration may be withdrawn during the period when the patient is actively dying and survival is measured in hours or a few days. Usually, at this point, medications are discontinued or doses are reduced (exclusive of planned sedation).

References

1. **Pennington CR.** Disease-associated malnutrition in year 2000. *Postgraduate Medical Journal* 1998;74:65–71.

2. **Barber MD; Ross JA; Voss AC; Tisdale MJ; Fearon KCH.** The effect of an oral nutritional supplement enriched with fish oil on weight-loss in patients with pancreatic cancer. *British Journal of Cancer* 1999;81(1):80–6.

3. **Winick M.** Nutrition education in medical schools. *American Journal of Clinical Nutrition* 1993;58:825–7.

4. Essentials of nutrition education in medical schools: a national consensus. Report of the American Medical Student Association's Nutrition Carriculum Project. *American Journal of Clinical Nutrition* 1997;65:1559–61.

5. **Gwatkin DR.** Health inequalities and the health of the poor: What do we know? What can we do? *Bulletin of the World Health Organization* 2000;78(1):3–17.

6. **Twycross R.** *Introducing Palliative Care.* Oxford: Radcliffe Medical Press, 1999.

7. **Jatoi A; Kumar S; Sloan JA; Nguyen PL.** On appetite and its loss. *Journal of Clinical Oncology* 2000;18(15):2930–2.
8. **Fearon KCH; Barber MD; Moses AGW.** The cancer cachexia syndrome. *Surgical Oncology Clinics of North America* 2001;10(1):109–21.
9. **Solomon MZ; O'Donnell L; Jenings B; Guilfoy V; Wolf SM; Nolan K., *et al.*** Decisions near the end of life: professional views on life-sustaining treatments. *American Journal of Public Health* 1993;83(1):14–23.
10. **Christakis NA; Asch DA.** Biases in how physicians choose to withdraw life support. *The Lancet* 1993;342:642–6.
11. **Claessens MT; Lynn J; Zhong A; Desbiens NA; Phillips RS; Wu AW., *et al.*** Dying with lung cancer or chronic obstructive pulmonary disease: insights from SUPPORT. *Journal of the American Geriatric Society* 2000;48(5)Supplement: S146–S153.
12. **Ahronheim JC; Morrison RS; Baskin SA; Morris J; Meier DE.** Treatment of the dying in the acute care hospital: advanced dementia and metastatic cancer. *Archives of Internal Medicine* 1996;156:2094–100.
13. **Winter SM.** Terminal nutrition: framing the debate for the withdrawal of nutritional support in terminally ill patients. *American Journal of Medicine* 2000;109:723–41.
14. **MacDonald N; Ayoub JP; Barkun A; Dalzell MA; Gagnon B; Rosenberg L.** Carcinoma of the pancreas: an integrated programme. *Cancer Strategy* 2000;2(1):17–24.
15. **Beale RJ; Bryg DJ; Bihari DJ.** Immunonutrition in the critically ill: a systematic review of clinical outcome. *Critical Care Medicine* 1999;27(12):2799–805.
16. **Gadek JM; DeMichele SJ; Karlstad MD; Pacht ER; Donahoe M; Albertson TE., *et al.*** Effect of enteral feeding with eicosapentaenoic acid, gamma-linolenic acid and antioxidants in patients with acute respiratory distress syndrome. *Critical Care Medicine* 1999;27(8):1409–20.
17. **McKenna K; Thompson C.** Osmoregulation in clinical disorders of thirst appreciation. *Clinical Endocrinology* 1998;49:139–52.
18. **Musgrave CF; Bartal N; Opstad J.** The sensation of thirst in dying patients receiving IV hydration. *Journal of Palliative Care* 1995;11(4):17–21.
19. **McCann RM; Hall WJ; Groth-Juncker A.** Comfort care for terminally ill patients: the appropriate use of nutrition and hydration. *Journal of the American Medical Association* 1994;272(16):1263–6.
20. **Ellershaw JE; Sutcliffe JM; Saunders CM.** Dehydration and the dying patient. *Journal of Pain and Symptom Management* 1995;10(3):192–7.
21. **De Conno F; Ventafridda V; Saita L.** Skin problems in advanced and terminal cancer patients. *Journal of Pain and Symptom Management* 1991;6(4):247–56.
22. **Sykes NP.** Constipation and diarrhoea. In: Doyle D; Hanks GWC; MacDonald N., editors. *The Oxford Textbook of Palliative Medicine*, 2nd edn. New York: Oxford University Press, 1998;513–26.
23. **Bruera E; Franco JJ; Maltoni M; Watanabe S., *et al.*** Changing pattern of agitated impaired mental status in patients with advanced cancer: association with cognitive monitoring, hydration and opioid rotation. *Journal of Pain and Symptom Management* 1995;10:287–91.
24. **Viola RA; Fainsinger R; Scott JF; Wells GA; Allston J; Bruera E.** A study of fluid therapy and mental status in palliative care patients. Manuscript submitted for publication.
25. **Burge FI; King DB; Wilson D.** Intravenous fluids and the hospitalized dying: a medical last rite? *Canadian Family Physician* 1990;86:883–6.
26. **Viola RA; Wells GA; Peterson J.** The effects of fluid status and fluid therapy on the dying: a systematic review. *Journal of Palliative Care* 1997;13(4):41–52.
27. **Bruera E; Schoeller T; Pruvost M.** Proctoclysis for hydration of terminal cancer patients. *The Lancet* 1994;344:1699.

28. **Fainsinger RL; MacEachern T; Miller MJ; Bruera E; Spachynski K; Kuehn N., *et al.*** The use of hypodermoclysis for rehydration in terminally ill cancer patients. *Journal of Pain and Symptom Management* 1994;9(5):298–302.
29. NHO paper on terminal sedation.
30. **Billings A; Block SD.** Slow euthanasia. *Journal of Palliative Care* 1994;1996;12(4):21–30.

Index